AF664657

Cancer Treatment and Research

Volume 167

Series editor

Steven T. Rosen, Duarte, CA, USA

More information about this series at http://www.springer.com/series/5808

Howard L. Kaufman · Janice M. Mehnert
Editors

Melanoma

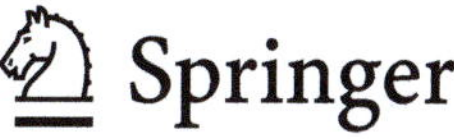

Editors
Howard L. Kaufman
Rutgers Cancer Institute of New Jersey
New Brunswick, NY
USA

Janice M. Mehnert
Robert Wood Johnson Medical School
Rutgers Cancer Institute of New Jersey
New Brunswick, NJ
USA

ISSN 0927-3042
Cancer Treatment and Research
ISBN 978-3-319-22538-8 ISBN 978-3-319-22539-5 (eBook)
DOI 10.1007/978-3-319-22539-5

Library of Congress Control Number: 2015946100

Springer Cham Heidelberg New York Dordrecht London

Printed on acid-free paper

Springer International Publishing AG Switzerland is part of Springer Science+Business Media
(www.springer.com)

Contents

Heterogeneity in Melanoma

Batool Shannan, Michela Perego, Rajasekharan Somasundaram and Meenhard Herlyn

Abstract

Melanoma is among the most aggressive and therapy-resistant human cancers. While great strides in therapy have generated enthusiasm, many challenges remain. Heterogeneity is the most pressing issue for all types of therapy. This chapter summarizes the clinical classification of melanoma, of which the research community now adds additional layers of classifications for better diagnosis and prediction of therapy response. As the search for new biomarkers increases, we expect that biomarker analyses will be essential for all clinical trials to better select patient populations for optimal therapy. While individualized therapy that is based on extensive biomarker analyses is an option, we expect in the future genetic and biologic biomarkers will allow grouping of melanomas in such a way that we can predict therapy outcome. At this time, tumor heterogeneity continues to be the major challenge leading inevitably to relapse. To address heterogeneity therapeutically, we need to develop complex therapies that eliminate the bulk of the tumor and, at the same time, the critical subpopulations.

Keywords

Melanoma · Heterogeneity · Therapy

Batool Shannan and Michela Perego have equally contributed.

B. Shannan · M. Perego · R. Somasundaram · M. Herlyn (✉)
Molecular and Cellular Oncogenesis Program, Melanoma Research Center,
The Wistar Institute, 3601 Spruce Street, Philadelphia, PA 19104, USA
e-mail: herlynm@wistar.org

H.L. Kaufman and J.M. Mehnert (eds.), *Melanoma*,
Cancer Treatment and Research 167, DOI 10.1007/978-3-319-22539-5_1

Abbreviations

ABCB5	ATP-binding cassette subfamily B5
AKT	V-akt murine thymoma viral oncogene homolog
ALCAM	Activated leukocyte cell adhesion molecule
ALDH1	Aldehyde dehydrogenase 1
ARID1A	AT-rich interactive domain-containing protein 1A
BRAF	V-raf murine sarcoma viral oncogene homolog B1
CD	Cluster differentiation
CDK	Cyclin-dependent Kinase
CDKN2A	Cyclin-dependent kinase inhibitor 2A
ERK	Extracellular signal-regulated kinase
Fbxw-7	F-box/WD repeat-containing protein 7
gp100	Glycoprotein 100
HGF	Hepatocyte growth factor
IGF	Insulin-like growth factor
JARID1B	Jumonji/ARID1 (JARID1) histone 3 K4 (H3K4) demethylases
Kit	C-kit tyrosine kinase receptor
MAPK	Mitogen-activated protein kinase
MART-1/Melan-A	Melanoma antigen recognized by T cells-1/melanoma antigen A
MCAM	Melanoma cell adhesion molecule
MEK	MAPK/ERK Kinase
MITF	Microphthalmia-associated transcription factor
mTOR	Mammalian target of Rapamycin
NF	Neurofibromatosis
NGF	Nerve growth factor
NGFR	Nerve growth factor receptor
NRAS	Neuroblastoma RAS viral (v-ras) oncogene homolog
PI3K	Phosphoinositide-3 Kinase
PTEN	Phosphatase and tensin homolog
Rac1	Ras-related C3 botulinum toxin substrate-1
RAF	RAS viral (v-raf) oncogene homolog
RAS	RAS viral (v-ras) oncogene homolog
SCF	Stem cell factor
SEER	Surveillance, epidemiology, end results
TGF-β	Transforming growth factor beta
TICs	Tumor-initiating cells
TME	Tumor microenvironment
TNF	Tumor necrosis factor
TP53	Tumor protein p53
UV	Ultraviolet

Contents

1 Introduction

Melanoma is the most aggressive form of skin cancer and incidences continue to rise worldwide. According to the American Cancer Society, an estimated 76,100 new cases of melanoma will be diagnosed in the USA and 9710 people are expected to die of metastatic disease [48]. SEER data indicate the prevalence of melanoma in the older age group, particularly men over the age of 65. However, in recent years, young adults, particularly women between the ages of 25–39 years, have pronounced increases in incidence rates, often with severe outcomes [4, 39, 71]. Although intense intermittent sun exposure is a major risk factor for melanoma, family history of melanoma, genetic susceptibility, environmental factors, and immunosuppression are some of the other factors that influence incidence rates [48].

Efforts are underway to understand the biology of melanoma heterogeneity to better design strategies for more precise choices for targeting. In this chapter, we review clinical and genetic profiles in melanoma and discuss heterogeneity as one of the most significant causes for cancer therapy resistance.

2 Clinical and Molecular Classification of Melanoma

Clinical and histological classifications of melanoma have been extensively described (Fig. 1a, b). When dividing melanomas into those derived from cells within epithelia, there are four categories: (1) lentigo and desmoplastic melanomas (from areas on the head and neck with high ultraviolet (UV) exposure); (2) low UV exposure areas (gives rise to superficial spreading and spitzoid melanomas which also includes non-malignant lesions such as acquired and dysplastic nevi, Spitz nevi, and atypical Spitz tumors); (3) mucosal melanomas (those of the genital track); and (4) lesions of palms, soles, and nails giving rise to acral melanomas (Fig. 1a). Melanomas arising in areas outside of epithelia represent the second major group. The group is comprised of melanomas in the eye and internal organs such as the gut (Fig. 1b). Dermis-derived melanomas in the skin include blue nevus-like melanomas and those arising within congenital nevi. It is speculated that this latter group of lesions arise from neural crest-like stem cells in the dermis [70], but experimental proof has yet to be determined. Alternatively, findings in other cancers such as leukemia/lymphoma, breast cancer, or various brain tumors suggest

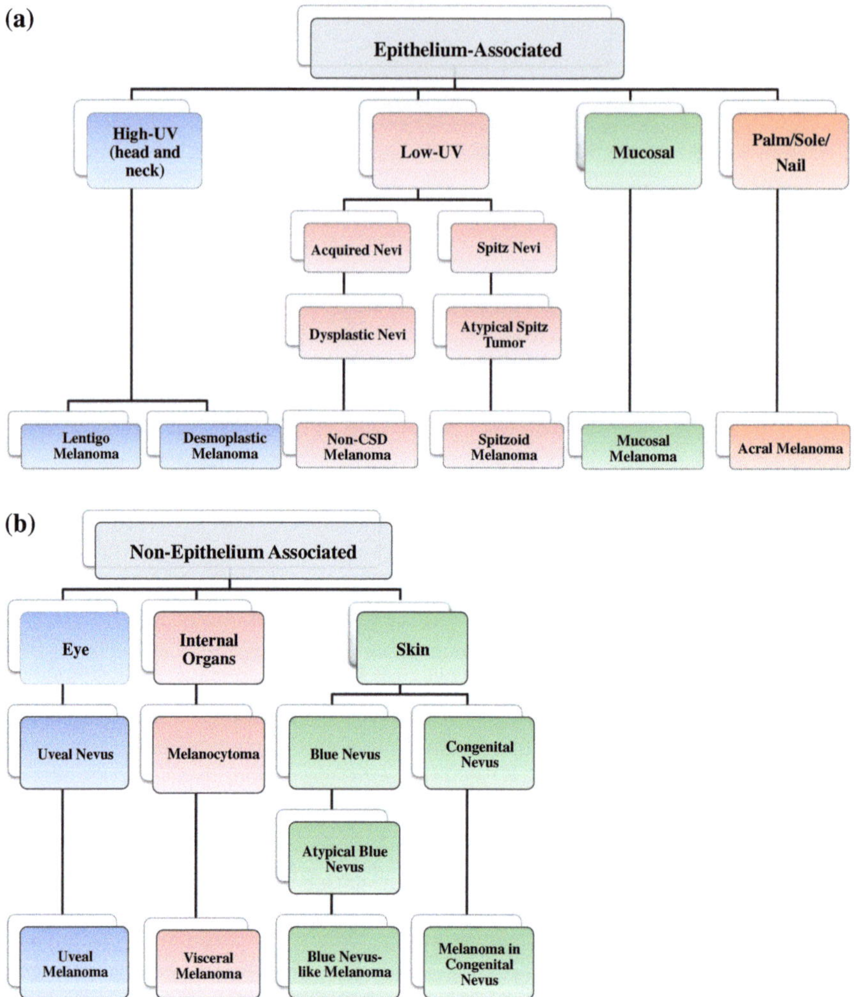

Fig. 1 Clinical grouping of melanoma. There are distinct patterns of clinical appearances of melanoma that led to the distinction of the *histogenetic* types in the first classification system in 1973. **a** Melanomas arising from epithelium-associated melanocytes. The relationship between sun exposure and melanoma has been established for decades (high UV melanoma); however, it was later discovered that melanomas can also occur in areas that are well-protected from UV exposure (low UV, mucosal, and palm/sole/nail melanomas). **b** Melanomas arising from non-epithelium-associated melanocytes. These melanomas fall into the categories of intradermal melanocytic neoplasms (blue nevi, uveal melanoma). These types of melanoma harbor mutations of G protein alpha subunits of Gq family. These mutations are virtually absent from epithelium-associated melanocytes. Melanocytomas are neoplasms of the central nervous system and they closely resemble blue nevi. However, they can pose differential problems to melanoma metastases diagnosis. *CSD* chronic sun damage. Adapted from Bastian [4]

that most, if not all, tumors arise from the respective stem cell populations. In human skin, there are two populations of neural crest-like stem cells, one in the dermis [28] and the other in the bulge region of the hair follicle [68]. Each stem cell can differentiate into multiple cell types including neuronal cells, melanocytes, smooth muscle cells, adipocytes, chondrocytes, osteoblasts, or Schwann cells [28]. Which of the two stem cells is more important in melanoma development is not clear, although there is a general lack of clinical and pathological information on melanomas arising from hair follicles. Interestingly, melanocytes can dedifferentiate to neural crest-like stem cells when Notch signaling is activated [42] suggesting a fluid transition from one state of cellular differentiation to the other, making it very difficult to trace the origin of melanomas. As tumors become more aggressive, they often lose their pigmentation markers and dedifferentiate acquiring stem cell features, which make them more resistant to therapy.

The clinical classifications are the results of long-standing observations. They have been critical in making therapy decisions, although their usefulness as guides has been controversial. For practicing oncologists, a distinction between benign and malignant has been most critical, with intermediate stages generating controversial discussions, some of which have been ongoing for decades without a clear resolution. One major reason for this is that any suspected lesion is surgically removed for extensive diagnostic evaluation. Thus, follow-up of existing lesions has rarely been done, leading to considerable variations in risk estimates for dysplastic nevi, as well as biologically early melanomas that progress to aggressive tumors. Genetic analyses of melanocytic lesions have for the first time allowed a more detailed classification, but such new classifications are at an early stage as we know of very few drivers in the disease. Still, the first genetic analyses are becoming routine in making clinical decisions for melanoma therapy.

It is important to discuss the major mutations in melanoma and their affected pathways, while acknowledging that of all human cancers, melanomas carry the most mutations, generally more than 10 per Mb with lung cancer following as the second most non-euploid tumor [33]. The mitogen-activated protein kinase (MAPK) pathway is one of the major signaling cascades involved in the control of cell growth and migration. The RAS/RAF/MEK/ERK pathway regulates cell properties downstream of tyrosine kinase receptors and heterodimeric G protein-coupled receptors. Melanomas are addicted to MAPK activation, regardless of whether or not tumors carry mutations in genes coding for proteins in this pathway. In normal melanocytes, the pathway is activated by growth factors/ligands such as stem cell factor (SCF), fibroblast growth factor, and hepatocyte growth factor (HGF). In melanoma, the same growth factors (except SCF) are produced for autocrine stimulation. Most important for melanoma cells is the constitutive activation of the MAPK pathway through activating mutations of BRAF ($\sim$50 % of melanomas) or NRAS (20–25 % of mutations; Fig. 2). This allows cells to vigorously grow, even in the absence of ligand. For example, the V600E mutation in BRAF upregulates the pathway 800-fold when compared to the inactive forms [63]. Mutations in BRAF can already occur in nevi, but they generally lead to the induction of senescence because cells are unable to cope with such tremendous

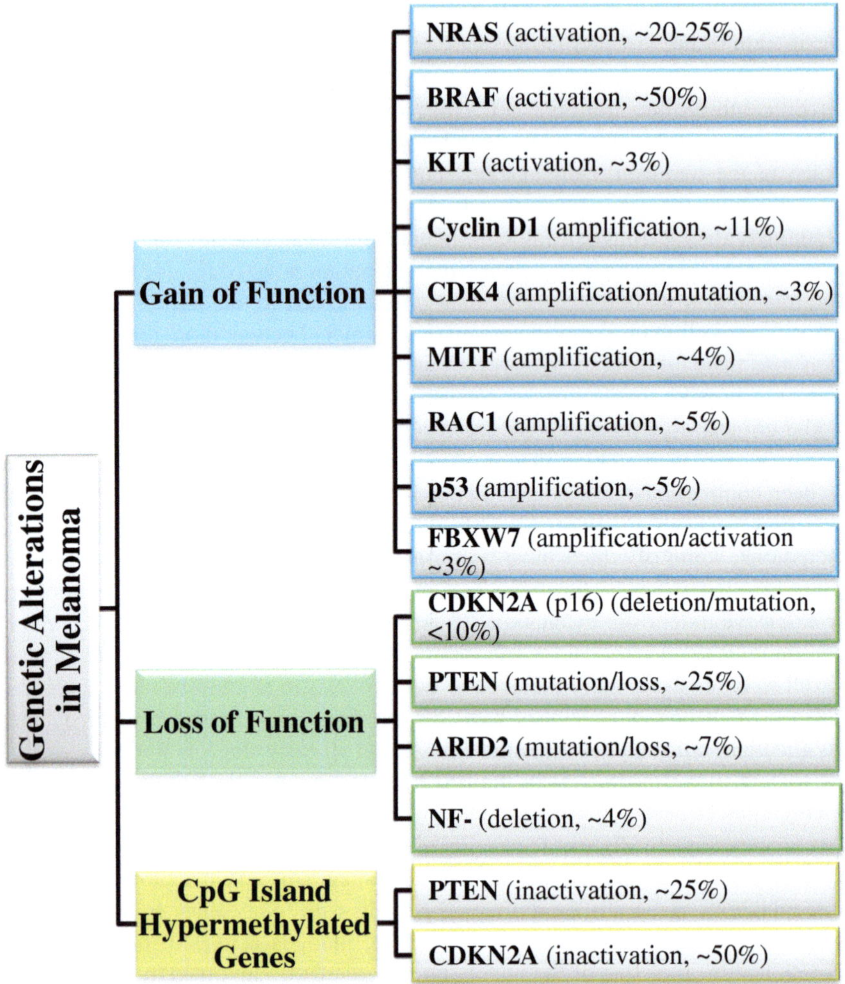

Fig. 2 Genetic mutations in melanoma. A landscape of the most frequently mutated driver mutations in melanoma. Genetic analyses have found that mutations in specific pathways are more prevalent in some melanoma subtypes than others. Moreover, whole-exome sequencing has enabled the discovery of several new melanoma genes with functionally consequential (and probably actionable) mutations, and the identification of many driver mutations directly attributed to UV mutagenesis

activation stress. NRAS mutations activate the pathway similarly to BRAFV600E. Those two genes are the most important drivers in melanoma, representing over 70 % of all melanomas because both mutations never occur in the same cell to avoid *overdrive*. However, they are not the only drivers in a given tumor as other codrivers are required for malignant transformation, including those for overcoming induced senescence. Such codrivers are likely highly heterogeneous, and we only know of a few (Fig. 2). Thus, codrivers can be oncogenes (CDK4, Cyclin D1) or inactivation of tumor suppressor genes (phosphatase and tensin homolog [PTEN]). Likely, cells carry more than one codriver, but their real number remains uncertain and will only be better understood in years to come. Gaining this knowledge is important because each codriver will likely constitutively activate additional pathways, which will require specific targeting for therapy.

Microphthalmia-associated transcription factor (MITF), a master regulator of melanocyte development, has different regulatory functions that are associated with the level of MITF protein expression. High levels of MITF protein exert an anti-proliferative activity by predisposing cells to cell cycle arrest and differentiation through cell cycle regulators (CDk2, p21, p16). Low levels of MITF can also lead to cell cycle arrest. PI3K and AKT mutations are relatively rare in melanomas, whereas those for the tumor suppressor PTEN, which negatively regulates the PI3K/AKT pathways, are more common. Many growth factors, such as IGF-1, also signal through PI3K/AKT leading to constitutive activation of the pathways in most, if not all, melanomas. Thus, therapy strategies in melanoma often involve targeting the PI3K pathway; however, the results are mixed. Inhibition of the pathway as a sole therapeutic strategy is insufficient. In all likelihood, a combination of MAPK inhibition (BRAF, MEK, or ERK targeting) together with PI3K/AKT/mTOR inhibition is most likely to succeed. Lastly, p53 plays an important role in suppressing progression of benign nevi to melanoma [59, 60]. The frequency of p53 mutations in melanoma is low (<10 %); however, p53 is not fully functional in many melanomas through yet-to-be-clarified mechanisms.

At this time, it is too early to develop a genetic classification of melanoma except the broad distinction between BRAF/NRAS/KIT mutant and wild-type (triple-negative) melanomas. Both groups will require major subdivisions to take into account the drivers/codrivers. The more detailed we can group the different melanomas, the better we can target the constitutively activated pathways at the same time, i.e., at the beginning of therapy and not just after resistance to the first drugs has developed. Our goal will be to hit the melanomas early and hard while taking into account the intratumoral heterogeneity that may be present. In the following section, we will briefly summarize the major findings in intratumor heterogeneity at the genetic level.

3 Genetic Heterogeneity in Melanoma

Intratumor genetic heterogeneity between both individual melanoma biopsies and spatially and temporarily parted biopsies of the same tumor has been documented [13, 66]. Such intratumor heterogeneity is not unique to melanoma and has been documented in a variety of human tumors including brain tumors [37, 40, 56], and cancers of the head and neck [35], kidney [16], thyroid [62], pancreas [9], breast [12], lung [61], and esophagus [32], as well as in some non-solid cancers [1, 13, 21]. In melanoma, it was possible to isolate single cells of BRAF V600E/wt-NRAS and wt-BRAF/NRASQ16R genotypes from the same lesion [53]. Also, BRAF genotyping from single melanoma cells showed heterogeneity between primary and metastatic lesions [29], or among metastatic lesions [30, 64, 67], raising the question of whether intratumor heterogeneity determines the efficacy of BRAFV600E-targeted therapies. In other studies, the presence of two different NRAS mutations (Q61K and Q61R) was found coexisting within the same metastatic lesion after therapy failure [36]. Considerable heterogeneity is also observed in relapsed tumors after BRAF inhibitor therapy. Shi et al. [54] developed a genetic tree, in which different metastases of the same patients could be traced according to the genetic profile of oncogenes and tumor suppressor genes.

4 Biological Heterogeneity in Melanoma

It is well documented that melanomas express heterogeneously tumor-associated antigens such as gp100 and melanoma antigen recognized by T cells-1 (MART-1; Fig. 3). Cells not expressing MART-1 and gp100 escape immune surveillance, which may explain past failures in passive and active immunotherapies [55]. MITF expression also varies within lesions and is inversely correlated to the differentiation status of melanoma cells with those expressing low MITF levels displaying a more undifferentiated phenotype [3, 8]. Intriguingly, melanoma cells can dynamically switch between a differentiated and undifferentiated state similar to the dynamic changes in epithelial cancers, such as head and neck squamous cell carcinoma, which switch between epithelial and mesenchymal phenotypes. Tumor cell subpopulations, initially characterized as tumor stem cells with tumor-initiating or tumor-maintaining properties, have been described for most human tumors, including melanomas. Table 1 summarizes the tumor subpopulations in melanoma, with a brief description of their phenotypic and biological characterization. Melanoma subpopulations are found across distinct patient samples, and the same markers identify a small percentage of cells in different patients (Fig. 3, bottom row, Fig. 4). The causes of differences in expression patterns are still unclear but likely not due to a hierarchical model of cancer stem cells. However, in melanoma, differences in subpopulations follow a more stochastic pattern. Potentially, there is a direct role of the tumor microenvironment (TME) in favoring the selection and expansion of a specific subpopulation [10, 17, 19, 38, 47, 58]. Host TME factors, including the presence of cytokines and growth factors secreted in the tumor milieu, also contribute to dynamic phenotypic changes of tumor cells as reported for breast, ovarian, and colon cancers [2, 23, 26, 52]. The role of growth factors and cytokines in phenotypic changes of melanoma is not well delineated. Some reports suggested a role of TNF-α, TGF-ß, and HGF in melanoma-targeted therapy resistance [18, 24, 25, 27, 57, 65] because they all change the phenotype of cells. Similarly, hypoxia can profoundly change the quantity of melanoma subpopulations. Our own experience points to multiple factors that control phenotypic heterogeneity, some of which may be active at the same time. Because of these dynamics and since every single melanoma cell is tumorigenic [46], we have replaced the term *melanoma stem cells* with *melanoma-initiating cells*. Our data support the earlier findings from

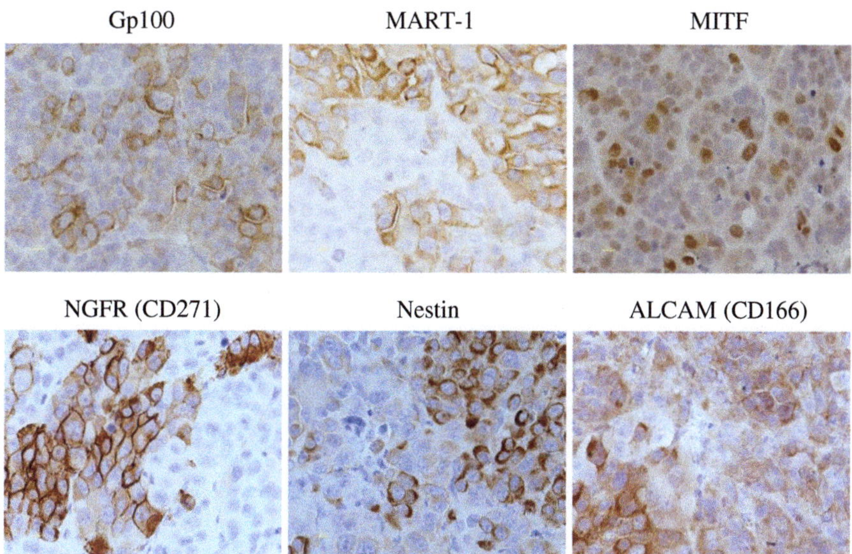

Fig. 3 Melanoma intratumor heterogeneity. Immunohistochemistry analysis of human melanoma xenografts. Melanoma xenografts display intratumor heterogeneity for gp100, MART-1, and MITF expression. Similar heterogeneity can be observed for neural crest-associated markers NGFR and Nestin and for ALCAM (CD166). Total magnification 400×

Table 1 Phenotypic characterization of melanoma subpopulations originally identified as melanoma stem cells

Marker	Biological role	Melanoma
CD20	B cell marker	Originally identified as melanoma stem cell marker [14]; associated with aggressive melanomas [5, 41, 51]
CD133	Transmembrane protein, hematopoietic and fetal brain stem cells, cancer stem cells	Tumor-initiating cells [34]; increased expression on poorly differentiated aggressive melanomas [22]
ABCB5	Intracellular and extracellular transmembrane transport	Chemoresistant cells [50]; involved in melanoma evasion of antitumor immunity [49] and in shaping vasculogenic mimicry supporting tumor growth [15]
CD271	NGF receptor; neural crest-derived tissues	Tumor-initiating cells [6]; correlation with poor prognosis and metastatic potential [11]
JARID1B	Histone demethylase	Slow-cycling TIC [46]; JARID1B+ cells are sensitive to mitochondrial respiration inhibition [47] and are sensitive to radioimmunotherapy [20]
ALDH1	Aldehyde dehydrogenase	Drug-resistant cells [7]; partially confirmed in the studies of Prasmickaite et al. [31, 43]

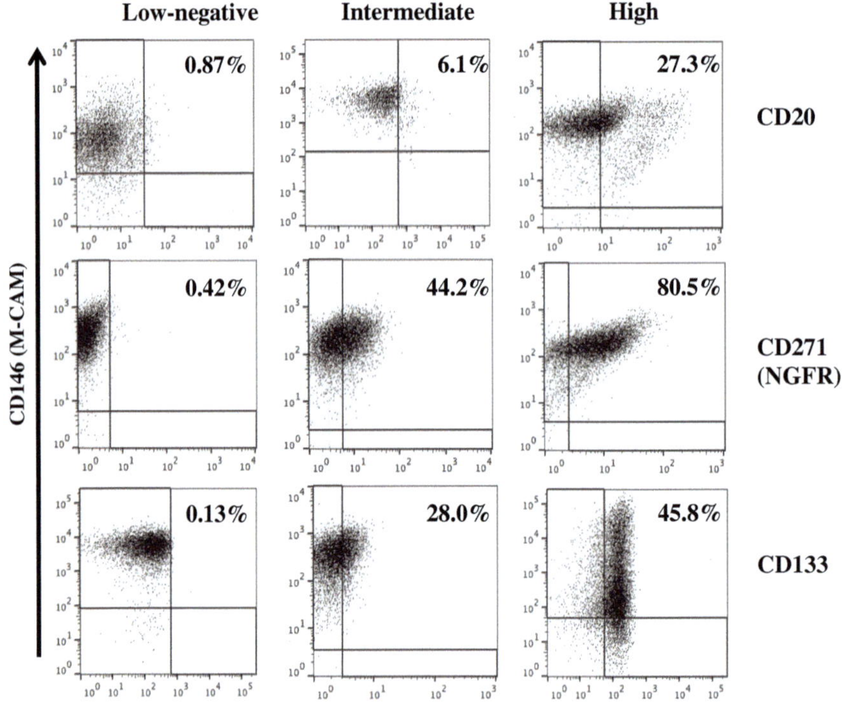

Fig. 4 Melanoma subpopulations are differentially represented in melanoma specimens. CD20, CD271 (NGFR), and CD133 biomarkers identify different subpopulation within melanoma xenografts. These subpopulations can be absent or very small (*left column*), present at intermediate (*middle column*) level or highly expressed (*right column*). Only live human cells isolated from xenografts are considered for the analysis; on *x*-axis, the marker of interest is shown, and on the *y*-axis, CD146 (MCAM) as a common marker. Percentages of CD146+ subpopulation cells are provided in the *upper right quadrant* in each graph

the Morrison group that single melanoma cells are capable of inducing tumors in highly immunodeficient animals [44, 45]. The subpopulations are critical for tumor maintenance as prolonged suppression decreases growth both in vitro and in vivo. They are also most critical for therapy resistance and require direct targeting [47]. Therefore, we propose that two different strategies are required, one to eliminate the bulk of the tumor and the other to target these minor, but biologically important subpopulations.

5 Conclusions

Recent advances in molecular medicine have identified melanoma as a complex, heterogeneous disease comprised of several distinct genotypes and phenotypes. The issue of tumor heterogeneity has posed a significant challenge in the goal of curing

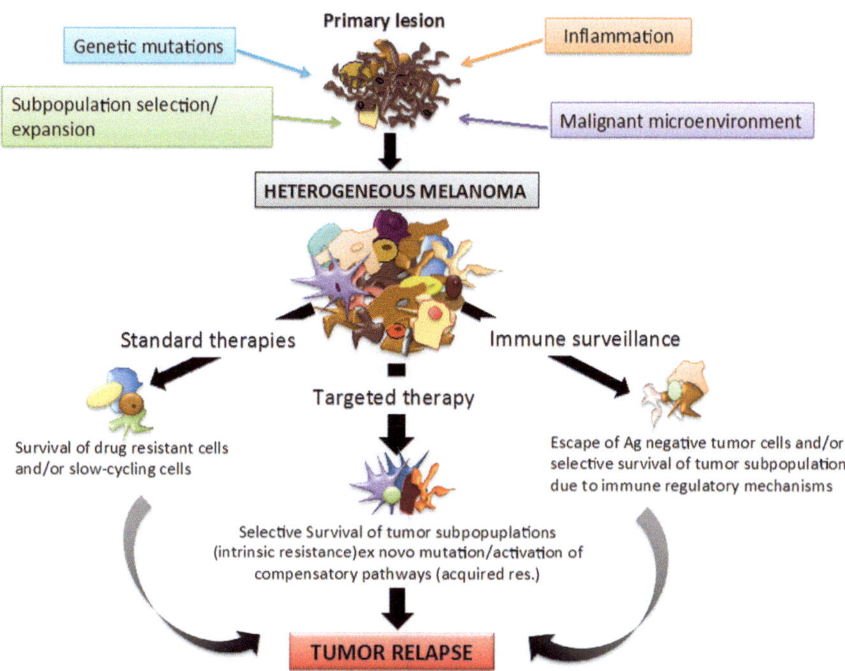

Fig. 5 Melanoma heterogeneity and clinical implication. Primary melanoma cells respond to different stimuli from the TME generating a heterogeneous tumor. Different subpopulations within melanoma lesions can survive to different therapeutic treatments and sustain the tumor for the development of relapse

melanoma as even recently identified targeted therapies fail to provide long-lasting remission in patients. We have briefly summarized the current clinical knowledge and major challenges in melanoma biology with the goal of identifying possible causes of melanoma heterogeneity (Fig. 5). The primary tumor cells are exposed to a variety of signals that all contribute to heterogeneity. Relapse during standard, targeted, and immunotherapies is nearly inevitable; we have to learn to either accommodate the heterogeneity with complex therapies or drive the malignant cells into a phenotype that is more uniform and can be attacked with single therapies. Additional studies are needed to better understand the mechanism leading to the complex phenotypes in this malignancy. It will be necessary to investigate how the TME harbors and protects selective tumor subpopulations during therapies. Hence, understanding the complex nature of tumor cells with their microenvironment will provide clues to design better therapies with the aim of achieving long-lasting cures.

Acknowledgments The authors thank Jessica L. Kohn for editorial assistance. This work was partially funded by the PA Department of Health, NCI K01 CA175269, NIH grants P01

CA114046, P01 CA025874, P30 CA010815, and R01 CA047159, the V Foundation for Cancer Research (JV), and the Dr. Miriam and Sheldon G. Adelson Medical Research Foundation.

Conflict of Interest The authors declare no financial conflict of interest.

References

1. Anderson K, Lutz C, van Delft FW et al (2011) Genetic variegation of clonal architecture and propagating cells in leukaemia. Nature 469:356–361
2. Asiedu MK, Ingle JN, Behrens MD, Radisky DC, Knutson KL (2011) TGFbeta/TNF(alpha)-mediated epithelial-mesenchymal transition generates breast cancer stem cells with a claudin-low phenotype. Cancer Res 71:4707–4719
3. Bailey CM, Morrison JA, Kulesa PM (2012) Melanoma revives an embryonic migration program to promote plasticity and invasion. Pigm Cell Melanoma Res 25:573–583
4. Bastian BC (2014) The molecular pathology of melanoma: an integrated taxonomy of melanocytic neoplasia. Ann Rev Pathol 9:239–271
5. Bittner M, Meltzer P, Chen Y et al (2000) Molecular classification of cutaneous malignant melanoma by gene expression profiling. Nature 406:536–540
6. Boiko AD, Razorenova OV, van de Rijn M et al (2010) Human melanoma-initiating cells express neural crest nerve growth factor receptor CD271. Nature 466:133–137
7. Boonyaratanakornkit JB, Yue L, Strachan LR et al (2010) Selection of tumorigenic melanoma cells using ALDH. J Invest Dermatol 130:2799–2808
8. Borrull A, Ghislin S, Deshayes F, Lauriol J, Alcaide-Loridan C, Middendorp S (2012) Nanog and Oct4 overexpression increases motility and transmigration of melanoma cells. J Cancer Res Clin Oncol 138:1145–1154
9. Campbell PJ, Yachida S, Mudie LJ et al (2010) The patterns and dynamics of genomic instability in metastatic pancreatic cancer. Nature 467:1109–1113
10. Cheli Y, Giuliano S, Fenouille N et al (2012) Hypoxia and MITF control metastatic behaviour in mouse and human melanoma cells. Oncogene 31:2461–2470
11. Civenni G, Walter A, Kobert N et al (2011) Human CD271-positive melanoma stem cells associated with metastasis establish tumor heterogeneity and long-term growth. Cancer Res 71:3098–3109
12. Ding L, Ellis MJ, Li S et al (2010) Genome remodelling in a basal-like breast cancer metastasis and xenograft. Nature 464:999–1005
13. Ding L, Ley TJ, Larson DE et al (2012) Clonal evolution in relapsed acute myeloid leukaemia revealed by whole-genome sequencing. Nature 481:506–510
14. Fang D, Nguyen TK, Leishear K et al (2005) A tumorigenic subpopulation with stem cell properties in melanomas. Cancer Res 65:9328–9337
15. Frank NY, Schatton T, Kim S et al (2011) VEGFR-1 expressed by malignant melanoma-initiating cells is required for tumor growth. Cancer Res 71:1474–1485
16. Gerlinger M, Horswell S, Larkin J et al (2014) Genomic architecture and evolution of clear cell renal cell carcinomas defined by multiregion sequencing. Nat Genet 46:225–233
17. Ghislin S, Deshayes F, Lauriol J et al (2012) Plasticity of melanoma cells induced by neural cell crest conditions and three-dimensional growth. Melanoma Res 22:184–194
18. Gray-Schopfer V, Wellbrock C, Marais R (2007) Melanoma biology and new targeted therapy. Nature 445:851–857
19. Holzel M, Bovier A, Tuting T (2013) Plasticity of tumour and immune cells: a source of heterogeneity and a cause for therapy resistance? Nat Rev Cancer 13:365–376
20. Jandl T, Revskaya E, Jiang Z et al (2013) Melanoma stem cells in experimental melanoma are killed by radioimmunotherapy. Nucl Med Biol 40:177–181

21. Keats JJ, Chesi M, Egan JB et al (2012) Clonal competition with alternating dominance in multiple myeloma. Blood 120:1067–1076
22. Klein WM, Wu BP, Zhao S, Wu H, Klein-Szanto AJ, Tahan SR (2007) Increased expression of stem cell markers in malignant melanoma. Mod Pathol 20:102–107
23. Knutson KL, Lu H, Stone B et al (2006) Immunoediting of cancers may lead to epithelial to mesenchymal transition. J Immunol 177:1526–1533
24. Koefinger P, Wels C, Joshi S et al (2011) The cadherin switch in melanoma instigated by HGF is mediated through epithelial-mesenchymal transition regulators. Pigm Cell Melanoma Res 24:382–385
25. Krepler C, Chunduru SK, Halloran MB et al (2013) The novel SMAC mimetic birinapant exhibits potent activity against human melanoma cells. Clin Cancer Res 19:1784–1794
26. Kulbe H, Chakravarty P, Leinster DA et al (2012) A dynamic inflammatory cytokine network in the human ovarian cancer microenvironment. Cancer Res 72:66–75
27. Landsberg J, Kohlmeyer J, Renn M et al (2012) Melanomas resist T-cell therapy through inflammation-induced reversible dedifferentiation. Nature 490:412–416
28. Li L, Fukunaga-Kalabis M, Yu H et al (2010) Human dermal stem cells differentiate into functional epidermal melanocytes. J Cell Sci 123:853–860
29. Lin J, Goto Y, Murata H et al (2011) Polyclonality of BRAF mutations in primary melanoma and the selection of mutant alleles during progression. Br J Cancer 104:464–468
30. Long GV, Wilmott JS, Haydu LE et al (2013) Effects of BRAF inhibitors on human melanoma tissue before treatment, early during treatment, and on progression. Pigm Cell Melanoma Res 26:499–508
31. Luo Y, Dallaglio K, Chen Y et al (2012) ALDH1A isozymes are markers of human melanoma stem cells and potential therapeutic targets. Stem Cells 30:2100–2113
32. Maley CC, Galipeau PC, Finley JC et al (2006) Genetic clonal diversity predicts progression to esophageal adenocarcinoma. Nat Genet 38:468–473
33. Mar VJ, Wong SQ, Li J et al (2013) BRAF/NRAS wild-type melanomas have a high mutation load correlating with histologic and molecular signatures of UV damage. Clin Cancer Res 19:4589–4598
34. Monzani E, Facchetti F, Galmozzi E et al (2007) Melanoma contains CD133 and ABCG2 positive cells with enhanced tumourigenic potential. Eur J Cancer 43:935–946
35. Mroz EA, Tward AD, Pickering CR, Myers JN, Ferris RL, Rocco JW (2013) High intratumor genetic heterogeneity is related to worse outcome in patients with head and neck squamous cell carcinoma. Cancer 119:3034–3042
36. Nazarian R, Shi H, Wang Q et al (2010) Melanomas acquire resistance to B-RAF(V600E) inhibition by RTK or N-RAS upregulation. Nature 468:973–977
37. Nickel GC, Barnholtz-Sloan J, Gould MP et al (2012) Characterizing mutational heterogeneity in a glioblastoma patient with double recurrence. PLoS ONE 7:e35262
38. O'Connell MP, Marchbank K, Webster MR et al (2013) Hypoxia induces phenotypic plasticity and therapy resistance in melanoma via the tyrosine kinase receptors ROR1 and ROR2. Cancer Discov 3:1378–1393
39. O'Leary RE, Diehl J, Levins PC (2014) Update on tanning: more risks, fewer benefits. J Am Acad Dermatol 70:562–568
40. Piccirillo SG, Combi R, Cajola L et al (2009) Distinct pools of cancer stem-like cells coexist within human glioblastomas and display different tumorigenicity and independent genomic evolution. Oncogene 28:1807–1811
41. Pinc A, Somasundaram R, Wagner C et al (2012) Targeting CD20 in melanoma patients at high risk of disease recurrence. Mol Ther 20:1056–1062
42. Pinnix CC, Lee JT, Liu ZJ et al (2009) Active Notch1 confers a transformed phenotype to primary human melanocytes. Cancer Res 69:5312–5320
43. Prasmickaite L, Engesaeter BØ, Skrbo N et al (2010) Aldehyde dehydrogenase (ALDH) activity does not select for cells with enhanced aggressive properties in malignant melanoma. PLoS ONE 5:e10731

44. Quintana E, Shackleton M, Sabel MS, Fullen DR, Johnson TM, Morrison SJ (2008) Efficient tumour formation by single human melanoma cells. Nature 456:593–598
45. Quintana E, Shackleton M, Foster HR et al (2010) Phenotypic heterogeneity among tumorigenic melanoma cells from patients that is reversible and not hierarchically organized. Cancer Cell 18:510–523
46. Roesch A, Fukunaga-Kalabis M, Schmidt EC et al (2010) A temporarily distinct subpopulation of slow-cycling melanoma cells is required for continuous tumor growth. Cell 141:583–594
47. Roesch A, Vultur A, Bogeski I et al (2013) Overcoming intrinsic multidrug resistance in melanoma by blocking the mitochondrial respiratory chain of slow-cycling JARID1B(high) cells. Cancer Cell 23:811–825
48. Schadendorf D, Fisher DE, Garbe C et al (2015) Melanoma. Nature Rev Dis Primers 1:1–20
49. Schatton T, Schutte U, Frank NY et al (2010) Modulation of T-cell activation by malignant melanoma initiating cells. Cancer Res 70:697–708
50. Schatton T, Murphy GF, Frank NY et al (2008) Identification of cells initiating human melanomas. Nature 451:345–349
51. Schmidt P, Kopecky C, Hombach A, Zigrino P, Mauch C, Abken H (2011) Eradication of melanomas by targeted elimination of a minor subset of tumor cells. Proc Natl Acad Sci USA 108:2474–2479
52. Schwitalla S, Fingerle AA, Cammareri P et al (2013) Intestinal tumorigenesis initiated by dedifferentiation and acquisition of stem-cell-like properties. Cell 152:25–38
53. Sensi M, Nicolini G, Petti C et al (2006) Mutually exclusive NRASQ61R and BRAFV600E mutations at the single-cell level in the same human melanoma. Oncogene 25:3357–3364
54. Shi H, Hugo W, Kong X et al (2014) Acquired resistance and clonal evolution in melanoma during BRAF inhibitor therapy. Cancer Discov 4:80–93
55. Slingluff CL Jr, Colella TA, Thompson L et al (2000) Melanomas with concordant loss of multiple melanocytic differentiation proteins: immune escape that may be overcome by targeting unique or undefined antigens. Cancer Immunol Immunother 48:661–672
56. Sottoriva A, Spiteri I, Piccirillo SG et al (2013) Intratumor heterogeneity in human glioblastoma reflects cancer evolutionary dynamics. Proc Natl Acad Sci USA 110:4009–4014
57. Straussman R, Morikawa T, Shee K et al (2012) Tumour micro-environment elicits innate resistance to RAF inhibitors through HGF secretion. Nature 487:500–504
58. Sztiller-Sikorska M, Koprowska K, Jakubowska J et al (2012) Sphere formation and self-renewal capacity of melanoma cells is affected by the microenvironment. Melanoma Res 22:215–224
59. Terzian T, Torchia EC, Dai D et al (2010) P53 prevents progression of nevi to melanoma predominantly through cell cycle regulation. Pigm Cell Melanoma Res 23:781–794
60. Tsao H, Goel V, Wu H, Yang G, Haluska FG (2004) Genetic interaction between NRAS and BRAF mutations and PTEN/MMAC1 inactivation in melanoma. J Invest Dermatol 122:337–341
61. Turke AB, Zejnullahu K, Wu YL et al (2010) Preexistence and clonal selection of MET amplification in EGFR mutant NSCLC. Cancer Cell 17:77–88
62. Vitale M (2013) Intratumor BRAFV600E heterogeneity and kinase inhibitors in the treatment of thyroid cancer: a call for participation. Thyroid 23:517–519
63. Wan PT, Garnett MJ, Roe SM et al (2004) Mechanism of activation of the RAF-ERK signaling pathway by oncogenic mutations of B-RAF. Cell 116:855–867
64. Wilmott JS, Tembe V, Howle JR et al (2012) Intratumoral molecular heterogeneity in a BRAF-mutant, BRAF inhibitor-resistant melanoma: a case illustrating the challenges for personalized medicine. Mol Cancer Ther 11:2704–2708
65. Wilson TR, Fridlyand J, Yan Y et al (2012) Widespread potential for growth-factor-driven resistance to anticancer kinase inhibitors. Nature 487:505–509
66. Yachida S, Jones S, Bozic I et al (2010) Distant metastasis occurs late during the genetic evolution of pancreatic cancer. Nature 467:1114–1117

67. Yancovitz M, Litterman A, Yoon J et al (2012) Intra- and inter-tumor heterogeneity of BRAF (V600E))mutations in primary and metastatic melanoma. PLoS ONE 7:e29336
68. Yu H, Kumar SM, Kossenkov AV, Showe L, Xu X (2010) Stem cells with neural crest characteristics derived from the bulge region of cultured human hair follicles. J Invest Dermatol 130:1227–1236
69. Yue L, Huang ZM, Fong S et al (2015) Targeting ALDH1 to decrease tumorigenicity, growth and metastasis of human melanoma. Melanoma Res 25:138–148
70. Zabierowski SE, Fukunaga-Kalabis M, Li L, Herlyn M (2011) Dermis-derived stem cells: a source of epidermal melanocytes and melanoma? Pigm Cell Melanoma Res 24:422–429
71. Zhang M, Qureshi AA, Geller AC, Frazier L, Hunter DJ, Han J (2012) Use of tanning beds and incidence of skin cancer. J Clin Oncol 30:1588–1593

Melanoma Epidemiology and Prevention

Marianne Berwick, David B. Buller, Anne Cust, Richard Gallagher, Tim K. Lee, Frank Meyskens, Shaily Pandey, Nancy E. Thomas, Marit B. Veierød and Sarah Ward

Abstract

The epidemiology of melanoma is complex, and individual risk depends on sun exposure, host factors, and genetic factors, and in their interactions as well. Sun exposure can be classified as intermittent, chronic, or cumulative (overall) exposure, and each appears to have a different effect on type of melanoma. Other environmental factors, such as chemical exposures—either through occupation, atmosphere, or food—may increase risk for melanoma, and this area warrants further study. Host factors that are well known to be important are the numbers and types of nevi and the skin phenotype. Genetic factors are classified as

M. Berwick (✉)
Department of Internal Medicine, University of New Mexico, MSC10-5550, Albuquerque, NM 87131-0001, USA
e-mail: mberwick@salud.unm.edu

D.B. Buller
Klein Buendel, Inc., 1667 Cole Boulevard, Suite 225, Golden, CO 80401, USA
e-mail: dbuller@kleinbuendel.com

A. Cust
Sydney School of Public Health, Sydney Medical School, University of Sydney, Level 6, 119-143 Missenden Road, Camperdown, NSW 2050, Australia
e-mail: Anne.Cust@sydney.edu.au

R. Gallagher · T.K. Lee
Cancer Control Research Program, BC Cancer Agency, 675 West 10th Avenue, Vancouver, BC V5Z 1L3, Canada
e-mail: rgallagher@bccrc.ca

T.K. Lee
e-mail: tlee@bccrc.ca

F. Meyskens
Public Health and Epidemiology, University of California, Irvine, USA
e-mail: flmeyske@uci.edu

H.L. Kaufman and J.M. Mehnert (eds.), *Melanoma*,
Cancer Treatment and Research 167, DOI 10.1007/978-3-319-22539-5_2

high-penetrant genes, moderate-risk genes, or low-risk genetic polymorphisms. Subtypes of tumors, such as BRAF-mutated tumors, have different risk factors as well as different therapies. Prevention of melanoma has been attempted using various strategies in specific subpopulations, but to date optimal interventions to reduce incidence have not emerged.

Keywords
Epidemiology · Risk factors · Genetic factors · Host characteristics · Prevention

Contents

S. Pandey
Mount Sinai School of Medicine, One Gustave L. Levy Place, New York, NY 10029, USA
e-mail: shaily.pandey@gmail.com

N.E. Thomas
University of North Carolina, 413 Mary Ellen Jones Bldg. CB#7287, Chapel Hill, NC 275992, USA
e-mail: Nancy_Thomas@med.unc.edu

M.B. Veierød
Department of Biostatistics, Institute of Basic Medical Sciences, P.O. Box 1122 Blindern, 0317 Oslo, Norway
e-mail: m.b.veierod@medisin.uio.no

S. Ward
Centre for Genetic Origins of Health and Disease (GOHaD), The University of Western Australia, M409, 35 Stirling Hwy, Crawley, WA 6009, Australia
e-mail: Sarah.ward@uwa.edu.au

1 Epidemiology

1.1 Introduction

Melanoma incidence has increased dramatically over the last 50 years, rising from 8.2 to 9.4 cases per 100,000 population in 1975 (females and males, respectively), age-adjusted, to approximately 24.2 and 35.4 per 100,000 in 2010 (females and males, respectively), in the USA. Mortality has increased also, with a plateau among females being reached recently, but with continued increase among males. This chapter is designed to bring the most up-to-date and accurate knowledge about the epidemiology of melanoma and current preventive practices. The focus is mainly on risk factors with less attention to prevention because, surprisingly, there is no clear path to melanoma prevention. Although reduction of intermittent sun exposure seems the most logical way to prevent the disease, it has not produced robust evidence of reduced incidence and mortality, even in Australia where the most widely applied preventive work has been done over time. Clearly, there are some things we have yet to learn about melanoma in order to reduce morbidity and mortality from this lethal disease.

1.2 Risk Factors for Melanoma

1.2.1 Sun Exposure

Sun exposure is the major environmental cause of melanoma [111, 112]. The proportion of melanoma attributed to sun exposure has been estimated to more than 90 % in Australia, Canada, Nordic countries, Switzerland, and the USA [5, 72, 98, 245] and between 78 and 90 % in several other European countries [5] including the UK with a recent estimate of 86 % of melanoma due to sun exposure [192].

Our knowledge of the complex association between sun exposure and melanoma comes mainly from case-control and cohort epidemiological studies. The geographic distribution of melanoma and the results of migration studies also provide evidence for the importance of *ambient sun exposure* [90].

Measurements of individual exposure vary between studies but are commonly classified as *intermittent* (short, intense sun exposure through activities such as sunbathing, outdoor recreations, and holidays in sunny climates), *chronic* (more continuous, primarily occupational exposure), and *total* sun exposure (the sum of intermittent and chronic exposure). Several case-control and cohort studies have investigated the association between individual sun exposure and melanoma risk. Meta-analyses of these studies show consistent results [65, 75, 76, 178] that continue to be supported by the results of studies published after the meta-analyses were undertaken [112]. There is strong evidence that an intermittent pattern of sun exposure increases melanoma risk. Chronic sun exposure shows no association, or a weak inverse association with melanoma risk. Total lifetime sun exposure is positively associated with melanoma risk, but the relationship is weaker than that for intermittent sun exposure. *Sunburn* is a marker of an intermittent pattern of sun exposure, and there is a tendency for greater consistency of positive associations for sunburn than for intermittent exposure. The summary relative risks (RR) and 95 % confidence intervals (95 % CI) for highest versus lowest category of exposure in meta-analyses of more than 50 studies were RR 2.0 (95 % CI 1.7–2.4) for sunburn, RR 1.6 (95 % CI 1.3–2.0) for intermittent, RR 1.0 (95 % CI 0.9–1.0) for chronic, and RR 1.3 (95 % CI 1.0–1.8) for total sun exposure [75, 76]. Moreover, significantly higher risk was found for intermittent than chronic exposure among studies that published results for both exposures, RR 1.5 (95 % CI 1.2–1.8) and RR 1.1 (95 % CI 0.9–1.4), respectively.

The weak association with chronic sun exposure may be due to its promotion of epithelial thickening and this together with a tanning effect may offer a modest protection against later exposure to solar radiation. Some of the studies of chronic sun exposure reported risk estimates below 1.00 [75, 76], but these results should not be interpreted as a protective effect. Chronic exposure is mainly occupational exposure for outdoor workers, and in studies of the different types of sun exposure, the reference categories may have consisted of individuals with high intermittent exposure together with individuals with low sun exposure, thereby artifactually producing low-risk ratios in those with high chronic exposure [90]. A recent analysis of two large case-control studies found no association between occupational exposure and melanoma risk and no indication of confounding by recreational exposure [236]. Importantly, the presence of solar keratoses, a marker of high cumulative sun exposure, is consistently positively associated with melanoma risk [90, 186].

Melanoma risk differs not only by pattern of sun exposure, but also by *body site*, *age*, and *phenotype of the host* (Sect. 1.2.3). This indicates that melanoma may arise through multiple causal pathways [241]. Head and neck melanomas have been linked to chronic sun exposure, with older age at diagnosis and melanoma on the trunk and limbs to younger ages and intermittent exposure. Notably, the available evidence suggests that sun exposure can cause melanoma on all body sites, but risks tend to be higher for usually sun-exposed sites than occasionally exposed sites [47, 90]. For sunburn, strong positive associations have been found at all body sites (head/neck, trunk, arms, and legs) and with no significant site-specific differences in recent meta-analyses and pooled analyses [47, 186].

Early-life sun exposure, sometimes decades before diagnosis, is probably important. Migration studies have found that *childhood* is a sensitive period [90]. The current evidence also suggests that melanoma risk continues to increase with accumulating intermittent sun exposure. Meta-analyses have reported increased melanoma risk with increasing number of sunburns during *all life periods* (childhood, adolescence, adulthood, and lifetime) [59], with no significant differences between sunburns in childhood and adulthood [75, 76].

The entire ultraviolet (UV) spectrum is classified as carcinogenic to humans [82]. Since most of UVB (280–315 nm) and all UVC (100–280 nm) are removed by stratospheric ozone, about 95 % of the midday solar UV radiation reaching the Earth's surface is UVA (315–400 nm) and 5 % UVB. Because individuals are exposed simultaneously to UVA and UVB when outdoors, it is difficult to distinguish between the effects of UVA and UVB in human studies. UVB is an established risk factor for sunburn, while both UVB and UVA may cause melanoma [112].

1.2.2 Indoor Tanning

Several case-control and a few cohort studies have investigated indoor tanning in relation to melanoma [32], and a causal positive association has been established [112]. The summary relative risk in the most recent meta-analysis of cohort and population-based case-control studies was 1.3 (95 % CI 1.1–1.4) for ever versus never use [32] and increased to 1.6 (95 % CI 1.4–1.9) when first use was before 35 years of age [33]. Furthermore, the risk is found to increase with the number of sessions [32, 136]. There is no indication that the risk associated with indoor tanning is substantially confounded by sun exposure [32, 96, 233].

Indoor tanning is popular in many countries and has become an important source of UV exposure. Up to 95–100 % of the body is exposed in a sunbed compared to 15–50 % during outdoor activities [22]. Measurements of modern sunbeds show UV irradiance higher than midday summer sun in Southern Europe and Australia, and exceeding the limits allowed by safety standards/regulations [106] (IARC [111, 112]; Gies et al. [84]; Nilsen et al. [185]; Tierney et al. 229). We still do not know which UV wavelengths actually increase melanoma risk. The irradiance from modern sunbeds is mainly in the UVA range with a fraction of UVB [67, 106] (Gies et al. [84]; Nilsen et al. [185]), and this is alarming in light of the increased focus on UVA as a carcinogen [82].

1.2.3 Other Environmental Factors

While the overwhelming majority of epidemiologic research has properly focused on the relationship between host characteristics (including genetics), exposure to UV radiation, and risk of cutaneous melanoma, findings from a number of relatively small studies have suggested that there may be other factors influencing risk of the disease.

Occupation and Melanoma

Several studies have suggested that exposure to polycyclic aromatic hydrocarbons, benzene, or other chemicals used in the printing industry [3, 41, 142, 163, 183] are associated with the development of melanoma. Similarly, studies of chemical workers have also shown elevated risks of melanoma [171, 179, 224]. Cohort studies of electrical and electronics workers [146, 203, 220] along with at least one case-control study [179] have also shown elevated risks for melanoma. It has been hypothesized that workers in occupations exposed to ionizing radiation might also be at increased risk of melanoma [3, 71, 218, 238, 252].

A number of investigations [29, 91, 94, 196] of airline pilots and cabin crew who might presumably be routinely exposed to cosmic radiation during high-altitude flight have also produced results suggestive of an increase in risk of melanoma.

However, several cohort studies among airline crews have also proved negative for melanoma [197, 250]. A more detailed review of findings from occupational and environmental studies of melanoma is found in Fortes and de Vries [70].

It should be noted that not all studies show elevated risk in any of these industries or occupations. In addition, workers in chemical, electrical, and electronics industries are potentially exposed to a large number of agents in the workplace, making it difficult or impossible to relate the elevated risks to one or more specific chemicals. Most of the elevated risk estimates are based on relatively small numbers of melanoma cases, as the studies to date have been predominantly cohort investigations designed to evaluate incidence or mortality due to common cancers, and melanoma is still a relatively rare disease in most populations. Finally, these occupational studies are usually based only on employment records and thus cannot adjust for the major known risk factors for the disease including phenotypic characteristics, nevus density, and UV radiation exposure.

PCBs

Relatively few studies have been conducted to look for specific environmental risk factors for melanoma, but among these, a number of studies have shown an elevated risk in individuals with suspected exposure to organochlorine compounds, such as polychlorinated biphenyls (PCBs) and some chlorine-based pesticides [1, 146, 161, 198, 203, 207, 208, 220, 240, 248]. As noted above, although these studies have some significant limitations, the results, with few exceptions, for implied industrial PCB exposure have been fairly consistently positive.

PCBs are aromatic compounds containing between one and ten chlorine atoms attached to a biphenyl structure. There are 209 reported congeners or variants, and PCBs—used commercially initially as dielectric fluids in electrical capacitors and transformers—contain mixtures of many of the congeners [134]. As potential adverse effects of PCBs became clear, most countries banned their production and use—the USA, Canada, and Australia in the 1970s and the European Union in the 1980s. However, PCBs are extremely persistent organic pollutants and survive in the environment for many years. PCBs are known to bioaccumulate in adipose tissue, and most human exposure in developed countries is through dietary intake of fish and animal products. Animal studies have shown evidence of malignant and benign tumors in the liver, lung, and oral mucosa in rats [176, 177] for a number of PCB congeners. However, melanoma was not among the tumors assessed in these studies, as a suitable animal model for melanoma has not yet been found.

A number of carcinogenic mechanisms [127], including formation of reactive oxygen species [69, 145, 157], endocrine disruption [80, 180, 204], and immune compromise [50, 147, 162, 173, 174, 209, 219], are known to be activated by PCBs. The evidence that PCBs can cause immune suppression is of particular interest because melanoma risk is known to increase between threefold and fourfold in individuals who are immunosuppressed due to agents given for organ transplantation [104, 117, 138].

One of the major drawbacks of human studies of melanoma and PCBs noted above is that no direct biological measures have been made in study subjects. A recent case-control study [73] evaluated blood levels of 14 PCB congeners and 11 organochlorine pesticides in 80 melanoma cases and 310 controls, and these investigators found significantly increasing trends in risk for melanoma with increasing blood levels of total PCBs, non-dioxin-like PCBs, and dioxin-like PCBs. Significant but more modest positive relationships were also seen with levels of some chlorine-based pesticide residues. These results persisted after adjustment for phenotypic factors, sun sensitivity, and sun exposure. Although the results of this preliminary study need confirmation in other investigations, they suggest that further, more detailed studies of organic chlorine compounds and melanoma may be productive. Recently, the International Agency for Research on Cancer (IARC) has reclassified PCBs from Group 2 "probably carcinogenic to humans" to Group 1 "carcinogenic to humans" [134].

The information to date from studies of non-ultraviolet radiation (UVR)-related factors in relation to malignant melanoma is not strong. However, the more recent studies showing elevated risks in those with significant exposure through the workplace or with relatively high blood levels indicate that other factors aside from UVR may play a part in the etiology of the disease.

Chromium

As our understanding of the molecular changes that accompany melanomagenesis increases [14, 53], it has become apparent that in contrast to non-melanoma skin cancer, the singular role of UVR in melanomagenesis has become less certain [166, 167]. Not all of the attributable risk for cutaneous melanoma can be linked to UVR exposure, and the molecular pathology suggests that UVR alone may not be the etiologic agent [14]. Additionally, only about 10 % of melanomas have a strong Mendelian (heritable) component. Clearly, there are likely to be any number of cocarcinogens. A vexing and unexplained clinical observation is that Albino Africans develop multiple and often severe squamous cell carcinomas but very, very few melanomas [61], suggesting that melanin is necessary for the development of melanoma, and melanin interacts with heavy metals.

Chromium, specifically hexavalent chromium Cr(VI), has been classified as a class I human carcinogen for quite some time. Occupational epidemiology has strongly implicated exposure by welders and others as contributing to the pathogenesis of lung cancer [122, 123, 214]. There is also considerable data that document that Cr(VI) can cause lung tumors in mice [251] as well as a TH1-driven response indicative of type IV hypersensitivity [38].

The possible role of Cr(VI) in melanomagenesis was stimulated by participation in the CARET, in which it was demonstrated that β-carotene supplementation led to more, rather than fewer, lung cancers in smokers [187]. Redox metabolism is important in β-carotene and in melanocytes and melanoma cells; subsequently, the possible role of heavy metals was thus investigated as *a redox factor* [166].

Austin and Reynolds [8] were the first to point out the association between heavy metal exposure and an increase in risk for melanoma. Concern about the effect of metal shedding, both local and systemically, led to a seminal epidemiologic meta-analysis study of other diseases in patients receiving hip-on-hip metal arthroplasties [188]. The crucial observation was that only melanoma was increased in these patients and in a time-related manner. A complex Nordic study also suggested a marked increase in both melanoma and prostate cancer [235]. However, a large (40,576 patients with hip replacement with metal-on-metal bearing surfaces and 248,995 with alternative bearings) but short-term (7 years) study of risk of malignant melanoma, hematologic malignancies, and prostate and renal tract cancers has demonstrated no increase in these malignancies [222].

Case and colleagues [122] conducted extensive studies in patients, and these have led to the following general observations [122, 132]: (1) Cr(VI) and cobalt (Co) were shed into the bloodstream of patients with prior metal-on-metal hip arthroplasties, but not in non-metal or knee arthroplasties (in which there is no direct metal–metal contact). (2) The concentration of Cr(VI) in the blood of these patients peaked at 6–12 years at 10 times "normal" levels and was measurable up to 10 years later. (3) Prospective follow-up also showed that there was also a statistically significant increase of both chromosome translocations and aneuploidy in peripheral blood lymphocytes at 6, 12, and 24 months after surgery. The changes were generally progressive with time, but the change in aneuploidy was much greater than that in chromosome translocations. However, no statistically significant correlations were found in secondary analyses between chromosome translocation indices and cobalt or chromium concentration in whole blood.

Experimental evidence shows that Cr(VI) may be involved in melanomagenesis [167]. Prolonged incubation of human melanocytes with a wide variety of metals at low non-toxic doses produced no effects. However, exposure to Cr(VI) resulted in morphological changes, aneuploidy was detected, and when cells from primary colonies were replated, secondary colonies formed. Additionally, exposure of human melanocytes to UVR and some metals causes bleaching of melanosomes and a pro-oxidant state [83]. Other physical evidence suggests a role in melanomagenesis as a wide variety of insecticides, PCBs, and metals (including chromium) have been identified bound to melanin [211]. These substances can convert the natural antioxidant to a pro-oxidant after UVR exposure. A separate piece of experimental evidence has emanated from the sequencing of a human melanoma [193]. The genomic results strongly indicated that both UV-induced and non-UV-induced DNA damages [a type associated with CR(VI)] were present. The evidence for a cocarcinogenesis role of hexavalent chromium in melanomagenesis is compelling and suggests that further investigation should lead to new etiologic and mechanistic insights.

1.2.4 Host Factors

Host factors greatly modify an individual's response to UVR, the principal environmental risk factor for melanoma. Host factors in this section refer to pigmentation characteristics: nevi; skin, hair, and eye colors; ability to tan; and propensity to burn.

Nevi

A major risk factor for melanoma is number and type of nevi. Nevi are benign collections of melanocytes, and the numbers of nevi have been implicated in numerous studies as the most important risk factor for melanoma, with an increased number of nevi associated with an increased risk of disease [15, 24, 158, 230]. A meta-analysis has shown that individuals with more than 100 normal nevi are at an almost seven times greater risk than individuals with few (≤15) nevi [75, 76]. The increase in risk is also thought to be incremental and proportional to the number of nevi present [158, 159]. It has been shown that the presence of 11–25 nevi conferred a 1.5-fold increase in risk compared with fewer than 10 nevi, and this risk doubled with each additional 25 nevi [158]. The size of the actual nevus also increases the risk of melanoma, especially those greater than 2.0 mm in diameter. The role of nevi as precursors of melanoma or markers of melanoma risk is controversial. They are, however, common adjacent to thin melanomas (those less than 1.70 mm) and less common among the thicker melanomas [210]. Approximately 50 % of melanomas less than 1.0 mm have adjacent neval remnants [221]. Still, many melanomas arise de novo; it is clear that individuals with many nevi are at high risk for developing melanoma [159].

Dysplastic or atypical nevi are also associated with an increased risk of melanoma. This subset of nevi are typified by cytological abnormality, with one definition requiring a macular component to at least one area of the lesion and at least three of either: an ill-defined border, an uneven contour, the presence of erythema, and variations in color or size greater than 5 mm [75, 76, 158]. Individuals with only one atypical lesion are already at a 1.6 times greater risk of melanoma, increasing to a tenfold greater risk with the presence of five or more atypical nevi [75, 76].

Atypical mole syndrome (also known as dysplastic nevus syndrome or familial atypical multiple mole and melanoma syndrome) is a rare phenotype characterized by at least two atypical nevi, high numbers (>100) of normal nevi and nevi on unusual body sites, such as the scalp, soles of the feet, buttocks, or breasts [15, 158]. Individuals with atypical mole syndrome, especially in conjunction with a family history of melanoma, are at an even greater risk of developing melanoma.

The exact nature of the role of nevi in melanoma development and progression is yet to be fully understood. This is likely to be, in part, because the factors affecting nevus expression and development are also complex and yet to be fully elucidated. A twin study found that the contribution of genetic factors to nevus expression was mediated by sun exposure and that with age, the component due to sun exposure declined greatly, increasing the proportion of nevus expression due to genetics [16]. Nevi on body sites regularly exposed to the sun had a smaller genetic contribution to variance than nevi on sun-protected sites, suggesting a greater environmental effect of sun exposure on the development of nevi on exposed body sites.

An interaction between sun exposure and nevi has been observed in various other investigations [24]. A study of Australian children found that increased sun exposure in childhood was significantly associated with an increased number of nevi [97]. A separate study of German adults found that intense, intermittent sun exposure in childhood or adolescence, characterized by sunburn, was significantly associated with high nevus counts and the occurrence of atypical nevi [77]. The authors suggested that sun exposure might induce nevus development, which subsequently affects risk of melanoma [77].

As noted earlier in this chapter, Whiteman et al. [242] have put forward a hypothesis for two divergent pathways for melanoma development on differing body sites. They propose that some individuals are prone to melanoma due to chronic sun exposure and are therefore more likely to develop melanoma on body sites regularly exposed to the sun, like the face. Alternatively, other individuals with a propensity for melanocytic instability are at risk of developing melanoma via a proliferative melanocytic pathway, characterized by atypical nevi or high numbers of nevi [24, 242]. The authors predict that melanoma development in the latter group of individuals is instigated early in life by sun exposure and then driven by other risk factors. They are therefore more likely to develop melanoma on body sites not chronically exposed to sunlight, such as the trunk, perhaps due to unstable melanocytic development. Supporting this theory are findings from an Italian study [49]. These studies found individuals with melanoma on the head or face significantly more likely to have fewer nevi and, conversely, individuals with melanoma on the trunk more likely to have high nevus counts.

Other Pigmentation Factors

Pigmentation characteristics are well-established host risk factors for melanoma, with skin, eye, and hair colors all known to be associated with susceptibility. An inverse relationship has been consistently demonstrated between melanoma risk and degree of skin pigmentation [6, 24, 159]. Fair-skinned individuals have a much higher risk for developing melanoma than dark-skinned individuals, such that risk estimates in individuals of non-European descent, who are typically darker-skinned, are up to 10–20-fold less than those in individuals of European descent, who are typically lighter-skinned [15, 230].

Skin reaction to the sun is also a predictor of melanoma risk. Skin that freckles easily has a tendency to burn or an inability to tan, showing an increased propensity for the disease [37, 159, 230]. Some authors have hypothesized that skin reaction contributes less to melanoma risk than actual skin color, while others have postulated that skin reaction is a better predictor of risk than skin color [6, 159]. Analytically, skin reactivity has been shown to be a strong, independent predictor of susceptibility to melanoma and may also be a more robust measure of pigmentation due to the issues surrounding accurate measurement of skin pigmentation within and across studies [6, 230].

A pooled analysis of 10 case-control studies [30] showed that both fair skin types and a high degree of freckling were associated with a twofold increase in risk of developing melanoma, independent of each other, hair color and number of nevi. The effect of freckling on risk was notably mediated by age, with a much higher risk found in those less than 40 years of age. This could be related to the stronger predictive effect of sun exposure in childhood and adolescence, with degree of freckling acting as a marker for degree of sun exposure as well as an indicator of melanocyte instability.

This pooled analysis, along with numerous other epidemiological studies [158, 230], found an increased risk of melanoma among individuals with red or blonde hair, or blue or green eyes. While Bliss et al. [30] found hair and eye colors to be independent risk factors for melanoma, Gandini et al. [75, 76] have questioned whether the association between these traits is completely independent of skin color. While clearly associated with melanoma, they argue that it cannot be a causal relationship and that they appear to be risk factors for the disease simply due to their correlation with skin pigmentation. As a result, a number of investigators have formed indexes to avoid collinearity in pigmentation characteristics and risk. Furthermore, as eye and hair colors are less prone to misclassification or recall bias than measurements of skin color or skin reaction to the sun, they may represent a more accurate marker of overall pigmentation traits, strengthening their association with melanoma susceptibility [75, 76].

As with many factors affecting melanoma risk, the relationship with pigmentation characteristics is complicated and still not clearly understood. Further complexities lie in the known and potential underlying genetic variants associated with pigmentation.

1.2.5 Germline Genetic Factors and Genome-Wide Association Studies (GWAS)

Melanoma sometimes develops within families (about 10 % of people with melanoma report a first- or second-degree relative with melanoma [99]), but this occurrence may be due to relatives sharing either genetic risk factors or environmental risk factors such as excessive sun exposure, or both. A population-based study of Australian twins estimated that 55 % of the variation in susceptibility to melanoma is due to genetic influences [215]. Genetic factors have also been shown to contribute as much or more to melanoma risk prediction than classical risk factors, over and above pigmentary effects [57]. The discovery of melanoma susceptibility genes can improve our knowledge of the biological pathways involved in melanoma development. This knowledge can be translated into potential new targets for future therapies and more accurate melanoma prediction tools which can improve our identification of people at high risk for melanoma who might benefit from screening or targeted prevention strategies [57].

High-Penetrance Gene Mutations

CDKN2A on chromosome 9p21 was identified in 1994 as the first high-penetrance melanoma susceptibility gene [119, 165]. *CDKN2A* encodes two distinct proteins, p16INK4A and p14ARF, which are involved in cell cycle control, tumor suppression, and melanocyte senescence [165]. The p16INK4A protein binds to the cyclin-dependent kinases CDK4 and CDK6, inhibiting phosphorylation of the retinoblastoma protein and progression of the cell through the G1 cell cycle checkpoint. The p14ARF protein induces cell cycle arrest or apoptosis via the p53 pathway. Mutations in the *CDK4* gene are also associated with very high risk of melanoma, and the activities of *CDK4* and p16 have similar downstream effects [99]. However, *CDK4* mutations are very rare and only found in a handful of melanoma families worldwide [99].

Only about 2 % of all melanoma cases in the population carry a *CDKN2A* mutation, but the probability is much higher when a strong family history of melanoma or multiple primary tumors are present [26, 87]; as such, *CDKN2A* mutations are estimated to account for approximately 40 % of familial cases [87]. Carriers of a *CDKN2A* mutation have a substantial lifetime risk of developing cutaneous malignant melanoma; population-based estimates indicate that around 30–50 % of mutation carriers will develop melanoma by 80 years of age [20, 58], whereas lifetime risk estimates derived from clinic-based sampling (of families with multiple cases of melanoma) range from 58 to 90 % penetrance by 80 years of age [27].

Intermediate-Risk Gene Variants

The melanocortin-1 receptor (*MC1R*) gene, which encodes the melanocyte-stimulating hormone receptor, was identified as the first low- to medium-penetrance gene associated with melanoma risk [99, 232]. It is one of the major genes that determine skin and hair colors, although there is evidence that it acts via pigmentary and non-pigmentary pathways to influence melanoma development [56, 120, 201]. There are many common variants of *MC1R* [121], but only six of them are usually referred to as "red hair color phenotype" or "R" variants (associated with red hair, fair skin, freckling, poor sun sensitivity) and are associated with a greater-than-twofold increased risk of melanoma [56, 201, 243, 244]. The other *MC1R* variants (usually referred to as "r" or "non-RHC") generally have a relatively weak association with red hair color phenotype and have a weaker association with melanoma risk [56, 201, 243, 244]. Although each variant individually is associated with a small increase in risk of melanoma, some people carry more than one variant and the combined effect can be large (e.g., more than fourfold increased risk of melanoma for people carrying 2 "R" alleles compared to wild-type alleles). Also, since the prevalence of *MC1R* variants conveying elevated risk in populations of European origin is very high (ranging up to about 70 %) [56, 120], as a group they account for a substantial proportion of disease in the population [243, 244]. It is estimated that approximately 21 % of the familial aggregation of melanoma among those developing melanoma under the age of 40 is explained by MC1R variants, assuming a multiplicative polygenic risk model [56].

More recently, *MITF*, the microphthalmia-associated transcription factor, was identified as a medium-penetrance melanoma susceptibility gene through a candidate gene approach in individuals affected with melanoma and renal cell carcinoma [21] and whole-genome sequencing of melanoma-prone families [249]. *MITF* regulates several other genes whose functions in melanocytes range from development, differentiation, survival, cell cycle regulation, and pigment production [249]. The *MITF* E318K variant allele is relatively uncommon in the population (about 1 % prevalence) but is associated with a 2–3-fold increased risk of melanoma, which is higher for those with multiple primary melanomas [249]. The presence of the E318K variant allele is associated with a higher nevus count and non-blue eye color.

Of interest, it has been shown that variation in *MC1R* and *MITF* is more strongly associated with melanoma in people with darker phenotypic traits than those with fairer complexions [25, 56, 120] and that risk of melanoma among carriers with "low-risk" phenotypes was as great or greater than among those with "at-risk" phenotypes with few exceptions [25].

Low-Penetrance Gene Variants

Since 2008, a series of genome-wide association studies (GWAS) has led to a substantial increase in our understanding of melanoma genetics [2, 13, 28, 39, 135, 149]. While the discovery of high- and medium-penetrance susceptibility genes has used genetic linkage and candidate gene approaches in families with a strong family history, the discovery of low-penetrance susceptibility genes relies on large, often unselected case-control studies.

As expected, these GWAS have identified or confirmed variants in or near pigmentation genes as being associated with melanoma risk, including *MC1R*, *TYR*, *ASIP*, *SLC45A2*, *IRF4*, and *TYRP1*. Risk variants for melanoma also lie in or near *MTAP*, *PLA2G6*, and *IRF4*, *TERT/CLPTM1L*, loci that have been shown to be associated with nevus count variation. However, one of the most important developments to come from the GWAS approach is the identification of susceptibility genes that do not act via pigmentation pathways but instead are involved in other cellular processes such as DNA repair and cell cycle control; these include genes in or near *ATM*, *CASP8*, *CCND1*, *MX2* [2, 13, 135, 149], and *FTO*, which appear to have a broader function than its obesity-related effects [113]. The minor allele frequencies for these genomic variants are in the range of 1–49 %, and the risk of melanoma associated with the risk allele is in the range of a 1–2-fold increased risk [135]. On their own, each of these variants only slightly increases risk of melanoma; however, carrying several variants can significantly increase melanoma risk, which may also be further modified by environmental factors such as UV exposure.

Future Directions

Future directions in this field include determining which are the causal variants associated with melanoma risk, determining the biological mechanisms underlying the non-pigmentary associations, evaluating the gene–gene and gene-environment interactions, and incorporating genetic variants into melanoma risk prediction models and testing their effect on motivating risk-reducing behaviors as a cancer prevention strategy.

1.2.6 Somatic Genetic Factors: Tumor Subtypes

Another direction related to genetic analyses is based on tumor, or somatic, alterations. Melanoma is a heterogeneous disease with a variety of histologic subtypes and complex epidemiology. Age-specific incidence patterns display early- and late-onset peak frequencies for trunk and face/ear melanomas, respectively [130, 131], consistent with hypotheses that melanoma arises from more than one causal pathway and contain distinct melanoma genotypes [241]. *NRAS* and *BRAF* mutations, mutually exclusive of each other, are found, respectively, in 10–30 and 25–60 % of primary melanomas [60, 63, 64, 93, 228]. Less frequently, melanomas contain *KIT* mutations, particularly mucosal melanoma or melanomas arising on acral or on sun-damaged sites [53]. *GNAQ* and *GNA11* mutations were discovered in uveal and CNS melanomas, defining additional molecular melanoma subgroups [81, 129, 200]. Frequently, melanomas also contain *PTEN*, *CDKN2A*, *CDK4*, and *CCND1* copy number alterations that help to define molecular subgroups [54, 55].

Newer high-throughput sequencing methods for tumors have allowed studies to identify many additional somatic mutations in melanomas [103, 110, 128, 156, 239], including *NF1* and *RAC1* mutations (5 % of cases) and *BRAF* gene fusions [35, 110]. Recently, it was also discovered that 30–40 % of melanomas harbor mutations in the promoter region of the telomerase reverse transcriptase (*TERT*) gene, and these *TERT* promoter mutations were found to occur more frequently in *BRAF*-mutant melanomas [101, 105, 108, 107]. The contribution of these newly discovered mutations to melanoma subclassifications remains to be fully elucidated.

Clinical Characteristics of Tumor Subtypes

BRAF- and *NRAS*-mutant melanomas have been examined in several studies in relationship to their clinical characteristics. *BRAF*-mutant melanomas are associated with young age at diagnosis, intermittently sun-exposed sites such as the trunk, superficial spreading subtype, absence of solar elastosis, and presence of mitoses [17, 60, 63, 64, 93, 144, 155, 228]. *NRAS*-mutant melanomas are associated with older age at diagnosis, but less associated with specific anatomic location, are more likely to be nodular subtype, and show increased Breslow thickness and presence of mitoses [60, 63, 64, 86, 139, 228, 231, 234]. Interestingly, *RAC1*-mutant melanomas are more common in older men on the head and neck location [128], while *TERT* promoter mutations in melanomas are associated with older age, increased Breslow thickness, nodular subtype, and tumor ulceration [101].

BRAF-mutant melanomas were found to be more common in patients with increased numbers of nevi [93, 228] and with the presence of nevi adjacent to the melanomas [63, 195]. These findings are plausible as approximately 70 % of nevi contain *BRAF* mutations [194]. *BRAF* mutations were associated with the ability to tan but not with freckling or hair or eye color [93, 228]. *TERT* promoter mutations in melanoma were not associated with hair, skin, or eye color or number of nevi [101].

Sun Exposure and Tumor Subtypes

The mechanistic contribution of sun exposure to melanomagenesis remains to be elucidated. Most studies note indirect evidence, such as associations between mutations with anatomic site, to infer a relationship to UV exposure; however, body site alone may influence mutational status. Studies examining sun exposure questionnaire data found that *BRAF*-mutant melanoma was associated with high early-life ambient [228] and individual self-reported childhood sun exposure [144] and was less likely to occur in people with high cumulative sun exposure [92]. However, these results remain to be replicated. Of note, while the majority of *BRAF*-mutant melanomas harbor a single base change resulting in *BRAF*V600E alteration, approximately 10 % of *BRAF* mutations in melanoma contain two adjacent base changes, tandem mutations [226] that have not been found in *BRAF*-mutant tumors of other types, such as colon and lung cancers. It is possible that these tissue-specific tandem mutations arise related to UV exposure [227]. The *BRAF*V600K tandem mutation has engendered particular interest. Among a cohort of Australian patients with metastatic melanoma, the frequency of non-*BRAF*V600E, including V600K, mutations increased with older age and histologic solar elastosis at the primary melanoma site [164]. In a North European cohort, participants with *BRAF*V600K-mutated melanoma were significantly older at diagnosis than those with *BRAF*V600E-mutated melanoma [118]. In an Austrian cohort, *BRAF*V600K mutations were more frequent than *BRAF*V600E mutations in in situ lentigo maligna melanomas [223]. However, we are not aware of a study that has examined *BRAF*V600K-mutant melanoma in relationship to reported sun exposure.

A variety of evidence suggests that UVB exposure might be responsible for mutations in melanoma tumor suppressor genes. *PTEN*, *CDKN2A*, and *P53* harbor higher rates of UVB signature mutations than oncogenic *BRAF* and *NRAS* variants, and *TP53* and *CDKN2A* harbor higher rates of UVB signature mutations than non-skin cancers [102]. Furthermore, *PTEN* mutations occur in approximately 50 % of melanomas from xeroderma pigmentosum patients, who are susceptible to UV mutagenesis, while *BRAF*, *NRAS*, and *KIT* mutation frequencies were lower than *PTEN* [160]. Next-generation sequencing has more recently identified UVB signature hot spot mutations in putative oncogenes, including at *PPP6C* R264C, *STK19* D89N, and *RAC1* P29S [103, 128]. In addition, *TERT* promoter mutations in melanoma, also UVB signature mutations, are more frequent at both chronically and intermittently sun-exposed than non-exposed sites, although these mutations were not associated with reported sun behavior [101]. Additional work will be necessary to collect epidemiologic evidence, including from sun exposure questionnaires, as to whether these mutations are associated with ambient exposure, sun behaviors, and patterns of UV exposures.

Melanocortin-1 receptor (*MC1R*), which is a highly polymorphic gene whose variants are associated with red hair, fair traits, and melanoma risk, was found to be strongly associated with *BRAF*-mutant melanoma on non-chronically sun-damaged skin in US and Italian cohorts [133] and regardless of signs of chronic solar damage in a separate Italian cohort [68]. However, studies conducted in North Carolina and Australia found no association between carriage of *MC1R* variants and *BRAF*-mutant melanoma [93, 228], while a study conducted in Germany found *BRAF*-mutant melanoma to be less frequent among *MC1R* variant carriers than non-carriers, with the effect dependent entirely upon the nodular subtype [212]. A recent study in Spanish and Austrian populations found no association of *MC1R* status with *BRAF*-mutant melanoma across all tumor sites but a non-significant association for truncal melanoma and a significant inverse association between *MC1R* variants and *BRAF*-mutant melanomas of the head and neck [92]. Additional larger—perhaps international—studies seem necessary to provide any real understanding of the association of *MC1R* variants with *BRAF*-mutant melanoma in the context of possible anatomic site and histologic subtype dependencies.

In conclusion, it has become clear that *BRAF*, *NRAS*, *KIT*, *GNAQ*, and *GNA11* mutations in melanoma contribute to the definitions of melanoma subgroups. Additional mutations recently identified in tumor suppressor genes and oncogenes are expected to refine this classification. Much work is anticipated to determine the associations of these mutational subgroups with genetic risk factors, sun exposure, and outcomes. Understanding the risk based on mutation subgroups is ultimately expected to contribute to our understanding of how to design targeted prevention messages.

1.2.7 Gene-Environment Interaction

The interactions revealed through the Genes Environment and Melanoma study (GEM) analyses will identify some of the "missing heritability" that GWAS have not found [253]. Few new studies address the gaps or the need to identify risk for melanoma among those without traditional risk factors. Our GEM analysis of a rare MITF mutation shows significant interactions with low nevus density and dark hair color [25]. GWAS of melanoma have identified additional genetic risk factors but unfortunately have not yet been useful for public health interventions. It is critical to identify genetic factors in concert with the environmental factors, mainly UV exposure, and to be able to control for moderators, such as pigmentation and number of nevi, as did Thomas et al. [228] with risk in GEM for BRAF mutations. Approximately 10–15 % of individuals diagnosed with melanoma can expect to die from their disease. At this point in time, there are no reliable biomarkers to distinguish aggressive melanoma from a more indolent lesion. Exciting progress in treatment has been made in the last few years—using immunotherapy (anti-CTLA-4, anti-PD-1, chimeric antigen receptor therapy); however, life has not been significantly prolonged by treatment and still only one-third of patients respond. Researchers are largely clueless as to why more don't benefit [52]. If we could identify lesions that are aggressive at early stages of the disease, we could make a huge impact on disease-specific mortality.

1.3 Survival and Melanoma

1.3.1 Ecologic Studies

Ecologic studies are subject to many unknown biases. However, they can also provide insights into scientific problems and so have utility. In the area of melanoma mortality, there are few large studies that have been conducted, so the large databases maintained by the US SEER program and the WHO database can be helpful to evaluate trends over time and by latitude. Some time ago, Lemish et al. [141] observed that survival from melanoma increased with increasing melanoma incidence among several populations and suggested that high levels of ambient sun exposure might induce a more biologically benign type of melanoma. Recent data evaluating a very large number of populations support this association of the positive temporal and geographic association with incidence and survival [7].

Conflicting analyses, however, exist. For example, two studies have found no association between latitude or other measures of UV exposure and mortality from melanoma in the USA [116, 130, 131]; however, others have reported a positive association between increasing latitude (decreasing UV) and increasing melanoma mortality rates [46, 216] or a negative association between increasing latitude and melanoma mortality [34, 66, 78].

A different measure of previous sun exposure derived for ecologic study is season of diagnosis. Seasonality of diagnosis has been shown to be associated with melanoma mortality in one study. Boniol et al. [31] found that in Australia, those diagnosed in the summer had a significantly reduced risk of dying from melanoma compared to those diagnosed in the winter with a hazard ratio (HR) of 0.72 (95 % CI 0.65–0.81). Again, there are conflicting data. A report from Spain [172] showed a significant association between diagnosis in July and August (the Spanish summer) and mortality from melanoma. Finally, another report from Australia [115] found no association between season of diagnosis and survival from melanoma in Victoria. Clearly, the weight of the evidence for melanoma in these ecological studies does not support a role for diagnosis during the summer and improved survival.

So, in summary, the ecologic studies are mixed in their results, but the weight of the evidence no longer supports a strong positive association between latitude and UV exposure.

1.3.2 Analytic Studies

Unfortunately, few analytic studies have interviewed patients for sun exposure and residential histories and then followed subjects for mortality. Berwick et al. [23] reported an inverse association between measures of solar exposure and melanoma mortality. The authors suggested that this provocative finding might indicate a beneficial effect of sun exposure in relationship to survival with melanoma mediated by vitamin D produced by sun exposure. Alternative hypotheses were also offered that previous sun exposure might induce more indolent melanomas through increased melanization and DNA repair capacity.

Interestingly, Heenan et al. [100] published a somewhat similar analysis finding that solar elastosis was of borderline significance (P for trend = 0.07) and inversely associated with death from melanoma.

Rosso et al. [206] have also suggested that intense intermittent sun exposure prior to the diagnosis of melanoma is associated with an improved survival. A study from the UK measured serum vitamin D at diagnosis and found that those with the highest level of serum vitamin D had the best survival [181].

To add to the confusion, Berwick and colleagues [25] have now analyzed survival data from a very large international cohort of melanoma patients and find that there is little association between sun exposure prior to diagnosis and melanoma survival. This seems like a reasonable conclusion given the mixed evidence presented above.

In summary, the analytic studies evaluating mortality in relationship to solar exposure prior to diagnosis have quite mixed results. The discrepancy among studies is worthy of further investigation. Analytic studies are generally considered to be more valid than ecologic studies and could come up with different interpretations of data because they may suffer less from misclassification of solar UV. In addition, measures of individual sun exposure are likely to be more precise than those estimated by latitude or UV exposure, regardless of how measured.

2 Prevention and Evaluation of Efficacy

Prevention of sunburn and reduction of time spent in the sun has been the aim of many sun safety interventions. These interventions have focused on children and adults in settings ranging from childcare facilities, schools, and outdoor recreation sites to workplaces and community-wide campaigns that attempt to reach at-risk populations in a variety of venues. Interventions have primarily relied on training, education, and communication, with a few including distribution of sun protective products (e.g., sunscreen) and organizational actions and policies.

Metrics for both sunburn and time spent in the sun have varied. Sunburn has been measured as either any sunburn or number of sunburns. Time in the sun has been assessed through reported amount of time outdoors, with some studies focusing simply on time spent sunbathing for the purpose of getting a suntan and others distinguishing intentional exposure such as sunbathing from incidental sun exposure associated with outdoor recreation. Observational methods for assessing sun exposure have been used which include assessment of skin color change, measures of UV from polysulfone badges worn by respondents, and counts of melanocytic nevi. Unfortunately, there is no "gold standard" for assessing changes in solar UV exposure, rendering comparison of results from different prevention studies difficult.

The public commonly assumes that sunscreen is a good preventive measure against skin cancer, including melanoma. This assumption was confirmed by a randomized controlled trial (RCT) of regular sunscreen use among 1621 people aged 25–75 in Queensland, Australia, and demonstrated a 50 % reduction (hazard ratio 0.50; 95 % CI 0.24–1.02; $P = 0.051$) in melanoma incidence, particularly invasive melanomas (hazard ratio 0.27; 95 % CI 0.08–0.97) at a 10-year follow-up. This finding was echoed in an observational study [137] where they found that routine use of sunscreen and other sun protection methods was higher among controls than among cases ($P = 0.03$) and other sun protection methods ($P = 0.006$). However, in this study, the authors are cautious about the results as few used sunscreen routinely and the measures of other sun protection methods lacked specificity.

2.1 Interventions in Childcare and School Settings

Studies that evaluated sun safety interventions for children in childcare and school settings have provided mixed results on the effectiveness of these. In childcare settings, two studies reported no change in sun exposure measured by parent reports or by change in melanocytic nevi in the children's skin [18, 19, 246], but one study did find that children spent less time outdoors during peak sun hours at childcare centers with sun protection policies [124]. One study also failed to produce changes in sunburn prevalence after an educational intervention with parents [18, 19].

Several interventions directed at primary school-aged children have resulted in reduced sun exposure measured by self-reports, UVR (UV)-sensitive dosimeters, skin color change, or development of fewer melanocytic nevi [43, 44, 45, 51, 109, 126, 140, 169, 170], but a few did not affect sun exposure [85, 109, 205]. These interventions involved instructional materials inserted into the school curriculum or had dermatologists talk with staff and parents.

A limited number of interventions have been evaluated with secondary school-aged children. One intervention using instructional materials inserted into the school curriculum reduced sun exposure or sunbathing [213], but another study using school-based instruction did not [44, 45]. Also, a recent study of an Internet-delivered curriculum did not improve the frequency of sunbathing [40].

Interventions containing appearance-focused messaging or photo-aging information, including UV imaging, have reduced college students' time in the sun [114, 150], although regional differences have been seen in this effect [152]. Some interventions have failed to influence time in the sun [143, 151, 154, 202] or actually produced increased sun exposure on some measures [48]. In some of these interventions, college students were provided with sunscreen and UV monitors, too [48, 114, 202].

Studies on interventions in schools have also produced some evidence that they can reduce sunburn. Sunburn incidence has been reduced with interventions in primary schools [42], secondary schools [40], and college [143]. However, studies in these contexts have also failed to report change in sunburn [18, 19, 51, 175, 199], and one study found increased sunburn frequency post-intervention [48].

2.2 Interventions in Occupational Settings

Interventions targeting sun exposure and sunburn in workplaces have been less common than those delivered in school settings; however, they have generally been effective at improving both outcomes. Specifically, one study of a 10-year follow-up to yearly education and mandatory sun protection policy with road workers found reduced sun exposure measured by skin tanning and solar keratosis [247]. Another study on ski area employees found reduction in sunburns by employees immediately [42] although this reduction was no longer evident in the following summer [4] or when the intervention was distributed throughout the North American ski industry [4]. Finally, the sun protection program at ski areas did not affect sunburn prevalence among guests [237].

Likewise, an intervention for swimming pools that included signage, program guidebooks, and instructions on training lifeguards to teach sun safety to children reduced sunburns among lifeguards in a randomized trial [79]. This intervention remained effective at decreasing sunburns among lifeguards when disseminated nationwide to pools where lifeguards also reported the presence of pool policies to promote sun safety to children and parents and teaching sun safety to children [95].

2.3 Interventions in Outdoor Recreation

Sun safety interventions in outdoor recreation settings have able to reduce sun exposure and sunburn. One study delivering photo-aging information, photograph of UV damage, and free sunscreen did find some reduction in sunbathing but not in incidental sun exposure [153]. Another study on a similar intervention with beach visitors reduced their frequency of sunbathing and prevalence of sunburn at a 2-month follow-up but only sunbathing and not sunburn prevalence at a 1-year follow-up [191]. A third study conveying risk information and UV photographs did not affect sun exposure [190]. However, a fourth intervention that included information on the harms of sun exposure and benefits of protection on sunscreen labels decreased sunburn prevalence but not time in the intense sun [182].

2.4 Interventions on Dermatology Patients

Two recent evaluations have explored whether interventions with dermatology patients can decrease sun exposure and sunburns. One study in China did report decreased sun exposure following clinic-based education and provision of sunscreen [108, 107], but another study in the USA intervening with melanoma patients with the aim of improving protection of their children found no overall impact on children's time outdoors or sunburn [89]. Parents at moderate to high risk of developing skin cancer limited their time in the sun following an intervention using printed information and telephone contact but did not change their children's sun exposure [125].

2.5 Community-Wide Interventions

Finally, a small number of studies have examined the effect of community-wide interventions that convey sun protection messages through a variety of venues. The longest intervention is the SunSmart campaign in Australia. The latest time series evaluation showed that time spent outdoors in the sun and incidence of sunburn had declined over the years of the campaign [62]. A community-wide intervention in Falmouth, Massachusetts, also reported a reduction in painful sunburns in children but no change in their sun exposure [168]; however, this intervention was limited by the cross-sectional nature of the evaluation, so that the individuals responding at baseline were not the same individuals responding after the intervention.

2.6 Does Sun Safety Increase Time in the Sun?

A few studies mentioned earlier found that time in the sun increased following the prevention intervention, which raises concerns that people use sun protection and exposure to prolong intentionally their time in the sun. This same concern has been advanced in studies showing that population that used sunscreen had greater melanocytic nevi, an indicator of sun exposure [9, 10, 11, 12, 18, 19, 148], although a recent study from Canada found that sunscreen reduced nevi in a randomized prospective design [74]. The negative effects of sunscreen may be most evident when individuals choose to be outdoors in the sun rather than when their time in the sun is determined by factors out of their control such as work schedules. However, it is also possible that this effect arises from confounding by indication, where individuals who need and use sunscreens the most have sun-sensitive light skin and are at highest risk of more nevi, regardless of their amount of sun exposure. Individuals who engage in other sun safety practices may be able to spend extended time outside without obtaining high doses of solar UVR [36]. Also, sun exposure can have benefits, including the production of vitamin D. The aim is to achieve the right balance.

2.7 Limitations

A few limitations to the research on interventions to prevent sunburn and reduce time in the midday sun are worth noting. Some studies had poor-quality designs (e.g., lack of a control group, small samples). Many studies relied on self-report measures of sunburn and time in the midday sun. There is evidence that self-reports on sunburns can be valid [36, 189, 225], but an expert panel recommended that measures define sunburn (e.g., red and/or painful from exposure to the sun) and provide a specific recall period (e.g., past three months) [217]. Observational measures of time in the sun by colorimeter assessments of change in skin color have limitations, too (e.g., color can fade; precise amount of exposure is difficult to measure).

3 Conclusions

There is a great deal known about melanoma; however, there is much still to understand. A current trend is to evaluate “gene–environment interactions.” There are new genetic discoveries every day, and these may help to understand the etiology and factors important for melanoma progression. Environmental exposure is extremely difficult to measure, but measurement is likely an important problem that investigators may solve in the future. The best advice that can be given for prevention is the "precautionary principle," that is, individuals should avoid extreme exposure to UV light including tanning beds. Skin examination is a second piece of important advice for secondary prevention of melanoma, which is covered in the next chapter. Individuals should become "aware" of their skin—any unusual spots or nodules deserve the attention of a primary care physician or a dermatologist. Together, caution in the sun and awareness of one's skin are today the best advice for melanoma prevention.

References

1. Akhtar FZ, Garabrant DH, Ketchum NS et al (2004) Cancer in U.S. Air Force veterans of the Vietnam war. J Occup Environ Med 46:123–136
2. Amos CI, Wang LE, Lee JE et al (2011) Genome-wide association study identifies novel loci predisposing to cutaneous melanoma. Hum Mol Genet 20:5012–5023
3. Andersen A, Barlow L, Engeland A et al (1999) Work-related cancer in Nordic countries. Scand J Work Environ Health 15:1–116
4. Andersen PA, Buller DB, Walkosz BJ et al (2012) Expanding occupational sun safety to an outdoor recreation industry: a translational study of the go sun smart program. Trans Behav Med 2(1):10–18
5. Armstrong BK, Kricker A (1993) How much melanoma is caused by sun exposure? Melanoma Res 3:395–401
6. Armstrong BK, Kricker A (2001) The epidemiology of UV induced skin cancer. J Photochem Photobiol B 63:8–18
7. Armstrong BK (2006) Ch. 6. Epidemiology of melanoma and current trends. In: Dunitz M (ed) Textbook of melanoma, London
8. Austin DF, Reynolds P (1986) Occupation and malignant melanoma of the skin. Recent Results Cancer Res 102:98–107
9. Autier P, Boniol M, Dore JF (2007) Sunscreen use and increased duration of intentional sun exposure: still a burning issue. Int J Cancer 121(1):1–5
10. Autier P, Dore JF, Negrier S et al (1999) Sunscreen use and duration of sun exposure: a double-blind, randomized trial. J Natl Cancer Inst 91(15):1304–1309
11. Autier P, Dore JF, Reis AC et al (2000) Sunscreen use and intentional exposure to ultraviolet A and B radiation: a double blind randomized trial using personal dosimeters. Br J Cancer 83 (9):1243–1248
12. Autier P, Mezzetti M, Dore JF et al (1998) Sunscreen use, wearing clothes, and number of nevi in 6 to 7-year-old European children. J Natl Cancer Inst 90(24):1870–1872
13. Barrett JH, Iles MM, Harland M et al (2011) Genome-wide association study identifies three new melanoma susceptibility loci. Nat Genet 43:1108–1113
14. Bastian BC (2014) The molecular pathology of melanoma: an integrated taxonomy of melanocytic neoplasia. Annu Rev Pathol 9:239–271
15. Bataille V, de Vries E (2008) Melanoma—part 1: epidemiology, risk factors, and prevention. BMJ 337:1287–1291
16. Bataille V, Snieder H, MacGregor A et al (2000) Genetics of risk factors for melanoma: an adult twin study of nevi and freckles. J Natl Cancer Inst 92:457–463
17. Bauer J, Buttner P, Murali R et al (2011) BRAF mutations in cutaneous melanoma are independently associated with age, anatomic site of the primary tumor, and the degree of solar elastosis at the primary tumor site. Pigment Cell Melanoma Res 24:345–351
18. Bauer J, Buttner P, Wiecker TS et al (2005) Effect of sunscreen and clothing on the number of melanocytic nevi in 1812 German children attending day care. Am J Epidemiol 161(7): 620–627

19. Bauer J, Buttner P, Wiecker TS et al (2005) Interventional study in 1232 young German children to prevent the development of melanocytic nevi failed to change sun exposure and sun protective behavior. Int J Cancer 116(5):755–761
20. Begg CB, Orlow I, Hummer AJ et al (2005) Lifetime risk of melanoma in CDKN2A mutation carriers in a population-based sample. J Natl Cancer Inst 97:1507–1515
21. Bertolotto C, Lesueur F, Giuliano S et al (2011) A SUMOylation-defective MITF germline mutation predisposes to melanoma and renal carcinoma. Nature 480:94–98
22. Berwick M (2008) Are tanning beds "safe"? Human studies of melanoma. Pigment Cell Melanoma Res 21:517–519
23. Berwick M, Armstrong BK, Ben-Porat L et al (2005) Sun exposure and mortality from melanoma. J Natl Cancer Inst 97:195–199
24. Berwick M (2011) Melanoma Epidemiology. In: Bosserhoff A (ed) melanoma development. Springer, Vienna
25. Berwick M, Macarthur J, Orlow I et al (2014) MITF E318K's effect on melanoma risk independent of, but modified by, other risk factors. Pigment Cell Melanoma Res. doi:10.1111/pcmr.12215
26. Berwick M, Orlow I, Hummer AJ et al (2006) The prevalence of CDKN2A germ-line mutations and relative risk for cutaneous malignant melanoma: an international population-based study. Cancer Epidemiol Biomarkers Prev 15:1520–1525
27. Bishop DT, Demenais F, Goldstein AM et al (2002) Geographical variation in the penetrance of CDKN2A mutations for melanoma. J Natl Cancer Inst 94:894–903
28. Bishop DT, Demenais F, Iles MM et al (2009) Genome-wide association study identifies three loci associated with melanoma risk. Nat Genet 41:920–925
29. Blettner M, Zeeb H, Auvinen A et al (2003) Mortality from cancer and other causes among male airline cockpit crew in Europe. Int J Cancer 106:946–952
30. Bliss J, Ford D, Swerdow A et al (1995) Risk of cutaneous melanoma-associated with pigmentation characteristics and freckling—systematic overview of 10 case-control studies. Int J Cancer 61:367–376
31. Boniol M, Armstrong BK, Doré JF (2006) Variation in incidence and fatality of melanoma by season of diagnosis in new South Wales, Australia. Cancer Epidemiol Biomarkers Prev 15:524–526
32. Boniol M, Autier P, Boyle P et al (2012) Cutaneous melanoma attributable to sunbed use: systematic review and meta-analysis. BMJ 345:e4757
33. Boniol M, Autier P, Boyle P et al (2012) Correction. Cutaneous melanoma attributable to sunbed use: systematic review and meta-analysis. BMJ 345:e8503
34. Boscoe FP, Schymura MJ (2006) Solar ultraviolet-B exposure and cancer incidence and mortality in the United States, 1993–2002. BMC Cancer 6:624
35. Botton T, Yeh I, Nelson T et al (2013) Recurrent BRAF kinase fusions in melanocytic tumors offer an opportunity for targeted therapy. Pigment Cell Melanoma Res 26:845–851
36. Brandberg Y, Sjoden PO, Rosdahl I (1997) Assessment of sun-related behaviour in individuals with dysplastic naevus syndrome: a comparison between diary recordings and questionnaire responses. Melanoma Res 7(4):347–351
37. Bressac-de-Paillerets B, Avril M-F, Chompret A et al (2002) Genetic and environmental factors in cutaneous malignant melanoma. Biochimie 84:67–74
38. Brown C, Lacharme-Lora L, Mukonoweshuro B et al (2013) Consequences of exposure to peri-articular injections of micro- and nano-particulate cobalt-chromium alloy. Biomaterials 34(34):8564–8580
39. Brown KM, Macgregor S, Montgomery GW et al (2008) Common sequence variants on 20q11.22 confer melanoma susceptibility. Nat Genet 40:838–840
40. Buendia Eisman A, Arias Santiago S, Moreno-Gimenez JC et al (2013) An internet-based programme to promote adequate UV exposure behaviour in adolescents in Spain. J Eur Acad Dermatol Venereol 27(4):442–453

41. Bulbulyan MA, Ilychova SA, Zahm SH et al (1999) Cancer mortality among women in the Russian printing industry. Am J Ind Med 36:166–171
42. Buller DB, Andersen PA, Walkosz BJ et al (2005) Randomized trial testing a worksite sun protection program in an outdoor recreation industry. Health Educ Behav 32(4):514–535
43. Buller DB, Buller MK, Beach B et al (1996) Sunny days, healthy ways: evaluation of a skin cancer prevention curriculum for elementary school-aged children. J Am Acad Dermatol 35 (6):911–922
44. Buller DB, Reynolds KD, Yaroch A et al (2006) Effects of the sunny days, healthy ways curriculum on students in grades 6 to 8. Am J Prev Med 30(1):13–22
45. Buller DB, Taylor AM, Buller MK et al (2006) Evaluation of the sunny days, healthy ways sun safety curriculum for children in kindergarten through fifth grade. Pediatr Dermatol 23 (4):321–329
46. Bulliard JL (2000) Site-specific risk of cutaneous malignant melanoma and pattern of sun exposure in New Zealand. Int J Cancer 85:627–632
47. Caini S, Gandini S, Sera F et al (2009) Meta-analysis of risk factors for cutaneous melanoma according to anatomical site and clino-pathological variant. Eur J Cancer 45:3054–3063
48. Carli P, Crocetti E, Chiarugi A et al (2008) The use of commercially available personal UV meters does cause less safe tanning habits: a randomized controlled trial. Photochem Photobiol 84(3):758–763
49. Carli P, Palli D (2003) RE: Melanocytic nevi, solar keratosis, and divergent pathways to cutaneous melanoma. J Natl Cancer Inst 95:1801
50. Carpenter DO (2006) Polychlorinated biphenyls (PCBs): routes of exposure and effects on human health. Rev Environ Health 21:1–23
51. Cercato MC, Nagore E, Ramazzotti V et al (2013) Improving sun-safe knowledge, attitude and behaviour in parents of primary school children: a pilot study. J Cancer Educ 28(1):151–157
52. Couzin-Frankel J (2013) Cancer Immunother. Science 342:1432–1433
53. Curtin JA, Busam K, Pinkel D et al (2006) Somatic activation of KIT in distinct subtypes of melanoma. J Clin Oncol 24:4340–4346
54. Curtin JA, Fridly J, Kageshita T et al (2005) Distinct sets of genetic alternatives in melanoma. N Engl J Med 353(20):2135–2147
55. Curtin JA, Fridly J, Kageshita T et al (2005) Distinct sets of genetic alterations in melanoma. N Engl J Med 353:2135–2147
56. Cust AE, Goumas C, Holland EA et al (2012) MC1R genotypes and risk of melanoma before age 40 years: a population-based case-control-family study. Int J Cancer 131:E269–E281
57. Cust AE, Goumas C, Vuong K et al (2013) MC1R genotype as a predictor of early-onset melanoma, compared with self-reported and physician-measured traditional risk factors: an Australian case-control-family study. BMC Cancer 13:406
58. Cust AE, Harland M, Makalic E et al (2011) Melanoma risk for CDKN2A mutation carriers who are relatives of population-based case carriers in Australia and the UK. J Med Genet 48:266–272
59. Dennis LK, Vanbeek MJ, Beane Freeman LE et al (2008) Sunburns and risk of cutaneous melanoma: does age matter? A comprehensive meta-analysis. Ann Epidemiol 18:614–627
60. Devitt B, Liu W, Salemi R et al (2011) Clinical outcome and pathological features associated with NRAS mutation in cutaneous melanoma. Pigment Cell Melanoma Res 24:666–672
61. Diffey BL, Healy E, Thody AJ et al (1995) Melanin, melanocytes, and melanoma. Lancet 346:1713
62. Dobbinson SJ, Wakefield MA, Jamsen KM et al (2008) Weekend sun protection and sunburn in Australia trends (1987–2002) and association with SunSmart television advertising. Am J Prev Med 34(2):94–101
63. Edlundh-Rose E, Egyhazi S, Omholt K et al (2006) NRAS and BRAF mutations in melanoma tumours in relation to clinical characteristics: a study based on mutation screening by pyrosequencing. Melanoma Res 16:471–478

64. Ellerhorst JA, Greene VR, Ekmekcioglu S et al (2011) Clinical correlates of NRAS and BRAF mutations in primary human melanoma. Clin Cancer Res 17:229–235
65. Elwood JM, Jopson J (1997) Melanoma and sun exposure: an overview of published studies. Int J Cancer 73:198–203
66. Elwood JM, Lee JA, Walter SD et al (1974) Relationship of melanoma and other skin cancer mortality to latitude and ultraviolet radiation in the United States and Canada. Int J Epidemiol 3:325–332
67. Facta S, Fusette SS, Bonino A et al (2012) UV Emissions from artificial tanning devices and their compliance with the European technical standard. Health Phys 104:385–393
68. Fargnoli MC, Pike K, Pfeiffer RM et al (2008) MC1R variants increase risk of melanomas harboring BRAF mutations. J Invest Dermatol 128:2485–2490
69. Fornnum F, Mariussen E, Reistad T (2006) Molecular mechanisms involved in the toxic effects of polychlorinated biphenyls (PCBs) and brominated flame retardants (BFRs). J Toxicol Environ Health A 69:21–35
70. Fortes C, de Vries E (2008) Nonsolar occupational risk factors for cutaneous melanoma. Int J Dermatol 47(4):319–328. doi:10.1111/j.1365-4632.2008.03653.x
71. Freedman DM, Sigurdson A, Rao RS et al (2003) Risk of melanoma among radiology technologists in the United States. Int J Cancer 103:556–562
72. Gallagher RP, Lee TK, Bajdik CD et al (2010) Ultraviolet radiation. Chronic Dis Can 29: S51–S68
73. Gallagher RP, MacArthur A, Lee TK et al (2011) Plasma levels of polychlorinated biphenyls and risk of cutaneous malignant melanoma: a preliminary study. Int J Cancer 128:1872–1880
74. Gallagher RP, Rivers JK, Lee TK et al (2000) Broad-spectrum sunscreen use and the development of new nevi in white children: a randomized controlled trial. JAMA 283 (22):2955–2960
75. Gandini S, Sera F, Cattaruzza MS et al (2005) Meta-analysis of risk factors for cutaneous melanoma: I. Common and atypical naevi. Eur J Cancer 41:28–44
76. Gandini S, Sera F, Cattaruzza MS et al (2005) Meta analysis of risk factors for cutaneous melanoma: II. Sun exposure. Eur J Cancer 41:45–60
77. Garbe C, Buttner P, Weiss J et al (1994) Associated factors in the prevalence of more than 50 common melanocytic nevi, atypical melanocytic nevi and actinic lentigines: multicenter case-control study of the Central Malignant Melanoma Registry of the German Dermatological Society. J Invest Dermatol 102:700–705
78. Garland CF, Garland FC, Gorham ED (2003) Epidemiologic evidence for different roles of ultraviolet A and B radiation in melanoma mortality rates. Ann Epidemiol 13:395–404
79. Geller AC, Glanz K, Shigaki D et al (2001) Impact of skin cancer prevention on outdoor aquatics staff: the pool cool program in Hawaii and Massachusetts. Prev Med 33:155–161
80. Gellert RJ, Heinrichs WL, Swerdloff RS (1972) DDT homologues: estrogen-like effects on the vagina, uterus and pituitary of the rat. Endocrinologoy 91:1095–1100
81. Gessi M, Hammes J, Lauriola L et al (2013) GNA11 and N-RAS mutations: alternatives for MAPK pathway activating GNAQ mutations in primary melanocytic tumours of the central nervous system. Neuropathol Appl Neurobiol 39:417–425
82. El Ghissassi F, Baan R, Straif K et al (2009) A review of human carcinogens—part D: radiation. Lancet Oncol 10:751–752
83. Gidanian S, Mentelle M, Meyskesn FL et al (2008) Melanosomal damage in normal human melanocytes induced by UVB and metal uptake—a basis for the pro-oxidant state of melanoma. Photochem Photobiol 84(3):556–564
84. Gies P, Javorniczky J, Henderson S et al (2011) UVR emissions from solaria in Australia and implications for the regulation process. Photochem Photobiol 87(1):184–190. doi:10.1111/j.1751-1097.2010.00835.x
85. Giles-Corti B, English DR, Costa C et al (2004) Creating SunSmart schools. Health Educ Res 19(1):98–109

86. Goel VK, Lazar AJ, Warneke CL et al (2006) Examination of mutations in BRAF, NRAS, and PTEN in primary cutaneous melanoma. J Invest Dermatol 126:154–160
87. Goldstein AM, Chan M, Harland M et al (2007) Features associated with germline CDKN2A mutations: a GenoMEL study of melanoma-prone families from three continents. J Med Genet 44:99–106
88. Green AC, Williams GM, Logan V et al (2011) Reduced melanoma after regular sunscreen use: randomized trial follow-up. J Clin Oncol 29:257–263
89. Gritz ER, Tripp MK, Peterson SK et al (2013) Randomized controlled trial of a sun protection intervention for children of melanoma survivors. Cancer Epidemiol Biomark Prev 22(10):1813–1824
90. Gruber SB, Armstrong BK (2006) Cutaneous and ocular melanoma. In: Schottenfeld D, Fraumeni JF Jr (eds) Cancer epidemiology and prevention, 3rd edn. Oxford University Press, New York
91. Gundestrup M, Storm HH (1999) Radiation induced acute myeloid leukemia in commercial jet cockpit crew: a population-based cohort study. Lancet 354:2029–2031
92. Hacker E, Nagore E, Cerroni L et al (2013) NRAS and BRAF mutations in cutaneous melanoma and the association with MC1R genotype: findings from Spanish and Austrian populations. J Invest Dermatol 133(4):1027–1033
93. Hacker E, Hayward NK, Dumenil T et al (2009) The association between MC1R genotype and BRAF mutation status in cutaneous melanoma: findings from an Australian population. J Invest Dermatol 130:241–248
94. Haldorsen T, Reitan JB, Tventen U (2001) Cancer incidence among Norwegian cabin attendants. Int J Epidemiol 30:825–830
95. Hall DM, McCarty F, Elliott T et al (2009) Lifeguards' sun protection habits and sunburns: association with sun-safe environments and skin cancer prevention program participation. Arch Dermatol 145(2):139–144
96. Han J, Colditz GA, Hunter DJ (2006) Risk factors for skin cancers: a nested case-control study within the nurses' health Study. Int J Epidemiol 35:1514–1521
97. Harrison S, McLennan R, Spear R et al (1994) Sun exposure and melanocytic naevi in young Australian children. Lancet 344:1529–1532
98. Harvard Report on Cancer Prevention (1996) Causes of human cancer. Ultraviolet light Cancer Causes Control 7:S39–S40
99. Hayward NK (2003) Genetics of melanoma predisposition. Oncogene 22:3053–3062
100. Heenan PJ, English DR, Holman CD et al (1991) Survival among patients with clinical stage I cutaneous malignant melanoma diagnosed in Western Australia in 1975/76 and 1980/81. Cancer 68:2079–2087
101. Heidenreich B, Nagore E, Rachakonda PS et al (2014) Telomerase reverse transcriptase promoter mutations in primary cutaneous melanoma. Nat Commun 5:3401
102. Hocker T, Tsao H (2007) Ultraviolet radiation and melanoma: a systematic review and analysis of reported sequence variants. Hum Mutat 28:578–588
103. Hodis E, Watson IR, Kryukov GV et al (2012) A landscape of driver mutations in melanoma. Cell 150:251–263
104. Hollenbeak CS, Todd MM, Billingsley EM et al (2005) Increased incidence of melanoma in renal transplantation recipients. Cancer 104:1962–1967
105. Horn S, Figl A, Rachakonda PS et al (2013) TERT promoter mutations in familial and sporadic melanoma. Science 339:959–961
106. Hornung RL, Magee KH, Lee WJ et al (2003) Tanning facility use: are we exceeding food and drug administration limits? J Am Acad Dermatol 49:655–661
107. Huang FW, Hodis E, Xu MJ et al (2013) Highly recurrent TERT promoter mutations in human melanoma. Science 339:957–959
108. Huang C, Yan S, Ren J et al (2013) A quantitative assessment of the effects of formal sun protection education on photosensitive patients. Photodermatol Photoimmunol Photomed 29(5):261–265

109. Hunter S, Love-Jackson K, Abdulla R et al (2010) Sun protection at elementary schools: a cluster randomized trial. J Natl Cancer Inst 102(7):484–492
110. Hutchinson KE, Lipson D, Stephens PJ et al (2013) BRAF fusions define a distinct molecular subset of melanomas with potential sensitivity to MEK inhibition. Clin Cancer Res 19:6696–6702
111. IARC (1992) IARC monographs on the evaluation of carcinogenic risks to humans TARC 55: solar and ultraviolet radiation. IARC, Lyon
112. IARC (2012) IARC monographs on the evaluation of carcinogenic risks to humans. 100: a review of human carcinogens. Part D: radiation. IARC, Lyon
113. Iles MM, Law MH, Stacey SN et al (2013) A variant in FTO shows association with melanoma risk not due to BMI. Nat Genet 45:428–432
114. Jackson KM, Aiken LS (2006) Evaluation of a multicomponent appearance-based sun-protective intervention for young women: uncovering the mechanisms of program efficacy. Health Psychol 25(1):34
115. Jayasekara H, Karahalios E, Thursfield V et al (2009) Season of diagnosis has no effect on survival from malignant melanoma. Int J Cancer 125:488–490
116. Jemal A, Devesa SS, Fears TR et al (2000) Cancer surveillance series: changing patterns of cutaneous malignant melanoma mortality rates among whites in the United States. J Natl Cancer Inst 92:811–818
117. Jensen P, Hansen S, Moller B et al (1999) Skin cancer in kidney and heart transplant recipients and different long-term immunosuppressive therapy regimens. J Am Acad Dermatol 40:177–186
118. Jewell R, Chambers P, Harland M et al (2012) Clinicopathologic features of V600E and V600K melanoma-letter. Clin Cancer Res 18:6792–6793
119. Kamb A, Shattuck-Eidens D, Eeles R et al (1994) Analysis of the p16 gene (CDKN2) as a candidate for the chromosome 9p melanoma susceptibility locus. Nat Genet 8:23–26
120. Kanetsky PA, Panossian S, Elder DE et al (2010) Does MC1R genotype convey information about melanoma risk beyond risk phenotypes? Cancer 116:2416–2428
121. Kanetsky PA, Rebbeck TR, Hummer AJ et al (2006) Population-based study of natural variation in the melanocortin-1 receptor gene and melanoma. Cancer Res 66:9330–9337
122. Keegan GM, Learmonth ID, Case CP (2008) A systematic comparison of the actual, potential, and theoretical health effects of cobalt and chromium exposures from industry and surgical implants. Crit Rev Toxicol 38(8):645–674. doi:10.1080/10408440701845534
123. Kendzia B, Behrens T, Jocket KH et al (2013) Welding and lung cancer in a pooled analysis of case-control studies. Am J Epidemiol 178(10):1513–1525
124. Kenfield SA, Geller AC, Richter EM et al (2005) Sun protection policies and practices at child care centers in Massachusetts. J Community Health 30(6):491–503
125. Kim BH, Glanz K (2013) Text messaging to motivate walking in older African Americans: a randomized controlled trial. Am J Prev Med 44(1):71–75
126. Kimlin M, Parisi A (2001) Usage of real-time ultraviolet radiation data to modify the daily erythemal exposure of primary schoolchildren. Photodermatol Photoimmunol Photomed 17(3):130–135
127. Knerr S, Schrenk D (2006) Carcinogenicity of "non-dioxinlike" polychlorinated biphenyls. Crit Rev Toxicol 36:663–694
128. Krauthammer M, Kong Y, Ha BH et al (2012) Exome sequencing identifies recurrent somatic RAC1 mutations in melanoma. Nat Genet 44:1006–1014
129. Kusters-Vandevelde HV, Klaasen A, Kusters B et al (2010) Activating mutations of the GNAQ gene: a frequent event in primary melanocytic neoplasms of the central nervous system. Acta Neuropathol 119:317–323
130. Lachiewicz AM, Berwick M, Wiggins CL et al (2008) Epidemiologic support for melanoma heterogeneity using the surveillance, epidemiology, and end results program. J Invest Dermatol 128:1340–1342

131. Lachiewicz AM, Berwick M, Wiggins CL et al (2008) Survival differences between patients with scalp or neck melanoma and those with melanoma of other sites in the surveillance, epidemiology, and end results (SEER) program. Arch Dermatol 144:515–521
132. Ladon D, Doherty A, Newson R et al (2004) Changes in metal levels and chromosome aberrations in the peripheral blood of patients after metal-on-metal hip arthroplasty. J Arthroplasty 8(Suppl 3):78–83
133. Landi MT, Bauer J, Pfeiffer RM et al (2006) MC1R germline variants confer risk for BRAF-mutant melanoma. Science 313:521–522
134. Lauby-Secretan B, Loomis D, Bouvard V et al (2013) Carcinogenicity of polychlorinated biphenyls and polybrominated biphenyls. Lancet Onc 14:287–288
135. Law MH, Macgregor S, Hayward NK (2012) Melanoma genetics: recent findings take us beyond well-traveled pathways. J Invest Dermatol 132:1763–1774
136. Lazovich DA, Vogel RI, Berwick M et al (2010) Indoor tanning and risk of melanoma: a case-control study in a highly exposed population. Cancer Epidemiol Biomarkers Prev 19:1557–1568
137. Lazovich D, Vogel RI, Berwick M et al (2012) Melanoma risk in relation to use of sunscreen or other sun protection methods. Cancer Epidemiol Biomarkers Prev 20:2583–2593
138. LeMire L, Hollowood K, Gray D et al (2006) Melanomas in renal transplant recipients. Br J Dermatol 154:472–477
139. Lee JH, Choi JW, Kim YS (2011) Frequencies of BRAF and NRAS mutations are different in histological types and sites of origin of cutaneous melanoma: a meta-analysis. Br J Dermatol 164:776–784
140. Lee TK, Rivers JK, Gallagher RP (2005) Site-specific protective effect of broad-spectrum sunscreen on nevus development among white schoolchildren in a randomized trial. J Am Acad Dermatol 52(5):786–792
141. Lemish WM, Heenan PJ, Holman CD et al (1983) Survival from preinvasive and invasive malignant melanoma in Western Australia. Cancer 52:580–585
142. Linet M, Malker HS, Chow W et al (1995) Occupational risks for cutaneous melanoma among men in Sweden. J Occup Environ Med 37:1127–1135
143. Liu KE, Barankin B, Howard J et al (2001) One-year followup on the impact of a sun awareness curriculum on medical students' knowledge, attitudes, and behavior. JCMS 5(3): 193–200
144. Liu W, Kelly JW, Trivett M et al (2007) Distinct clinical and pathological features are associated with the BRAF(T1799A(V600E)) mutation in primary melanoma. J Invest Dermatol 127:900–905
145. Liu J, Song E, Liu L et al (2012) Polychlorinated biphenyl quinine metabolites lead to oxidative stress in HepG2 cells and the protective role of dihydrolipoic acid. Toxicol In Vitro 26:841–848
146. Loomis D, Browning SR, Schenck AP et al (1997) Cancer mortality among electric utility workers exposed to polychlorinated biphenyls. Occup Environ Med 54:720–728
147. Lu YC, Wu YC (1985) Clinical findings and immunological abnormalities in Yu-Cheng patients. Environ Health Perspect 59:17–29
148. Luther H, Altmeyer P, Garbe C et al (1996) Increase of melanocytic nevus counts in children during 5 years of follow-up and analysis of associated factors. Arch Dermatol 132(12): 1473–1478
149. Macgregor S, Montgomery GW, Liu JZ et al (2011) Genome-wide association study identifies a new melanoma susceptibility locus at 1q21.3. Nat Genet 43:1114–1118
150. Mahler HI, Kulik JA, Gerrard M et al (2007) Long-term effects of appearance-based interventions on sun protection behaviors. Health Psychol 26(3):350–360
151. Mahler HI, Kulik JA, Gerrard M et al (2010) Effects of upward and downward social comparison information on the efficacy of an appearance-based sun protection intervention: a randomized, controlled experiment. J Behav Med 33(6):496–507

152. Mahler HI, Kulik JA, Gerrard M et al (2013) Effects of photoaging information and UV photo on sun protection intentions and behaviours: a cross-regional comparison. Psychol Health 28(9):1009–1031
153. Mahler HI, Kulik JA, Gibbons FX et al (2003) Effects of appearance-based interventions on sun protection intentions and self-reported behaviors. Health Psychol 22(2):199–209
154. Mahler HI, Kulik JA, Harrell J et al (2005) Effects of UV photographs, photoaging information, and use of sunless tanning lotion on sun protection behaviors. Arch Dermatol 141(3):373–380
155. Maldonado JL, Fridlyand J, Patel H et al (2003) Determinants of BRAF mutations in primary melanomas. J Natl Cancer Inst 95:1878–1890
156. Mar VJ, Wong SQ, Li J et al (2013) BRAF/NRAS wild-type melanomas have a high mutation load correlating with histologic and molecular signatures of UV damage. Clin Cancer Res 19:4589–4598
157. Marabini L, Calo R, Fucile S (2011) Genotoxic effects of polychlorinated biphenyls (PCB 153, 138, 101, 118) in a fish cell line (RTG-2). Toxicol In Vitro 25:1045–1052
158. Markovic S, Erickson L, Rao R et al (2007) Malignant melanoma in the 21st century, part 1: epidemiology, risk factors, screening, prevention and diagnosis. Mayo Clin Proc 82:365–380
159. Marks R (2002) Epidemiology of melanoma. Clin Exp Dermatol 25:459–463
160. Masaki T, Wang Y, Digiovanna JJ et al (2014) High frequency of PTEN mutations in nevi and melanomas from xeroderma pigmentosum patients. Pigment Cell Melanoma Res 27:454–464
161. Mazzuckelli LF, Schulte PA (1993) Notification of workers about an excess of malignant melanoma. Am J Ind Med 23:85–91
162. McFarland VA, Clarke JU (1989) Environmental occurrence, abundance, and potential toxicity of polychlorinated biphenyl congeners: considerations for a congener-specific analysis. Environ Health Perspect 81:225–239
163. McLaughlin JK, Malker HS, Blot WJ et al (1988) Malignant melanoma in the printing industry. Am J Ind Med 13:301–304
164. Menzies AM, Haydu LE, Visintin L et al (2012) Distinguishing clinicopathologic features of patients with V600E and V600K BRAF-mutant metastatic melanoma. Clin Cancer Res 18:3242–3249
165. Meyle KD, Guldberg P (2009) Genetic risk factors for melanoma. Hum Genet 126:499–510
166. Meyskens FL, Berwick M (2008) UV or not UV: metals are the answer. Cancer Epidemiol Bio Prev 17:268–270
167. Meyskens FL, Yang S (2011) Thinking about the role (largely ignored) of heavy metals in cancer prevention: hexavalent chromium and melanoma as case in point. Recent Results Cancer Res 188:65–74
168. Miller DR, Geller AC, Wood MC et al (1999) The Falmouth safe skin project: evaluation of a community program to promote sun protection in youth. Health Educ Behav 26(3):369–384
169. Milne E, Jacoby P, Giles-Corti B et al (2006) The impact of the Kidskin sun protection intervention on summer suntan and reported sun exposure: was it sustained? Prev Med 42(1): 14–20
170. Milne E, Simpson JA, Johnston R et al (2007) Time spent outdoors at midday and children's body mass index. Am J Public Health 97(2):306–310
171. Moore DH, Patterson WH, Hatch F et al (1997) Case-control study of malignant melanoma among employees of the Laurence Livermore National Laboratory. Am J Ind Med 32: 377–391
172. Morales Suárez-Varela M, Llopis-González A, Lacasaña-Navarro M et al (1990) Trends in malignant skin melanoma and other skin cancers in Spain, 1975–1983, and their relation to solar radiation intensity. J Environ Pathol Toxicol Oncol 10:245–253
173. Moysich KB, Mendola P, Schisterman EF et al (1999) An evaluation of proposed frameworks for grouping polychlorinated biphenyl (PCB) congener data into meaningful analytic units. Am J Ind Med 35:223–231

174. Nakanishi Y, Shigematsu N, Kurita Y et al (1985) Respiratory involvement and immune status in yusho patients. Environ Health Perspect 59:31–36
175. Naldi L, Chatenoud L, Bertuccio P et al (2007) Improving sun-protection behavior among children: results of a cluster-randomized trial in Italian elementary schools. The "SoleSi SoleNo-GISED" Project. J Invest Dermatol 127(8):1871–1877
176. National Toxicology Program (2006) NTP Toxicology and carcinogenesis studies of 3.3′, 4.4′, 5 pentachlorobiphenyl (PCB126) in female Harlan Sprague-Dawley rats (Gavage studies). Natl Toxicol Program Tech Rep Ser 520:244–246
177. National Toxicology Program (2010) NTP toxicology and carcinogenesis studies of 2.3′, 4.4′, 5-pentachlorobiphenyl (PCB118) in female Harlan Sprague-Dawley rats (Gavage studies). Natl Toxicol Program Tech Rep Ser 559:1–174
178. Nelemans PJ, Rampen FHJ, Ruiter DJ et al (1995) An addition to the controversy on sunlight exposure and melanoma risk: a meta-analytical approach. J Clin Epidemiol 48:1331–1342
179. Nelemans PJ, Scholte R, Groenendal H et al (1993) Melanoma and occupation-results of a case-control study in Netherlands. Br J Ind Med 50:642–646
180. Nelson JA (1974) Effects of DDT analogues and PCB mixtures on 17-beta estradiol binding to the rat uterine receptor. Biochem Pharmacol 23:447–451
181. Newton-Bishop JA, Beswick S, Randerson-Moor J et al (2009) Serum 25-hydroxyvitamin D3 levels are associated with Breslow thickness at presentation and survival from melanoma. J Clin Oncol 27:5339–5344
182. Nicol I, Gaudy C, Gouvernet J et al (2007) Skin protection by sunscreens is improved by explicit labeling and providing free sunscreen. J Invest Dermatol 127(1):41–48
183. Nielsen H, Henriksen L, Olsen JH (1996) Malignant melanoma among lithographers. Scand J Work Environ Health 22:108–111
184. Nielsen K, Måsbäck A, Olsson H et al (2012) A prospective population-based study of 40,000 women regarding host factors, UV exposure and sunbed use in relation to risk and anatomic site of cutaneous melanoma. Int J Cancer 42:319–324
185. Nilsen LT, Aalerud TN, Hannevik M et al (2011) UVB and UVA irradiances from indoor tanning devices. Photochem Photobiol Sci 10(7):1129–1136. doi:10.1039/c1pp05029j
186. Olsen CM, Zens MS, Green AC et al (2011) Biologic markers of sun exposure and melanoma risk in women: pooled case-control analysis. Int J Cancer 129:713–723
187. Omenn GS, Goodman GE, Thornquist MD et al (1996) Effects of a combination of beta carotene and vitamin A on lung cancer and cardiovascular disease. N Engl J Med 334(18): 1150–1155
188. Onega T, Baron J, MacKenzie T et al (2006) Cancer after total joint arthroplasty: a meta-analysis. Cancer Epidemiol Biomarkers Prev 15(8):1532–1537
189. O'Riordan DL, Lunde KB, Steffen AD et al (2006) Validity of beachgoers' self-report of their sun habits. Arch Dermatol 142(10):1304–1311
190. Pagoto S, McChargue D, Fuqua RW (2003) Effects of a multicomponent intervention on motivation and sun protection behaviors among midwestern beachgoers. Health Psychol 22(4):429
191. Pagoto SL, Schneider KL, Oleski J et al (2010) The sunless study: a beach randomized trial of a skin cancer prevention intervention promoting sunless tanning. Arch Dermatol 146(9):979
192. Parkin DM, Mesher D, Sasieni P (2011) Cancers attributable to solar (ultraviolet) radiation exposure in the UK 2010. Br J Dermatol 105:S66–S69
193. Pleasance ED, Cheetham RK, Stephens PJ et al (2010) A comprehensive catalogue of somatic mutations from a human cancer genome. Nature 463:191–196
194. Pollock PM, Harper UL, Hansen KS et al (2003) High frequency of BRAF mutations in nevi. Nat Genet 33:19–20
195. Poynter JN, Elder JT, Fullen DR et al (2006) BRAF and NRAS mutations in melanoma and melanocytic nevi. Melanoma Res 16:267–273
196. Pukkala E, Aspholm R, Auvinen A et al (2002) Incidence of cancer among Nordic airline pilots over five decades: occupational cohort study. Br Med J 325:567–569

197. Pukkala E, Auvinen A, Wahlberg G et al (1995) Incidence of cancer among Finnish airline cabin attendants 1967–1992. Br Med J 311:649–652
198. Purdue MP, Hoppin JA, Blair A et al (2006) Occupational exposures to organochlorine insecticides and cancer incidence in the agricultural health study. Int J Cancer 120:642–649
199. Quereux G, Nguyen JM, Volteau C et al (2009) Prospective trial on a school-based skin cancer prevention project. Eur J Cancer Prev 18(2):133–144
200. Van Raamsdonk CD, Griewank KG, Crosby MB et al (2010) Mutations in GNA11 in uveal melanoma. N Engl J Med 363:2191–2199
201. Raimondi S, Sera F, Gandini S et al (2008) MC1R variants, melanoma and red hair color phenotype: a meta-analysis. Int J Cancer 122:2753–2760
202. Roberts DC, Black D (2009) Comparison of interventions to reduce sun exposure. Behav Med 35(2):67–76
203. Robinson CF, Petersen M, Palu S (1999) Mortality patterns among electrical workers employed in the U.S. construction industry. Am J Ind Med 36:630–637
204. Robinson PE1, Mack GA, Remmers J et al (1990) Trends of PCB, hexachlorobenzene, and betabenzene hexachloride levels in the adipose tissue of the U.S. population. Environ Res 53:175–92
205. Roetzheim RG, Love-Jackson KM, Hunter SG et al (2011) A cluster randomized trial of sun protection at elementary schools: results from year 2. Am J Prev Med 41(6):615–618
206. Rosso S, Sera F, Segnan N et al (2008) Sun exposure prior to diagnosis is associated with improved survival in melanoma patients: results from a long-term follow-up study of Italian patients. Eur J Cancer 44:1275–1281
207. Ruder AM, Hein MJ, Nilsen N et al (2006) Mortality among workers exposed to polychlorinated biphenyls (PCB) in an electrical capacitor manufacturing plant in Indiana: an update. Environ Health Perspect 114:18–23
208. Ruder AM, Hein MJ, Hopf NB et al (2014) Mortality among 24,865 workers exposed to polychlorinated biphenyls (PCBs) in three electrical capacitor manufacturing plants: a ten-year update. Int J Hyg Environ Health 217(2-3):176–187. doi:10.1016/j.ijheh.2013.04.006
209. Safe S (1993) Toxicology, structure-function relationship, and human and environmental health impacts of polychlorinated biphenyls: progress and problems. Environ Health Perspect 100:259–268
210. Sagebiel RW (1993) Melanocytic nevi in histologic association with primary cutaneous melanoma of superficial spreading and nodular types: effect of tumor thickness. J Invest Dermatol 100:322S324S
211. Sarna T, Schwartz HA (2006) The physical properties of melanin. In: Nordlund JJ, Boissy R, Hearing VJ et al (eds) The pigmentary system, 2nd edn. Blackwell Publishing, New York
212. Scherer D, Rachakonda PS, Angelini S et al (2010) Association between the germline MC1R variants and somatic BRAF/NRAS mutations in melanoma tumors. J Invest Dermatol 130:2844–2848
213. Schuz N, Eid M (2013) Beyond the usual suspects: target group- and behavior-specific factors add to a theory-based sun protection intervention for teenagers. J Behav Med 36 (5):508–519
214. Seidler A, Janichen S, Hegewaled J et al (2013) Systematic review and quantification of respiratory cancer risk from occupational exposure to hexavalent chromium. Int Arch Occup Environ Health 86(8):957–960
215. Shekar SN, Duffy DL, Youl P et al (2009) A population-based study of Australian twins with melanoma suggests a strong genetic contribution to liability. J Invest Dermatol 129:2211–2219
216. Shipman AR, Clark AB, Levell NJ (2011) Summier European countries have lower melanoma mortality. Clin Exp Dermatol 36:544–547
217. Shoveller JA, Lovato CY (2001) Measuring self-reported sunburn: challenges and recommendations. Chronic Dis Can 22(3–4):83–98
218. Sigurdson AJ, Doody MM, Rao RS et al (2003) Cancer incidence in the US radiology technologists health study 1983–1988. Cancer 97:3080–3089

219. Silberhorn EM, Glauert HP, Robertson LW (1990) Carcinogenicity of polyhalogenated biphenyls: PCBs and PBBs. Crit Rev Toxicol 20:440–496
220. Sinks T, Steele G, Smith AB et al (1992) Mortality among workers exposed to polychlorinated biphenyls. Am J Epidemiol 136:389–398
221. Skender-Kalnenas TM, English DR, Hennan PJ (1995) Benign melanocytic lesions: risk markers or precursors of cutaneous melanoma? J Am Acad Dermatol 33:1000–1007
222. Smith AJ, Dieppe P, Porter M et al (2012) Risk of cancer in first seven years after metal-on-metal hip replacement compared with other bearings and general population: linkage study between the National Joint Registry of England and Wales and hospital episode statistics. Brit Med. doi:10.1136/bmj.e2383
223. Stadelmeyer E, Heitzer E, Resel M et al (2014) The BRAF V600 K mutation is more frequent than the BRAF V600E mutation in melanoma in situ of lentigo maligna type. J Invest Dermatol 134:548–550
224. Teta J, Schnatter R, Ott GM et al (1990) Mortality surveillance in a large chemical company: the Union Carbide Corporation experience. Am J Ind Med 17:435–447
225. Thieden E, Philipsen PA, Sandby-Moller J et al (2005) Sunburn related to UV radiation exposure, age, sex, occupation, and sun bed use based on time-stamped personal dosimetry and sun behavior diaries. Arch Dermatol 141(4):482–488
226. Thomas NE, Alexander A, Edmiston SN et al (2004) Tandem BRAF mutations in primary invasive melanomas. J Invest Dermatol 122:1245–1250
227. Thomas NE, Berwick M, Cordeiro-Stone M (2006) Could BRAF mutations in melanocytic lesions arise from DNA damage induced by ultraviolet radiation? J Invest Dermatol 126:1693–1696
228. Thomas NE, Edmiston SN, Alexander A et al (2007) Number of nevi and early-life ambient UV exposure are associated with BRAF-mutant melanoma. Cancer Epidemiol Biomarkers Prev 16:991–997
229. Tierney P, Ferguson J, Ibbotson S et al (2013) Nine out of 10 sunbeds in England emit ultraviolet radiation levels that exceed current safety limits. Br J Dermatol 168(3):602–608. doi:10.1111/bjd.12181
230. Tucker M, Goldstein A (2003) Melanoa etiology: where are we? Oncogene 22:3042–3052
231. Uribe P, Wistuba II, Gonzalez S (2009) Allelotyping, microsatellite instability, and BRAF mutation analyses in common and atypical melanocytic nevi and primary cutaneous melanomas. Am J Dermatopathol 31:354–363
232. Valverde P, Healy E, Sikkink S et al (1996) The Asp84Glu variant of the melanocortin 1 receptor (MC1R) is associated with melanoma. Hum Mol Genet 5:1663–1666
233. Veierød MB, Adami HO, Lund E et al (2010) Sun and solarium exposure and melanoma risk: the effects of age, pigmentary characteristics and nevi. Cancer Epidemiol Biomarkers Prev 19:111–120
234. Viros A, Fridlyand J, Bauer J et al (2008) Improving melanoma classification by integrating genetic and morphologic features. PLoS Med 5:e120
235. Visuri TI, Pukkala E, Pulkkinen P et al (2006) Cancer incidence and causes of death among total hip replacement patients: a review based on Nordic cohorts with a special emphasis on metal-on-metal bearings. Proc Inst Mech Eng H 220(2):399–407
236. Vuong K, McGeechan K, Armstrong BK et al (2013) Occupational sun exposure and risk of melanoma according to anatomical site. Int J Cancer. doi:10.1002/ijc.28603
237. Walkosz BJ, Buller DB, Andersen PA et al (2008) Increasing sun protection in winter outdoor recreation: a theory-based health communication program. Am J Prev Med 34(6): 502–509
238. Wang JX, Zhang LA, Li BX et al (2002) Cancer incidence and risk estimate among medical X-ray workers in China 1950–1995. Health Phys 82:455–466
239. Wei X, Walia V, Lin JC et al (2011) Exome sequencing identifies GRIN2A as frequently mutated in melanoma. Nat Genet 43:442–446

240. Wesseling C, Antich D, Hogstedt C et al (1999) Geographical differences of cancer incidence in Costa Rica in relation to environmental and occupational pesticide exposure. Int J Epidemiol 28:365–374
241. Whiteman DC, Pavan WJ, Bastian BC (2011) The melanomas: a synthesis of epidemiological, clinical, histopathological, genetic, and biological aspects, supporting distinct subtypes, causal pathways, and cells of origin. Pigment Cell Melanoma Res 24:879–897
242. Whiteman D, Watt P, Purdie D et al (2003) Melanocytic nevi, solar keratosis, and divergent pathways to cutaneous melanoma. J Natl Cancer Inst 95:806–812
243. Williams PF, Olsen CM, Hayward NK et al (2011) Melanocortin-1-receptor and risk of cutaneous melanoma: a meta-analysis and estimates of population burden. Int J Cancer 129:1730–1740
244. Williams LH, Shors AR, Barlow WE et al (2011) Identifying persons at highest risk of melanoma using self-assessed risk factors. J Clin Exp Dermatol Res 2
245. Winther JF, Ulbak K, Dreyer L et al (1997) Avoidable cancers in the Nordic countries. Radiation APMIS Suppl 76:83–99
246. Wollina U, Heim C, Bennewitz A et al (2014) Interventional three-year longitudinal study of melanocytic naevus development in pre-school children in Dresden. Saxony Acta Derm Venereol 94(1):63–67
247. Woolley T, Lowe J, Raasch B et al (2008) Workplace sun protection policies and employees' sun-related skin damage. Am J Health Behav 32(2):201–208
248. Wright WE, Peters JM, Mack TM (1983) Organic chemicals and malignant melanoma. Am J Ind Med 4:577–581
249. Yokoyama S, Woods SL, Boyle GM et al (2011) A novel recurrent mutation in MITF predisposes to familial and sporadic melanoma. Nature 480:99–103
250. Zeeb H, Belttner M, Hammer GP et al (2002) Cohort mortality study of German cockpit crew 1960–1997. Epidemiology 13:693–699
251. Zeidler-Erdely PC, Meighan TG, Erdely A et al (2013) Lung tumor promotion by chromium-containing welding particulate matter in a mouse model. Part Fibre Toxicol 5: 10–45
252. Zielinski JM, Garner MJ, Krewski D et al (2005) Decreases in occupational exposure to ionizing radiation among Canadian dental workers. J Can Dent Assoc 71:29–33
253. Zuk O, Hechter E, Sunyaev SR et al (2012) The mystery of missing heritability: genetic interactions create phantom heritability. PNAS 109:1193–1198

Methods of Melanoma Detection

Sancy A. Leachman, Pamela B. Cassidy, Suephy C. Chen, Clara Curiel, Alan Geller, Daniel Gareau, Giovanni Pellacani, James M. Grichnik, Josep Malvehy, Jeffrey North, Steven L. Jacques, Tracy Petrie, Susana Puig, Susan M. Swetter, Susan Tofte and Martin A. Weinstock

Abstract

Detection and removal of melanoma, before it has metastasized, dramatically improves prognosis and survival. The purpose of this chapter is to (1) summarize current methods of melanoma detection and (2) review state-of-the-art detection methods and technologies that have the potential to reduce melanoma mortality. Current strategies for the detection of melanoma range from population-based educational campaigns and screening to the use of algorithm-driven imaging technologies and performance of assays that identify markers of transformation.

S.A. Leachman (✉)
Department of Dermatology and Knight Cancer Institute, Oregon Health and Science University, 3303 SW Bond Avenue, CH16D, Portland, OR 97239, USA
e-mail: leachmas@ohsu.edu

P.B. Cassidy
Department of Dermatology and Knight Cancer Institute, Oregon Health and Science University, 3125 SW Sam Jackson Park Road, L468R, Portland, OR 97239, USA
e-mail: cassidyp@ohsu.edu

S.C. Chen
Department of Dermatology, Emory University School of Medicine, 1525 Clifton Road NE, 1st Floor, Atlanta, GA 30322, USA
e-mail: schen2@emory.edu

C. Curiel
Department of Dermatology and Arizona Cancer Center, University of Arizona, 1515 N Campbell Avenue, Tucson, AZ 85721, USA
e-mail: ccuriel@email.arizona.edu

A. Geller
Department of Dermatology, Harvard School of Public Health and Massachusetts General Hospital, Landmark Center, 401 Park Drive, 3rd Floor East, Boston, MA 02215, USA
e-mail: ageller@hsph.harvard.edu

H.L. Kaufman and J.M. Mehnert (eds.), *Melanoma*,
Cancer Treatment and Research 167, DOI 10.1007/978-3-319-22539-5_3

This chapter will begin by describing state-of-the-art methods for educating and increasing awareness of at-risk individuals and for performing comprehensive screening examinations. Standard and advanced photographic methods designed to improve reliability and reproducibility of the clinical examination will also be reviewed. Devices that magnify and/or enhance malignant features of individual melanocytic lesions (and algorithms that are available to interpret the results obtained from these devices) will be compared and contrasted. In vivo confocal microscopy and other cellular-level in vivo technologies will be compared to traditional tissue biopsy, and the role of a noninvasive "optical biopsy" in the clinical setting will be discussed. Finally, cellular and molecular methods that have been applied to the diagnosis of melanoma, such as comparative genomic hybridization (CGH), fluorescent in situ hybridization (FISH), and quantitative reverse transcriptase polymerase chain reaction (qRT-PCR), will be discussed.

D. Gareau
Laboratory of Investigative Dermatology, The Rockefeller University, 1230 York Avenue, New York, NY 10065, USA
e-mail: daniel.gareau@rockefeller.edu

G. Pellacani
Department of Dermatology, University of Modena and Reggio Emilia, Via del Pozzo 71, Modena, Italy
e-mail: giovanni.pellacani@unimore.it

J.M. Grichnik
Department of Dermatology and Cutaneous Surgery, University of Miami School of Medicine, Room 912, BRB (R-125), 1501 NW 10th Avenue, Miami, FL 33136, USA
e-mail: grichnik@miami.edu

J. Malvehy · S. Puig
Melanoma Unit, Dermatology Department, Hospital Clinic Barcelona, Villarroel 170, 08036 Barcelona, Spain
e-mail: jmalvehy@clinic.ub.es

S. Puig
e-mail: spuig@clinic.ub.es

J. North
University of California, San Francisco, 1701 Divisadero Street, Suite 280, San Francisco, CA 94115, USA
e-mail: jeffrey.north@ucsf.edu

S.L. Jacques
Department of Biomedical Engineering and Dermatology, Oregon Health and Science University, 3303 SW Bond Avenue, CH13B, Portland, OR 97239, USA
e-mail: jacquess@ohsu.edu

Keywords
Melanoma detection · In vivo confocal microscopy · Hyperspectral imaging · Melanoma screening · Dermoscopy · Gene expression profiling · Optical coherence tomography · Melanoma prevention · Atypical nevi · Melanoma digital photography · Optical biopsy · Quantitative real-time PCR (qRT-PCR) · Fluorescence in situ hybridization (FISH)

Contents

T. Petrie
Department of Biomedical Engineering, Oregon Health and Science University,
3303 SW Bond Avenue, CH13B, Portland, OR 97239, USA
e-mail: petrie@ohsu.edu

S.M. Swetter
Department of Dermatology/Cutaneous Oncology, Stanford University, 900 Blake Wilbur Drive, W3045, Stanford, CA 94305, USA
e-mail: sswetter@stanford.edu

S. Tofte
Department of Dermatology, Oregon Health and Science University, 3303 SW Bond Avenue, CH16D, Portland, OR 97239, USA
e-mail: toftes@ohsu.edu

M.A. Weinstock
Departments of Dermatology and Epidemiology, Brown University,
V A Medical Center 111D, 830 Chalkstone Avenue, Providence, RI 02908, USA
e-mail: maw@brown.edu

1 Background

Incidence and mortality rates for melanoma have increased steadily since the 1900s. Melanoma estimates for 2014 in the US include 76,100 new invasive and 63,770 new in situ cases, along with 9710 anticipated deaths [190]. The probability of developing melanoma from birth to death is now estimated to be 1 in 34 in men and 1 in 53 in women [190]. In the latest version of the AJCC staging guidelines [25], a total of 38,918 cases of melanoma are staged: 18,370 (47.2 %) Stage I; 9269 (23.8 %) Stage II; 3307 (8.5 %) Stage III; and 7972 (20.5 %) Stage IV. The 5- and 10-year survival rates decrease with advancing stage. For example, 10-year survival rates for localized (Stages I and II) melanoma range from 93 % for Stage IA to 39 % for Stage IIC. Reported ten-year survival rates for regionally metastatic (Stage III) disease range from 68 % for Stage IIIA to 24 % for Stage IIIC, and the 10-year survival rate for Stage IV disease is only 10–15 % [25]. It is not possible to determine from these data how many lives might have been saved if patients with metastatic disease had been detected at Stage IA. However, a "back of the envelope" estimate would suggest that of the almost 8000 Stage IV patients diagnosed, only about 10 % (800) would be predicted to be alive at 10 years. If 50 % of these 8000 patients had been diagnosed earlier with Stage IA disease, the estimate of living patients at 10 years would be increased to approximately 4120 (4000 patients X 10 % + 4000 X 93 %), potentially saving 3320 lives. This rough estimate is only intended to be illustrative of the concept that ***early detection of melanoma has the potential to dramatically reduce death due to this disease***.

In addition to mortality increases, the cost of treatment of melanoma increases dramatically with the stage of disease [104]. Six independent studies of the cost of melanoma treatment in the US conclude that the direct cost of melanoma care increases with increasing stage of disease [11, 57, 108, 188, 201, 213]. A summary of annual per-patient medical costs for melanoma in 2010 US dollar equivalents published by Guy et al. demonstrated a range from $2169 to $31,032/year to treat local disease, $31,778 to $69,006/year to treat regionally metastatic disease, and $34,103 to $152,244/year to treat distant metastatic disease [104]. These numbers do not take into consideration the escalation of cost for metastatic disease in the current era of targeted immunotherapies, which cost approximately $60,000–$120,000 per course of therapy for the drug alone, and do not include the costs of administration and management of side effects or associated hospitalization costs. Detection of melanoma at the earliest stages has the potential for substantial reduction in healthcare costs.

The capacity of early melanoma detection to save lives and dollars will depend on the application of a variety of detection methods. In this chapter, a full spectrum of detection methods will be reviewed, including (1) population and public health approaches, (2) skin cancer screening and self-skin examination approaches, (3) photographic methods,

(4) dermoscopic methods, (5) spectral imaging methods, (6) in vivo confocal microscopy methods, (7) optical coherence tomography methods, (8) electrical impedance and ultrasound detection methods, and (9) molecular methods to improve the diagnosis of melanoma. Each detection method has costs and opportunities associated with application to patient care, and the ultimate goal is to optimize the use of each method in a context that will provide the greatest reduction of melanoma-related death at the lowest cost.

2 Population-Level Approaches to Early Detection

2.1 The Role of Public Health Campaigns in the Early Detection of Melanoma

Screening for melanoma generally occurs in two venues—clinic-based (performed by dermatologists or primary care physicians) and mass screening, often led by the American Academy of Dermatology [83, 85] or similar organizations such as Euromelanoma in Europe [196]. A third form of melanoma screening that has recently emerged combines screening and educational awareness, including publicity on behavioral risks and training of physicians in behavior modification skills, and takes place in a given state or workplace. These population-based programs bear some resemblance to large-scale, statewide public health efforts to reduce rates of smoking in Massachusetts and California, which led to dramatic decreases in smoking rates and concomitant reduction of tobacco-related disease [122, 176].

American Academy of Dermatology Mass Screening Programs
The American Academy of Dermatology has conducted free skin cancer screening programs since 1985. Although screenees that are identified as possibly having a melanoma are not frequently followed up for histologic outcome, among the 242,374 skin cancer screenings conducted during the period 1992–1994, 363 screenees had histologically proven melanoma. Middle-aged and older men (age ≥50 years) comprised only 25 % of persons screened but comprised 44 % of those with a confirmed diagnosis of melanoma. The overall yield of melanoma (the number of confirmed diagnoses per the number of screenees) was 1.5 per 1000 screenings compared with a yield of 2.6 per 1000 screenings among men age ≥50 years. The yield was improved further for men age ≥50 years who reported either a changing mole (4.6 per 1000 screenings) or skin types I and II (3.8 per 1000 screenings) [83, 85]. The authors of AAD studies and those from the Euromelanoma screening programs agreed that the yield of mass screening for melanoma would be improved by outreach to middle-aged and older men, with particular focus on men with changing moles or with skin types I and II. Messages to primary care physicians illustrated that they should be attuned to the risk factors among all of their patients but should be alerted in particular to the heightened risk of melanoma for men age ≥50 years.

Training of Primary Care Physicians
Given that most Americans will not see a dermatologist during their lifetime but make frequent visits to primary care physicians (PCPs), it is necessary to train PCPs

in minimal triage of at-risk individuals requiring further expert dermatologist consultation. To this end, Eide et al. developed a 1- to 2-h interactive, Web-based course in skin cancer detection for practicing board-certified PCPs (http://www.skinsight.com/info/for_professionals/dermatology-education-resources) and evaluated its use and success with 54 PCPs at 2 US sites using pretests, immediate tests, and 6 month posttests [63].

The mean score for appropriate diagnosis and management increased from 36.1 to 46.7 % (odds ratio (OR) 1.6; 95 % confidence interval (CI), 1.4–1.9), with strongest improvement found for benign lesions from 32.1 to 46.3 % (OR 1.9; 95 % CI, 1.6–2.4). Dermatology referrals for suspicious lesions or new visits by participants' patients decreased at both sites after the course (from 630 to 607 and from 726 to 266, respectively) [63]. Ongoing efforts are underway to train medical students in the basic elements of the skin cancer screening examination [82].

Status of Major Skin Cancer Screening Efforts

In 2009, the United States Preventive Services Task Force (USPSTF), utilizing studies through 2006, concluded that the current evidence for skin cancer screening is insufficient to assess the balance of benefits and harms of the service. Since 2006, two major non-randomized studies have demonstrated the potential benefit of screening and education. At the same time, the USPSTF has given greater attention to a balance of evidence from observational studies and randomized studies rather than to the latter alone. Mounting evidence of the benefit to harm ratio is of crucial importance as preventive services that have a rating of A (high) or B (moderate) from the USPSTF will be relevant to the application of the Affordable Care Act [186].

In response to apparently high rates of melanoma at the Lawrence Livermore National Laboratory (LLNL), Schneider et al. designed an educational campaign to promote self-examination and targeted screening. This first non-randomized study monitored thickness and crude incidence of melanomas detected during three phases of increasing melanoma surveillance. These periods were as follows: (1) pre-awareness (1969–1975), (2) early awareness of increased melanoma risk (1976–1984), and (3) screening program (1984–1996). Crude incidence of melanomas thicker than 0.75 mm decreased during the 3 periods from 22.1 to 15.13 to 4.62 cases per 100,000 person-years ($p = 0.001$ by chi-square for trend) with the larger decrease from the active screening program. No eligible melanoma deaths occurred among LLNL employees during the screening period, whereas the expected number of deaths was calculated to be 3.39 deaths ($p = 0.034$) [182].

In the second non-randomized study, fueled by a large public awareness initiative, more than 360,000 residents of Schleswig-Holstein (a northern state in Germany) ages 20 and above received full-body skin examinations from dermatologists and trained PCPs. PCPs were trained in mandatory 8-hour programs and reimbursed the equivalent of $25 for screening and recording of the skin cancer examination. Twenty-seven percent of female and 10 % of male residents received screenings between July 1, 2003, and June 30, 2004. Incidence and mortality rates for Schleswig-Holstein and adjacent regions were compared for the period 2000–2009, encompassing a period prior to screening, during screening, and post-screening. Incidence rates were greater as recorded in the Cancer Registry of Schleswig-Holstein than Saarland (control state), and mortality rates dropped an estimated 45 % for men and women, while adjacent areas such as Denmark and the rest of Germany experienced little change during this 10-year period [64, 118, 205].

On the heels of this statewide effort, a nationwide screening program with no preceding educational campaign is currently taking place in Germany. Reports indicate that more than 75 % of primary care physicians have received the same 8-h training program and more than 30 million screenings have taken place (2008–2013). Comparisons in incidence and mortality rates between Germany and their nine adjacent countries are being planned.

Potential Harms of Skin Cancer Screening

While demonstrating screening-associated reductions in mortality is paramount, the USPSTF is also interested in assessing the potential harms associated with melanoma screening. Such harms may include pre- or post-screening anxiety, embarrassment encountered during screening, unnecessary excisions, costs, and scarring associated with biopsies and excisions. Future research should seek to assess harms from skin cancer screening in large-scale efforts such as the nationwide campaign in Germany or in healthcare system-led efforts currently underway at the University of Pittsburgh Medical Center.

With respect to data on screening anxiety, a study of 324 patients undergoing investigation of a suspicious skin lesion in the UK at a Pigmented Lesion Clinic consented to complete a baseline and 6-month survey. Using recognized cutoff scores, 27 % of women reported clinically high levels of anxiety at the time of clinic arrival, in comparison with 10 % of men ($p < 0.0001$). Patients given an immediate benign post-clinical diagnosis reported a reduction in anxiety ($p < 0.0001$), but patients requiring a biopsy reported elevated levels of anxiety. Approximately 30 % of these biopsy patients reported clinically high levels of anxiety both before and after diagnosis [8].

Expanding Population-Based Approaches to High-Risk States

Statewide efforts in the US and elsewhere are needed to replicate findings from Schleswig-Holstein. In particular, in states with high melanoma mortality rates, prescreening campaigns could be launched to promote public awareness of the importance of skin self-examination and physician examination. Cancer registry and vital statistics data can be utilized to compare states with high screening penetration versus unscreened states, and routinely administered surveys such as the Behavioral Risk Factor Surveillance System can measure awareness, exposure to screening information, intentions to screen, self-efficacy for skin cancer screening, and actual practice of the skin self-examination and receipt of a skin cancer screening. Additionally, cost studies should be incorporated.

2.2 Effects of Skin Self-examination and Clinician Skin Examination on Early Melanoma Detection

Multiple studies support the value of early detection of melanoma through skin self-examination (SSE) and clinician skin examination, though evidence that this translates into reduced population-based melanoma mortality has thus far been insufficient for the USPSTF to recommend skin screening as part of primary care practice. Ample data suggest that melanomas detected by clinicians through directed skin examinations or during the course of routine physical examinations (e.g., "opportunistic screening") are thinner than those found by patients or their significant others [5, 66, 116, 125, 197]. In an analysis of 9 worldwide studies of over 7500 patients, a mean decreased tumor thickness of 0.55 mm was found when comparing melanomas initially detected by physicians versus by patients or significant others [200]. Thus, peer-reviewed data and observational evidence support the efficacy of SSE in detecting thinner melanomas and reducing mortality.

Skin Self-Examination

In 1996, Berwick et al. [32] reported a 63 % reduction in lethal or advanced melanoma associated with SSE in a population-based, case-control study of Connecticut residents. The mean thickness of melanomas was reduced, though not significantly, in the 15 % of patients who performed SSE, compared with those who did not (OR 0.58; 95 % CI, 0.31–1.11). Subsequent analysis of the study population at a median of 5.4 years demonstrated lower risk of death from melanoma in patients with increased skin screening practices (inferred from a combination of skin awareness, SSE, and physician skin examination), although reported SSE itself was not associated with reduced melanoma mortality [31]. A 2003 study found that regular performance of SSE was associated with a significantly reduced likelihood of melanomas >1 mm at diagnosis (covariate-adjusted OR 0.65; 95 % CI, 0.45–0.93), although details regarding the thoroughness and frequency of SSE were not reported [47].

Improved understanding of the effectiveness of SSE has been hindered by variable study definitions of SSE, including the number or percent of body sites examined and the frequency and method of examination [152, 209] and the small number of studies examining the reported benefits of techniques such as the use of photographs to supplement SSE [153]. In a study of 321 recently diagnosed cutaneous melanoma patients, Pollitt et al. [163] showed that the thoroughness of SSE, as measured by the number of body sites examined and use of a picture aid illustrating a melanoma, was the best predictor of reduced melanoma thickness, with thinner tumors observed in patients who frequently examined at least some of their skin in the year prior to melanoma diagnosis (OR 2.66; 95 % CI, 1.48–4.80). The effect of SSE was even greater in men and in older patients (>60 years).

Despite the potential benefit of self-inspection of the skin for early melanoma detection, the prevalence of SSE in the general population is low. It is estimated that only 10–25 % of individuals in the US practice regular, thorough SSE [210]. Effective self-identification of melanoma is dependent on several factors, including increased awareness and knowledge of SSE practices, health provider teaching of SSE to patients, and consistent performance of SSE by patients [53]. The American Cancer Society recommends thorough SSE of all body areas, including the back, back of the legs, and scalp [192] areas that are typically difficult to self-inspect. While the USPSTF described insufficient evidence to recommend SSE for the general population in its 2009 report, the potential benefit in high-risk groups such as older men was noted [186].

However, a population-based telephone survey in Queensland, Australia, demonstrated that only 20 % of men 50 years or older examined the skin of their whole body at least once in the past year [6]. For higher risk populations, various educational programs have successfully increased SSE performance [153, 173, 174]. Other studies have demonstrated that patient and partner intervention with specialized information, such as using videos and telephone reminders, may increase the prevalence of SSE [113]. Other interventions, such as use of mole-mapping images during self-examination, can increase the accuracy of SSE [50].

Efforts have been made to better understand the psychosocial factors that affect skin examination behaviors in an attempt to identify mechanisms to improve compliance with skin examination recommendations. In an international Web-based survey of the general population, it was demonstrated that self- and professional skin examinations were associated with (1) a perceived risk of developing melanoma; (2) perceived benefits of, and barriers to, skin examination; and (3) perceived confidence in one's ability to engage in screening. Additionally, among those with no history of melanoma, higher cancer-related worry was associated with greater frequency of SSE [117]. Self-skin examination practices and seeking of physician skin examinations have also been evaluated in high-risk *CDKN2A/p16* mutation carrying families [21, 22, 199]. These studies confirm a relatively low baseline compliance with skin examination recommendations, despite counseling of risk. However, following provision of genetic test results and counseling, unaffected carriers demonstrated a significantly improved compliance in skin examination practices for as long as two years following the test reporting session. These data suggest that individually tailored risk messaging may improve compliance with early detection recommendations.

Clinical Skin Examination

While numerous worldwide studies have demonstrated that physician detection of melanoma is associated with thinner tumors at diagnosis [200], no randomized trials have established the efficacy of clinician screening for melanoma on mortality reduction. The 2009 USPSTF statement found insufficient evidence to recommend for or against routine skin cancer screening of the general population by primary care providers [186]. Since that time, however, evidence for improved melanoma outcomes with clinician skin screening was reported in a population-based case-control study by Aitken et al. of Queensland residents aged 20–75 years with histologically confirmed first primary invasive melanoma diagnosed between January 2000 and December 2003 [5]. This study demonstrated a 14 % lower risk of being diagnosed with a thick (>0.75 mm) melanoma following a clinician skin examination within 3 years of diagnosis (OR 0.86; 95 % CI, 0.75–0.98). The decrease in risk was greatest for the thick melanomas (risk reduction 40 % for lesions ≥3 mm), resulting in a projected 26 % fewer melanoma deaths in screened cases versus unscreened cases within 5 years.

A subsequent US study of 566 adults with invasive melanoma assessed the role of physician skin examination in the year prior to diagnosis and found that men over age 60 appeared to benefit the most from this practice [198]. Thinner tumors (≤1 mm) were significantly associated with physician discovery ($p \leq 0.0001$), though this was reported by only 19 % of patients. However, patients who had a full-body skin examination by a physician in the year prior to diagnosis were more than twice as likely to have a thinner melanoma (OR 2.51; 95 % CI, 1.62–3.87), largely due to the effect of the physician skin examination in men >60 years, who had four times the odds of a thinner melanoma (OR 4.09; 95 % CI, 1.88–8.89).

These studies, along with the aforementioned Lawrence Livermore National Laboratory cohort time series, the German SCREEN population-based time series, and ongoing nationwide skin screening program in Germany (discussed in Sect. 2.1), suggest that integration of the skin examination into a routine physical assessment by primary care providers may be a practical strategy for reducing skin cancer mortality. Clinician skin examination should be synergistic with skin self-examination for early melanoma detection. However, the documented prevalence of annual clinician skin examination ranges from only 8–21 % and varies according to the type of health provider [7, 114, 129, 175, 180]). Studies have demonstrated that dermatologists are significantly better than non-dermatologist physicians at diagnosing melanoma [92], although most suggest that tumor thickness does not appear to substantially differ by provider type. Since Americans make an average of 1.7 visits to primary care providers each year, they can serve as an important source of skin cancer diagnosis and triage.

Indeed, most physician-detected melanomas are found by primary care providers, not dermatologists, a statistic related to national shortages in the dermatology workforce, and primary care providers perform the initial biopsy of 1.4–13 % of all melanomas [98]. Therefore, dermatologists and primary care providers must work in tandem to promote early melanoma detection. However, published data suggest that primary care providers in the US may not be adequately trained to identify early skin cancer [84, 148]. Many physicians have minimal exposure to skin cancer examination practices during medical school and residency, resulting in lack of knowledge and confidence in skin cancer diagnosis and effective patient assessment, thereby creating barriers to routine skin exams by primary care providers.

Factors that promote and/or prevent skin cancer screening among US primary care providers and dermatologists were evaluated in a survey study of >1600 randomly selected physicians [189]. More dermatologists (81 %) reported performing whole body skin examination on patients than did family practitioners (59.6 %) ($p < 0.05$) or internists (56.4 %) ($p < 0.05$). Among all physicians, time constraints, competing comorbidities, and patient embarrassment were reported as the top 3 barriers to performing full skin examinations. Factors that facilitated skin screening among all physicians included having patients at high risk for skin cancer, patient demand for complete examination/mole check, and the influence of specialty medical training.

Effective educational and training programs are essential to increase the efficacy and implementation of comprehensive skin examinations by healthcare providers in at-risk populations. A number of Web-based educational programs have been designed for this purpose [63], including a 1.5-h Web-based, interactive training program called INFORMED (INternet-based program FOR Melanoma Early Detection), available at http://www.skinsight.com/info/for_professionals/skin-cancer-detection-informed/skin-cancer-education. As mentioned above, a recent US study evaluated the effect of INFORMED on 54 primary care providers at two integrated healthcare delivery systems on practice patterns, including referral or visits to dermatology and skin biopsies during the six months following training [63]. Scores for appropriate diagnosis and management increased from 36 % pre-training to 47 % post-training (OR 1.6; 95 % CI 1.4–1.9), with greatest improvement for benign skin lesions. Rates of dermatology utilization decreased without any change in biopsies performed or skin cancers diagnosed, suggesting that primary care provider training in skin cancer did not increase specialty referrals or over-biopsy/treatment, likely due to the improvement in diagnosis and management of benign lesions.

3 The Role of Clinical Examination-Based Detection Methods for Melanoma

3.1 The Comprehensive Skin Examination

A screening examination for skin lesions by a trained practitioner takes only a few minutes and can reveal melanomas in areas not easily viewed by the patient such as the back and posterior legs. The clinician skin examination allows for the assessment of melanoma risk factors such as fair skin phenotype/sun sensitivity, increased nevus count, and/or clinically atypical nevi. It requires few materials, namely adequate examination lighting and possible use of a magnifying lens or dermatoscope, though this latter tool requires appropriate training. The INFORMED Web-based curriculum provides clinical guidance for early detection of melanoma (as well as other common skin cancers) by primary care providers, although it is available for the lay public to use, as well.

For either self-examination or clinician examination, it is important to be systematic and thorough. One suggested physical examination procedure uses a standard sequence of "down and back" (down the anterior body, then back up the posterior). A specific algorithm for clinicians is as follows: (1) examination of the face and rest of the head and neck while the patient is sitting on the examination table; (2) examination of the scalp, which is particularly important in men with thinning hair; (3) examination of all surfaces of the arms and hands; (4) having the patient to lie down on his/her back for viewing of the chest, abdomen, anterior thighs, anterior legs, dorsal feet, soles, and toe webs; and (5) having the patient turn over for examination of the calves, posterior thighs, buttocks, and back if this permits optimal examination over a standing position. The upper body could also be examined when the patient is sitting or standing. Additionally, an examination of the genitals should be offered to patients as part of the total body skin examination. Physician inspection of skin, especially high-risk melanoma sites (trunk for men, legs and trunk for women), should be encouraged during routine examinations, and simply looking at the back (the site of over 30 % of melanomas in men) would be a useful first step in promoting early melanoma detection. Early detection of a melanoma during a clinical examination can be lifesaving as well as a highly rewarding experience for the provider. Increasing the efficacy and implementation of clinician skin examination, skin self-examination, and targeted population screening may provide the greatest immediate impact the medical community can have on reduction of melanoma mortality.

3.2 Use of Longitudinal Photography for Early Detection of Melanoma

It is often a challenge for a clinician to distinguish an early cutaneous melanoma from an atypical but benign nevus during the clinical examination. The overlap of benign and malignant clinical features may lead to overlooking melanoma and/or excising an excessive number of benign lesions [130]. This clinical scenario applies to both unaided visual and dermoscopic examinations [120, 164].

Digital photography optimizes the monitoring of skin lesion features over time through clinical comparison with baseline and serial photographic documentation. Total body digital photography (TBDP) has been shown to be helpful in the detection of changes in shape, color, or surface eventually occurring in any lesion, and for the identification of new or regressing lesions aided by baseline and subsequent imaging sessions (Fig. 1) [26, 97, 105, 132, 172, 208]. This technique is particularly helpful in the surveillance of individuals with numerous melanocytic nevi, including but not limited to atypical mole syndrome, or other high-risk cohorts such as patients with a personal or family history of multiple cutaneous melanomas, xeroderma pigmentosum, or patients undergoing metastatic melanoma treatment with B-Raf inhibitors.

One metric of the utility of TBDP is in the benign to malignant biopsy ratio. Feit et al. [69] reported 93 lesions biopsied in 576 patients undergoing TBDP. Twenty-seven (35 %) of 77 melanocytic lesions were diagnosed as melanoma, translating to a benign to malignant ratio of 3:1. Banky et al. reported similar benign to malignant ratios using TBDP [26]. These ratios compare very favorably

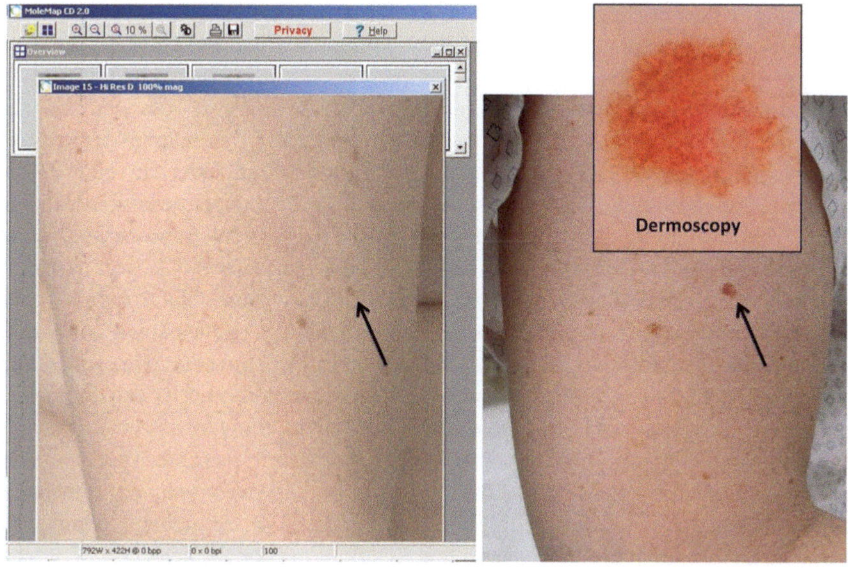

Fig. 1 Total body digital photography is helpful in detecting changes in shape, color, or surface in any lesion. Total body images are obtained for patients at high risk from melanoma, and these patients are then on follow-up. The lesion on the patient's right arm appeared distinctly different than his/her other moles. In addition, some erythema was noted on the subsequent visit (*right panel*). The follow-up dermoscopic image (*inset*) was not entirely diagnostic for melanoma. However, when compared to the baseline image (*left panel*), the lesion had clearly changed. The observed interval change increased the clinical concern for melanoma prompting a skin biopsy. Histological evaluation confirmed the diagnosis of in situ melanoma

with the ratios of 12:1 or 30:1 reported for unaided examination by dermatologists and general physicians, respectively [26]. Of note, while the benign to malignant ratio of biopsies is a useful indicator of diagnostic accuracy, it is also somewhat dependent on the patient mix seen by each individual physician (e.g., a dedicated pigmented lesion clinic in an academic dermatology department will have a different patient mix than that of a primary care provider). Another benefit to TBDP is that the melanomas detected when using this technique tend to be thinner. Banky found that 44 % of melanomas were in situ (vs. 35 % in regional controls) and that the median thickness of the invasive tumors was 0.39 mm (vs. 0.60 mm). Lastly, usage of TBDP can prevent unnecessary biopsies as well as decrease patient's worry. Hanrahan et al. conducted a randomized prospective trial evaluating the effect of photography in the hands of PCPs and found that while there was no difference in melanoma detection, fewer benign pigmented lesions, such as seborrheic keratoses, were removed when using photography [106]. Risser et al. [172] found no difference in the rate of biopsy in a pigmented lesion specialty clinic when photographs were used, but pointed out that the benefit from TBDP most likely lies in patients who are not already "de-moled," with most of the atypical nevi removed prior to the photographs.

Sequential digital dermoscopy imaging (SDDI) involves the capture and assessment of successive dermoscopic images separated by an interval of time and can include single or multiple melanocytic lesions that warrant surveillance for suspicious changes. This imaging is performed in two settings: short-term digital monitoring (usually over a period of 3 months) for suspicious melanocytic lesions and long-term surveillance (in most instances at intervals of 6–12 months) [143]. A recent meta-analysis grouped both short- and long-term SDDI together and showed that the number of lesions needed to monitor one detected melanoma ranged from 31 to 1008 depending on the clinical setting (lower numbers of lesions were needed to find a melanoma with short-term monitoring) [179]. For every additional month of monitoring, one additional melanoma was detected, with the chances to detect a melanoma during surveillance shown to increase as the length of follow-up extended. Furthermore, the proportion in situ melanoma and thin melanomas detected by SDDI were higher than expected in the general population. Taken together, the literature suggests that SDDI allows for the detection of at least a portion of dermoscopically featureless or otherwise occult melanomas. When used in high-risk patients or on individual suspicious melanocytic lesions, SDDI demonstrates a significant clinical impact with melanomas detected exclusively using SDDI in 34–61 % of these patients (Fig. 2).

The combined use of TBDP and digital dermoscopy, also known as the "two-step method of digital follow-up," has been primarily implemented for the surveillance of patients at high risk for cutaneous melanoma [139]. This method has been proposed as a more sensitive strategy in cutaneous melanoma screening, by allowing not only the detection of dermoscopic changes over time but also detection of macroscopic changes and the occurrence of new lesions not previously identified for follow-up [178].

In the largest retrospective "two-step method" study published to date, 1152 lesions were excised during the surveillance of 779 monitored lesions in 618 patients at high risk for melanoma. A total of 98 melanomas were detected: 60 in the monitored lesions and 38 among the 373 lesions that were new or undetected on previous TBDP. The most frequent dermoscopic changes detected were asymmetric enlargement in almost 60 % ($n = 418$), focal changes in structure in 197 (27 %), and pigmentation in 122 (17 %), the latter two identified more frequently in melanomas than in nevi ($p < 0.001$). No significant differences were detected between dermoscopic and histopathological characteristics of the melanomas in each group, with a considerable proportion of melanomas misclassified as benign in both groups (26.3 and 38.3 %, respectively). Almost 40 % of cutaneous melanomas diagnosed in the study corresponded to lesions that were not under dermoscopic surveillance [177].

Challenges in the selection of lesions for SDDI include the variability in the expertise of the clinicians, the heterogeneous appearance of the lesions, and a broad

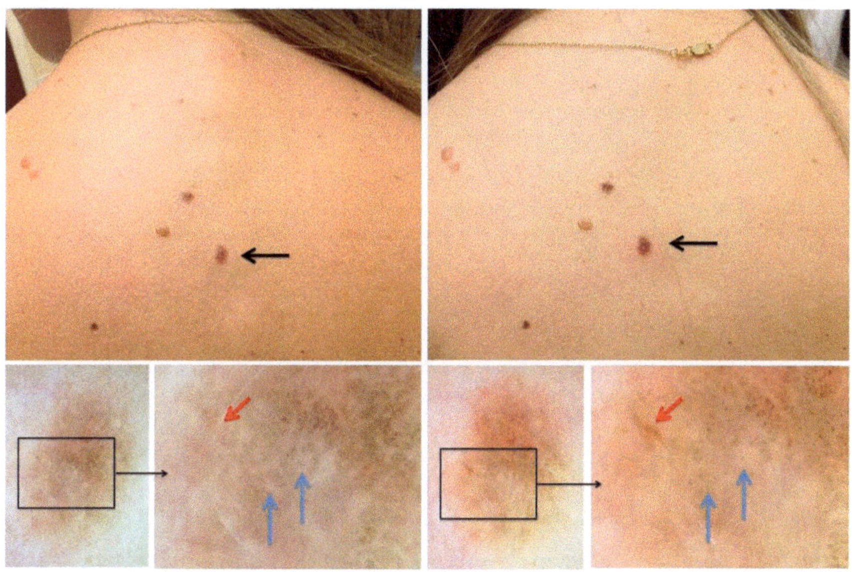

Fig. 2 Sequential digital dermoscopy imaging has significant clinical impact when used in high-risk patients or on individual suspicious melanocytic lesions. Dermoscopic monitoring may be used in limited circumstances when it is unclear whether a lesion is problematic. In this case, the lesion had negative network features but otherwise clinically appeared benign in a patient who had not noted changes and wished to avoid biopsy. At 3-month follow-up, architectural changes were noted dermoscopically. The red arrow points to a new structure, and blue arrows indicate one area where changes have occurred in the distribution of globules and negative network structures. The lesion proved to be a Breslow's 0.45-mm melanoma

range of risk of cutaneous melanoma development across high-risk cohorts. Some authors have suggested an individualized surveillance plan, with digital dermoscopy performed at follow-up intervals of 3 months for patients with familial multiple mole and melanoma (FAMMM) syndrome and 6–12 months (depending on additional risk factors) for those with atypical mole syndrome [12].

Another challenge is represented by patients' compliance. During SDDI, the risk of missing a melanoma (estimated in approximately 4 % of patients) [179] during the baseline visit should be considered relative to the benefit of a more accurate diagnosis at the follow-up examination, with consequent detriment of sensitivity at baseline compensated by higher overall specificity [119]. However, most melanomas detected during follow-up in patients with multiple nevi were false negatives in the clinical and dermoscopical examination at the first visit [178]. In this context, the lack of patient compliance should be carefully considered, since low adherence to digital dermoscopy follow-up could compromise the efficacy of this approach [17].

Given the above listed benefits of longitudinal use of TBDP and dermoscopy, one may wonder why the technology is not utilized more widely. In 2010, Rice et al. [170] surveyed academic pigmented lesion centers and found that approximately 67 % of the 49 respondents utilized photography to monitor pigmented lesions. The rate is lower for dermatologists who do not practice in pigmented lesion centers. The primary reason for not using photography in the study was logistical constraints. There is no doubt that adjuvant diagnostic tools add more time to the already busy clinic, and they may take additional training by both the dermatologist and staff to efficiently and effectively incorporate these useful imaging modalities into the daily workflow. Incentives for providers to utilize such tools should be considered, particularly for patients who are at risk for melanoma.

3.3 Use of Dermoscopy as an Adjunct to Skin Examination

Dermoscopy, also known as dermatoscopy or epiluminescence microscopy, is a noninvasive technique that uses a dermatoscope for the diagnosis of skin tumors and other skin diseases [15, 19]. Evidence-based data of the highest level support the use of dermoscopy in the diagnosis of skin cancer, including melanoma, basal cell carcinoma, and squamous cell carcinoma [24, 121, 204]. Because of the strength of this data, most clinical guidelines in melanoma include dermoscopy as an essential tool for the examination of pigmented and non-pigmented skin tumors to detect melanoma [23, 78]. This tool is most relevant and useful in clinically equivocal cases and in the early recognition of difficult-to-recognize melanomas [20, 46, 164] (Figs. 3, 4, and 5). Dermatologists worldwide are familiar with dermoscopy, though effective application of the technique requires training [34, 154] and experience. In a prospective randomized study by Argenziano et al. [18], a 4-hour course on dermoscopy increased the ability of trainees to detect skin cancer, including melanoma, in actual clinical settings. The use of dermoscopy has more recently expanded outside the practice of dermatology and is now being incorporated into the diagnostic armamentarium of general physicians. In Australia and Europe, teaching of the method has become standard practice for primary healthcare providers. Moreover, a study in students showed a significant, positive impact in the recognition of melanoma after a short course on dermoscopy [112]. The authors of the study concluded that dermoscopy should be included in medical student education.

Basics of Dermoscopy

Dermoscopy is based on careful observation of the architecture of a selected skin lesion via the use of an optical instrument and illumination. The instrument allows the observer to examine the pigment (melanin, blood, or other) in the epidermis and dermis. With the dermatoscope, it is possible to minimize the reflection of light from the surface of the skin that would otherwise obscure the underlying structures and limit the optimal perception of colors. Two main types of dermatoscopes are available: polarized and non-polarized (depending on their capacity to integrate

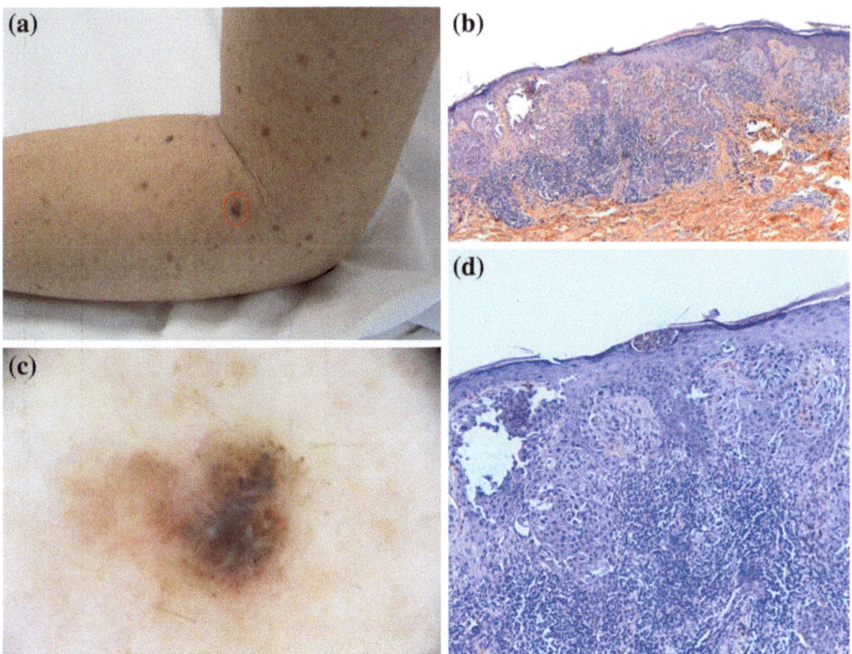

Fig. 3 Clinical, dermoscopic, and histologic images of a superficial spreading melanoma, Breslow thickness 0.9 mm. Clinical image (**a**). Dermoscopy (**c**) shows an asymmetric lesion with multiple colors (*light brown*, *dark brown*, *blue*, *black*, and *white*), global globular pattern, with presence of atypical globules, *black dots*, and *white shiny streaks*. H&E histology ×100 (**b**). The presence of pigmented melanoma nests in the upper epidermis in (**d**, H&E histology ×200) corresponds to black dots in dermoscopy

cross-polarization filters). Non-polarized dermoscopy requires direct contact with the skin and immersion liquid, including water, mineral oil, or gel. Polarized dermoscopy does not require immersion liquid, and contact is not mandatory due to the optical properties of the two polarization filters adapted in the dermatoscope. Although most features observed with polarized and non-polarized dermoscopy are similar, specific differences have been described [207].

In the case of digital dermoscopy, the optical instrument is connected to a video or photographic camera to obtain digital images that can be visualized on a computer screen. Some commercial devices have been introduced for the acquisition and storage of images through the use of dedicated software for clinical practice. With digital dermoscopy devices, follow-up comparisons of atypical lesions are possible in high-risk patients, which have the potential to improve early detection of melanoma and reduction of unnecessary biopsies, particularly in patients with multiple atypical moles [178, 179].

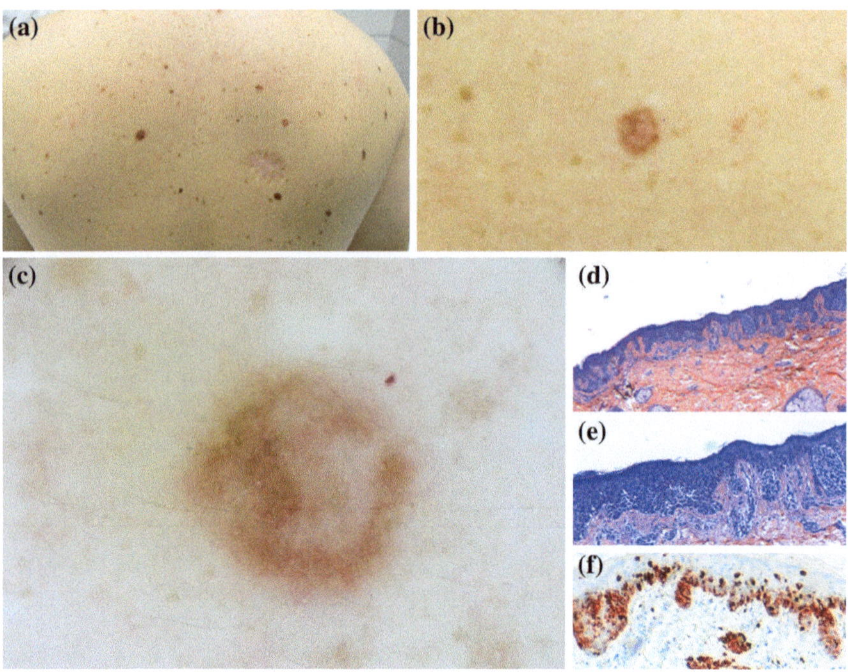

Fig. 4 Clinical, dermoscopic, and histologic images of an early invasive superficial spreading melanoma, Breslow thickness 0.4 mm located on the back. Clinical views in (**a**) and (**b**). Under dermoscopy (**c**), the lesion shows asymmetry, atypical pigment network, few globules irregularly distributed, erythema with some dotted vessels, and short white streaks. H&E histology ×40 (**d**) and ×100 (**e**). The double staining with MelanA and Ki67 shows pagetoid growth and proliferating melanocytes in the dermis (**f**)

Diagnosis with Dermoscopy

A variety of methods for the dermoscopic diagnosis of melanoma and other skin tumors have been proposed by different authors in the last 30 years [16, 33, 39, 193]. These methods use a combination of features of pigmentation, patterns, and structures of the lesion to distinguish between benign and malignant tumors. In general, melanoma exhibits more colors and structures relative to benign lesions, and these features are more likely to be asymmetrically distributed in the lesion. In order to achieve the greatest diagnostic accuracy with dermoscopy, it is essential to be aware of the histopathological correlations associated with the dermoscopic features. The presence or absence of the structures, their distribution in the lesion, and the presence of colors are strictly correlated to pathology with one main difference: Dermoscopy is the examination in the horizontal plane, whereas pathology works in the vertical section of the tissue [137]. It has been postulated that pathology and dermoscopy are particularly complementary for this reason [70]. Dermoscopy has also been effectively utilized to guide gross pathology of melanocytic lesions and for sampling of archived samples in melanoma [137, 185].

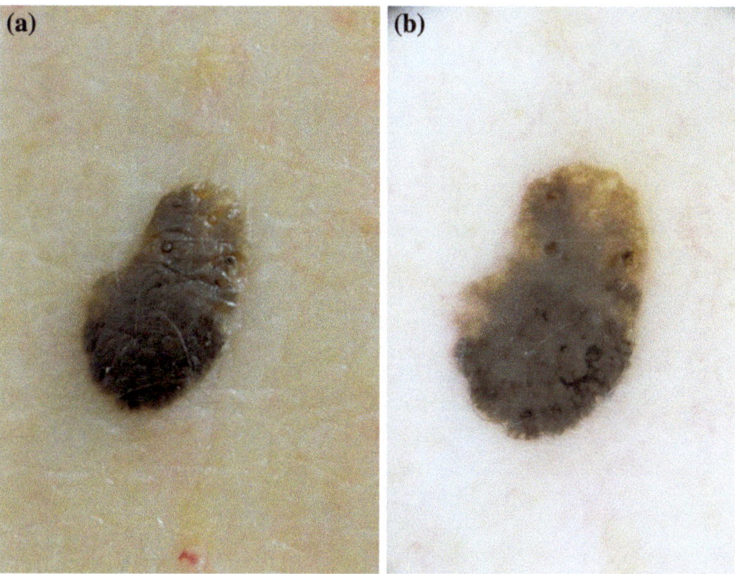

Fig. 5 Clinical and dermoscopic images of a suspicious lesion, asymmetric with black and blue colors. Clinical image (**a**). Under dermoscopy (**b**), the lesion shows abrupt cutoff of the border, presence of fat fingers at the periphery, comedolike openings, and milialike cysts, which favor a diagnosis of benign seborrheic keratosis

Dermoscopic Features in Melanoma

Specific dermoscopic features are associated with melanoma [140]. Depending on the subtype of melanoma and location on the body, different patterns can be observed. In melanomas arising in special locations such as face, acral sites, mucosa, or nails, dermoscopic patterns tend to be influenced by the special anatomy of the skin and the particular growth of the tumors. During the progression of melanoma, new features progressively appear due to the architectural disorganization and bizarre distribution of pigment and vessels associated with neovascularization. In thick tumors, asymmetry in color and structures, presence of multiple colors (blue-gray, brown, black, red, white), complex patterns (combination of many structures in the same lesion), and particular structures characteristic of melanoma are frequent. In contrast, in very early melanomas, dermoscopic features of melanoma tend to be less evident and can be similar to atypical nevi. In Table 1, we summarize the dermoscopic criteria for melanoma.

Recently, dermoscopy utilized in conjunction with other imaging techniques, such as longitudinal digital photography or reflectance confocal microscopy, permitted detection of new melanomas associated with the use of BRAF inhibitors in the treatment of BRAF-mutated metastatic melanomas [60] (Fig. 6).

Table 1 Dermoscopic criteria for melanoma

Pattern	Definition
Dermoscopic global pattern	
Multicomponent pattern	Combination of 3 or more distinctive dermoscopic structures (pigment network, globules, streaks, blotches)
Nonspecific pattern	Pigmented lesion lacking sufficient criteria to meet a reticular, globular, homogenous, or starburst pattern definition
Starburst pattern	–
Multiple colors	The presence of 5 colors in a melanocytic lesion is a sufficient criterion for melanoma diagnosis The combination of black and blue is a criterion for nodular melanoma Pink and red in a melanocytic lesion are suspicious for malignancy
Dermoscopic specific criteria	
Atypical pigment network	Black, brown, or gray network with irregular holes and thick lines
Irregular dots/globules	Irregularly distributed black, brown round to oval, variously sized structures
Irregular streaks (pseudopods and radial streaming)	Irregularly distributed bulbous and often kinked or fingerlike projections seen at the edge of the lesion. They arise from network structures or the body of the tumor. Colors range from tan to black
Blue-whitish veil	Irregular, structureless area of confluent blue pigmentation with an overlying white "ground glass" film. Pigmentation cannot occupy entire lesion and usually corresponds to a clinically elevated part of the lesion
Regression structures	White scarlike depigmentation and/or blue pepperlike granules usually corresponding to a clinically flat part of the lesion
Vascular structures	Irregularly distributed hairpin vessels, dotted vessels, linear irregular vessels, vessels and/or erythema within regression structures
Blotches	Darkly pigmented homogeneous areas irregularly distributed in melanoma
Shiny white streaks (chrysalids)	Short white lines in polygonal distribution only visible with cross-polarized dermoscopy associated with malignancy, with melanoma, and with invasive melanoma
Rosettes	Four white dots in a rhomboidal distribution, arranged as a four-leaf clover, only visible with cross-polarized dermoscopy

(continued)

Table 1 (continued)

Pattern	Definition
Dermoscopic specific criteria/patterns in special locations	
Acral lentiginous melanoma	
Parallel ridge pattern	Pigmentation in the ridges of the fingerprints associated with acral melanoma
Diffuse irregular pigmentation	Geographic pigmentation in different shades of brown with ill-defined border
Lentigo maligna and lentigo maligna melanoma	
Irregular peri-follicular pigmentation	Irregular pigmentation around follicular openings with a c-shape
Granular annular pattern	Blue-gray spots around hair follicles creating an annular pattern
Rhomboidal structures	Confluent pigment around hair follicles that with progression may also invade follicular areas
Isobars	A circle in a circle surrounding a follicular opening
Pink-red rhomboidal structures	Erythema around follicular openings focally seen in early invasive lentigo maligna or amelanotic melanoma

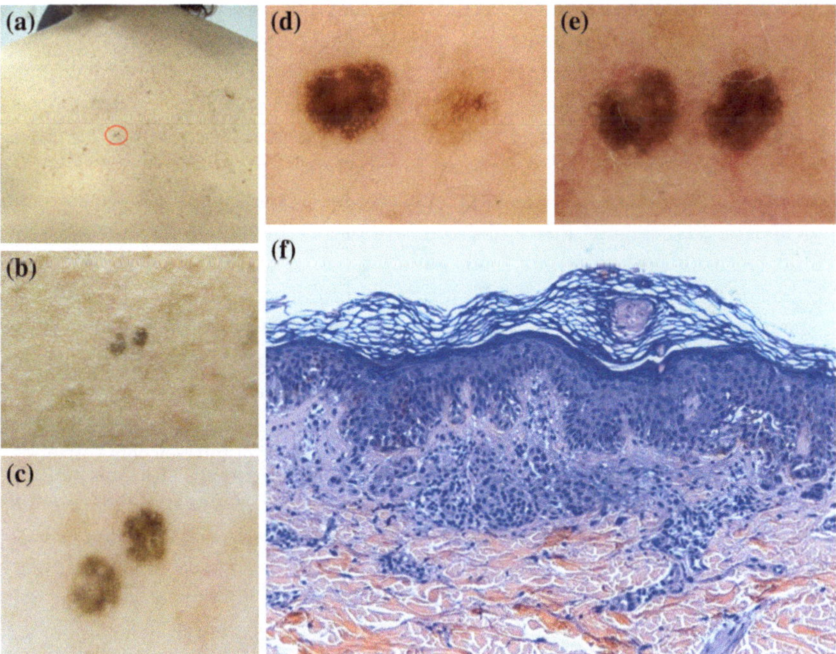

Fig. 6 Clinical, dermoscopic, and histologic images of a cutaneous lesion on a metastatic melanoma patient undergoing treatment with a BRAF inhibitor. Clinical (**a** and **b**) and dermoscopic (**c**, **d**, and **e**) images of two lesions on the back that presented with changes over a 1-month period of digital follow-up. Dermoscopy in November 2013 (**d**) and dermoscopy in December 2013 (**e**). Both lesions were excised. The lesion on the right showed growth and increase in pigmentation and was diagnosed as a severely dysplastic nevus, but melanoma in situ arising in a nevus could not be ruled out. H&E histology ×200 (**f**)

4 Advanced Technological Methods for Melanoma Detection

4.1 Beyond Visual Dermoscopy: Machine Vision in Melanoma Detection

Machine vision here refers to optical imaging and image processing, which extends the vision of the dermatologist. Machine vision is an area of technological growth in dermatology. Optical imaging can use light outside the visible spectrum to see what the eye cannot see. For example, near-infrared light can probe deeply into darkly pigmented lesions that appear black to the eye. Optical imaging can also use visible light with spectral analysis to quantify skin constitution that the eye cannot easily recognize. For example, spectral analysis can distinguish the amount of blood perfusion despite variation in melanin pigmentation or dermal scattering. Analysis of optical images can detect patterns and statistical metrics that are not easily recognized by the brain, for example, the statistics that characterize the branching of melanin pigment networks to recognize melanoma.

Machine vision can be based either (1) on a priori understanding of the mechanism underlying the spectrum or image or (2) on statistical development of a discriminator between two tissue states. The first approach is based on an understanding of how the measurement or image features depend on the tissue composition or structure. The advantage is that variation in observations can be interpreted in terms of variation in tissue composition or structure. The second approach correlates measurements or image features with tissue status, based on a training set of tissue types known by gold standard histopathological, biochemical, or clinical diagnosis to be either in one state or another, for example, normal versus pathological. The advantage is that a discriminator can be identified that optimally discriminates between a normal and pathological state, even when the tissue composition or structure responsible for the discrimination is not understood.

Two aspects of machine vision are illustrated here by examples. They include (1) image acquisition through hyperspectral imaging, reflectance confocal microscopy, and photoacoustic imaging; and (2) image analysis.

Hyperspectral Imaging

The term "hyperspectral imaging" refers to the use of wavelengths beyond the visible spectrum seen by the eye. Images acquired using two or more wavelengths can be algebraically combined to yield a new image sensitive to a particular tissue component. For example, Kollias and Baqer [124] showed that the metric log(R(650 nm)/R(720 nm)), where R denotes reflectance, 650 nm is deep red light, and 720 nm is deeper red light, was proportional to the epidermal melanin content. Thus, two images at these 2 wavelengths can be combined to map the x,y spatial distribution of melanin in the skin.

Ultraviolet A (UVA) light penetrates skin only superficially and is strongly absorbed by melanin. Hence, images of superficial skin structure are acquired (~upper 100 μm). Near-infrared light penetrates skin deeply and is absorbed by melanin, blood, and water. Hence, images of the deeper skin structure are acquired (~upper 1 mm).

Figure 7 shows a multispectral image set acquired using 4 differently colored light-emitting diodes (LEDs) to provide illumination, from invisible UVA to visible deep red. The UVA-illuminated image (Fig. 7 at 364 nm wavelength) clearly displays the superficial pigment, while in longer wavelength images (Fig. 7b–d using blue 488, red orange 598, and deep red 678 nm light), the pigmented lesion fades. Nevertheless, the image taken with deep red light illumination (Fig. 7d) reveals the thicker, denser, and/or deeper pigment.

While melanin absorption is an obvious marker for melanoma, light scattering may also prove useful. Garcia-Uribe et al. [79] have reported that light scattering increases in melanoma (benign nevi < dysplastic nevi < melanoma); hence, light scattering may be an additional metric for discriminating melanoma versus benign nevi.

When imaging pigmented lesions, hyperspectral imaging primarily utilizes photons that have penetrated into the skin, backscattered from the dermis, and transmitted through epidermis to escape at the skin surface. Thus, it is a form of transmission imaging where the light source originates in the dermis. The key

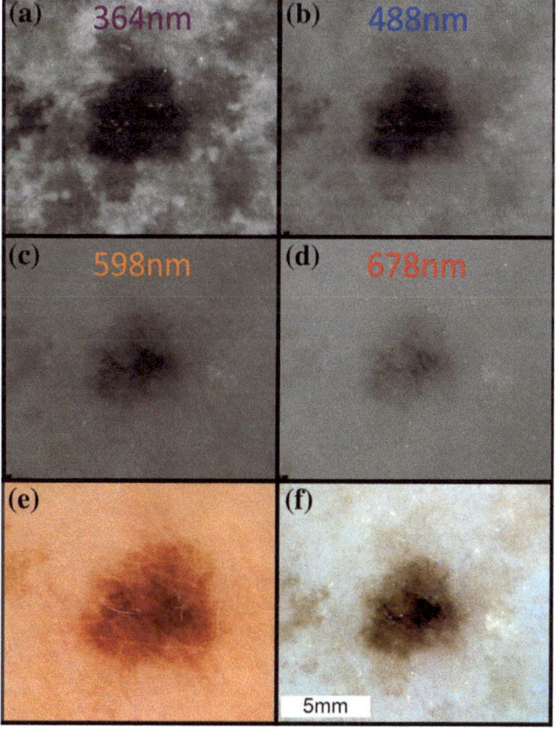

Fig. 7 Multispectral imaging of a common nevus in sun-damaged skin. Imaging at the wavelengths 364 nm (**a**), 488 nm (**b**), 598 nm (**c**), and 678 nm (**d**) with correlating standard dermoscopy (**e**) as well as a reconstruction of the *red/green/blue* image from the multispectral data (**f**) that is calibrated in reflectance units (Images by D. Gareau)

advantages of hyperspectral imaging are its ability to rapidly survey macroscopic fields of view and its relatively low cost.

Reflectance Confocal Microscopy (RCM)
Reflectance confocal microscopy (RCM), or confocal laser scanning microscopy (CLSM), is sensitive to backscatter of light by melanosomes, which are highly reflective [168]. RCM can detect pagetoid melanocytes in the epidermis, which correlate with melanoma, and a disorganized melanosome distribution along the epidermal–dermal junction (DEJ) that sometimes occurs in melanoma [80, 156]. Busam et al. [45] offered a commentary on the strengths and weaknesses of RCM for the detection of melanoma. Scope et al. [184] provided a glossary of terminology for RCM.

Wiltgen et al. [212] studied 50 malignant melanomas and 50 benign pigmented nevi and reported that RCM images of common benign nevi showed more architectural structures and contrast than images of malignant melanoma, which appeared more homogeneous. Guitera et al. [101] described a study of melanoma lesions versus nevi, basal cell carcinoma, and other skin tumors, which cited seven RCM features (cerebriform nests, atypical cobblestone pattern with small nucleated cells in the epidermis, marked cytological atypia, pagetoid cells, and disarranged epidermal layer with no honeycomb pattern) that associated with melanoma. They reported 87.6 % sensitivity and 70.8 % specificity. Braga et al. presented a comparison in six cases of RCM features versus dermoscopic and histopathologic features [40]. Pellacani et al. reported on RCM of 100 melanoma lesions, distinguishing four types of melanoma: (1) "dendritic cell melanomas," (2) melanomas typified by roundish melanocytes, (3) melanomas characterized by dermal nesting proliferation, and (4) combined-type melanomas [158].

Photoacoustic Imaging (PAI)
Photoacoustic imaging (PAI) uses a focused pulsed laser to deliver light to a focal spot within the skin and detects the sound generated by thermoelastic expansion due to absorption of light. Scanning the laser focus in x, y, and z throughout the volume of a pigmented lesion yields a 3D image of the lesion [68]. Hence, PAI is especially sensitive to melanin, which strongly absorbs light. PAI is a rapidly developing imaging modality that will likely contribute significantly to noninvasive in vivo imaging of the 3D structure of pigmented lesions.

Image Analysis
Automated image analysis can recognize edges for segmentation of tissue types and detect spatial patterns and textures in existing images to yield new images that enhance contrast of optically perturbing structures such as cancer or pigmented lesions. Image analysis algorithms can be applied to dermoscopic images to reveal pathological versus normal morphology or to generate a quantitative end point metric for classification, that is, the percent chance that a pigmented lesion is melanoma.

Early work by Cascinelli et al. [48] quantitatively analyzed image features such as lesion edge, morphology, texture, and color to obtain a positive predictive value of 0.45 and a negative predictive value of 0.95. Subsequent analytical methods included the use of geometries and Burroni's islands of colors [14]. Bauer et al. [30] used such features to obtain a positive predictive value of 0.87 and a negative predictive value of 0.99. Table 2 compares the sensitivities and specificities of recent computational approaches in comparison with algorithms used in dermoscopy with visual inspection.

Wiltgen et al. [212] discussed the classes of image analysis features in RCM images for discriminating malignant and benign melanocytic lesions. Koller et al. [123] studied a large number of RCM images (10,122 test images, after 6147 images in a training set) using CART (Classification and Regression Trees) analysis software (Salford Systems, San Diego, CA). They reported rather poor discrimination of melanoma versus benign nevi, which they attributed to non-standardized image acquisition, and cautioned that better results may rely on standardized acquisition. Gareau et al. [80] reported an image analysis algorithm for using RCM images to detect a disrupted dermal–epidermal junction (DEJ) in melanoma. Kurugol et al. [127] developed an algorithm incorporating texture analysis to use RCM images to localize the DEJ, which may prove useful in identifying a disrupted DEJ.

An example of image analysis is the skeletonization of the pigmented network in dermoscopic images of pigmented lesions. Statistical analysis of the branches in the pigmented network can yield the regularity among branch segments as a quantifiable metric. Figure 8 shows the use of an algorithm to find a diagnostically relevant feature, the coefficient of variation (COV) of branch lengths in the pigmented network. The standard deviation of the branch lengths divided by the average branch length (the COV) is 0.312 for Fig. 8b but 1.077 for Fig. 8d, indicating that the second lesion has more branch length variability. This COV metric is expected to grow with increasing atypical pigmented network features and may prove to be a useful quantitative descriptor indicating a suspicious lesion.

Table 2 Sensitivity (Se) and specificity (Sp) of melanoma detection reported for various algorithms in research studies

	Se (%)	Sp (%)
Pattern analysis [171]	85	79
ABCD [171]	84	75
7-point checklist [171]	78	65
CASH [171]	98	68
Menzies method [171]	85	85
*SIAscopy (European cohort) [65]	50	84
*SIAscopy (Australian cohort) [65]	44	95
*Solar scan [144]	91	68
*Pre-melafind 1 [72]	98	44
*Pre-melafind 2 [72]	91	38

Computer-automated analyses are marked (*). Visual analyses are unmarked

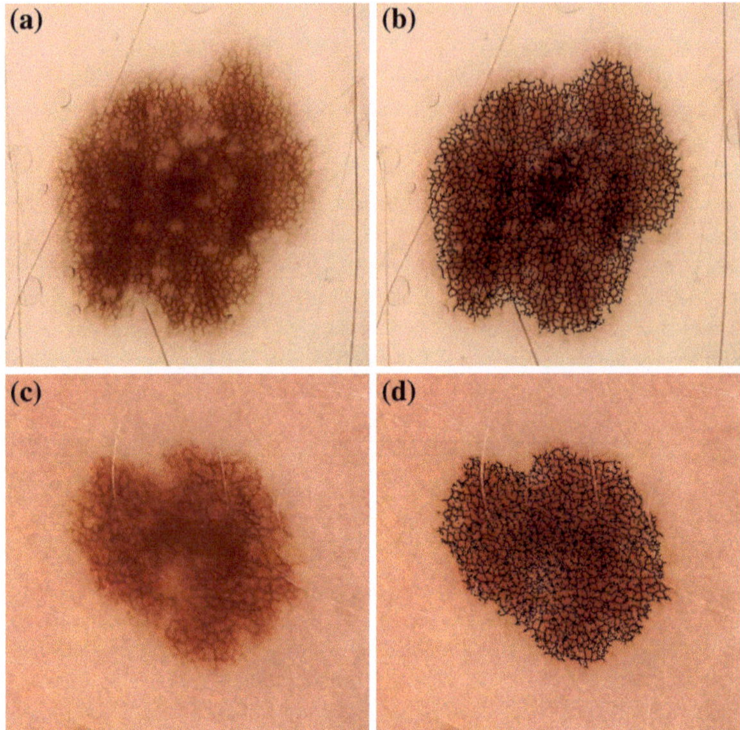

Fig. 8 Computer-automated identification of the pigmented network in two lesions. The original images are (**a**) and (**c**), and the images with computer-identified networks superimposed are (**b**) and (**d**) (Images by D. Gareau)

In summary, optical imaging and image analysis can characterize pigmented skin lesions and contribute to the discrimination of benign nevi, dysplastic nevi, and melanoma. Dermoscopy, hyperspectral imaging, confocal reflectance microscopy, and photoacoustic imaging are examples of image formation. Image analysis can use such images to yield new images based on spectral behavior, spatial patterns, and textures that characterize pigmented lesions.

4.2 In Vivo Confocal Microscopy

Historical Development

The microscope (invented in the 1500s in the Netherlands) was developed by Galileo. Galileo created the first compound microscope in 1625, enabling the discovery of the cell by Robert Hooke in 1665. The LASER, demonstrated in 1960 and reported in 1962 [135], became a powerful tool in combination with the confocal microscope [145], though initial optical sectioning of biological tissue used white light [161]. Rapid laser scanning microscopy was demonstrated for noninvasive skin imaging in 1995 [168] and improved to video rate in 1999 [166].

The reflectance confocal microscope has potential for clinical translation in dermatology thanks to engineering of rapid polygon scanning, which enabled video rate imaging [166–168] and a stable mechanical interface for skin coupling. The commercialized VivaScope (Caliber ID, Rochester, NY), which has 1 micrometer lateral resolution, 0.75 mm field of view, and temporal resolution of ~10 image frames per second, achieves excellent resolution and contrast in epidermis. Reflectance mode confocal scanning laser microscopy (RCM) enables en-face (horizontal plane) dynamic visualization of cellular and architectural morphology in vivo. The ability to observe cellular details is a key advantage of RCM over other noninvasive skin imaging techniques such as high-frequency ultrasound [115, 126] and magnetic resonance imaging [194]. Recent advances in optical coherence tomography [55] are beginning to improve the resolution to the cellular level. Though promising, these results are not widely confirmed, and it remains to be seen whether optical coherence tomography will undergo the massive clinical translation seen with RCM since 1995.

Resolution

RCM implements optical sectioning (instead of conventional physical cryostat sectioning) by measuring the light that reflects off a 1 μm spot where the laser focuses. The 1 μm laser spot size dictates the spatial resolution, which is about 1 μm. The time resolution is about 10 Hertz, which is 10 frames per second on a monitor screen.

Penetration

In RCM, light penetrates to a subsurface focus of the laser and reflects back from that focus out of the skin and into a detector in the microscope. Light that reflects superficially to the focus is eliminated, and so if the focus is too deep, there will be no signal. Because the laser must propagate into the skin and from the subsurface focus back to the detector in the microscope, the depth penetration of RCM is limited to 100–200 μm in human skin at the 830 nm laser wavelength used in the commercial system. Longer wavelengths (e.g., 1064 nm) penetrate more deeply, and shorter wavelengths (e.g., 488 nm) offer superior resolution at the cost of resolution or penetration, respectively. The variability in the imaging penetration depth also depends on natural variation in the concentration of reflective components composing skin such as keratin, collagen, and melanin.

This process is (1) noninvasive, as enabled by the optical sectioning confocal principle; (2) painless because the laser power is <10 milliwatts; (3) safe because the laser wavelength, 830 nm, is near-infrared light that does not damage DNA; and (4) rapid compared to biopsy and histological analysis, requiring a few seconds for the acquisition of single images (up to 0.75 × 0.75 mm) up to 10–20 min for the acquisition of 3–5 full mosaics at different depths covering an area up to 8 × 8 square mm, which is usually needed for melanoma differential diagnosis.

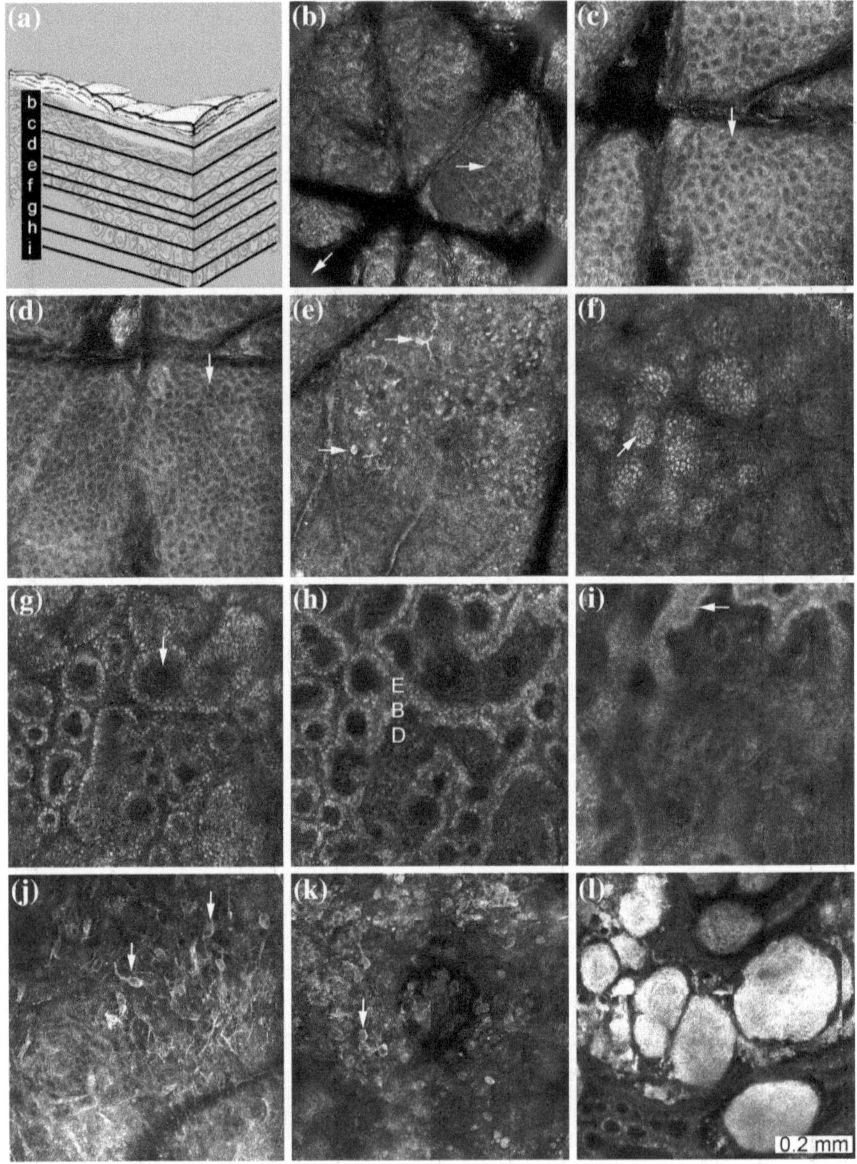

In the commercialized VivaScope® 1500, which is mounted on an articulating arm, a plastic window with an adhesive outer ring is affixed to the skin, enabling large mosaics which effectively increase the field of view from a single 0.75-mm image to up to 8 mm. The handheld version of the device (VivaScope® 3000) only affords a series of 0.75 × 0.75 mm images. Figure 9 shows a representative set of images.

◀ **Fig. 9** Confocal reflectance microscopy images (0.75 × 0.75 mm each) of skin. The layered skin architecture (**a**) is shown in sequentially deeper optical sections (**b–i**). The superficial section (**b**) shows the bright peripheral ring of the plastic window surface; bright, stratified keratin structure; and faint dark nuclei in the stratum granulosum (*arrow*, 25–35 μm diameter). The upper stratum spinosum (**c**) contains keratinocytes (12–25 μm diameter) in a honeycomb pattern. The deeper stratum spinosum (**d**) has a greater number of smaller keratinocytes. Suspected pagetoid melanocytes (**e**) lie above surface of the stratum basale (**f**), where basal cells form a cobblestone appearance. Basal cells (**g**) form bright rings around dim reticulated fibers around *dark circles* that are capillaries (*arrow*). The optical section (**h**) that bisects the rete pegs shows the spinous epidermis (E), basal layer (B), and papillary dermis (D). In the deep optical section (**i**), the collagen dermis that would show individual fibers is blurred. The arrow indicates the deepest basal layer cells. Additional images shown here include pagetoid pleomorphic melanocytes in the epidermis in a melanoma (**j**), junctional aggregates and sheets of pleomorphic malignant melanocytes in a melanoma (**k**), and compact nests of melanocytes in a nevus (**l**). *Note* Confocal images not all from the same patient

Contrast

The appearance of normal skin in RCM is characterized by similarly sized and shaped cells, whether appearing in the honeycomb pattern in the spinous and granular layers or the cobblestone pattern of the basal layer. Additionally, the appearance varies according to Fitzpatrick skin type, sun exposure, age, and physiological condition [110, 131]. The RCM features of a wide range of pathologies [96, 109] have been described in the literature. However, new imaging modalities require training that can be supported by understanding the mechanism of contrast. The mechanism of contrast in reflectance confocal microscopy is the naturally occurring microscopic differences in refractive index that exist in biological tissue. The advantage of this contrast mechanism is that it is endogenous, but the disadvantage is that it is nonspecific, which means pattern recognition is required to interpret the biological meaning of the anatomical features observed in confocal micrographs. Reflectance (optical scattering) occurs when microscopic components of high refractive index (n) lie in surrounding media of low refractive index. One example is keratin ($n1 = 1.40$) in cytoplasm ($n2 = 1.34$). An even stronger scattering component is melanin because its refractive index is $n1 = 1.72$. The difference in refractive index $\Delta n = n1 - n2$ is larger (0.38) for melanin in cytoplasm than (0.06) for keratin in cytoplasm or collagen in the dermis. Therefore, melanin appears brighter than keratin or collagen.

Melanoma Pathology

Clinical melanoma diagnosis is exceptionally challenging, and the use of confocal microscopy has been extensively researched [42, 44, 94, 128, 159]. The key diagnostic RCM melanoma features in the epidermal layers are enlarged atypical cells with pleomorphic morphology including stellate, oval, and fusiform types, nuclei that are enlarged, and coarse dendritic processes. These features have also been reported in clinically amelanotic melanomas [44]. Alteration of the architecture at the dermal–epidermal junction and aggregates of atypical cells clustering into nests at the junction and in the dermis are also clues for melanoma identification [157]. In the case of small melanomas, which are particularly difficult to diagnose with dermoscopy, one report [165] suggested that RCM microscopic morphologies, such as the presence of at least five pagetoid cells per mm^2, tangled lines within the epidermis, and atypical roundish cells at the dermoepidermal junction, were characteristics of melanoma. The diagnostic sensitivity and specificity of RCM reported in the literature is widely variable because each study reports on a data set selected by particular researchers and has been analyzed by clinicians and pathologists with particular training. Table 3 provides an overview of the published reports.

In clinical practice, RCM should be considered as an adjunct to dermoscopy, since it should be performed on selected lesions, and feature interpretation should consider the dermoscopic background. Systematic use of RCM in a prospective cohort of over 1000 patients reduced the number of excisions needed (as determined by the number of benign lesions removed to find one melanoma) from 14.6 to 6.8, also reducing the number of lesions requiring referral for digital dermoscopy monitoring [160].

Future Directions

Challenges to the clinical utility of RCM include the time required to acquire confocal images, the awkwardness of the physical device, and the fact that confocal images are both difficult and time-consuming to read. The hardware issues are being addressed by investigation of line scanning as a rapid and simpler (i.e., smaller package) alternative to point scanning [4, 62, 81].

Image interpretation remains difficult because of qualitative and quantitative challenges, both of which will likely be eased by computer vision approaches in the future. To qualitatively assess tissue morphology, extensive training is required. Although the number of healthcare professionals trained to read RCM is growing and consensus terminology [184] is taking root, RCM remains slow to expand to its full diagnostic promise in dermatology. Automated computer image analysis has great potential to guide novice readers by illustrating features that it can quantitatively identify through image processing. RCM images should be standardized by the absolute reflectance from the window surface that contacts the skin and then processed digitally to generate metrics that can be numerically compared to a threshold to generate a diagnostic classification such as nevus, dysplastic nevus, or melanoma. Ultimately, it will likely be shown that the threshold will be nebulous and that dysplasia can be quantitatively scored on a scale from benign to malignant. A convenient property of digitally rendered diagnoses is that they can be rapidly evaluated against a set of "melanoma diagnosis threshold" scores to generate the receiver–operator characteristic of the diagnostic. Such a system would allow dermatologists to "dial in" their desired level of conservative tendency when choosing how aggressively to biopsy.

Preliminary works have included automated identification of pagetoid melanoma cells [80], identification of the dermal/epidermal junction [80, 127], and the identification of the honeycomb keratinocyte pattern in the spinous and granular epidermis. Though sensitivity/specificity studies have not yet tested these three

Table 3 Summary of diagnostic sensitivity and specificity reported in the literature

Author	Year	Journal	Nevi/Melanomas	Sensitivity	Specificity	Note
Gerger	2005 [94]	J Invest Dermatol	90/27	88.1–98.1	97.6–98.9	Selected images in clinically equivocal and non-equivocal cases
Pellacani	2005 [157]	J Am Acad Dermtol	65/37	97.3	82.6	Dermoscopically equivocal lesions
Bono	2006 [35]	Br J Dermatol	183/23	83	69	Dermoscopically equivocal small (<3 mm) lesions
Gerger	2006 [95]	Cancer	90/27	90.74	98.89	–
Pellacani	2007 [159]	J Invest Dermatol	215/136	77.9–89.7	69.7–52.1	Dermoscopically equivocal lesions
Gerger	2008 [93]	Br J Dermatol	20/50	97.5	99	–
Guitera	2009 [103]	J Invest Dermatol	203/123	91	68	Dermoscopically equivocal lesions
Segura	2009 [187]	J Am Acad Dermtol	92	86.1–100	57.1–95.3	–
Guitera	2010 [102]	J Invest Dermatol	203/81	93	82	Lentigo maligna and pigmented macules
Curchin	2011 [52]	Australas J Dermatol	29/13	92.3	75	Difficult lesions
Guitera	2012 [101]	J Invest Dermatol	375/216 (+119 BCC)	87.6	70.8	Consecutive dermoscopically equivocal lesions including non-melanoma skin cancers
Stevenson	2013 [195]	Dermatol Pract Concept	5 studies	93	76	Meta-analysis
Alarcon	2014 [9]	Br J Dermatol	172/92	97.8	92.8	Excision rate

characteristics for computer-automated diagnostic purposes, a study that used human analysis [159] achieved sensitivity/specificity of 78/70, 90/59, and 88/52 % based on the three single characteristics, respectively. Future work will undoubtedly develop computer vision metrics that attempt to mimic the human-documented [184] patterns. Perhaps the most exciting potential is that of machine vision as instructive and educational, elucidating morphological patterns that sensitively and specifically detect melanomas that are not easily perceived by humans.

4.3 Optical Coherence Tomography

How It Works and the Gaps It Fills

Optical coherence tomography (OCT) is a safe, fast, noninvasive, cross-sectional in situ imaging system. It is commonly compared to ultrasound because both techniques use reflected waves to reconstruct an image. While ultrasound can measure the time of flight of sound waves, the speed of light is too fast and therefore interferometry methods are used. Interferometry splits a light source into two paths, and differences in the lengths of the two paths cause the two light sources to interfere with each other when recombined. In OCT, one part traverses a *reference* path terminated with a mirror and the other traverses a *sample* path where the tissue structures absorb or scatter the light.

For the near-infrared wavelengths typically used, scattering and not absorption is the dominant effect, resulting in a sufficient number of photons being reflected back. These reflected photons from the tissue sample constructively and destructively interfere with the reflected photons from the reference arm to generate the interference signal. This interference signal can be measured by a variety of sensing devices depending on system design and the principal wavelength of the light source.

Most OCT systems use broadband light sources to create one-dimensional images of reflecting structures in tissue at a given spot. These are sometimes called *axial scans* or *A-scans*. Sets of A-scans are typically acquired in a raster scanning pattern and assembled into 2D cross-sectional images that can then be stacked to form 3D volumes. Capturing multiple A-scans at a single location over time is used to create functional images involving dynamic tissue properties. Measuring blood flow [49] and the mechanical response to vibration [206] are two examples of functional imaging.

Two broad classes of OCT are in use today (Fig. 10): time domain OCT (TD-OCT) and Fourier domain OCT (FD-OCT). TD-OCT was the first to be widely deployed in ophthalmology settings and uses a moving reference arm mirror and a photodetector to identify reflections in tissue samples. FD-OCT measures the interference at each frequency of light and uses the Fourier transform to convert frequency domain measurements into spatial domain values. FD-OCT itself has two principal variants: spectral domain OCT (SD-OCT), which uses a diffraction grating

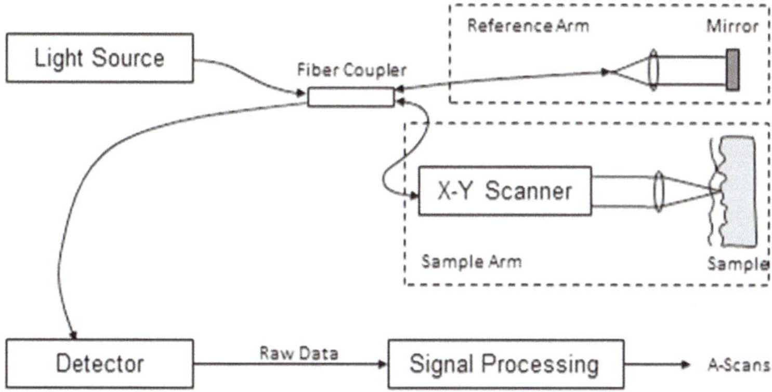

Fig. 10 Generic fiber-based OCT schematic. For TD-OCT and SD-OCT, the light source is usually a super-luminescent diode (SLD), while for SS-OCT, it is usually a tunable laser. In TD-OCT, the reference arm mirror moves; for other types, it is fixed. The detector in SD-OCT is a spectrometer, and in others, it is usually a balanced photodetector. Details of the optics and components, such as optical circulators and polarization controllers, vary significantly between designs and have not been included

and a line scan camera to measure all the frequencies at once, and swept-source OCT (SS-OCT), which uses a tunable light source and a balanced detector to measure each frequency individually. Both FD-OCT methods are faster than TD-OCT and have a better signal-to-noise ratio [58].

Many further variations on these general classes of OCT exist. Polarization-sensitive OCT detects birefringence changes in tissue. Microscopy variants, called optical coherence microscopy (OCM), add transverse resolution enhancements to increased axial resolution abilities. Full-field versions blend the best parts of reflectance confocal microscopy with OCM. These are just some examples of the OCT innovation that continue to grow at a rapid pace.

In all of these designs, the axial resolution is proportional to the square of the center wavelength of the light source and inversely proportional to the bandwidth of the light source: $\Delta z = 2\ \ln(2)\lambda^2/(\pi\Delta\lambda)$ where Δz is the axial resolution and $\Delta\lambda$ is the light source full-width half-maximum (FWHM) bandwidth. Broadband light sources are therefore used to create good axial resolutions. Smaller center or principal wavelengths also contribute to better axial resolution. Most of the initial work in OCT has been based on available light sources and optics developed for the telecommunications industry [181], which means the most common principal wavelengths are around 800, 1300, or 1550 nm. With the increased attention on OCT, new light sources, sensors, and optics are now in development driven by the biological application. However, because of its availability and its ability to penetrate more deeply [13], OCT systems using light sources with a center wavelength of around 1300 nm are most commonly reported in dermatology applications. Axial resolutions for commercially available systems now range from 5.5 to 16 μm.

Lateral resolutions are dictated by the optics of each system. One of the benefits of OCT is the ability to obtain good axial resolution while positioning the optics a distance away from the sample. This is accomplished using low numerical aperture (NA) sample optics and facilitates, for instance, imaging retinas from several centimeters away. For dermatology applications, this creates a trade-off: Low NAs create a more uniform lateral resolution through the tissue sample at depths of up to 2 mm, while higher NAs are used to create better lateral resolution at the expense of imaging depth. For low NA systems, this lateral resolution is typically between 5 and 15 μm [61, 202]. Recent interest in OCM, which uses high NA optics coupled with very broadband light sources, yields both high axial and high lateral resolutions at the expense of depth of field [111]. A variation on this idea is full-field OCT (FF-OCT), which creates en-face images similar to confocal microscopy but with the ability to image more deeply [55]. Recently, a high-definition OCT (HD-OCT) has been introduced with cellular resolution [36]. Different non-melanocytic and melanocytic skin tumors have been described with HD-OCT with histopathological correlation [37, 38, 133, 134].

This ability to image up to 1 mm in HD-OCT and 2 mm with HD of tissue coupled with axial and lateral resolutions measured in microns positions OCT between confocal laser scanning microscopy (CSLM) and high-frequency ultrasound (HFUS) in terms of resolution and depth penetration. OCT has better resolution than HFUS but worse resolution than CSLM. OCT has better depth penetration than CSLM but worse than HFUS.

For more details on how OCT works, see [41, 73, 162].

Strengths/Weaknesses

For dermatology applications, OCT has long been heralded as a potential diagnostic solution that does not require invasive surgery, does not alter the sample morphology, and can be repeated over time for the same suspicious lesion. Unfortunately, the resolution of OCT is still insufficient to replace histopathology where cellular differentiation is required [59]. In the case of HD-OCT, cellular resolution is achieved but with some limitations (compared to confocal microscopy) that are critical in the recognition of melanocytic lesions, such as the possibility of differentiating dendritic cells. At the same time, the field of view compared to confocal microscopy with HD-OCT is reduced to 1.3 mm that in the study of melanocytic lesions makes a diagnostic conclusion difficult. These limitations may be not relevant in the recognition of epidermal tumors including actinic keratosis, squamous cell carcinoma, or basal cell carcinoma. Future integration of OCT, HD-OCT, and confocal microscopy may be very promising due to the complementary information that they allow one to visualize. In the case of OCT, even though the histopathology correlates may be missing, several studies suggest OCT is capable of revealing microstructures in skin that correlate well with known morphological changes introduced by various diseases [51, 141, 146, 147, 215]. Most of the promising research thus far has been in the area of non-melanoma skin cancers. A cautionary study showed basal cell carcinomas could be differentiated from normal skin, but the subtypes could not be discerned [75].

Melanoma detection is still an area of active investigation and will remain so as the resolution of OCT continues to improve. On the one hand, de Giogi et al. [59] attempted to correlate histology, dermoscopy, and OCT on 10 patients without significant success. They concluded that a differential diagnosis between melanoma and benign melanocytic nevus using OCT was not possible. In contrast, another group attempted to characterize melanocytic skin lesions using OCT in vivo as either melanoma or benign nevus. They assessed 92 lesions from 75 patients and carefully validated the results histologically [75]. The most significant differences found were that melanomas showed marked architectural disarray and lacked clear dermoepidermal borders compared to benign nevi. Other differences were identified in the study, and their conclusion was that micromorphologic features visible in OCT have the potential to be used as discriminating features. Caveats included the inability to subclassify the benign nevi and the need for further sensitivity and specificity studies with other types of skin tumors.

Availability/Usability

The general assessment for using OCT to diagnose melanoma is that it is still in the "promising stage" and will continue to improve, but it is not quite ready for clinical practice [142, 147, 155, 191].

At present, OCT is limited to assessment of tissue microstructures and cannot provide cellular features visible in traditional histopathology or CSLM, though it can provide in situ imaging at deeper depths than CSLM. Nevertheless, the clinical community continues to wait for significant advances before adopting OCT as a diagnostic tool. Meanwhile, vendors are beginning to produce tools so providers can at least begin experimenting and learning more about the capabilities and limitations of OCT [74, 142].

OCT and HD-OCT have become a very active area of research, especially in the last decade [216]. There has been a proliferation of novel enhancements and advances, from the significant improvements in light sources and sensing devices to the introduction of new designs and software processing algorithms. Despite the current limitations, most authors continue to be optimistic that continued improvements will finally enable OCT to fulfill its promise as a vital tool in clinical practice.

4.4 Electrical Impedance and Ultrasound Detection Technologies

This section presents an introduction to two modalities for detecting and/or imaging melanoma. These include (1) electrical impedance spectroscopy (EIS) and (2) high-frequency ultrasound (HUS).

Electrical Impedance Spectroscopy (EIS)

The electrical impedance of a tissue largely depends on (1) ions and (2) membranes. More specifically, the key factors are (1) the concentration and mobility of charged ions and (2) the presence of tight junction membranes, cellular membranes, and macromolecular surfaces against which the ions can move to capacitively store energy. Hence, electrical impedance can characterize both the extracellular matrix and the intracellular matrix within which ions move as well as the membranes (and surfaces) that can support charge separation. The influence of ion mobility will decrease if the tissue is less hydrated, the matrix is denser, or the number of ions is low. The capacitive effect will decrease if the membranes are leaky or there are fewer membranes.

The electrical impedance of skin when measured by topical application of electrodes is dominated by the high resistance of the stratum corneum. Changes in stratum corneum hydration or structure can be followed by electrical measurements at low frequencies (<1 kHz). To measure the living epidermis and dermis, the stratum corneum must be bypassed. Tape stripping can remove the stratum corneum to allow electrical measurements of the underlying skin layers. Alternatively, microneedles serving as electrodes can penetrate the stratum corneum, thereby placing the electrodes in direct contact with the underlying skin layers [100]. The SciBase system uses such microneedles (SciBase Inc., http://www.scibase.se). For the detection of melanoma, the influence of the stratum corneum must be bypassed.

Electrical measurements in tissues have been studied for some time [71, 183, 214]. Plus and minus charges that accumulate on either side of a membrane will store electrostatic energy, which can be described as a capacitance C [Farads]. The movement of ions imparts a loss of energy due to frictional forces that heats the tissue. The mobility of the ions can be described by conductance, and the inverse of conductance is resistance R [ohms]. There is a time constant for charging of a capacitor, τ = RC [s]. If an alternating current (AC) is applied to the skin, the capacitance due to membranes and macromolecular surfaces will charge to 63 % of maximum in a time period of τ seconds. If the frequency (f [Hz] or [cycles/s]) of the AC is low ($f\tau \ll 1$), the capacitance will fully charge. If the frequency of the AC is high ($f\tau \gg 1$), the capacitance will not charge because the ions will just jiggle in place but not move over any appreciable distance. The energy loss due to heating (which is negligible in diagnostic measurements) is maximum when the frequency matches the time constant ($f\tau \approx 1$), since the ions are constantly moving to charge and then discharge the membrane capacitors. So the time constant τ or the center frequency $f_c = \tau/(2\pi)$ is a key parameter that characterizes the frequency dependence of electrical impedance.

There can be a variety of local domains with distinct membrane surfaces and ion mobilities, which have distinct values of $f_{c,\mathrm{domain}}$. Hence, the observed dispersion centered around the f_c of the population of domains will broaden as the heterogeneity of local domains increases. This broadening is described by the factor a, where the capacitive energy storage, expressed as the real permittivity (ε'), behaves proportional to $1/(1 + (f/f_c)^{1-a})$, which equals 1 at low f and zero at high f. Figure 11 shows the behavior of a generic dispersion centered at f_c and the effect of increasing heterogeneity (a increasing from 0 to 0.5). The real permissivity (ε') describes capacitive energy storage, and the imaginary permissivity (ε'') describes the dissipative frictional losses of ion movement.

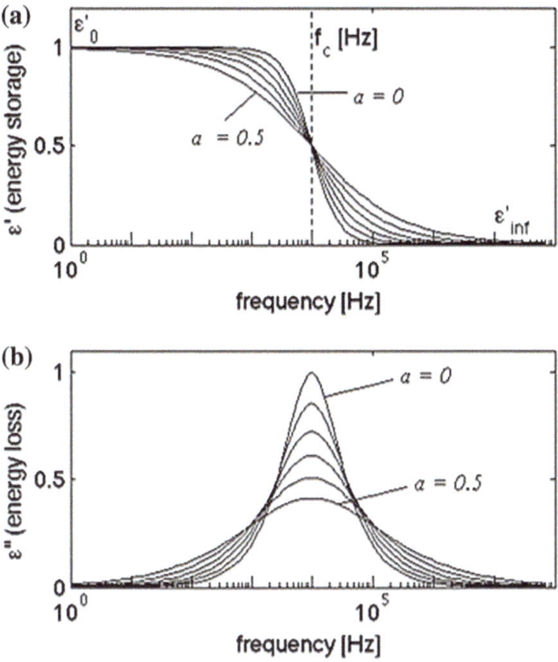

Fig. 11 A generic dispersion of electrical impedance. This example shows a central frequency (f_c) of 10^4 Hz. **a** The real permittivity (ε') is high at low frequencies, where membranes block DC current and capacitive charging of membranes by ions stores energy. At high frequencies, the impedance is low where ions are free to move, but they oscillate so fast and cannot charge the membranes, so energy storage is low. **b** The imaginary permittivity (ε'') shows the energy losses maximizing at the central frequency f_c, where the rate of charging and discharging the membranes by ion movement optimizes the energy dissipation by frictional losses. The factor a characterizes the heterogeneity of the dispersion. Each local domain has its own local unique $f_{c.\text{domain}}$, and a distribution of domains will have a net broadened f_c. As the heterogeneity increases, the a increases from 0 to 0.5

There are several types of capacitive charging with different characteristic f_c, called *dispersions*. The movement of ions up against tight junction membranes or other rather macroscopic membrane surfaces (including electrodes) involves large ion movements through the extracellular matrix, and hence, the time constant of charging (τ) is large and f_c is low, approximately in the 1 Hz to 10 kHz range. This process is called the *α dispersion*. The movement of intracellular ions up against cell membranes and macromolecular surfaces involves shorter range ion movements; hence, the τ is short and f_c is high, approximately in the 1 kHz to 100 MHz range. This process is called the *β dispersion*. The rotation of dipoles, such as bound water, amino acid side groups, and other small molecules, occurs at very high frequencies, approximately in the 100–1000 MHz range, and is called the *δ dispersion*. At ~10 GHz, the rotation of free water occurs and is called the *γ dispersion*.

Most studies on skin are conducted in the frequency range of the α and β dispersions. Figure 12 shows a typical dispersion spectrum of the real permissivity versus frequency for tape-stripped skin. The frequency ranges for the α and β dispersions of skin are much lower than the ranges for soft tissues. The α of skin is ~11 Hz, while the α for soft tissue is in the range 100 Hz to 10 kHz. The β of skin is ~64 kHz, while the β for soft tissue is in the range 100 kHz to 1 MHz. Not shown are data reported using the SciBase system [3], which are similar to the β dispersion data in Fig. 12.

Clinical EIS Studies of Melanoma

The use of electrical impedance spectroscopy (EIS) to detect skin cancer followed early work by Stig Ollmar on using EIS to detect effects on the skin barrier function. Additionally, the thesis by Åberg is recommended [1]. There is significant inter-subject variability in the parameters that describe the permissivity dispersion of skin sites. Therefore, comparisons are always made relative to a nearby normal skin site on a subject. Investigators using the SciBase system use principal component analysis (PCA) to analyze data, relying on training sets to train the algorithm. For example, the sensitivity to malignant melanoma was reported to be 95 % (59/62) and specificity to be 49 % (72/148) [2]. However, the PCA description does not inform about the variation in tissue structure caused by melanoma. Such clinical studies report only the PCA analysis and do not report the dispersion spectra that might inform about mechanism of contrast. In a recently published multicenter

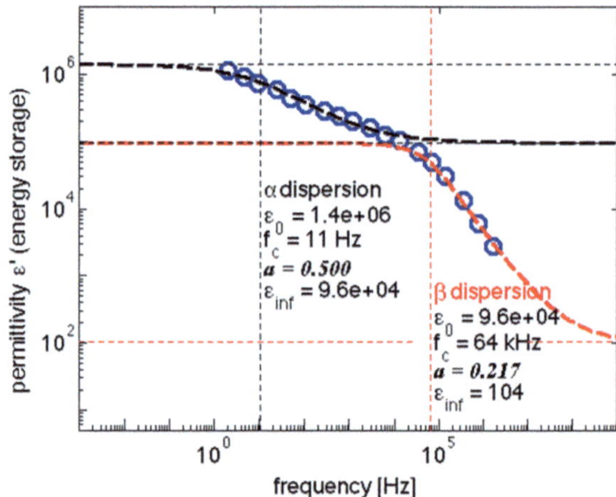

Fig. 12 Measurements of the permittivity of tape-stripped skin show the electrical behavior of the viable skin tissue. The data (*blue circles*) are from [214]. There are two apparent dispersions. In this particular skin site, the α dispersion (*black dashed line*) is centered around 11 Hz (and a potential contribution from polarization of the electrodes is not clear) and is attributed to ions moving through the extracellular space to charge tight junction membranes. The β dispersion (*red dashed line*) is centered around 64 kHz and is attributed to intracellular ion movement to charge cellular membranes. The data measured by the SciBase system (not shown) [3] aligns with the β dispersion data in this figure but with a lower f_c

prospective blinded study with SciBase, 1951 subjects with 2416 lesions were enrolled; 1943 lesions were eligible and evaluable for the primary efficacy end point (including 265 melanomas—112 in situ and 153 invasive melanomas with a median Breslow thickness of 0.57 mm, 48 basal cell carcinomas, and 7 squamous cell carcinomas). The observed sensitivity of Nevisense was 96.6 % (256 of 265 melanomas) with an exact one-sided 95 % lower confidence bound estimated at 94.2 % and an observed specificity of 34.4 % with an exact two-sided 95 % confidence bound estimated at 32.0–36.9 %. The positive and negative predictive values of Nevisense were 21.1 and 98.2 %, respectively. The observed sensitivity for non-melanoma skin cancer was 100 % (55 of 48 BCC and 7 SCC) with an exact two-sided 95 % confidence bound estimated at 93.5–100 % [138].

In summary, EIS is a low-cost and simple measurement for topical assessment of skin and is reported to be responsive to the changes in skin properties caused by melanoma. The ion mobilities of the extracellular and intracellular spaces, the status of membranes that can be charged by ions, and the heterogeneity of local domains contribute to the signals. The use of microneedles for perforating the stratum corneum and serving as electrodes in direct contact with the epidermis is an especially welcome innovation. More reports of the frequency spectra data from the EIS measurements would be welcomed and potentially could elucidate the contrast mechanisms underlying melanoma detection.

Ultrasound detection of melanoma

High-frequency ultrasound (HUS) is another method for detecting melanoma. An ultrasound transducer delivers high frequency pressure waves to the skin and collects time-delayed reflected waves. The time delay corresponds to the round-trip propagation of the waves to some depth and then back to the surface for detection. Like a radar system, the ultrasound signal can create depth-resolved images. The mechanism of the reflected ultrasound signal is based on the presence of variations in tissue density, which yields variations in the impedance of the tissue that cause reflections. A tissue that is very homogenous will be *anechoic*. A tissuelike dermis has significant fluctuations in mass and hence is highly *echogenic*. The attenuation of ultrasound is very frequency dependent, falling roughly as the square of frequency, f^2. Low-frequency ultrasound can image many centimeters into a tissue. However, ultrasound in the 10–30 MHz range can only image to a depth of $\sim$10 mm. Because of the high frequency, the spatial resolution (10 s of μm) is much better than for low-frequency ultrasound (mm).

The method was first demonstrated as skin ultrasonography [10]. It can detect the thickness of melanoma and is used for detecting melanoma in lymph nodes. But the challenge is to use HUS to discriminate benign from pigmented lesions in situ in the skin.

A study using 20 MHz HUS [107] compared the 25 melanoma lesions (MM) versus 29 basal cell papillomas (BCP) and 15 benign melanocytic nevi (BN). The study compared the echogenicity of the dermis below the tested lesion. MM showed low attenuation of ultrasound such that the high echogenic dermis was clearly seen. In contrast, BCP showed higher attenuation of ultrasound, so there was an apparent shadow cast into the dermis. The shadowing was reported to correlate most significantly with histological extent of hyperkeratosis, and three cases of non-keratotic acanthotic BCP were noted to be classified as MM by the method. Nevertheless, melanoma was discriminated from BCP with 100 % sensitivity and 79 % specificity. With addition of entry echo line enhancement (EEE), the specificity was improved to 93 %. BN demonstrated patchy shadowing as a result of being keratotic, indicating a more spatially heterogeneous lesion than MM. The specificity for discriminating BN from MM was low (30 %). HUS shows promise for discriminating MM from BCP, while the discrimination of BN and MM needs some improvements.

Toward this end, the use of focused ultrasound that creates an image at a restricted depth was developed so as to increase the sensitivity of the signal contrast between BN and MM [169]. The method is called retroflex transmission imaging (RTI) [99]. In the ultrasound application of RTI to skin, HUS is focused to a small spot near the surface, and the transmitted signal propagates into the tissue volume. The total volumetric backscatter is detected, but the magnitude of this signal is sensitive to the attenuation properties of the small focused spot. Hence, higher contrast for the surface spot is achieved. Scanning the focused spot yields an image that can take advantage of the increased spatial variation in attenuation in BN relative to MM. The method was tested on 25 MM, 24 seborrheic keratosis (SK), and 38 BN. The differentiation of SKs from melanoma showed specificity of 79 % and sensitivity of 100 %. The differentiation of BN and MM showed specificity of 30 % and sensitivity of 100 % without RTI and 55 % specificity with RTI and EEE. This improvement in specificity is encouraging and argues for continued work on novel approaches to HUS imaging.

In summary, HUS is an imaging modality useful for assessing melanoma thickness. It also reveals the anechoic nature of melanoma and its uniformity in attenuation properties.

4.5 Molecular Assays for the Detection of Melanoma

Over the past decade, molecular assessment of the tumor genome has been increasingly utilized as a diagnostic adjunct in the evaluation of histopathologically ambiguous melanocytic tumors. While the majority of melanocytic neoplasms can be accurately diagnosed through routine histopathologic analysis by a properly trained pathologist, a significant minority of cases have conflicting histopathologic features that result in diagnostic discordance, even between expert dermatopathologists [67]. As histopathologic assessment of these difficult tumors often yields equivocal diagnoses, ancillary tests are needed to better direct patient care. Early cytogenetic analysis of melanocytic nevi and melanomas demonstrated that 96 % of unequivocal melanomas have detectable chromosomal gains or losses [28]. In contrast, melanocytic nevi, with the exception of a subset of Spitz nevi with chromosome 11p gain, do not exhibit such aberrations. Chromosomal gains and losses in melanoma are not randomly distributed in the genome. They occur repeatedly at chromosomal loci that provide a selective growth advantage for the tumor. This fundamental difference in the genomes of melanomas and nevi facilitated the development of molecular assays that can assist in the diagnosis of melanocytic tumors.

4.6 Fluorescent In Situ Hybridization (FISH)

Fluorescent in situ hybridization (FISH) employs fluorescently labeled oligonucleotide probes targeting specific chromosomal loci to assess for copy number changes in tumor cells. Multi-probe FISH assays can simultaneously detect copy number changes at multiple chromosomal loci and are currently clinically available to assist in the diagnosis of melanocytic tumors. Utilizing previous cytogenetic data of recurrent chromosomal aberrations in melanoma, a 4-probe FISH assay was developed in 2009 targeting three loci on chromosome 6 (6q23, 6p25, and CEP6) and one at locus 11q13 that discriminated unequivocal melanocytic nevi from melanomas with a sensitivity and specificity of 87 and 95 %, respectively [89]. Subsequent studies of this probe set involving specific types of melanocytic tumors yielded similar sensitivity and specificity, including:

- Distinguishing nevoid melanoma from mitotically active nevi [91]
- Distinguishing conjunctival melanoma from conjunctival nevi [43]
- Distinguishing metastatic melanoma in lymph nodes from nodal nevi [56]
- Distinguishing blue nevuslike melanoma from cellular blue nevi [76]
- Diagnosing atypical junctional melanocytic proliferations [86, 149]

A lower sensitivity of 47 % was found for discriminating desmoplastic melanomas from sclerosing nevi [87].

Most studies of FISH in melanocytic tumors have involved unambiguous melanocytic nevi and melanomas. However, the clinical utility of FISH as a diagnostic aid is contingent on its ability to discriminate between benign and malignant tumors with ambiguous histopathologic features. Ambiguous spitzoid neoplasms are the most frequent tumors for which FISH is utilized [150]. Other frequent tumor types for which FISH is ordered include atypical blue nevuslike proliferations, dysplastic nevuslike neoplasms, biphasic tumors (i.e., combined nevus or melanoma arising in a nevus), possible nevoid melanoma, and acral or mucosal tumors. Difficulty in collecting large cohorts of ambiguous melanocytic tumors with long-term follow-up has resulted in a paucity of FISH studies in such tumors. The largest study of the chromosome 6 and 11 FISH assay in ambiguous melanocytic tumors yielded a lower sensitivity of 43 % (9/21) for the detection of ambiguous tumors with lymph node or distant metastasis [203], raising concern about the generalizability of prior FISH studies to ambiguous tumors for which the test is clinically used.

A more recent study found increased sensitivity for the detection of spitzoid melanoma with the addition of probes detecting homozygous loss of 9p21 where the *CDKN2A* gene resides [77]. Chromosome 9p21 loss has also been associated with increased risk for metastasis in atypical spitzoid tumors in children [88].

A new FISH assay including probes targeting chromosomal loci 9p21, 6p25, 8q24, and 11q13 reportedly has increased sensitivity and specificity of 94 and 98 %, respectively, in distinguishing unequivocal melanomas and nevi [90].

4.7 Comparative Genomic Hybridization (CGH)

Comparative genomic hybridization (CGH) involves extraction and fluorescent labeling of tumor DNA, with subsequent competitive hybridization against control DNA to metaphase chromosomes or DNA microarrays to detect chromosomal gains or losses. Array-based CGH offers higher resolution of the genome and is considered by many to be the current method of choice in melanoma diagnostics. Compared to FISH, which targets a limited number of chromosomal loci, CGH provides a representative view of the entire genome and thus has greater potential to detect multiple chromosomal aberrations. With the vast majority of melanomas possessing multiple chromosomal gains and losses in their genomes, CGH can provide valuable diagnostic information to assist pathologists in the diagnosis of melanocytic tumors with conflicting histopathologic findings.

Past CGH analysis of melanomas demonstrated different patterns of chromosomal aberrations between melanomas arising in chronically sun-damaged skin, intermittently sun-exposed skin, and acral and mucosal melanomas [54]. Acral and mucosal melanomas arise through a non-UV light-dependent pathway that is characterized by marked genomic instability with chromosomal amplifications. Such amplifications are presented to a much lesser extent in the other two categories. In addition, these amplifications occur early in tumorigenesis in many acral melanomas preceding the invasive stage of disease [151] and can be relatively easily detected with CGH or FISH if the diagnosis is in question.

CGH in Blue, Spitz, and Congenital Melanocytic Nevi and Their Histopathologic Mimics

CGH studies of the spectrum of melanocytic tumors resembling blue nevi, Spitz nevi, and congenital nevi have found unique genomic alterations in these types of neoplasms that assist in differentiating benign and malignant tumors. Cellular blue nevi and the majority of ambiguous blue nevuslike proliferations do not have chromosomal aberrations detectable by CGH [136]. In contrast, blue nevuslike melanomas have ≥3 chromosomal aberrations. Similarly, routine congenital melanocytic nevi do not exhibit chromosomal aberrations. Benign hypercellular proliferations within congenital nevi ("proliferative nodules") can clinically and histopathologically mimic melanoma. CGH analysis of such proliferations shows gain or loss of entire chromosomes, particularly loss of chromosome 7, 9, or 10, which is distinct from the multiple gains and losses of chromosomal fragments that typify melanoma arising in congenital melanocytic nevi [29].

Spitz tumors often exhibit the greatest degree of histopathologic ambiguity. The majority of Spitz nevi do not have detectable chromosomal aberrations by CGH, excluding a subset of desmoplastic Spitz nevi that harbor *HRAS* mutations and/or isolated gain of chromosome 11p where *HRAS* resides [27]. Another subset of apparently benign spitzoid neoplasms has chromosome 3p21 loss (*BAP1* tumor suppressor gene locus), which can be associated with a *BAP1*-mutant germline syndrome of amelanotic spitzoid nevi, cutaneous and uveal melanomas, and mesothelioma [211]. Chromosomal aberrations other than isolated 3p loss or isolated 11p gain are concerning for spitzoid melanoma, especially if multiple chromosomal gains or losses are detected.

4.8 Quantitative Real-Time Polymerase Chain Reaction (qRT-PCR) and Next-Generation Sequencing

Currently, FISH and CGH are the primary molecular tests clinically available to assist in the diagnosis of histopathologically ambiguous melanocytic tumors. A 23-gene expression signature utilizing qualitative reverse transcriptase polymerase chain reaction (qRT-PCR) has also recently been developed for this purpose. Gene expression measurements from the assay are analyzed to generate a score that reports a lesion as being consistent with a benign nevus or a malignant melanoma. The signature is marketed under the name Myriad myPath™ Melanoma and is undergoing clinical validation to differentiate benign nevi from malignant melanoma across a variety of histological subtypes. Other molecular techniques are currently utilized for prognosis and directing treatment. A qRT-PCR expression profile assay has been developed by Castle Biosciences© as a prognostic tool for predicting metastatic risk in Stages I or II melanoma and is marketed under the test name DecisionDx-Melanoma. Based on analysis of the expression of 31 genes, tumors are classified as low (3 %) or high (69 %) risk for developing metastasis within 5 years. The validation studies for these tests were presented at the 2013 (Castle) and 2014 (Myriad) American Society of Clinical Oncology meetings, but as of June 2014, neither has been published in a peer-reviewed journal.

Next-generation sequencing (NGS) is widely employed in research of melanocytic neoplasia and has many potential exciting uses in the diagnostic setting, but it has not yet transitioned into clinical practice for melanoma diagnostics. Foundation Medicine© currently offers the NGS clinical test FoundationOne™ for solid tumors, which can be used to characterize the spectrum of possible mutations in melanoma and help guide selection of mutation-specific treatments (e.g., BRAF inhibitors for BRAF mutant melanoma). This test uses NGS to sequence all exons of 236 cancer-related genes, including BRAF, HRAS, GNAQ, GNA11, KIT, BAP1, CDKN2A, and PTEN, as well as 47 introns from 19 genes often altered in cancers. However, as mutations in these genes can be seen in both melanomas and nevi, this test does not provide useful diagnostic information for ambiguous melanocytic tumors.

Table 4 compares the tests described above.

Table 4 Clinically available molecular tests for melanocytic tumors

	FISH	CGH	DecisionDx-Melanoma™	FoundationOne™	Myriad myPath™
Clinical use	Diagnostic test	Diagnostic test	qRT-PCR-based prognostic test	NGS mutation detection	qRT-PCR-based diagnostic test
Advantages of technique	– Minimal tissue required – Single cell resolution with intact tumor architecture permitting detection of intratumoral genetic heterogeneity – Ability to detect translocations	– Ability to assess all 23 chromosomes – No proficiency in fluorescent microscopy required	Reportedly provides additional prognostic value beyond the current AJCC staging data	– Single test providing full sequencing of genes associated with melanoma – Can assist in identifying potential treatments for advanced melanomas	– Reportedly provides additional diagnostic value in discriminating benign versus malignant melanocytic lesions
Limitations of technique	– Only visualizes a tiny fraction of the genome – Technical expertise in fluorescent microscopy required	– Limited ability to assess for intratumoral heterogeneity – Potential for dilution of test results from non-neoplastic DNA in sample (e.g., lymphocytes and fibroblasts)	– Limited to early Stages I–II melanoma – New test with little evidence published	– No diagnostic or prognostic value – High cost	– New test with little evidence published – Unclear if diagnostic accuracy is as reproducible in difficult histological cases – No correlation with outcome

All 4 platforms use formalin-fixed, paraffin-embedded tissue samples from routine biopsies. *FISH* fluorescent in situ hybridization, *CGH* comparative genomic hybridization, *qRT-PCR* qualitative reverse transcriptase polymerase chain reaction, and *NGS* next-generation sequencing

5 Conclusion

Effective melanoma early detection methods and technologies are likely to become increasingly available and useful, but one of the key challenges faced in the clinic is the integration of these modalities into current practice. In addition to describing current methods of melanoma detection, which include population-level approaches to early detection, the role of clinical examination-based methods, advanced technological detection methods, and molecular assay detection methods, a secondary purpose of this chapter has been to outline a rational approach to the use of these methods in the context of patient care. A pragmatic approach to maximize the strengths and minimize the weaknesses of the various technologies and methods is needed. We conclude that to be effective, this pragmatic approach must take into consideration logistical clinical issues related to the time, equipment, and expertise requirements for each technology as well as the cost and convenience for the patient. Developing creative strategies to utilize the most appropriate technology or method in the most cost- and time-effective manner is a critical step toward making early detection of virtually all melanomas a reality. Perhaps as never before, through the development of a comprehensive strategy to detect melanoma early, we have the opportunity to reduce suffering secondary to melanoma through early detection. Although there are some rapidly progressive forms of melanoma that are unlikely to be detectable prior to metastasis (e.g., aggressive nodular melanomas), successful application of early detection technologies and methods has enormous potential to save the lives of individuals with melanoma and reduce the costs associated with melanoma treatment.

References

1. Åberg P (2004) Skin cancer as seen by electrical impedance. Ph.D. thesis dissertation, Karolinska Institutet, Stockholm http://publications.ki.se/xmlui/bitstream/handle/10616/40085/thesis.pdf?sequence=1. Accessed 27 Feb 2014
2. Åberg P, Birgersson U, Elsner P et al (2011) Electrical impedance spectroscopy and the diagnostic accuracy for malignant melanoma. Exp Dermatol 20(8):648–652
3. Åberg P, Geladi P, Nicander I et al (2002) Variation of skin properties within human forearms demonstrated by non-invasive detection and multi-way analysis. Skin Res Technol 8(3):194–201
4. Abeytunge S, Li Y, Larson B et al (2013) Confocal microscopy with strip mosaicing for rapid imaging over large areas of excised tissue. J Biomed Opt 18(6):61227
5. Aitken JF, Elwood M, Baade PD et al (2010) Clinical whole-body skin examination reduces the incidence of thick melanomas. Int J Cancer 126(2):450–458
6. Aitken JF, Janda M, Lowe JB et al (2004) Prevalence of whole-body skin self-examination in a population at high risk for skin cancer (Australia). Cancer Causes Control 15(5):453–463
7. Aitken JF, Youl PH, Janda M et al (2006) Increase in skin cancer screening during a community-based randomized intervention trial. Int J Cancer 118(4):1010–1016
8. Al-Shakhli H, Harcourt D, Kenealy J (2006) Psychological distress surrounding diagnosis of malignant and nonmalignant skin lesions at a pigmented lesion clinic. J Plast Reconstr Aesthet Surg 59(5):479–486

9. Alarcon I, Carrera C, Palou J et al (2014) Impact of in vivo reflectance confocal microscopy on the number needed to treat melanoma in doubtful lesions. Br J Dermatol 170(4):802–808
10. Alexander H, Miller DL (1979) Determining skin thickness with pulsed ultra sound. J Invest Dermatol 72(1):17–19
11. Alexandrescu DT (2009) Melanoma costs: a dynamic model comparing estimated overall costs of various clinical stages. Dermatol Online J 15(11):1
12. Altamura D, Avramidis M, Menzies SW (2008) Assessment of the optimal interval for and sensitivity of short-term sequential digital dermoscopy monitoring for the diagnosis of melanoma. Arch Dermatol 144(4):502–506
13. Anderson RR, Parrish JA (1981) The optics of human skin. J Invest Dermatol 77(1):13–19
14. Andreassi L, Perotti R, Rubegni P et al (1999) Digital dermoscopy analysis for the differentiation of atypical nevi and early melanoma: a new quantitative semiology. Arch Dermatol 135(12):1459–1465
15. Argenziano G, Albertini G, Castagnetti F et al (2012) Early diagnosis of melanoma: what is the impact of dermoscopy? Dermatol Ther 25(5):403–409
16. Argenziano G, Catricala C, Ardigo M et al (2011) Seven-point checklist of dermoscopy revisited. Br J Dermatol 164(4):785–790
17. Argenziano G, Mordente I, Ferrara G et al (2008) Dermoscopic monitoring of melanocytic skin lesions: clinical outcome and patient compliance vary according to follow-up protocols. Br J Dermatol 159(2):331–336
18. Argenziano G, Puig S, Zalaudek I et al (2006) Dermoscopy improves accuracy of primary care physicians to triage lesions suggestive of skin cancer. J Clin Oncol 24(12):1877–1882
19. Argenziano G, Soyer HP, Chimenti S et al (2003) Dermoscopy of pigmented skin lesions: results of a consensus meeting via the Internet. J Am Acad Dermatol 48(5):679–693
20. Argenziano G, Zalaudek I, Ferrara G et al (2007) Dermoscopy features of melanoma incognito: indications for biopsy. J Am Acad Dermatol 56(3):508–513
21. Aspinwall LG, Leaf SL, Dola ER et al (2008) CDKN2A/p16 genetic test reporting improves early detection intentions and practices in high-risk melanoma families. Cancer Epidemiol Biomarkers Prev 17(6):1510–1519
22. Aspinwall LG, Taber JM, Leaf SL et al (2013) Melanoma genetic counseling and test reporting improve screening adherence among unaffected carriers 2 years later. Cancer Epidemiol Biomarkers Prev 22(10):1687–1697
23. Australian Cancer Network Melanoma Guidelines Revision Working Party (2008) Clinical practice guidelines for the management of melanoma in Australia and New Zealand. Cancer Council Australia and Australian Cancer Network, Sydney and New Zealand Guidelines Group. https://www.nhmrc.gov.au/_files_nhmrc/publications/attachments/cp111.pdf. Accessed 21 May 2014
24. Bafounta ML, Beauchet A, Aegerter P et al (2001) Is dermoscopy (epiluminescence microscopy) useful for the diagnosis of melanoma? Results of a meta-analysis using techniques adapted to the evaluation of diagnostic tests. Arch Dermatol 137(10):1343–1350
25. Balch CM, Gershenwald JE, Soong SJ et al (2009) Final version of 2009 AJCC melanoma staging and classification. J Clin Oncol 27(36):6199–6206
26. Banky JP, Kelly JW, English DR et al (2005) Incidence of new and changed nevi and melanomas detected using baseline images and dermoscopy in patients at high risk for melanoma. Arch Dermatol 141(8):998–1006
27. Bastian BC, LeBoit PE, Pinkel D (2000) Mutations and copy number increase of HRAS in Spitz nevi with distinctive histopathological features. Am J Pathol 157(3):967–972
28. Bastian BC, Olshen AB, LeBoit PE et al (2003) Classifying melanocytic tumors based on DNA copy number changes. Am J Pathol 163(5):1765–1770
29. Bastian BC, Xiong J, Frieden IJ et al (2002) Genetic changes in neoplasms arising in congenital melanocytic nevi: differences between nodular proliferations and melanomas. Am J Pathol 161(4):1163–1169

30. Bauer P, Cristofolini P, Boi S et al (2000) Digital epiluminescence microscopy: usefulness in the differential diagnosis of cutaneous pigmentary lesions. A statistical comparison between visual and computer inspection. Melanoma Res 10(4):345–349
31. Berwick M, Armstrong BK, Ben-Porat L et al (2005) Sun exposure and mortality from melanoma. J Natl Cancer Inst 97(3):195–199
32. Berwick M, Begg CB, Fine JA et al (1996) Screening for cutaneous melanoma by skin self-examination. J Natl Cancer Inst 88(1):17–23
33. Binder M, Kittler H, Steiner A et al (1999) Reevaluation of the ABCD rule for epiluminescence microscopy. J Am Acad Dermatol 40(2 Pt 1):171–176
34. Binder M, Puespoeck-Schwarz M, Steiner A et al (1997) Epiluminescence microscopy of small pigmented skin lesions: short-term formal training improves the diagnostic performance of dermatologists. J Am Acad Dermatol 36(2 Pt 1):197–202
35. Bono A, Tolomio E, Trincone S et al (2006) Micro-melanoma detection: a clinical study on 206 consecutive cases of pigmented skin lesions with a diameter < or = 3 mm. Br J Dermatol 155(3):570–573
36. Boone M, Jemec GB, Del Marmol V (2012) High-definition optical coherence tomography enables visualization of individual cells in healthy skin: comparison to reflectance confocal microscopy. Exp Dermatol 21(10):740–744
37. Boone MA, Norrenberg S, Jemec GB et al (2012) Imaging of basal cell carcinoma by high-definition optical coherence tomography: histomorphological correlation. A pilot study. Br J Dermatol 167(4):856–864
38. Boone MA, Norrenberg S, Jemec GB et al (2014) High-definition optical coherence tomography imaging of melanocytic lesions: a pilot study. Arch Dermatol Res 306(1):11–26
39. Bowling J, Argenziano G, Azenha A et al (2007) Dermoscopy key points: recommendations from the international dermoscopy society. Dermatology 214(1):3–5
40. Braga JC, Macedo MP, Pinto C et al (2013) Learning reflectance confocal microscopy of melanocytic skin lesions through histopathologic transversal sections. PLoS ONE 8(12): e81205
41. Brezinski ME (2006) Optical coherence tomography: principles and applications. Academic Press, Amsterdam
42. Busam KJ, Charles C, Lohmann CM et al (2002) Detection of intraepidermal malignant melanoma in vivo by confocal scanning laser microscopy. Melanoma Res 12(4):349–355
43. Busam KJ, Fang Y, Jhanwar SC et al (2010) Distinction of conjunctival melanocytic nevi from melanomas by fluorescence in situ hybridization. J Cutan Pathol 37(2):196–203
44. Busam KJ, Hester K, Charles C et al (2001) Detection of clinically amelanotic malignant melanoma and assessment of its margins by in vivo confocal scanning laser microscopy. Arch Dermatol 137(7):923–929
45. Busam KJ, Marghoob AA, Halpern A (2005) Melanoma diagnosis by confocal microscopy: promise and pitfalls. J Invest Dermatol 125(3): vii
46. Carli P, De Giorgi V, Argenziano G et al (2002) Pre-operative diagnosis of pigmented skin lesions: in vivo dermoscopy performs better than dermoscopy on photographic images. J Eur Acad Dermatol Venereol 16(4):339–346
47. Carli P, De Giorgi V, Palli D et al (2003) Dermatologist detection and skin self-examination are associated with thinner melanomas: results from a survey of the Italian Multidisciplinary Group on Melanoma. Arch Dermatol 139(5):607–612
48. Cascinelli N, Ferrario M, Bufalino R et al (1992) Results obtained by using a computerized image analysis system designed as an aid to diagnosis of cutaneous melanoma. Melanoma Res 2(3):163–170
49. Chen Z, Milner TE, Srinivas S et al (1997) Noninvasive imaging of in vivo blood flow velocity using optical doppler tomography. Opt Lett 22(14):1119–1121
50. Chiu V, Won E, Malik M et al (2006) The use of mole-mapping diagrams to increase skin self-examination accuracy. J Am Acad Dermatol 55(2):245–250

51. Coleman AJ, Richardson TJ, Orchard G et al (2013) Histological correlates of optical coherence tomography in non-melanoma skin cancer. Skin Res Technol 19(1):10–19
52. Curchin CE, Wurm EM, Lambie D et al (2011) First experiences using reflectance confocal microscopy on equivocal skin lesions in Queensland. Australas J Dermatol 52(2):89–97
53. Curiel-Lewandrowski C, Chen SC, Swetter SM (2012) Screening and prevention measures for melanoma: is there a survival advantage? Curr Oncol Rep 14(5):458–467
54. Curtin JA, Fridlyand J, Kageshita T et al (2005) Distinct sets of genetic alterations in melanoma. N Engl J Med 353(20):2135–2147
55. Dalimier E, Salomon D (2012) Full-field optical coherence tomography: a new technology for 3D high-resolution skin imaging. Dermatology 224(1):84–92
56. Dalton SR, Gerami P, Kolaitis NA et al (2010) Use of fluorescence in situ hybridization (FISH) to distinguish intranodal nevus from metastatic melanoma. Am J Surg Pathol 34 (2):231–237
57. Davis KL, Mitra D, Kotapati S et al (2009) Direct economic burden of high-risk and metastatic melanoma in the elderly: evidence from the SEER-Medicare linked database. Appl Health Econ Health Policy 7(1):31–41
58. De Boer JF (2008) Spectral/Fourier domain optical coherence tomography. In: Drexler W, Fujimoto JG (eds) Optical coherence tomography: technology and applications. Springer, Berlin
59. de Giorgi V, Stante M, Massi D et al (2005) Possible histopathologic correlates of dermoscopic features in pigmented melanocytic lesions identified by means of optical coherence tomography. Exp Dermatol 14(1):56–59
60. Debarbieux S, Dalle S, Depaepe L et al (2013) Second primary melanomas treated with BRAF blockers: study by reflectance confocal microscopy. Br J Dermatol 168(6):1230–1235
61. Drexler W (2004) Ultrahigh-resolution optical coherence tomography. J Biomed Opt 9 (1):47–74
62. Dwyer PJ, DiMarzio CA, Rajadhyaksha M (2007) Confocal theta line-scanning microscope for imaging human tissues. Appl Opt 46(10):1843–1851
63. Eide MJ, Asgari MM, Fletcher SW et al (2013) Effects on skills and practice from a web-based skin cancer course for primary care providers. J Am Board Fam Med 26(6): 648–657
64. Eisemann N, Waldmann A, Geller AC et al (2014) Non-melanoma skin cancer incidence and impact of skin cancer screening on incidence. J Invest Dermatol 134(1):43–50
65. Emery JD, Hunter J, Hall PN et al (2010) Accuracy of SIAscopy for pigmented skin lesions encountered in primary care: development and validation of a new diagnostic algorithm. BMC Dermatol 10:9
66. Epstein DS, Lange JR, Gruber SB et al (1999) Is physician detection associated with thinner melanomas? JAMA 281(7):640–643
67. Farmer ER, Gonin R, Hanna MP (1996) Discordance in the histopathologic diagnosis of melanoma and melanocytic nevi between expert pathologists. Hum Pathol 27(6):528–531
68. Favazza CP, Jassim O, Cornelius LA et al (2011) In vivo photoacoustic microscopy of human cutaneous microvasculature and a nevus. J Biomed Opt 16(1):016015
69. Feit NE, Dusza SW, Marghoob AA (2004) Melanomas detected with the aid of total cutaneous photography. Br J Dermatol 150(4):706–714
70. Ferrara G, Argenziano G, Soyer HP et al (2002) Dermoscopic and histopathologic diagnosis of equivocal melanocytic skin lesions: an interdisciplinary study on 107 cases. Cancer 95 (5):1094–1100
71. Foster KR, Schwan HP (1989) Dielectric properties of tissues and biological materials: a critical review. Crit Rev Biomed Eng 17(1):25–104
72. Friedman RJ, Gutkowicz-Krusin D, Farber MJ et al (2008) The diagnostic performance of expert dermoscopists vs a computer-vision system on small-diameter melanomas. Arch Dermatol 144(4):476–482

73. Fujimoto J, Drexler W (2008) Introduction to optical coherence tomography. In: Drexler W, Fujimoto JG (eds) Optical coherence tomography: technology and applications. Springer, Berlin
74. Gambichler T, Moussa G, Sand M et al (2005) Applications of optical coherence tomography in dermatology. J Dermatol Sci 40(2):85–94
75. Gambichler T, Orlikov A, Vasa R et al (2007) In vivo optical coherence tomography of basal cell carcinoma. J Dermatol Sci 45(3):167–173
76. Gammon B, Beilfuss B, Guitart J et al (2011) Fluorescence in situ hybridization for distinguishing cellular blue nevi from blue nevus-like melanoma. J Cutan Pathol 38(4): 335–341
77. Gammon B, Beilfuss B, Guitart J et al (2012) Enhanced detection of spitzoid melanomas using fluorescence in situ hybridization with 9p21 as an adjunctive probe. Am J Surg Pathol 36(1):81–88
78. Garbe C, Peris K, Hauschild A et al (2012) Diagnosis and treatment of melanoma. European consensus-based interdisciplinary guideline–Update 2012. Eur J Cancer 48(15):2375–2390
79. Garcia-Uribe A, Zou J, Duvic M et al (2012) In vivo diagnosis of melanoma and nonmelanoma skin cancer using oblique incidence diffuse reflectance spectrometry. Cancer Res 72(11):2738–2745
80. Gareau D, Hennessy R, Wan E et al (2010) Automated detection of malignant features in confocal microscopy on superficial spreading melanoma versus nevi. J Biomed Opt 15 (6):061713
81. Gareau DS, Abeytunge S, Rajadhyaksha M (2009) Line-scanning reflectance confocal microscopy of human skin: comparison of full-pupil and divided-pupil configurations. Opt Lett 34(20):3235–3237
82. Garg A, Wang J, Reddy SB et al (2014) The Integrated Skin Exam film: an educational intervention to promote early detection of melanoma by medical students. J Am Acad Dermatol 70(1):115–119
83. Geller AC, Sober AJ, Zhang Z et al (2002) Strategies for improving melanoma education and screening for men age > or = 50 years: findings from the American Academy of Dermatological National Skin Cancer Sreening Program. Cancer 95(7):1554–1561
84. Geller AC, Venna S, Prout M et al (2002) Should the skin cancer examination be taught in medical school? Arch Dermatol 138(9):1201–1203
85. Geller AC, Zhang Z, Sober AJ et al (2003) The first 15 years of the American Academy of Dermatology skin cancer screening programs: 1985–1999. J Am Acad Dermatol 48(1):34–41
86. Gerami P, Barnhill RL, Beilfuss BA et al (2010) Superficial melanocytic neoplasms with pagetoid melanocytosis: a study of interobserver concordance and correlation with FISH. Am J Surg Pathol 34(6):816–821
87. Gerami P, Beilfuss B, Haghighat Z et al (2011) Fluorescence in situ hybridization as an ancillary method for the distinction of desmoplastic melanomas from sclerosing melanocytic nevi. J Cutan Pathol 38(4):329–334
88. Gerami P, Cooper C, Bajaj S et al (2013) Outcomes of atypical spitz tumors with chromosomal copy number aberrations and conventional melanomas in children. Am J Surg Pathol 37(9):1387–1394
89. Gerami P, Jewell SS, Morrison LE et al (2009) Fluorescence in situ hybridization (FISH) as an ancillary diagnostic tool in the diagnosis of melanoma. Am J Surg Pathol 33(8): 1146–1156
90. Gerami P, Li G, Pouryazdanparast P et al (2012) A highly specific and discriminatory FISH assay for distinguishing between benign and malignant melanocytic neoplasms. Am J Surg Pathol 36(6):808–817
91. Gerami P, Wass A, Mafee M et al (2009) Fluorescence in situ hybridization for distinguishing nevoid melanomas from mitotically active nevi. Am J Surg Pathol 33 (12):1783–1788

92. Gerbert B, Maurer T, Berger T et al (1996) Primary care physicians as gatekeepers in managed care. Primary care physicians' and dermatologists' skills at secondary prevention of skin cancer. Arch Dermatol 132(9):1030–1038
93. Gerger A, Hofmann-Wellenhof R, Langsenlehner U et al (2008) In vivo confocal laser scanning microscopy of melanocytic skin tumours: diagnostic applicability using unselected tumour images. Br J Dermatol 158(2):329–333
94. Gerger A, Koller S, Kern T et al (2005) Diagnostic applicability of in vivo confocal laser scanning microscopy in melanocytic skin tumors. J Invest Dermatol 124(3):493–498
95. Gerger A, Koller S, Weger W et al (2006) Sensitivity and specificity of confocal laser-scanning microscopy for in vivo diagnosis of malignant skin tumors. Cancer 107 (1):193–200
96. González S, Gill M, Halpern AC (2008) Reflectance confocal microscopy of cutaneous tumors: an atlas with clinical, dermoscopic, and histological correlations. Informa Healthcare; distributed in North and South America. Taylor & Francis, London
97. Goodson AG, Florell SR, Hyde M et al (2010) Comparative analysis of total body and dermatoscopic photographic monitoring of nevi in similar patient populations at risk for cutaneous melanoma. Dermatol Surg 36(7):1087–1098
98. Goulart JM, Quigley EA, Dusza S et al (2011) Skin cancer education for primary care physicians: a systematic review of published evaluated interventions. J Gen Intern Med 26 (9):1027–1035
99. Green PS, Arditi M (1985) Ultrasonic reflex transmission imaging. Ultrason Imaging 7 (3):201–214
100. Griss P, Enoksson P, Tolvanen-Laakso HK et al (2001) Micromachined electrodes for biopotential measurements. J Microelectromech Syst 10:10–16
101. Guitera P, Menzies SW, Longo C et al (2012) In vivo confocal microscopy for diagnosis of melanoma and basal cell carcinoma using a two-step method: analysis of 710 consecutive clinically equivocal cases. J Invest Dermatol 132(10):2386–2394
102. Guitera P, Pellacani G, Crotty KA et al (2010) The impact of in vivo reflectance confocal microscopy on the diagnostic accuracy of lentigo maligna and equivocal pigmented and nonpigmented macules of the face. J Invest Dermatol 130(8):2080–2091
103. Guitera P, Pellacani G, Longo C et al (2009) In vivo reflectance confocal microscopy enhances secondary evaluation of melanocytic lesions. J Invest Dermatol 129(1):131–138
104. Guy GP Jr, Ekwueme DU, Tangka FK et al (2012) Melanoma treatment costs: a systematic review of the literature, 1990-2011. Am J Prev Med 43(5):537–545
105. Halpern AC (2003) Total body skin imaging as an aid to melanoma detection. Semin Cutan Med Surg 22(1):2–8
106. Hanrahan PF, D'Este CA, Menzies SW et al (2002) A randomised trial of skin photography as an aid to screening skin lesions in older males. J Med Screen 9(3):128–132
107. Harland CC, Kale SG, Jackson P et al (2000) Differentiation of common benign pigmented skin lesions from melanoma by high-resolution ultrasound. Br J Dermatol 143(2):281–289
108. Hillner BE, Kirkwood JM, Agarwala SS (2001) Burden of illness associated with metastatic melanoma: an audit of 100 consecutive referral center cases. Cancer 91(9):1814–1821
109. Hofmann-Wellenhof R, Pellacani G, Malvehy J et al (eds) (2012) Reflectance confocal microscopy for skin diseases. Springer, Berlin
110. Huzaira M, Rius F, Rajadhyaksha M et al (2001) Topographic variations in normal skin, as viewed by in vivo reflectance confocal microscopy. J Invest Dermatol 116(6):846–852
111. Izatt JA, Choma MA (2008) Theory of optical coherence tomography. In: Drexler W, Fujimoto JG (eds) Optical coherence tomography: technology and applications. Springer, Berlin
112. Jaimes N, Dusza SW, Quigley EA et al (2013) Influence of time on dermoscopic diagnosis and management. Australas J Dermatol 54(2):96–104

113. Janda M, Neale RE, Youl P et al (2011) Impact of a video-based intervention to improve the prevalence of skin self-examination in men 50 years or older: the randomized skin awareness trial. Arch Dermatol 147(7):799–806
114. Janda M, Youl PH, Lowe JB et al (2004) Attitudes and intentions in relation to skin checks for early signs of skin cancer. Prev Med 39(1):11–18
115. Jemec GB, Gniadecka M, Ulrich J (2000) Ultrasound in dermatology. Part I. High frequency ultrasound. Eur J Dermatol 10(6):492–497
116. Kantor J, Kantor DE (2009) Routine dermatologist-performed full-body skin examination and early melanoma detection. Arch Dermatol 145(8):873–876
117. Kasparian NA, Branstrom R, Chang YM et al (2012) Skin examination behavior: the role of melanoma history, skin type, psychosocial factors, and region of residence in determining clinical and self-conducted skin examination. Arch Dermatol 148(10):1142–1151
118. Katalinic A, Waldmann A, Weinstock MA et al (2012) Does skin cancer screening save lives? An observational study comparing trends in melanoma mortality in regions with and without screening. Cancer 118(21):5395–5402
119. Kittler H, Binder M (2002) Follow-up of melanocytic skin lesions with digital dermoscopy: risks and benefits. Arch Dermatol 138(10):1379
120. Kittler H, Guitera P, Riedl E et al (2006) Identification of clinically featureless incipient melanoma using sequential dermoscopy imaging. Arch Dermatol 142(9):1113–1119
121. Kittler H, Pehamberger H, Wolff K et al (2002) Diagnostic accuracy of dermoscopy. Lancet Oncol 3(3):159–165
122. Koh HK, Judge CM, Robbins H et al (2005) The first decade of the Massachusetts Tobacco Control Program. Public Health Rep 120(5):482–495
123. Koller S, Wiltgen M, Ahlgrimm-Siess V et al (2011) In vivo reflectance confocal microscopy: automated diagnostic image analysis of melanocytic skin tumours. J Eur Acad Dermatol Venereol 25(5):554–558
124. Kollias N, Baqer A (1986) On the assessment of melanin in human skin in vivo. Photochem Photobiol 43(1):49–54
125. Kovalyshyn I, Dusza SW, Siamas K et al (2011) The impact of physician screening on melanoma detection. Arch Dermatol 147(11):1269–1275
126. Kumagai K, Koike H, Nagaoka R et al (2012) High-resolution ultrasound imaging of human skin in vivo by using three-dimensional ultrasound microscopy. Ultrasound Med Biol 38 (10):1833–1838
127. Kurugol S, Dy JG, Brooks DH et al (2011) Pilot study of semiautomated localization of the dermal/epidermal junction in reflectance confocal microscopy images of skin. J Biomed Opt 16(3):036005
128. Langley RG, Rajadhyaksha M, Dwyer PJ et al (2001) Confocal scanning laser microscopy of benign and malignant melanocytic skin lesions in vivo. J Am Acad Dermatol 45(3):365–376
129. LeBlanc WG, Vidal L, Kirsner RS et al (2008) Reported skin cancer screening of US adult workers. J Am Acad Dermatol 59(1):55–63
130. Lindelöf B, Hedblad MA (1994) Accuracy in the clinical diagnosis and pattern of malignant melanoma at a dermatological clinic. J Dermatol 21(7):461–464
131. Longo C, Farnetani F, Ciardo S et al (2013) Is confocal microscopy a valuable tool in diagnosing nodular lesions? A study of 140 cases. Br J Dermatol 169(1):58–67
132. Lucas CR, Sanders LL, Murray JC et al (2003) Early melanoma detection: nonuniform dermoscopic features and growth. J Am Acad Dermatol 48(5):663–671
133. Maier T, Braun-Falco M, Hinz T et al (2013) Morphology of basal cell carcinoma in high definition optical coherence tomography: en-face and slice imaging mode, and comparison with histology. J Eur Acad Dermatol Venereol 27(1):e97–e104
134. Maier T, Braun-Falco M, Laubender RP et al (2013) Actinic keratosis in the en-face and slice imaging mode of high-definition optical coherence tomography and comparison with histology. Br J Dermatol 168(1):120–128
135. Maiman T (1962) Solid state laser and iraser studies. Solid State Electron 4 (Oct): 236–249

136. Maize JC Jr, McCalmont TH, Carlson JA et al (2005) Genomic analysis of blue nevi and related dermal melanocytic proliferations. Am J Surg Pathol 29(9):1214–1220
137. Malvehy J, Aguilera P, Carrera C et al (2013) Ex vivo dermoscopy for biobank-oriented sampling of melanoma. JAMA Dermatol 149(9):1060–1067
138. Malvehy J, Hauschild A, Curiel-Lewandrowski C et al (2014) Clinical performance of the Nevisense system in cutaneous melanoma detection: an international, multi-centre, prospective and blinded clinical trial on efficacy and safety. Br J Dermatol
139. Malvehy J, Puig S (2002) Follow-up of melanocytic skin lesions with digital total-body photography and digital dermoscopy: a two-step method. Clin Dermatol 20(3):297–304
140. Marghoob AA, Malvehy J, Braun RP (2012) Atlas of dermoscopy, 2nd edn. Informa Healthcare, London
141. Marghoob AA, Swindle LD, Moricz CZ et al (2003) Instruments and new technologies for the in vivo diagnosis of melanoma. J Am Acad Dermatol 49(5):777–797; quiz 798–779
142. Marschall S, Sander B, Mogensen M et al (2011) Optical coherence tomography-current technology and applications in clinical and biomedical research. Anal Bioanal Chem 400 (9):2699–2720
143. Menzies SW (2013) Evidence-based dermoscopy. Dermatol Clin 31(4):521–524, vii
144. Menzies SW, Bischof L, Talbot H et al (2005) The performance of SolarScan: an automated dermoscopy image analysis instrument for the diagnosis of primary melanoma. Arch Dermatol 141(11):1388–1396
145. Minsky M (1957) Microscopy apparatus. US patent 3,013,467, 19 Dec 1961
146. Mogensen M, Morsy HA, Thrane L et al (2008) Morphology and epidermal thickness of normal skin imaged by optical coherence tomography. Dermatology 217(1):14–20
147. Mogensen M, Thrane L, Jorgensen TM et al (2009) OCT imaging of skin cancer and other dermatological diseases. J Biophotonics 2(6–7):442–451
148. Moore MM, Geller AC, Zhang Z et al (2006) Skin cancer examination teaching in US medical education. Arch Dermatol 142(4):439–444
149. Newman MD, Mirzabeigi M, Gerami P (2009) Chromosomal copy number changes supporting the classification of lentiginous junctional melanoma of the elderly as a subtype of melanoma. Mod Pathol 22(9):1258–1262
150. North JP, Garrido MC, Kolaitis NA et al (2014) Fluorescence in situ hybridization as an ancillary tool in the diagnosis of ambiguous melanocytic neoplasms: a review of 804 cases. Am J Surg Pathol 38(6):824–831
151. North JP, Kageshita T, Pinkel D et al (2008) Distribution and significance of occult intraepidermal tumor cells surrounding primary melanoma. J Invest Dermatol 128(8): 2024–2030
152. Oliveria SA, Christos PJ, Halpern AC et al (1999) Evaluation of factors associated with skin self-examination. Cancer Epidemiol Biomarkers Prev 8(11):971–978
153. Oliveria SA, Dusza SW, Phelan DL et al (2004) Patient adherence to skin self-examination: effect of nurse intervention with photographs. Am J Prev Med 26(2):152–155
154. Pagnanelli G, Soyer HP, Argenziano G et al (2003) Diagnosis of pigmented skin lesions by dermoscopy: web-based training improves diagnostic performance of non-experts. Br J Dermatol 148(4):698–702
155. Patel JK, Konda S, Perez OA et al (2008) Newer technologies/techniques and tools in the diagnosis of melanoma. Eur J Dermatol 18(6):617–631
156. Pellacani G, Cesinaro AM, Seidenari S (2005) Reflectance-mode confocal microscopy for the in vivo characterization of pagetoid melanocytosis in melanomas and nevi. J Invest Dermatol 125(3):532–537
157. Pellacani G, Cesinaro AM, Seidenari S (2005) Reflectance-mode confocal microscopy of pigmented skin lesions—improvement in melanoma diagnostic specificity. J Am Acad Dermatol 53(6):979–985
158. Pellacani G, De Pace B, Reggiani C et al (2014) Distinct melanoma types based on reflectance confocal microscopy. Exp Dermatol 23(6):414

159. Pellacani G, Guitera P, Longo C et al (2007) The impact of in vivo reflectance confocal microscopy for the diagnostic accuracy of melanoma and equivocal melanocytic lesions. J Invest Dermatol 127(12):2759–2765
160. Pellacani G, Pepe P, Casari A et al (2014) Reflectance confocal microscopy as a second-level examination in skin oncology improves diagnostic accuracy and saves unnecessary excisions: a longitudinal prospective study. Br J Dermatol
161. Petran M, Hadravsky M, Egger MD et al (1968) Tandem-scanning reflected-light microscope. J Opt Soc Am 58(5):661–664
162. Podoleanu AG (2005) Optical coherence tomography. Br J Radiol 78(935):976–988
163. Pollitt RA, Geller AC, Brooks DR et al (2009) Efficacy of skin self-examination practices for early melanoma detection. Cancer Epidemiol Biomarkers Prev 18(11):3018–3023
164. Puig S, Argenziano G, Zalaudek I et al (2007) Melanomas that failed dermoscopic detection: a combined clinicodermoscopic approach for not missing melanoma. Dermatol Surg 33 (10):1262–1273
165. Pupelli G, Longo C, Veneziano L et al (2013) Small-diameter melanocytic lesions: morphological analysis by means of in vivo confocal microscopy. Br J Dermatol 168 (5):1027–1033
166. Rajadhyaksha M, Anderson RR, Webb RH (1999) Video-rate confocal scanning laser microscope for imaging human tissues in vivo. Appl Opt 38(10):2105–2115
167. Rajadhyaksha M, Gonzalez S, Zavislan JM et al (1999) In vivo confocal scanning laser microscopy of human skin II: advances in instrumentation and comparison with histology. J Invest Dermatol 113(3):293–303
168. Rajadhyaksha M, Grossman M, Esterowitz D et al (1995) In vivo confocal scanning laser microscopy of human skin: melanin provides strong contrast. J Invest Dermatol 104(6): 946–952
169. Rallan D, Bush NL, Bamber JC et al (2007) Quantitative discrimination of pigmented lesions using three-dimensional high-resolution ultrasound reflex transmission imaging. J Invest Dermatol 127(1):189–195
170. Rice ZP, Weiss FJ, DeLong LK et al (2010) Utilization and rationale for the implementation of total body (digital) photography as an adjunct screening measure for melanoma. Melanoma Res 20(5):417–421
171. Rigel DS, Russak J, Friedman R (2010) The evolution of melanoma diagnosis: 25 years beyond the ABCDs. CA Cancer J Clin 60(5):301–316
172. Risser J, Pressley Z, Veledar E et al (2007) The impact of total body photography on biopsy rate in patients from a pigmented lesion clinic. J Am Acad Dermatol 57(3):428–434
173. Robinson JK, Turrisi R, Mallett K et al (2010) Comparing the efficacy of an in-person intervention with a skin self-examination workbook. Arch Dermatol 146(1):91–94
174. Robinson JK, Turrisi R, Stapleton J (2007) Efficacy of a partner assistance intervention designed to increase skin self-examination performance. Arch Dermatol 143(1):37–41
175. Rodriguez GL, Ma F, Federman DG et al (2007) Predictors of skin cancer screening practice and attitudes in primary care. J Am Acad Dermatol 57(5):775–781
176. Roeseler A, Burns D (2010) The quarter that changed the world. Tob Control 19(Suppl 1): i3–i15
177. Salerni G, Carrera C, Lovatto L et al (2012) Characterization of 1152 lesions excised over 10 years using total-body photography and digital dermatoscopy in the surveillance of patients at high risk for melanoma. J Am Acad Dermatol 67(5):836–845
178. Salerni G, Carrera C, Lovatto L et al (2012) Benefits of total body photography and digital dermatoscopy ("two-step method of digital follow-up") in the early diagnosis of melanoma in patients at high risk for melanoma. J Am Acad Dermatol 67(1):e17–e27
179. Salerni G, Terán T, Puig S et al (2013) Meta-analysis of digital dermoscopy follow-up of melanocytic skin lesions: a study on behalf of the International Dermoscopy Society. J Eur Acad Dermatol Venereol 27(7):805–814

180. Saraiya M, Hall HI, Thompson T et al (2004) Skin cancer screening among U.S. adults from 1992, 1998, and 2000 National Health Interview Surveys. Prev Med 39(2):308–314
181. Schmitt J (1999) Optical coherence tomography (OCT): a review. IEEE J Sel Top Quantum Electron 5:1205–1215
182. Schneider JS, Moore DH 2nd, Mendelsohn ML (2008) Screening program reduced melanoma mortality at the Lawrence Livermore National Laboratory, 1984–1996. J Am Acad Dermatol 58(5):741–749
183. Schwan HP (1957) Electrical properties of tissue and cell suspensions. Adv Biol Med Phys 5:147–209
184. Scope A, Benvenuto-Andrade C, Agero AL et al (2007) In vivo reflectance confocal microscopy imaging of melanocytic skin lesions: consensus terminology glossary and illustrative images. J Am Acad Dermatol 57(4):644–658
185. Scope A, Busam KJ, Malvehy J et al (2007) Ex vivo dermoscopy of melanocytic tumors: time for dermatopathologists to learn dermoscopy. Arch Dermatol 143(12):1548–1552
186. U.S. Preventive Services Task Force (2009) Screening for skin cancer: U.S. Preventive Services Task Force recommendation statement. Ann Intern Med 150(3):188–193
187. Segura S, Puig S, Carrera C et al (2009) Development of a two-step method for the diagnosis of melanoma by reflectance confocal microscopy. J Am Acad Dermatol 61(2):216–229
188. Seidler AM, Pennie ML, Veledar E et al (2010) Economic burden of melanoma in the elderly population: population-based analysis of the Surveillance, Epidemiology, and End Results (SEER)–Medicare data. Arch Dermatol 146(3):249–256
189. Shaikh WR, Geller A, Alexander G et al (2012) Developing an interactive web-based learning program on skin cancer: the learning experiences of clinical educators. J Cancer Educ 27(4):709–716
190. Siegel R, Ma J, Zou Z et al (2014) Cancer statistics. CA Cancer J Clin 64(1):9–29
191. Smith L, Macneil S (2011) State of the art in non-invasive imaging of cutaneous melanoma. Skin Res Technol 17(3):257–269
192. Smith RA, Brooks D, Cokkinides V et al (2013) Cancer screening in the United States, 2013: a review of current American cancer society guidelines, current issues in cancer screening, and new guidance on cervical cancer screening and lung cancer screening. CA Cancer J Clin 63(2):88–105
193. Soyer HP, Argenziano G, Zalaudek I et al (2004) Three-point checklist of dermoscopy. A new screening method for early detection of melanoma. Dermatology 208(1):27–31
194. Stefanowska J, Zakowiecki D, Cal K (2010) Magnetic resonance imaging of the skin. J Eur Acad Dermatol Venereol 24(8):875–880
195. Stevenson AD, Mickan S, Mallett S et al (2013) Systematic review of diagnostic accuracy of reflectance confocal microscopy for melanoma diagnosis in patients with clinically equivocal skin lesions. Dermatol Pract Concept 3(4):19–27
196. Stratigos AJ, Forsea AM, van der Leest RJ et al (2012) Euromelanoma: a dermatology-led European campaign against nonmelanoma skin cancer and cutaneous melanoma. Past, present and future. Br J Dermatol 167 Suppl 2:99–104
197. Swetter SM, Johnson TM, Miller DR et al (2009) Melanoma in middle-aged and older men: a multi-institutional survey study of factors related to tumor thickness. Arch Dermatol 145(4): 397–404
198. Swetter SM, Pollitt RA, Johnson TM et al (2012) Behavioral determinants of successful early melanoma detection: role of self and physician skin examination. Cancer 118(15):3725–3734
199. Taber JM, Aspinwall LG, Leaf SL et al (2013) Partner involvement in conduct of skin self-examinations remains low following CDKN2A/p16 genetic test reporting and counseling. J Am Acad Dermatol 69(5):842–844
200. Terushkin V, Halpern AC (2009) Melanoma early detection. Hematol Oncol Clin North Am 23(3):481–500, viii
201. Tsao H, Rogers GS, Sober AJ (1998) An estimate of the annual direct cost of treating cutaneous melanoma. J Am Acad Dermatol 38(5 Pt 1):669–680

202. Vakoc BJ, Fukumura D, Jain RK et al (2012) Cancer imaging by optical coherence tomography: preclinical progress and clinical potential. Nat Rev Cancer 12(5):363–368
203. Vergier B, Prochazkova-Carlotti M, de la Fouchardiere A et al (2011) Fluorescence in situ hybridization, a diagnostic aid in ambiguous melanocytic tumors: European study of 113 cases. Mod Pathol 24(5):613–623
204. Vestergaard ME, Macaskill P, Holt PE et al (2008) Dermoscopy compared with naked eye examination for the diagnosis of primary melanoma: a meta-analysis of studies performed in a clinical setting. Br J Dermatol 159(3):669–676
205. Waldmann A, Nolte S, Weinstock MA et al (2012) Skin cancer screening participation and impact on melanoma incidence in Germany–an observational study on incidence trends in regions with and without population-based screening. Br J Cancer 106(5):970–974
206. Wang RK, Nuttall AL (2010) Phase-sensitive optical coherence tomography imaging of the tissue motion within the organ of Corti at a subnanometer scale: a preliminary study. J Biomed Opt 15(5):056005
207. Wang SQ, Dusza SW, Scope A et al (2008) Differences in dermoscopic images from nonpolarized dermoscope and polarized dermoscope influence the diagnostic accuracy and confidence level: a pilot study. Dermatol Surg 34(10):1389–1395
208. Wang SQ, Kopf AW, Koenig K et al (2004) Detection of melanomas in patients followed up with total cutaneous examinations, total cutaneous photography, and dermoscopy. J Am Acad Dermatol 50(1):15–20
209. Weinstock MA, Martin RA, Risica PM et al (1999) Thorough skin examination for the early detection of melanoma. Am J Prev Med 17(3):169–175
210. Weinstock MA, Risica PM, Martin RA et al (2007) Melanoma early detection with thorough skin self-examination: the "check it out" randomized trial. Am J Prev Med 32(6):517–524
211. Wiesner T, Obenauf AC, Murali R et al (2011) Germline mutations in BAP1 predispose to melanocytic tumors. Nat Genet 43(10):1018–1021
212. Wiltgen M, Gerger A, Wagner C et al (2008) Automatic identification of diagnostic significant regions in confocal laser scanning microscopy of melanocytic skin tumors. Methods Inf Med 47(1):14–25
213. Yabroff KR, Lamont EB, Mariotto A et al (2008) Cost of care for elderly cancer patients in the United States. J Natl Cancer Inst 100(9):630–641
214. Yamamoto T, Yamamoto Y (1976) Electrical properties of the epidermal stratum corneum. Med Biol Eng 14(2):151–158
215. Ziolkowska M, Philipp C, Liebscher J et al (2009) OCT of healthy skin, actinic skin and NMSC lesions. Med Laser Appl 24:256–264
216. Zysk AM, Nguyen FT, Oldenburg AL et al (2007) Optical coherence tomography: a review of clinical development from bench to bedside. J Biomed Opt 12(5):051403

Melanoma: Clinical Presentations

Nour Kibbi, Harriet Kluger and Jennifer Nam Choi

Abstract

The malignant cell in melanoma is the melanocyte. Because melanocytes are located in the basal layer of the epidermis, melanoma is most commonly seen on the skin. However, melanoma can also arise on mucosal surfaces such as the oral cavity, the upper gastrointestinal mucosa, the genital mucosa, as well as the uveal tract of the eye and leptomeninges. Melanomas tend to be pigmented but can also present as pink or red lesions. They can mimic benign or other malignant skin lesions. This chapter presents the spectrum of typical and less typical presentations of melanoma, as well as patterns of spread. It is divided into (1) cutaneous lesions; (2) patterns of regional spread, (3) non-cutaneous lesions; and (4) distant metastases.

Keywords

Atypical pigmented cutaneous lesions · Non-cutaneous melanoma · Melanoma of unknown primary site

Contents

N. Kibbi · H. Kluger (✉) · J.N. Choi
Departments of Dermatology and Medicine, Yale University School of Medicine, New Haven, USA
e-mail: harriet.kluger@yale.edu

H.L. Kaufman and J.M. Mehnert (eds.), *Melanoma*,
Cancer Treatment and Research 167, DOI 10.1007/978-3-319-22539-5_4

1 Cutaneous Tumors

Cutaneous melanomas are classified on the growth pattern into superficial spreading, nodular, lentigo maligna, and acral. Growth is typically described in two planes: Radial (horizontal) growth refers to melanocytic proliferation limited to the epidermis or focally as single cells or small nests within the papillary dermis, whereas vertical growth describes deeper invasion of nests or nodules of atypical melanocytes that are often larger than their counterparts in the superficial skin [1]. In certain instances, it is useful to think of these as "phases" of growth, such that the radial growth phase (RGP) may sometimes precede a vertical growth phase (VGP). The typical lesion of cutaneous melanoma is an asymmetric macule or nodule with irregular borders, frequently with variations in color within the lesion. On histology, it reveals nests of melanocytes within the epidermis that varies in size, shape, spacing, and display pagetoid spread, or a pattern of focal confluence [2]. Architectural patterns and cytomorphological features have been studied and are reviewed extensively by [3].

Alternative ways of classification have been proposed based on rate of growth [4]. In this schema based on trends in melanoma epidemiology, there are three subtypes of lesions: (1) slow-growing, located on intermittently sun-exposed areas with a sharply rising incidence; (2) very slow-growing on sun-exposed skin with moderate increase in incidence; and (3) fast-growing, arising in any body part with stable incidence and high mortality. Any scheme can be adopted so long as it is helpful in stratifying risk, rationalizing therapy, and predicting prognosis.

1.1 Superficial Spreading Melanoma

Superficial spreading melanoma (SSM) is the most common subtype of cutaneous melanoma, particularly in individuals with Skin Phototypes I and II, accounting for 60–70 % of all melanomas. It is typically diagnosed between the ages of 40 and 60 (see Table 1). The association between the number of nevi and SSM has been established [5, 6]. This subtype typically arises on the trunk in men and on the

Table 1 Clinical subtypes and classical feature of cutaneous melanoma

Clinical subtype	Percentage[a] (%)	Median age (years)	Frequent location	Precursor lesion	Growth pattern	Dermoscopy	Histopathology
Superficial spreading melanoma	57.4	51	Trunk in men, lower legs in women [2]	Can arise de novo or in preexisting nevus [5, 6]	Begins as <5 mm macule with notched borders; slow RGP limited to epidermis or focally in papillary dermis; develops into papule or nodule with a rapid VGP [2]	Broad network of multiple brown dots with pseudopods, color variation (red and blue), a sharp cutoff, and possible depigmentation [7]	Asymmetric, poorly circumscribed, irregular nests of melanocytes within the epidermis; with pagetoid spread [2]
Nodular melanoma	21.4	56	Trunk, head, neck in men more than women [2]	De novo, less commonly in preexisting nevus [8]	Begins as a blue to black, or pink to red nodule which may ulcerate or bleed; rapid VGP [9]	Individual globules with color variation (blue-gray), white streaks and irregular vessels [7]	Similar to superficial spreading melanoma [9]
Lentigo maligna melanoma	8.8	68	Nose, cheek, or any sun-damaged skin (including neck, scalp, and ears in men) [2]	Lentigo maligna [10]	Begins as a brown-to-black macule with variegated color and irregular indented border [7, 11]	Asymmetric, hyperpigmented follicular openings slowly overgrown by irregular pigmented dots [7]	Solitary tumor cells within epidermis, epithelium of adnexal structures; epidermal atrophy and signs of elastosis [2]
Acral lentiginous melanoma	4	63	Soles, most commonly, also palms, within or around nail apparatus [12]		Brown-to-black macule with color variegation and irregular borders [2]	Irregular, gray-brown polygons, multiple hypopigmented areas [7]	Proliferating, atypical melanocytes within basal layer of hyperplastic dermis either arranged solitary or in irregular nests [13]

RGP radial growth phase; *VGP* vertical growth phase

[a]Percentages are based on all cases of cutaneous, ocular, and mucosal melanoma. Percentages do not add up to 100, because unclassified melanomas (3.5 %) and other (5 %) were not included in the table

lower extremities in women. Depending on the location, the differential diagnosis might include atypical nevus, common benign nevus, seborrheic keratosis, or basal cell carcinoma. Classically, SSM begins as an asymmetric, irregularly scalloped macule or papule, usually <5 mm with mottled variegated color, and a central elevation with some surface distortion [2]. Over time, the lesion can grow to be significantly larger (Fig. 1a, b). Initially, the lesion behaves indolently, proliferating within the epidermis or superficial papillary dermis. However, for unknown

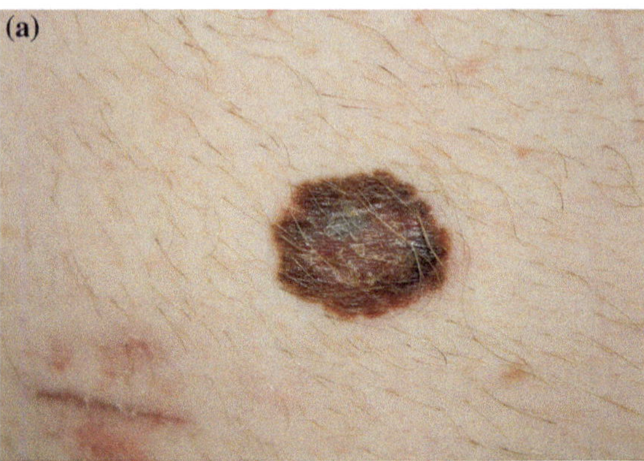

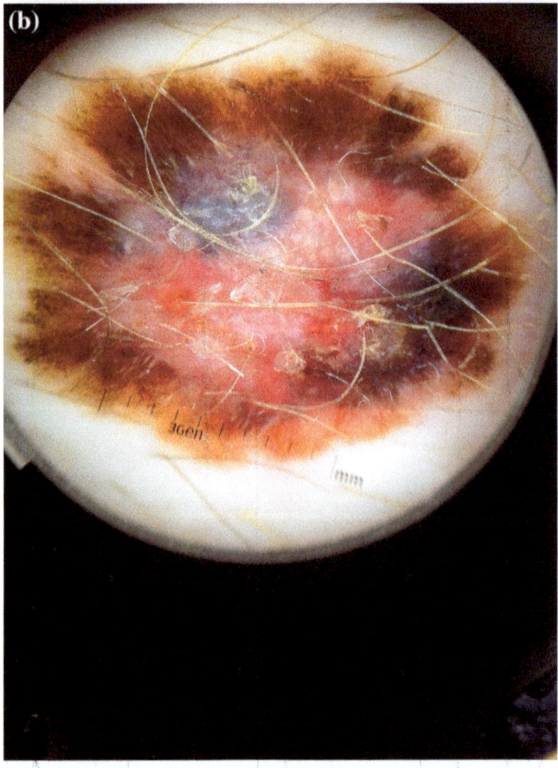

Fig. 1 **a** A superficial spreading melanoma presenting as a 1.9 × 1.7 cm *pink/brown/black* patch with a 7-mm *red* papule at the 5 o'clock location of the lesion. Histology revealed a 1.0 mm Breslow depth. **b** Dermoscopy showed prominent variegation in color and central haziness with pink, purplish, and gray discoloration

reasons, the malignant melanocytes invade the dermis and a more rapid VGP ensues, leading to a papule or nodule.

Although SSM is often associated with transformed nevi because of the association with nevi counts, it is estimated that approximately half of these lesions arise de novo. In fact, the likelihood that an individual nevus will progress to malignancy is low [14]: The risk of malignant transformation for common melanocytic nevi is one in thousands, while the risk for atypical melanocytic nevi is in the order of one in hundreds [15, 16]. Whereas the risk of SSM arising from common nevi increases with nevi counts [5, 6], for atypical nevi, the risk beyond five nevi does not accrue [17].

1.1.1 Melanoma In Situ

Melanoma in situ (MIS) is thought to precede more invasive melanoma. MIS refers to solitary melanocytes or nests of melanocytes found above the dermal–epidermal junction (DEJ) and extending into the uppermost layers of the epidermis. Melanocytes can involve the adnexal epithelium of pilosebaceous units and other structures. These nests do not mature as they cross into the dermis, but instead, retain the same size as their epidermal counterparts [2].

1.1.2 Host Immune Response in Melanoma

More so than any other malignant neoplasm, melanoma antigens are highly immunogenic [18]. To demonstrate the role of the immune system in melanoma, it was shown that melanoma incidence was higher in immunosuppressed individuals [19]. It is no surprise, therefore, that many melanomas display immune escape mechanisms: For instance, they may selectively lose or mutate known immunogenic antigens, down-regulate MHC class I molecules on antigen presenting cells, and change the cytokine milieu toward a tolerizing environment [20].

Up to two-thirds of patients show signs of partial regression, a phenomenon which may represent an immune response. Macroscopically, this is seen by focal areas in the lesion of gray, hypo-, or depigmented structures, which can be mistaken for vitiligo or halo nevi, while histopathological examinations reveal accumulated melanin-laden macrophages and infiltrating lymphocytes, often arranged in a bandlike pattern in the dermis [21, 22]. Spontaneous regression inversely correlates with tumor thickness; as such, up to two-thirds of the thinnest melanomas (0.75 mm or less in thickness) show partial regression [23, 24]. The mechanism of regression is unclear, though assumed to be immune-mediated, given the infiltrate of lymphocytes and plasma cells [25, 26]. Some have even proposed a contact sensitizer to be the cause for recruiting the adaptive immune system to the tumor environment [27].

The prognostic significance of regression is not well understood: A recent study demonstrated increased risk of metastases in 43 cases of melanoma with extensive but partial regression compared with matched controls [28]. To explain this, it is thought that regression signifies the presence of deeper invasion that may have already led "the horse out of the barn," so to speak. Although some investigations have confirmed that partial regression is an adverse prognostic factor [29, 30], others have failed to demonstrate this [31, 32]. To complicate matters further, melanoma of unknown primary (MUP), in which the primary lesion is assumed to be regressed, appears to have survival advantage as compared to patients with positive nodes and a known primary tumor [33, 34]. This would suggest that lymph node infiltration triggers the immune response against melanoma. The conflicting data may indicate the instances of success and failure of the immune system at attacking the tumor.

Besides spontaneous partial regression, which is common, complete regression is rare, and until 2005, only 38 cases were reported [35]. There is a marked predilection in males, with a male to female ratio of approximately 2:1, and an average age of onset of 48. Survival is variable, but poor, ranging from 6 weeks to 11 years. Among those that died of metastatic disease, the average survival was 13 months. Similar to partial regression, in complete regression, the patient often describes a change in a preexisting nevus: enlargement, friability, hypopigmentation, hyperpigmentation, bleeding, and eventual regression. Histology of the reviewed case reports by High et al. mostly showed epidermal attenuation, decreased epidermal melanocytes, papillary dermal fibrosis, a chronic inflammatory infiltrate, telangiectasia, and presence of dermal melanophages. The authors point out that requiring melanophages in the diagnostic criteria may exclude amelanotic melanoma lesions that have regressed, but without including this feature, the positive predictive value of diagnosis is too low, given that the prevalence of complete regression is low. One rare form of complete tumor regression is known as tumoral melanosis (TM). TM presents as a 1–5 cm blue-black nodule, suspicious for a primary invasive melanoma [22]. However, histology reveals dense dermal or dermal and subcutaneous melanophage infiltrates.

1.2 Nodular Melanoma

Nodular melanoma (NM) is the second most common type in fair-skinned individuals, representing approximately 15–20 % of melanomas. It commonly presents on the trunk, head, or neck, with a greater incidence in men (Fig. 2). This subtype is thought to arise de novo over a period of weeks to months as a vertically infiltrating tumor without much of a RGP. For this reason, they tend to be diagnosed at a thicker, more advanced stage [8]. Early on, the lesion is classically an asymmetric blue or black nodule with regular borders. Two to eight percent of such tumors, however, can be pink or red in coloration and in those instances are termed "amelanotic" [9]. Because they lack pigment and are often smaller in diameter, 70 % of the time, melanoma is not initially considered in the diagnosis [36]. Whether pink or pigmented, NM may ulcerate or bleed. Depending on the presence or absence of pigmentation, the differential diagnosis includes the following: (1) for pigmented lesions: blue nevi, pigmented basal cell carcinoma, common benign nevus, and pigmented Spitz nevus; and (2) for amelanotic lesions: basal cell carcinoma, pyogenic granuloma, and atypical fibroxanthoma.

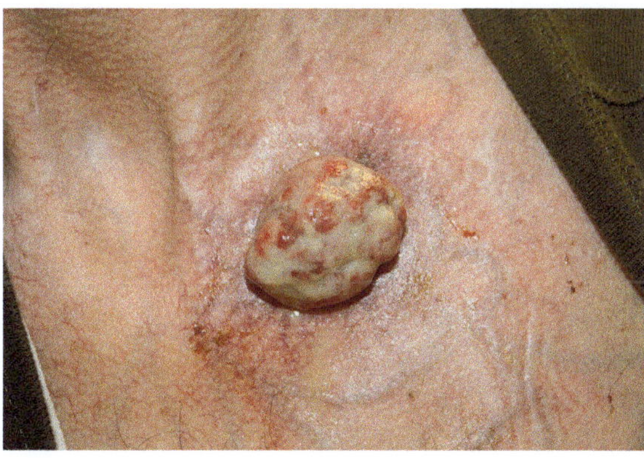

Fig. 2 A nodular melanoma presenting as a 4 cm fungating mass with purulent drainage. This nodule grew in size for over 2 years before the patient presented to the physician. Upon diagnosis, he was found to have lymph node involvement and died within 1 year from distant metastatic disease

1.2.1 Spitzoid Melanoma

Spitzoid melanoma can be mistaken early on for a Spitz nevus. On histology, both reveal a dermal nodule with overall symmetry of epithelioid melanocytes that do not mature with deeper extension. However, clues to the malignant nature of the lesion include arrangement into sheets of atypical melanocytes in the dermis and mitotic figures at the base of the lesion. Additional methods such as immunohistochemistry (IHC), fluorescence in situ hybridization (FISH), and comparative genomic hybridization (CGH) have had variable rates of success in distinguishing melanoma from nevus [37]. For instance, melanomas, unlike benign nevi, show gains or losses of particular segments or whole chromosomes, while approximately 20 % of benign Spitz nevi show increase in copy number of chromosome 11p, not typically found in melanoma [38].

1.2.2 Atypical Fibroxanthoma-Like Melanoma

NM can also be mistaken for atypical fibroxanthoma (AFX), the former being a diagnosis more dangerous to miss. Sangueza and Zelger report 4 cases of melanoma in 3 patients whose diagnosis was mistaken initially due to the unusual clinical presentation and pathological correlation, as well as negative melanin staining on IHC [39]. However, others have reported that AFX can present as a pseudopigmented lesion that can be mistaken for melanoma on clinical and pathological evaluation [40]. To circumvent this, the authors recommend iron stains to diagnose AFX, because degraded erythrocytes following ulceration and hemorrhage are ingested and appear as accumulated hemosiderin in neoplastic cells.

1.2.3 Collision (Contiguous) Tumors

The skin, more than any other organ, is exposed to extensive DNA damage. In the right host, multiple contiguous tumors may arise. Clinical examination may reveal an atypical lesion, which on histology shows multiple etiologies. One such report involves 2 cases: one of a BCC, which ultimately revealed an underlying amelanotic melanoma, and another of an amelanotic melanoma that concealed an AFX [41]. Collision tumors can also arise in skin grafts [42]; however, the significance of that observation has not been found.

1.3 Lentigo Maligna Melanoma

Lentigo maligna melanoma (LMM) is a less common subtype, comprising approximately 9 % of all cutaneous melanomas. Typically, lesions occur in older, chronically sun-damaged individuals, with a predilection for the nose and cheek in women, and neck, scalp, and ears in men. Unlike other subtypes, it is thought that LMM arises from cumulative sun exposure rather than intermittent sun damage. Although LMM is associated with fair skin phototypes, unlike SSM, it is not correlated with nevus counts [5, 6]. The precursor lesion in LMM is a form of in situ melanoma, known as lentigo maligna (LM) (Fig. 3). There is a considerable risk—estimated at 5 %—for progression of LM into LMM [10]. Because it develops on a background of sun damage, the differential diagnosis for LMM includes lesions of sun damage (solar lentigo, pigmented actinic keratosis) as well as lentiginous nevus, macular seborrheic keratosis, and pigmented basal cell carcinoma. Of note, lentiginous junctional nevi are described in the elderly, especially on a background of poikilodermic skin, but they are located—unlike LM and LMM—on the trunk and limbs. Needless to say, they may transform into LM and small cell melanomas [43].

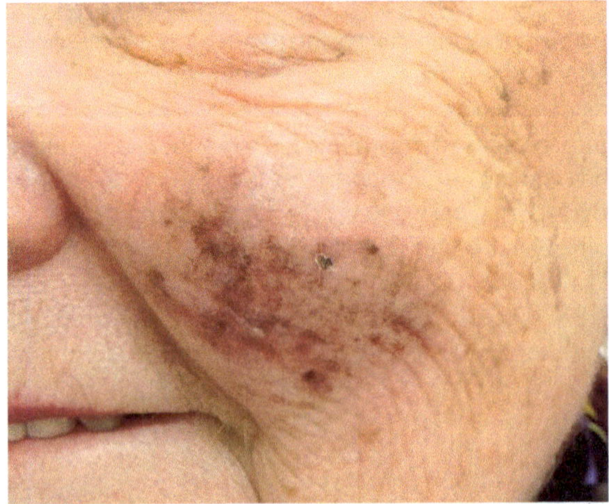

Fig. 3 Lentigo maligna (melanoma in situ) on the cheek of an elderly Caucasian woman. Site of hemorrhagic crust represents a recent biopsy site confirming the diagnosis. Full resection revealed no invasive component of melanoma

The lesion usually begins as an indolent, asymmetric brown-to-black macule with color variegation and an irregular indentation. On dermoscopy, these areas appear as hyperpigmented follicular openings that are overgrown by irregular pigmented dots arranged in an annular granular pattern [7, 11]. Stolz et al. estimated that 87 % of LMM presents with those features on dermoscopy. Others have tried to identify novel features, including increased density in the vascular network, and presence of rhomboidal structures and targetlike patterns [44]. Additionally, LMM may display subclinical levels of radial growth, resulting in incomplete excision, and high rates of recurrence. Later on, lesions may develop a nodular portion.

Microscopically, LMM exhibits lentiginous spread, in which solitary tumor cells, rather than tumor nests, extend into the epidermal and dermal layers [2]. Atypical melanocytes can be found in the epithelium of adnexal structures, particularly along the outer root sheath of hair follicles. An invasive component is often present and composed of spindle cells. Moreover, epidermal atrophy, signs of solar elastosis, and desmoplastic stromal change are not uncommon with LMM. Finally, work by King et al. suggests that atypical lentiginous proliferations may look similar to benign lentiginous junctional nevi in their retiform epidermal pattern; however, they also present with confluent growth of atypical melanocytes flanking the site of biopsy, which is more akin to atypical proliferative lesions (2005). Seeing as these lentiginous proliferations progress if left untreated, the authors suggest that they might be early LMM and therefore should be treated as such.

1.3.1 Desmoplastic Melanoma

LMM is associated with the highest rates of desmoplastic melanoma (DM). DM is a histological diagnosis that comprises 4 % of cutaneous melanomas and is found more commonly in older males and on sun-exposed skin [45, 46]. It can arise in LMM, acral melanoma (AM, see Sect. 1.4), or in the RGP of mucosal lymphoma [2]. The classic lesion is a skin-colored, red, or brown-black nodule or plaque in a sun-exposed site. Histologically, malignant melanocytes take on a spindle shape, separated by collagen fibers or fibrous stroma, which are present in foci or throughout the tumor. Cytologically, melanocytes appear bland, with visible atypia and stromal fibrosis [47]. The diagnosis requires deep tissue samples because superficial findings are nonspecific for scar or spindle cell neoplasms. The source of desmoplasia and increased collagen deposition is unknown. Some have postulated that the malignant melanocytes induce host responses leading to fibroblast proliferation and deposition of collagen [48, 49]. Others have argued that the melanocytes themselves undergo adaptive fibroplasia, allowing them to deposit collagen in the deeper dermal layers [50, 51].

DM is rarely metastatic but often highly infiltrative and locally aggressive, and approximately 30 % of cases display neurotropism. Of note, conventional staging has been shown to overestimate the likelihood of metastasis of these tumors [52, 53].

1.4 Acral Melanoma

AM is the least common subtype, comprising <5 % of cutaneous melanomas. It presents with equal incidence in all skin types and as such is the most common subtype in darker pigmented individuals. It constitutes 60–70 % of melanomas in black-skinned individuals [54] and 50 % in Asians [55–57]. Typically, AM occurs on the soles, but can also commonly occur on the palms and in or around the nail apparatus [12]. AM is difficult to diagnose because, especially when it is amelanotic, it can look like a benign lesion, such as a plantar wart or hematoma, or a squamous cell carcinoma.

Classically, AM begins as an asymmetric brown-to-black macule with variegated color and irregular borders. When involving the nail bed, it can present with longitudinal melanonychia extending onto the hyponychium or beyond the lateral or proximal nail fold, the latter referred to as Hutchinson's sign. Histologically, lesions begin as atypical single melanocytes or nests of melanocytes, sometimes displaying dendrites, and are present within all layers of a hyperplastic epidermis, in what is known as pagetoid scatter [13]. In the stratum corneum, numerous melanocytes and melanin granules are diffusely scattered.

The genetic markers of AM are different from the other subtypes of melanoma. Activating KIT mutations in exons 11, 13, and 17 is common, making the tumor susceptible to KIT inhibitors, such as imatinib [58, 59].

1.4.1 Subungual Melanoma

AM of the matrix is known as subungual melanoma (SUM) and represents 1–3 % of all cutaneous melanomas. Unlike any other melanoma type, SUM is not related to sun exposure. Because the nail plate is so dense, it is estimated that less than 2 % of UVA, and no UVB, is transmitted to the matrix [60].

SUM presents commonly with melanonychia striata, which are widening dark or irregularly pigmented longitudinal nail streaks with possible nail dystrophy and onycholysis [2]. Hyperpigmentation of the nail bed or matrix is concerning when it extends to the cuticle or hyponychium, and when the pigment is dark, irregular, or the width of the area involved is >3 mm. Nail pathologies to consider in that case are as follows: benign longitudinal melanonychia, subungual hematoma, pyogenic granuloma, onychomycosis with pigmentation, or hemorrhage.

SUM is misdiagnosed 85 % of the time, with the mean diagnostic delay being 30 months [61]. This is perhaps the case because approximately 23–44 % of patients with SUM reported local trauma to the nail [62]. It is unclear whether trauma draws attention to the area or whether post-traumatic inflammation induces carcinogenesis [63]. In favor of the latter, an analogous relationship exists between chronic skin wounds and the emergence of aggressive ulcerating forms of squamous cell carcinoma.

2 Regional Metastases

Regional metastases refer to the proximal spread of a melanoma within the skin and lymphatic vessels of the regional lymphatic system, including the regional lymph node. It is estimated that two-thirds of patients with clinical metastases following treatment of primary melanoma present initially with loco-regional metastases [64]. Regional metastases are classified into satellite, in-transit, and nodal based on the level of involvement within the lymphatic chain. As such, it relies on the premise that melanoma cells travel proximally in the lymphatic system. However, it is also known that melanoma can spread hematogenously and iatrogenically [65]. True hematogenous spread is confirmed by the development of metastases at the donor site of split thickness grafts and has been reported [66, 67]. That melanoma cells can spread in the blood vessels is no surprise, as tumor cells can express levels of tissue factor 1000-fold higher than normal tissue [68, 69]. The natural history of melanoma and patterns of spread can help guide treatment and set survival expectations.

2.1 Satellite and In-Transit Metastasis

Satellite metastases (SM) are metastatic nodules that appear within 2 cm of the primary tumor. In-transit metastasis (ITM) represent intralymphatic tumor invasion in the regional skin or subcutaneous tissue between the primary tumor site and the draining lymph node basin. Clinically, SM and ITM appear as cutaneous or subcutaneous tumors or, when present in the upper dermis, may present as dome-shaped papules or nodules, which may be brown, skin-colored, or pink (Fig. 4a, b). The reported 5-year survival rates of ITM are approximately 69 % without lymph node involvement and drop to 46 % with regional node involvement [70–72]. SM and ITM have been associated with thicker primary tumors, ulceration, primary lesions on the lower extremities, and regional lymph node metastasis [73–76]. In fact, second only to lymph node status, Weide et al. identified tumor thickness, not ulceration, as the greatest independent prognostic factor for melanoma patients with SM and ITM [71]. It is unclear whether the interval between primary diagnoses and emergence of regional disease is a prognostic factor, as studies report variable results [77–79].

The natural history and progression of melanoma to ITM is not understood. One theory postulates that melanoma cells enter the superficial and deep lymphatic vessels but, along the way, become lodged—as an embolus might—in the lymphatic channels, either due to obstructing nodal disease or due to impaired lymphatic drainage from the removal of lymph nodes [80]. This second explanation is based on a study in which patients with ITM who had undergone wide local excision (WLE) with elective lymph node dissection (ELND) were compared to those that underwent WLE only (and lymph node dissection if lymph nodes became clinically palpable) [75]. ITM incidence was 27 and 10 %, respectively, in those

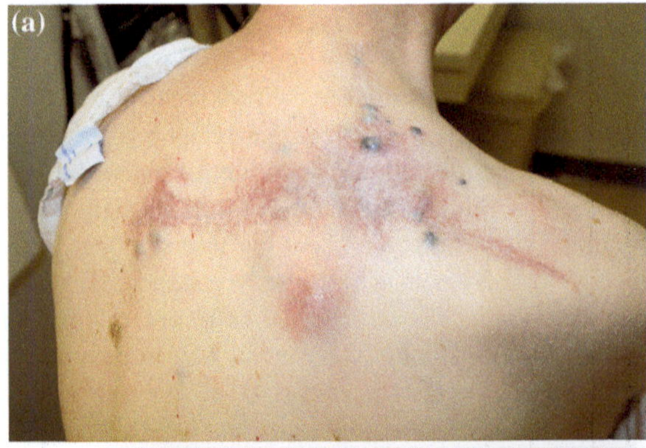

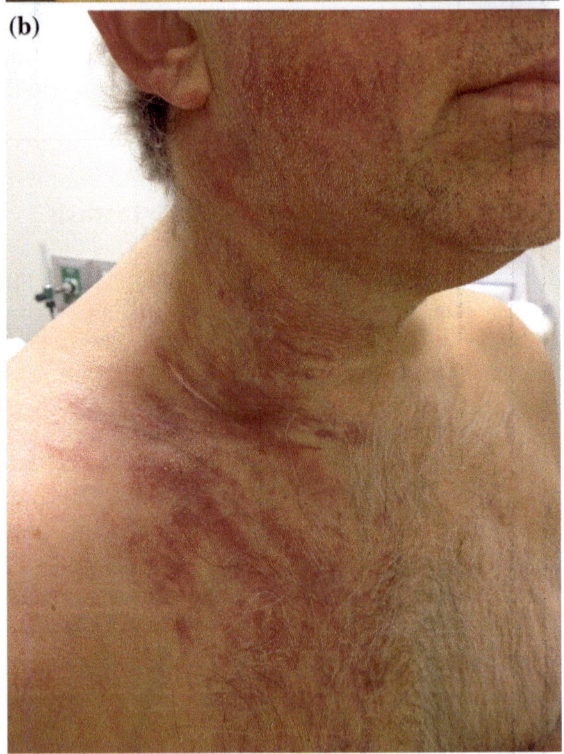

Fig. 4 **a** Numerous melanoma satellite metastases presenting as 0.3–1 cm subcutaneous blue-black nodules emanating from the original melanoma surgical site, in addition to a large 4-cm subcutaneous firm erythematous nodule inferior to the surgical site. **b** Satellite melanoma metastases presenting as streaklike erythematous plaques and nodules on the right neck and shoulder

groups, suggesting that surgical manipulation of regional nodes increased the risk of ITM. Other more recent studies have also suggested that ELND or SLND increases the risk of ITM [81, 82]. That being said, Pawlik et al. [83] are critical of these studies. They suggest that the comparison is unfair as most patients who undergo SLND or ELND have unfavorable tumor characteristics. In fact, a recent review of over 2000 patients with primary melanomas more accurately matched the two groups for tumor characteristics. The results showed that the rate of ITM in patients treated with WLE alone was 4.9 % and not significant from those who underwent WLE and SLND, which was 3.6 % [84]. Another German study compared the 5-year overall ITM rate and showed no difference between the SLND and delayed lymphadenectomy groups [85].

2.2 Nodal Metastases

Before sentinel lymph nodes were introduced as part of the staging evaluation of solid tumors, the concept of "orderly progression of nodal metastases" was attractive in melanoma, since cutaneous lymphatic flow was better defined than any other solid organ. However, data suggest that 34–84 % of sentinel nodes are located in unexpected (discordant) sites [86]. Lymph node mapping is important as the presence of lymph node metastases, as well as the number of nodes involved, remains the single most important prognostic factor for patients with stages I, II, or III disease [71].

In a study of 466 patients with known primary cutaneous melanoma who developed metastases, 50 % metastasized to the regional lymph node, 22 % to loco-regional sites, and 28 % to distant sites [87]. The median latency period for nodal metastases, similar to loco-regional spread, was found to be approximately a year and a half.

MUP is a unique and not uncommon phenomenon, occurring in 10–20 % of patients presenting with palpable regional disease [33]. The clinical presentation of MUP with nodal metastases is characterized by palpable lymphadenopathy without evidence of further metastatic disease and without apparent primary melanoma. Prognostic significance is unclear compared with melanoma of known primary (MKP), largely due to studies with small sample sizes and lack of control for prognostic variables. In a large single institution study, Lee et al. found improved overall survival after appropriate lymphadenectomy in patients with MUP as compared to MKP [65], which suggests that, in the absence of distant metastases, surgical excision of the positive nodes may have been curative for some MUP patients.

Besides external factors, proposed causes of MUP include de novo transformation of ectopic nodal melanocytes or spontaneous regression of a primary lesion. In support of the first hypothesis, benign nevus cells have been found in lymph nodes [88, 89]. These melanocytes may originate from benign metastasis or differentiated neural crest cells [90]. The problem with this hypothesis, as Lee et al. point out, is that it does not explain the survival benefit in patients with MUP. The second explanation suggests immune-mediated regression of the primary tumor. Circulating factor has been found to be present in regressed melanomas and is important in mediating cytotoxic responses [91], and anti-melanoma antibodies are more prevalent in MUP than in MKP [92]. Moreover, the presence of tumor infiltrating lymphocytes has been associated with regression patterns [93]. These results suggest that a combination of humoral and cytotoxic responses is involved in melanoma rejection. Finally, the most obvious explanation for improved survival in MUP is reduced disease burden, as patients with MUP undergo lymphadenectomy, which may also act to drive the activated immune system.

3 Non-cutaneous Melanomas

Normal melanocytes can be found in non-cutaneous sites, including the eye and mucosal tissues, such as the oral cavity, esophagus, nasal cavity and sinuses, genitals, and anus. Malignant transformation can occur in any of these sites. These subtypes of melanoma are less common than cutaneous melanoma and appear to be biologically distinct as well, given their patterns of spread and response to systemic therapy.

3.1 Uveal Melanomas

Two thousand new cases of uveal melanoma are diagnosed annually in the USA, an incidence that is much lower than cutaneous melanoma, and the incidence of uveal melanoma has been stable for the past decades, unlike cutaneous disease [94, 95]. This is the most common form of intraocular malignancy. The median age at presentation is in the 6th decade of life; however, it can also be diagnosed in young adults and children. The incidence does not differ between the genders, unlike cutaneous melanoma, which is more common in males. Familial cases of uveal melanoma are rarely reported. Only rare cases of uveal melanoma might have a heritable component, while family history is positive in 10 % of patients with cutaneous melanoma (Eagan et al. 1998). More recently, germline mutations in the BAP1 gene have been shown to be associated with uveal melanoma [96]. Approximately 50 % of patients with uveal melanoma will develop distant metastases, an incidence that is significantly higher than that of cutaneous melanoma [94].

Melanoma can arise in any of the three components of the uvea—the iris, the ciliary body, or the choroid. The latter is the most common site and represents the site of origin in 80 % of cases. The most common symptom at presentation is visual; patients typically report blurry vision or floaters when the disease is more advanced. However, uveal melanoma is often found on routine eye examination. Confirmation is accurately done by ultrasound and fluorescein angiography; fine needle aspiration biopsy is rarely needed and is no longer the standard of care to establish the diagnosis [97].

Staging of uveal melanoma is based on thickness and diameter, and these parameters correlate with survival. Given the lack of lymphatic drainage in the eye, dissemination to distant organs is hematogenous. Uveal melanomas appear to have a predilection to metastasizing to the liver more frequently than cutaneous melanomas and tend to have different driver mutations than cutaneous melanomas [97]. Gene expression assays and cytogenetics play a role in determining the prognosis for non-metastatic uveal melanoma and are currently widely used in combination with measures of depth, location, and diameter to determine whether surveillance for distant disease is warranted [98].

Most frequently, metastatic uveal melanomas home to the liver and are diagnosed due to ascites, right upper quadrant pain or jaundice. Typically, at this point, the disease is very advanced and the prognosis is often poor, as the liver metastases are difficult to control with local or systemic therapy. Less frequently, the primary site of metastases is the lungs or skin. Under these circumstances, patients present either with lung nodules incidentally found on surveillance imaging or imaging done for other purposes or with respiratory symptoms, or cutaneous or subcutaneous nodules. Given that spread is hematogenous, metastatic uveal melanoma is typically not diagnosed by lymphadenopathy as the presenting sign.

In the era of targeted therapies, metastatic uveal melanoma is treated with different drugs than metastatic melanoma of cutaneous origin. Overall, the prognosis for metastatic uveal melanoma is worse than for metastatic cutaneous melanoma, as this disease is less responsive to immune therapy and currently available targeted therapies [99]. It similarly responds poorly to chemotherapy. A recent trial demonstrated superiority of an inhibitor of MEK over standard chemotherapy—dacarbazine or temozolomide—in progression-free survival [100]. Disease presentation is dependent on the location of metastases.

3.2 Mucosal Melanomas

Similar to uveal melanoma, mucosal melanomas are substantially less common than their cutaneous counterparts [101]. These tumors can arise from any mucosal surface, and their presentation depends largely on the site of origin. Just over half the cases originate in the head and neck region (oral, nasal, and sinus mucosa), while the other half originate in the anal/genital mucosal surfaces. Rare sites of origin of mucosal melanoma include the lower urinary tract, esophagus, small intestine, and gallbladder [102]. The presentation of mucosal melanomas depends on the site of origin. Clearly, mucosal melanoma originating in the oral cavity, anus, and vulva is less likely to go undetected for a prolonged period of time than that originating in internal sites.

Unlike cutaneous melanoma, mucosal melanomas are found with similar frequency in patients of Black, Hispanic, or Asian origin, compared to non-Hispanic Caucasians. The incidence of mucosal melanoma increases substantially with age, and the likelihood of developing metastatic disease is higher than for cutaneous melanoma. Specifically, the survival is particularly poor for melanomas that arise in the pharynx, gastrointestinal tract (including anus), urinary tract, and vagina. This appears to be independent of the stage at diagnosis [103].

Primary mucosal melanomas of the head and neck can be divided into two major categories: melanoma of the sino-nasal cavities and melanoma of the oropharynx. The majority of case series are fairly small, and the data on presentation are sparse. For example, in a series of patients with mucosal melanoma of the head and neck seen at Emory University during a 20-year period, only 30 cases were identified. Just over half the patients (53 %) presented with early-stage disease. Mucosal melanoma was more prevalent in men (60 % of patients), and the median age was in the late 60s [104]. In a series from the Royal Marsden Hospital, 89 patients were identified during a period of 50 years [105].

Data on the presentation of melanomas that arise in the genitalia are similarly sparse. In a review of gynecologic melanoma cases seen at Duke University, 43 cases were seen during a 25-year period. Most other published case series involve a similar or smaller number of patients [106]. Of the 43 cases identified at Duke, 70 % were vulvar in origin, 21 % vaginal, and 9 % cervical. Most of the patients were older (median age 61 years) and about two-thirds presented with localized disease only. Most of the patients were diagnosed upon routine gynecological examination and were treated with radical surgical procedures, which did not appear to improve the outcome. The prognosis was poor overall, with less than half the patients alive at 5 years. The prognosis, however, has been reported to be slightly superior in melanomas arising in the vulva than those arising in other sites [107]. Given the sparse data (110 cases in this series of mucosal melanomas from all origins), it is unclear whether the improved survival in vulvar melanomas is independent of thickness and other prognostic variables, as these melanomas are more likely to be seen on routine gynecologic examination.

Anal or anorectal mucosal melanomas are similarly rare, although the incidence appears to be increasing [108]. In a series from Memorial Sloan Kettering Cancer Center of 96 patients seen over a 17-year period, 43 % had anal melanoma, 33 % anorectal melanoma, and 24 % rectal melanoma. Overall, anal lesions tended to be thinner than lesions that were more proximal and tended to be of earlier stage with a lower likelihood of lymph node involvement. Interestingly, patterns of recurrence also differed based on anatomic location. However, the rates of recurrence and overall survival were not significantly different between the groups. The diagnosis of anal and anorectal melanoma is often delayed because these tumors can be amelanotic; 20–25 % of cases have no pigment and can be difficult to distinguish from benign masses [109].

4 Presentation of Metastatic Cutaneous Melanoma

4.1 Presentation of Metastatic Cutaneous Melanoma of Known Primary Site

The rate of metastatic relapse among patients with early-stage melanoma varies depending on key prognostic factors: Breslow depth, mitotic rate, presence of ulceration, and lymph node involvement. These factors make up the current

American Joint Committee on Cancer staging system. The likelihood of metastatic dissemination in patients with stage I–III melanoma is between 10 and 80 %, depending on these prognostic variables. For example, a patient with stage IA disease has a 10 % chance of developing metastatic disease over 15 years, a patient with stage IIA disease has a 40 % chance, and a patient with stage IIIC disease has approximately a 80 % chance of developing metastatic disease over a similar period [70, 72].

Patients with a history of primary melanoma are typically monitored for disease recurrence. Other than pathologic staging at diagnosis, blood tests and imaging are used to verify that a patient does not have stage IV disease. Patients are then followed with serial physical examinations, blood tests, and imaging. There is no consensus regarding which imaging studies to do and when to do them. The National Comprehensive Cancer Network (NCCN) recommends imaging for stage I patients only if they have symptoms. For stage II patients, a chest X-ray is optional; and for stage IIB and IIC and III, CT scans, PET scans, and MRI are recommended as clinically indicated (www.NCCN.org). Surveillance practices are therefore highly variable.

Presentation of metastatic cutaneous melanoma varies based on the location of metastases. Approximately half the patients have a single site of distant metastasis at initial presentation. Common sites of distant disease include cutaneous and subcutaneous tissues (approximately 20 %), lungs, liver, and brain (approximately 50 % each). Less common sites of metastatic dissemination include the bones, bowels, adrenal glands, and heart [110, 111].

The time to development of metastatic disease is highly variable. In a series of patients undergoing surveillance at Yale University, the majority of recurrences occurred by the end of the third year of follow-up, with 47 % recurring in the first year and 32 % in the second year. Median interval between the first visit and time to recurrence was 10.6 months, suggesting that follow-up should be more frequent and involve additional laboratory and imaging studies in the initial years after diagnosis [112].

4.2 Presentation of Metastatic Cutaneous Melanoma of Unknown Primary Site

Metastatic melanoma of unknown primary can present in lymph nodes alone or in distant organs as well as in lymph nodes. Nodal disease alone or limited dermal metastases alone are thought to be stage III melanoma of unknown primary, described in Sect. 3.2. This section focuses on stage IV metastatic melanoma of unknown primary.

Up to 20 % of metastatic melanomas are of unknown primary site, depending on the series [113]. Genotyping of metastatic melanomas of unknown primary indicates a mutational pattern similar to that of cutaneous melanoma, rather than other melanoma subtypes such as mucosal melanoma [114]. A number of potential etiologies for melanoma of unknown primary site have been proposed; the most likely etiology is the regression of melanocytes at the primary site due to activity of tumor infiltrating lymphocytes, as reviewed by Lee et al. Other plausible explanations for melanoma of unknown primary site include malignant transformation of ectopic melanocytes, inability to differentiate a primary melanoma from benign nevi based on appearance, and resection of the primary lesion without pathologic examination of the biopsy site [33].

Presentation of stage IV melanoma of unknown primary is dependent on the site of metastasis. In a series of 398 cases from the John Wayne Cancer Center, over half had stage M1C disease at presentation (involvement of visceral organs other than the lungs and/or elevation of lactate dehydrogenase levels). Over half had more than one site of metastatic involvement, similar to the presentation of metastatic cutaneous MKP site. The prognosis in this series, as in other series of melanoma of unknown primary, appears to be superior to that of melanoma of known primary site, when adjusted for stage at presentation of metastatic disease [33] and [88, 115–118].

5 Summary

In this chapter, we summarized the clinical presentation of cutaneous, uveal, and mucosal melanomas. Each of these categories includes a mixed group of primary sites of origin, as melanoma can originate in pigmented cells at any physical location. The extent of disease at presentation influences the signs and symptoms with which patients will present. Overall, less extensive disease is associated with improved survival. Given the increasing incidence of this disease, heightened awareness is warranted, as it might lead to earlier detection.

References

1. Clemente C, Cook M, Ruiter D, Mihm M (2001) Histopathologic diagnosis of melanoma. World Health Organization melanoma programme publications, Milan, Trezzano SN
2. Bolognia JB, Jorizzo JL, Schaffer JV (2012) Dermatology. Saunders, Philadelphia
3. Ackerman A, Cerroni L, Kerl H (1994) Pitfalls in histopathologic diagnosis of malignant melanoma. Lea & Febiger, Philadelphia
4. Lipsker D, Engel F, Cribier B et al (2007) Trends in melanoma epidemiology suggest three different types of melanoma. Br J Dermatol 157(2):338–343
5. Swerdlow AJ, English J, Mackie RM et al (1986) Benign melanocytic naevi as a risk factor for malignant melanoma. Br Med J (Clin Res Ed) 292:1555–1559
6. Weiss J, Bertz J, Jung EG (1991) Malignant melanoma in southern Germany: different predictive value of risk factors for melanoma subtypes. Dermatologica 183:109–113
7. Argenziano G, Soyer HP, Chimenti S et al (2003) Dermoscopy of pigmented skin lesions: results of a consensus meeting via the internet. J Am Acad Dermatol 48:679–693
8. Demierre MF et al (2005) Early detection of thick melanomas in the United States: beware of the nodular subtype. Arch Dermatol 141(6):745–750
9. Koch SE, Lange JR (2000) Amelanotic melanoma: the great masquerader. J Am Acad Dermatol 42:731–734

10. Weinstock MA, Sober AJ (1987) The risk of progression of lentigo maligna to lentigo maligna melanoma. Br J Dermatol 116:303–310
11. Stolz W, Schiffner R, Burgdorf WH (2002) Dermatoscopy for facial pigmented skin lesions. Clin Dermatol 20:276–278
12. Shaw JH, Koea JB (1988) Acral (volar-subungual) melanoma in Auckland New Zealand. Br J Surg 75:69–72
13. Phan A, Touzet S, Dalle S et al (2007) Acral lentiginous melanoma: histopathological prognostic features of 121 cases. Br J Dermatol 157(2):311–318
14. Skender-Kalnenas TM, English DR, Heenan PJ (1995) Benign melanocytic lesions: risk markers or precursors of cutaneous melanoma? J Am Acad Dermatol 33:1000–1007
15. Bauer J, Garbe C (2004) Risk estimation for malignant transformation of melanocytic nevi. Arch Dermatol 140:127
16. Tsao H, Bevona C, Goggins W, Quinn T (2003) The transformation rate of moles (melanocytic nevi) into cutaneous melanoma. A population based estimate. Arch Dermatol 139:282–288
17. Garbe C, Buttner P, Weiss J et al (1994) Risk factors for developing cutaneous melanoma and criteria for identifying persons at risk: multicenter case-control study of the central malignant melanoma registry of the German Dermatological Society. J Invest Dermatol 102:695–699
18. Caballos P, Barnhill R (1993) Spontaneous regression of cutaneous tumors. Adv Dermatol 8:229–261
19. Nestle FO, Burg G, Dummer R (1999) New perspectives on immunobiology and immunotherapy of melanoma. Immunol Today 20:5–7
20. Marincola FM, Jaffee EM, Hicklin DJ, Ferrone S (2000) Escape of human solid tumors from T-cell recognition: molecular mechanisms and functional significance. Adv Immunol 74:181–273
21. Barr RJ (1994) The many faces of completely regressed malignant melanoma. Pathology (Phila) 2(2):359–370
22. Hayes PJ, Malone JC, Brown TC (2014) New blue-black nodule in a patient with a history of melanoma. JAMA Dermatol 150:767–768
23. McGovern VJ, Shaw HM, Milton GW (1983) Prognosis in patients with thin malignant melanoma: influence of regression. Histopathology 7:673–680
24. Abramova L, Slingluff CLJR, Patterson JW (2002) Problems in the interpretation of apparent "radial growth phase" malignant melanomas that metastasize. J Cutan Pathol 29:407–414
25. Ceballos PI, Barnhill RL (1993) Spontaneous regression of cutaneous tumors. Adv Dermatol 8:229–261
26. Boon T, Cerottini JC, Van den Eynde B et al (1994) Tumor antigens recognized by T lymphocytes. Annu Rev Immunol 12:337–365
27. Menzies SW, McCarthy WH (1997) Complete regression of primary cutaneous malignant melanoma. Arch Surg 132:553–556
28. Guitart J, Lowe L, Piepkorn M et al (2002) Histological characteristics of metastasizing thin melanomas. Arch Dermatol 138:603–608
29. Clark WH, Elder DE, Guerry D et al (1989) Model predicting survival in stage I melanoma based on tumor progression. J Natl Cancer Inst 81:1893–1904
30. Ronan SG, Eng AM, Briele HA et al (1987) Thin malignant melanomas with regression and metastases. Arch Dermatol 123:1326–1330
31. Fontaine D, Parkhill W, Greer W et al (2003) Partial regression of primary cutaneous melanoma. Am J Dermatopathol 25:371–373
32. Shaw HM, McCarthy WH, McCarthy SW et al (1987) Thin malignant melanomas and recurrence potential. Arch Surg 122:1147–1150
33. Lee CC, Faries MB, Wanek LA, Morton DL (2008) Improved survival after lymphadenectomy for nodal metastasis from an unknown primary melanoma. J Clin Oncol 26:535–541

34. Prens SP, van der Ploeg AP, van Akkooi AC, van Montfort CA, van Geel AN et al (2011) Outcome after therapeutic lymph node dissection in patients with unknown primary melanoma site. Ann Surg Oncol 13:3586–3592
35. High WA, Steward D, Wilbers CRH et al (2005) Completely regressed primary cutaneous malignant melanoma with nodal and/or visceral metastases: a report of 5 cases and assessment of the literature and diagnostic criteria. J Am Acad Dermatol 53(1):89–100
36. McClain SE, Mayo KB, Shada AL et al (2012) Amelanotic melanomas presenting as red skin lesions: a diagnostic challenge with potentially lethal consequences. Int J Dermatol 51 (4):420–426
37. Bastian BC (2002) Molecular cytogenetics as a diagnostic tool for typing melanocytic tumors. Recent Results Cancer Res 160:92–99
38. Bauer J, Bastian BC (2006) Distinguishing melanocytic nevi from melanoma by DNA copy number changes: comparative genomic hybridization as a research and diagnostic tool. Dermatol Ther 19:40–49
39. Sangüeza M, Zelger B (2007) Melanoma simulating atypical fibroxanthoma. Am J Dermatopathol 29(6):551–554
40. Diaz-Cascajo C, Weyers W, Borghi S (2003) Pigmented atypical fibroxanthoma: a tumor that may be easily mistaken for malignant melanoma. Am J Dermatopathol 25:1–5
41. McGregor DH, Cherian R, Romanas MM et al (2008) Amelanotic malignant melanoma: two collision tumors presenting as basal cell carcinoma and atypical fibroxanthoma. Ann Clin Lab Sci 38(2):157–162
42. Hiscutt EL, Adams JR, Ryan JM, Langtry JA et al (2009) Atypical fibroxanthoma, lentigo maligna melanoma and squamous cell carcinoma arising in the site of a thermal burn treated with skin grafts. Br J Oral Maxillofac Surg 47(2):157–158
43. Kossard S (2002) Atypical lentiginous junctional naevi of the elderly and melanoma. Aust J Dermatol 43(2):93–101
44. Pralong P, Bathelier E, Dalle S et al (2012) Dermoscopy of lentigo maligna melanoma: report of 125 cases. Br J Dermatol 167(2):280–287
45. Quinn MJ, Crotty KA, Thompson JF, et al (1998) Desmoplastic and desmoplastic neurotropic melanoma: experience with 280 patients. Cancer 83:1128–35
46. Jaimes N, Chen L, Dusza SW, Carrera C et al (2013) Clinical and dermoscopic characteristics of desmoplastic melanomas. JAMA Dermatol 149(4):413–421
47. McCarthy SW, Scolyer RA, Palmer AA (2004) Desmoplastic melanoma: a diagnostic trap for the unwary. Pathology 36(5):445–451
48. Gartner MF, Fearns C, Wilson EL, et al (1992) Unusual growth characteristics of human melanoma xenografts in the nude mouse: a model for desmoplasia, dormancy and progression. Br J Cancer 65:487–90
49. Fearns C, Dowdle EB The desmoplastic response: induction of collagen synthesis by melanoma cells in vitro. Int J Cancer 50:621–7
50. Bryant E, Ronan SG, Felix EL, Manaligod JR (1982) Desmoplastic malignant melanoma: a study by conventional and electron micro-scopy. Am J Dermatopathol 4:467–474
51. From L, Hanna W, Kahn HJ, Gruss J, Marks A, Baumal R (1983) Origin of the desmoplasia in desmoplastic malignant melanoma. Hum Pathol 14:1072–1080
52. De Almeida LS, Requena L, Rutten A et al (2008) Desmoplastic malignant melanoma: a clinicopathologic analysis of 113 cases. Am J Dermatopathol 30:207–215
53. Zettersten E, Sagebiel RW, Miller III Jr et al (2002) Prognostic factors in patients with thick cutaneous melanoma (>4 mm). Cancer 94:1049–1056
54. Hudson DA, Krige JE (1995) Melanoma in black South Africans. J Am Coll Surg 180:65–71
55. Chang JW, Yeh KY, Wang CH et al (2004) Malignant melanoma in Taiwan: a prognostic study of 181 cases. Melanoma Res 14:537–541
56. Cress RD, Holly EA (1997) Incidence of cutaneous melanoma among non-Hispanic whites, Hispanics, Asians, and blacks: an analysis of California cancer registry data, 1988–93. Cancer Causes Control 8:246–252

57. Cress RD, Holly EA (1997) Incidence of cutaneous melanoma among non-Hispanic whites, Hispanics, Asians and blacks: an analysis of California cancer registry data, 1988–93. Cancer Causes Control 8:246
58. Curtin JA, Fridlyand J, Kageshita T et al (2005) Distinct sets of genetic alterations in melanoma. N Engl J Med 353:2135–2147
59. Torres-Cabala CA, Wang WL, Trent J et al (2009) Correlation between KIT expression and KIT mutation in melanoma: a study of 173 cases with emphasis on the acral-lentiginous/mucosal type. Mod Pathol 22:1446–1456
60. Stern DK, Creasey AA, Quijije J et al (2011) UVA and UVB penetration of normal human cadaveric fingernail plate. Arch Dermatol 147(4):439–441
61. Gosselink CP, Sindone JL, Meadows BJ et al (2009) Amelanotic subungual melanoma: a case report. J Foot Ankle Surg 48(2):220–224
62. Mohrle M, Hafner HM (2002) Is subungual melanoma related to trauma? Dermatology 204 (4):259–261
63. Bormann G, Marsch WC, Haerting J et al (2006) Concomitant traumas influence prognosis in melanomas of the nail apparatus. Br J Dermatol 155(1):76–80
64. Reintgen DS, Cox C, Slingluff CLJ, Seigler HF (1992) Recurrent malignant melanoma: the identification of prognostic factors to predict survival. Ann Plast Surg 28:45–49
65. Mathes SJ and Hentz VR (2006) Malignant melanoma. Saunders, Philadelphia
66. Erol B, Ufuk U, Husamettin T et al (2008) True hematogenous metastases of melanoma on contralateral skin graft donor site: a case report. Melanoma Res 18(6):443–446
67. Hall JG, Herman C, Cook JL et al (2005) Melanoma arising in a skin graft. Ann Plast Surg 54:92–96
68. Mueller BM, Reisfeld RA, Edgington TS et al (1992) Expression of tissue factor by melanoma cells promotes efficient hematogenous metastasis. Proc Natl Acad Sci USA 89:11832–11836
69. Bromberg ME, Konigsberg WH, Madison JF et al (1995) Tissue factor promotes melanoma metastasis by a pathway independent of blood coagulation. Proc Natl Acad Sci USA 92:8205–8209
70. Balch CM, Gershenwald JE, Soong SJ, Thompson JF, Atkins MB et al (2009) Final version of 2009 AJCC melanoma staging and classification. J Clin Oncol 27:6199–6206
71. Weide B, Faller C, Büttner P, Pflugfelder A et al (2013) Prognostic factors of melanoma patients with satellite or in-transit metastasis at the time of stage III diagnosis. PLoS One 8 (4):e63137
72. Balch CM, Gershenwald JE, Soong SJ, Thompson JF, Atkins MB, Byrd DR, Buzaid AC, Cochran AJ, Coit DG, Ding S, Eggermont AM, Flaherty KT, Gimotty PA, Kirkwood JM, McMasters KM, Mihm MC Jr, Morton DL, Ross MI, Sober AJ, Sondak VK (2009) Final version of 2009 AJCC melanoma staging and classification. J Clin Oncol 27(36):6199–6206. doi:10.1200/JCO.2009.23.4799 Epub 2009 Nov 16
73. Wong JH, Cagle LA, Kopald KH et al (1990) Natural history and selective management of in transit melanoma. J Surg Oncol 44:146–150
74. Cascinelli N, Bufalino R, Marolda R et al (1986) Regional non-nodal metastases of cutaneous melanoma. Eur J Surg Oncol 12:175–180
75. Calabro A, Singletary SE, Balch CM (1989) Patterns of relapse in 1001 consecutive patients with melanoma nodal metastases. Arch Surg 124:1051–1055
76. Zogakis TG, Bartlett DL, Libutti SK et al (2001) Factors affecting survival after complete response to isolated limb perfusion in patients with in-transit melanoma. Ann Surg Oncol 8:771–778
77. Francken AB, Accortt NA, Shaw HM, Wiener M, Soong SJ et al (2008) Prognosis and determinants of outcome following locoregional or distant recurrence in patients with cutaneous melanoma. Ann Surg Oncol 15:1476–1484
78. Roses DF, Karp NS, Oratz R, Dubin N, Harris MN et al (1991) Survival with regional and distant metastases from cutaneous malignant melanoma. Surg Gynecol Obstet 172:262–268

79. Kretschmer L, Preusser KP, Marsch WC, Neumann C (2000) Prognostic factors of overall survival in patients with delayed lymph node dissection for cutaneous malignant melanoma. Melanoma Res 10:483–489
80. Karakousis CP, Choe KJ, Holyoke ED (1980) Biologic behavior and treatment of intransit metastasis of melanoma. Surg Gynecol Obstet 150:29–32
81. Estourgie SH, Nieweg OE, Valdes Olmos RA et al (2003) Review and evaluation of sentinel node procedures in 250 melanoma patients with a median follow-up of 6 years. Ann Surg Oncol 10:681–688
82. Estourgie SH, Nieweg OE, Kroon BB (2004) High incidence of in-transit metastases after sentinel node biopsy in patients with melanoma. Br J Surg 91:1370–1371
83. Pawlik TM, Ross MI, Thompson JF et al (2005) The risk of in-transit melanoma metastasis depends on tumor biology and not the surgical approach to regional lymph nodes. J Clin Oncol 23(21):4588–4590
84. Van Poll D, Thompson JF, McKinnon JG et al (2005) A sentinel node biopsy does not increase the incidence of in-transit metastasis in patients with primary cutaneous melanoma. Ann Surg Oncol 12(8):597–608
85. Kretschmer L, Beckmann I, Thoms KM et al (2005) Sentinel lymphonodectomy does not increase the risk of loco-regional cutaneous metastases of malignant melanomas. Eur J Cancer 41:531–538
86. Thompson JF, Uren RF, Shaw HM et al (1999) Location of sentinel lymph nodes in patients with cutaneous melanoma: new insights into lymphatic anatomy. J Am Coll Surg 189:195–204
87. Meier F, Will S, Ellwanger U et al (2002) Metastatic pathways and time courses in the orderly progression of cutaneous melanoma. Br J Dermatol 147:62–70
88. Das Gupta T, Bowden L, Berg JW (1963) Malignant melanoma of unknown primary origin. Surg Gynecol Obstet 117:341–345
89. Ridolfi RL, Rosen PP, Thaler H (1977) Nevus cell aggregates associated with lymph nodes: Estimated frequency and clinical significance. Cancer 39:164–171
90. Shenoy BV, Fort L 3rd, Benjamin SP (1987) Malignant melanoma primary in lymph node: the case of the missing link. Am J Surg Pathol 11:140–146
91. Maurer H, McIntyre OR, Rueckert F (1974) Spontaneous regression of malignant melanoma: pathologic and immunologic study in a ten year survivor. Am J Surg 127:397–403
92. Giuliano AE, Moseley HS, Irie RF et al (1980) Immunologic aspects of unknown primary melanoma. Surgery 87:101–105
93. Tefany FJ, Barnetson RS, Halliday GM et al (1991) Immunocytochemical analysis of the cellular infiltrate in primary regressing and non-regressing malignant melanoma. J Invest Dermatol 97:197–202
94. Singh AD, Topham A (2003) Incidence of uveal melanoma in the United States: 1973–1997. Ophthalmology 110:956–961
95. Jemal A, Siegel R, Xu J, Ward E (2010) Cancer statistics, 2010. CA Cancer J Clin 60:277–300
96. Battaglia A (2014) The importance of multidisciplinary approach in early detection of BAP1 tumor predisposition syndrome: clinical management and risk assessment. Clin Med Insights Oncol 28(8):37–47
97. Materin MA, Faries M, Kluger HM (2011) Molecular alternations in uveal melanoma. Curr Probl Cancer 35(4):211–224
98. Field MG, Harbor JW (2014) Recent developments in prognostic and predictive testing in uveal melanoma. Curr Opin Ophthalmol 25(3):234–239
99. Luke JJ, Triozzi PL, McKenna KC, Van Meir EG, Gershenwald JE, Bastian BC, Gutkind JS, Bowcock AM, Streicher HZ, Patel PM, Sato T, Sossman JA, Sznol M, Welch J, Thurin M, Selig S, Flaherty KT, Carvajal RD (2014) Biology of advanced uveal melanoma and next steps for clinical therapeutics. Pigment Cell Melanoma Res 28:135–147

100. Carvajal RD, Sosman JA, Quevedo JF, Milhem MM, Joshua AM, Kudchadkar RR, Linette GP, Gajewski TF, Lutzky J, Lawson DH, Lao CD, Flynn PJ, Albertini MR, Sato T, Lewis K, Doyle A, Ancell K, Panageas KS, Bluth M, Hedvat C, Erinjeri J, Ambrosini G, Marr B, Abramson DH, Dickson MA, Wolchok JD, Chapman PB, Schwartz GK (2014) Effect of **selumetinib** vs chemotherapy on progression-free survival in uveal melanoma: a randomized clinical trial. JAMA 311(23):2397–2405
101. Chang AE, Karnell LH, Menck HR (1998) The national cancer data base report on cutaneous and noncutaneous melanoma: a summary of 84,836 cases from the past decade. The American College of surgeons commission on cancer and the American Cancer Society. Cancer 83:1664
102. Patrick RJ, Fenske NA, Messina JL (2007) Primary mucosal melanoma. J Am Acad Dermatol 56(5):828–834
103. Bishop KD, Olszewski AJ (2014) Epidemiology and survival outcomes of ocular and mucosal melanomas: a population-based analysis. Int J Cancer 134(12):2961–2971
104. McLean N, Tighiouart M, Muller S (2008) Primary **mucosal melanoma** of the head and neck. Comparison of clinical **presentation** and histopathologic features of oral and sinonasal **melanoma**. Oral Oncol 44(11):1039–1046. doi:10.1016/j.oraloncology.2008.01.014
105. Yii NW, Eisen T, Nicolson M, A'Hern R, Rhys-Evans P, Archer D, Henk JM, Gore ME (2003) **Mucosal** malignant **melanoma** of the head and neck: the Marsden experience over half a century. Clin Oncol (R Coll Radiol) 15(4):199–204
106. DeMatos P, Tyler D, Seigler HF (1998) Mucosal melanoma of the female genitalia: a clinicopathologic study of forty-three cases at Duke University Medical Center. Surgery 124 (1):38–48
107. Mehra T, Grözinger G, Mann S, Guenova E, Moos R, Röcken M, Claussen CD, Dummer R, Clasen S, Naumann A, Garbe C (2014) Primary localization and tumor thickness as prognostic factors of survival in patients with mucosal melanoma. PLoS One 9(11):e112535
108. Cagir B, Whiteford MH, Topham A, Rakinic J, Fry RD (1999) Changing epidemiology of anorectal melanoma. Dis Colon Rectum 42:1203–1208
109. Brady MS, Kavolius JP, Quan SH (1995) Anorectal melanoma: a 64-year experience at Memorial Sloan-Kettering Cancer Center. Dis Colon Rectum 38:146–151
110. Tas F (2012) Metastatic behavior in melanoma: timing, pattern, survival, and influencing factors. J Oncol 2012(647684)
111. Flanigan JC, Jilaveanu LB, Faries M, Sznol M, Ariyan S, Yu JB, Knisely JP, Chiang VL, Kluger HM (2011) Melanoma brain metastases: is it time to reassess the bias? Curr Probl Cancer 35(4):200–210
112. Poo-Hwu WJ, Ariyan S, Lamb L, Papac R, Zelterman D, Hu GL, Brown J, Fischer D, Bolognia J, Buzaid AC (1999) Follow-up recommendations for patients with American Joint Committee on cancer stages I-III malignant melanoma. Cancer 86:2252–2258
113. Lee CC, Faries MB, Wanek LA et al (2009) Improved survival for stage IV melanoma from an unknown primary site. J Clin Oncol 27:3489–3495
114. Egberts F, Bergner I, Krüger S, Haag J, Behrens HM, Hauschild A, Röcken C (2014) Metastatic melanoma of unknown primary resembles the genotype of cutaneous melanomas. Ann Oncol 25(1):246–250
115. King R, Page RN, Googe PB et al (2005) Lentiginous melanoma: a histologic pattern of melanoma to be distinguished from lentiginous nevus. Mod Pathol 18(10):1397–1401
116. Satzger I, Völker B, Kapp A, Gutzmer R (2007) Tumoral melanosis involving the sentinel lymph nodes: a case report. J Cutan Pathol 34(3):284–286
117. Essner R, Lee JH, Wanek LA, Itakura H, Morton DL (2004) Contemporary surgical treatment of advanced-stage melanoma. Arch Surg 139:961–966
118. Egan KM, Seddon JM, Glynn RJ, Gragoudas ES, Albert DM (1988) Epidemiologic aspects of uveal melanoma. Surv Ophthalmol 32:239–251

Principles of Melanoma Staging

Genevieve M. Boland and Jeffrey E. Gershenwald

Abstract

Although now commonplace in contemporary cancer care, the systematic approach to classification of disease-specific cancers into a formalized staging system is a relatively modern concept. Overall, the goals of cancer staging are to characterize the status of cancer at a specific moment in time, risk stratify, facilitate prognostication, and inform clinical decision making. The revisions to the American Joint Committee on Cancer (AJCC) melanoma staging system over time reflect changes in our understanding of the biology of the disease. Since the 1st edition, where tumor thickness was defined anatomically by its relationship to the reticular or papillary dermis (Clark level) as well as tumor thickness (Breslow thickness), there have been significant strides in our use of clinicopathological variables to stratify low- versus high-risk patients. Management of the regional nodal basin has also changed dramatically over time, impacted by techniques such as lymphatic mapping and sentinel lymph node biopsy (SLNB) and changes in pathological evaluation of the regional lymph nodes. Additionally, stratification of distant metastases has evolved as survival outcomes have been shown to vary based upon anatomic site of metastases and serum lactate dehydrogenase levels. The variables in use in the current

G.M. Boland (✉) · J.E. Gershenwald
Department of Surgical Oncology, The University of Texas MD Anderson Cancer Center, Houston, TX, USA
e-mail: gmboland@mdanderson.org

J.E. Gershenwald
e-mail: jgershen@mdanderson.org

H.L. Kaufman and J.M. Mehnert (eds.), *Melanoma*,
Cancer Treatment and Research 167, DOI 10.1007/978-3-319-22539-5_5

(7th edition) AJCC staging system are surrogate markers of biology with validated impact of survival outcomes. Going forward, it is likely that these and additional clinicopathological factors will be integrated with molecular and other correlates of melanoma tumor biology to further refine and personalize melanoma staging.

Contents

1 Introduction and History

Although now commonplace in contemporary cancer care, the systematic approach to classification and description of tissue-specific cancers into a formalized staging system is a relatively modern concept. The first approach to oncologic staging was undertaken by the League of Nations Health Organization in the 1920s, by creating a Cancer Commission to examine cancer-related mortality and begin to catalogue the incidence and mortality of cancer from specific organs [1]. The International Union against Cancer (UICC) in Europe created a Committee on Clinical Stage Classification and Applied Statistics in 1952, while in the USA, the American Joint Committee on Cancer (AJCC) was founded in 1959 for a similar purpose. The first edition of the AJCC Cancer Staging Manual was published in 1977, and the UICC and AJCC established a formal relationship in 1987 [2–4].

In 1947, Ackerman and Del Regato described a four-tier system for staging of cutaneous melanoma based upon observed differences in death rates for these separate groups and included patients with (1) distant metastases, (2) clinically positive, histologically positive regional nodal metastases, (3) clinically negative, histologically positive regional nodal metastases, and (4) clinically and pathologically negative regional nodes [5]. This preceded the official TNM staging system for melanoma, which was established in the early 1960s. Inadequacies of the original TNM classification prompted transition to the three-stage clinicopathological system proposed by McNeer and Das Gupta from Memorial Sloan-Kettering Cancer Center in 1964 [6]. In the late 1970s, a four-stage system was developed at the University of Texas MD Anderson Cancer Center to specifically address the subset of patients with local, intransit, and satellite lesions who may be appropriate for limb perfusion [7]. Up to this point, the staging systems were based primarily upon clinical criteria that failed to further-stage patients with isolated primary melanoma, a group that comprises the largest clinical group of patients with newly diagnosed melanoma.

In 1970, Breslow defined microstaging in a quantitative way by defining the maximal thickness of the tumor [8], and in 1978, Breslow et al. [9] and Balch et al. [10] independently compared Breslow depth and Clark level and showed that Breslow depth was a more powerful and reproducible prognostic factor in melanoma. This allowed classification of the primary lesion based upon microscopic assessment of tumor depth of invasion. This technique requires identification of the deepest part of the tumor by the pathologist and measurement of the thickness in millimeters (mm), as defined by Breslow [8, 11]. According to College of American Pathologists (CAP) 2011 guidelines, "Maximum tumor thickness is measured with a calibrated ocular micrometer at a right angle to the adjacent normal skin. The upper point of reference is the granular layer of the epidermis of the overlying skin or, if the lesion is ulcerated, the base of the ulcer. The lower reference point is the deepest point of tumor invasion (i.e., the leading edge of a single mass or an isolated group of cells deep to the main mass)." (http://www.cap.org/apps/docs/committees/cancer/cancer_protocols/2011/SkinMelanoma_11protocol.pdf.) In multiple studies using multifactorial analysis, tumor thickness remains the most powerful predictor of survival [10, 12–15] and is the dominant variable in assigning patients to a T stage.

The AJCC published the first formalized staging system incorporating microstaging of the primary tumor in 1977 [16]. Stage I was classified by primary lesions and was divided into subgroups based upon the spread into the papillary dermis (level II) and/or ≤0.75 mm thick (IA) versus the papillary–reticular dermal interface (level III) and/or if 0.76–1.5 mm thick (IB). Stage II included patients with first station regional nodal spread or satellites within 2 cm of the primary lesion. Stage III included patients with massive or fixed regional lymph nodes or contralateral/bilateral nodal involvement. Stage IV included patients with distant metastases (Table 1). However, this staging system was not well received due to the over-simplification of stage I and II criteria and the vague nature of the definition of stage III disease [16–18]. In 1983, the AJCC melanoma staging system was updated to include more meaningful points for tumor thickness, a transition of intransit metastases from stage II to stages III or IV, and a restructuring of nodal disease into the appropriate stage categories based upon regional nodal versus distant nodal spread. At that time, it was appreciated that the concept of nodal burden was important and the new system included quantification of node size and number of intransit metastases. While more precise than the previous system, the staging system remained quite complex and did not gain popularity for this reason [17].

In 2001, the 6th edition of the AJCC staging manual for cancer included significant revisions based upon the analysis of 17,600 patients in the AJCC melanoma staging database [15]. T-category criteria were narrowed to include only Breslow

Table 1 1977 (1st edition) AJCC staging system for melanoma [16] (need to obtain permission)

Primary tumor	
T1	Invasion of papillary dermis and/or <0.75 mm thickness Tla: Satellite(s) within immediate or regional area of the primary lesion Tib: Intransit metastasis directed towards lymph node-draining basin
T2	Papillary-reticular dermis interface and/or 0.75–1.5 mm thickness Tla: Satellite(s) within immediate or regional area of the primary lesion Tib: Intransit metastasis directed towards lymph node-draining basin
T3	Reticular dermis and/or 1.51–3.0 mm thickness Tla: Satellite(s) within immediate or regional area of the primary lesion Tib: Intransit metastasis directed towards lymph node-draining basin
T4	Subcutaneous tissue and/or greater than 3 mm thickness Tla: Satellite(s) within immediate or regional area of the primary lesion Tib: Intransit metastasis directed towards lymph node-draining basin
Nodal involvement	
N0	No regional lymph node involvement
N1	Regional lymph node involvement of first station nodes only
N2	Lymph node involvement other than first station nodes
Distant metastasis	
Mx	Not assessed
M0	No known distant metastases
Ml	Distant metastasis present: specify site

thickness with thresholds of 1.0, 2.0, and 4.0 mm. The stage IV data cohort was expanded fivefold and contained data relating to the prognostic value of serum lactate dehydrogenase (LDH) level [15]. In 2009, the 7th edition of the AJCC system was published and included formal evaluation of the role of mitotic rate as a prognostic factor and assessment of nodal tumor burden to assess the role of lymphatic mapping and sentinel lymph node biopsy (SLNB) for staging of regional nodes. The criteria used for stage III was re-assessed and re-evaluated [19].

The revisions of the AJCC melanoma staging system reflect changes in our understanding of the biology of melanoma. The first edition defined tumor thickness anatomically, by Clark level and Breslow thickness. Over time, primary tumor criteria have become progressively more refined with the inclusion of an assessment of primary tumor ulceration and mitotic activity. Management of the regional nodal basin has also evolved significantly. For example, patients with primary cutaneous melanoma and clinically negative regional nodes deemed to have sufficient risk of occult microscopic regional metastasis are offered surgical evaluation of these regional nodal basins at risk using techniques such as lymphatic mapping and sentinel lymph node biopsy (SLNB) and more enhanced pathological evaluation of the sentinel nodes [20, 21]. Finally, stratification of distant metastases has evolved, as survival outcome analyses have demonstrated differences based upon site(s) of distant metastases and the presence of elevated serum LDH [19].

Overall, the goals of cancer staging are to characterize and communicate cancer status at a specific time, risk stratify, offer prognostic insight, and inform our clinical treatment decision-making process. The variables included in the current AJCC staging system reflect surrogate markers of biology with validated impact of survival outcomes. A vision for the future is to combine these and additional clinicopathological factors with new data analytics and molecular data to better personalize prognostic information and to distinguish differences in tumor biology with associated clinical impact.

2 TNM Classification (Table 1)

2.1 Primary Tumor (T)

Currently, TX indicates that the tumor cannot be assessed, whereas T0 means there is no evidence of primary tumor. Tis represents melanoma in situ, a situation in which abnormal melanocytes are present, but are confined to the epidermis of the skin. The remaining T classifications (T1–T4) collectively describing invasive melanomas (i.e., with dermal involvement) are defined by tumor thickness (Breslow) measured in mm (T1 ≤ 1 mm; T2 1.01–2.00 mm; T3 2.01–4.00; T4 > 4.0 mm) (Table 2). Multivariate analyses from multiple studies have demonstrated that Breslow tumor thickness is the most powerful predictor of survival among patients with early-stage melanoma [10, 12–15]. Since the 6th edition of the AJCC staging manual, these tumor thickness cut points have been defined as integers (i.e., 1, 2, and 4 mm).

Primary tumor ulceration was also included as a T classification and staging criterion beginning with the 6th edition of the AJCC melanoma staging system, based on its independent adverse prognostic significance with respect to survival in many studies [14, 15, 22–26]. As per 2009 CAP guidelines, it is defined as the combination of a full-thickness epidermal defect, evidence of reactive changes, and thinning, effacement, or reactive hyperplasia of the surrounding epidermis without trauma or evidence of a recent surgical procedure (http://www.cap.org/apps/docs/committees/cancer/cancer_protocols/2011/SkinMelanoma_11protocol.pdf). Ulcerated primary tumors are designated with a "b" suffix (e.g., T1b), and non-ulcerated primary tumors are designated with an "a" suffix (e.g., T1a) (Table 2).

An additional pathological variable utilized in the T1 classification is primary tumor mitotic rate (units, mitoses per mm^2). Mitotic rate is determined using the dermal "hotspot" approach by assessing for the area of vertical growth phase containing the most mitotic figures, with inclusion of adjacent fields until an area of 1 mm^2 has been assessed (please refer to 7th edition AJCC melanoma staging system chapter for further details) [19, 27]. Multiple studies have demonstrated a lower survival for patients whose primary tumor has mitotic activity compared to those without mitoses [28–31]. In a multifactorial analysis of over 10,000 patients with localized melanoma, the AJCC melanoma staging database demonstrated that mitotic rate, when dichotomized as <1 mitosis/mm^2 versus ≥ 1 mitosis/mm^2, was

Table 2 AJCC 7th edition TNM staging categories for cutaneous melanoma [19]

Melanoma TNM classification		
Classification	Thickness (mm)	Ulceration Status/Mitoses
T		
Tis	NA	NA
T1	≤1.00 mm	a: Without ulceration and mitosis <1/mm^2
		b: With ulceration or mitoses ≥1/mm^2
T2	1.01–2.00 mm	a: Without ulceration
		b: With ulceration
T3	2.01–4.00 mm	a: Without ulceration
		b: With ulceration
T4	>4.00 mm	a: Without ulceration
		b: With ulceration
N	No. of metastatic nodes	Nodal metastatic burden
N0	0	NA
N1	1	a: Micrometastasis[a]
		b: Macrometastasis[b]
N2	2–3	a: Micrometastasis[a]
		b: Macrometastasis[b]
		c: In transit metastases/satellites without metastatic nodes
N3	4 + metastatic nodes, or matted nodes, or in transit metastases/satellites with metastatic nodes	
M	Site	Serum LDH
M0	No distant metastases	NA
M1a	Distant skin, subcutaneous, or nodal mets	Normal
M1b	Lung metastases	Normal
M1c	All other visceral metastases	Normal
	Any distant metastasis	Elevated
M	Site	Serum LDH
M0	No distant metastases	NA
M1a	Distant skin, subcutaneous, or nodal mets	Normal
M1b	Lung metastases	Normal
M1c	All other visceral metastases	Normal
	Any distant metastasis	Elevated

Abbreviations: *NA* not applicable; *LDH* lactate dehydrogenase

[a]Micrometastases are diagnosed after sentinel lymph node biopsy

[b]Macrometastases are defined as clinically detectable nodal metastases confirmed pathologically

From Balch et al. [19] with permission

second only to tumor thickness as a predictor of survival ($p < 0.0001$), especially among patients with T1 melanomas [19]. Therefore, in the AJCC 7th edition staging manual, mitotic rate replaced level of invasion in defining the T1b category, except in the rare circumstances when mitotic rate cannot be accurately determined

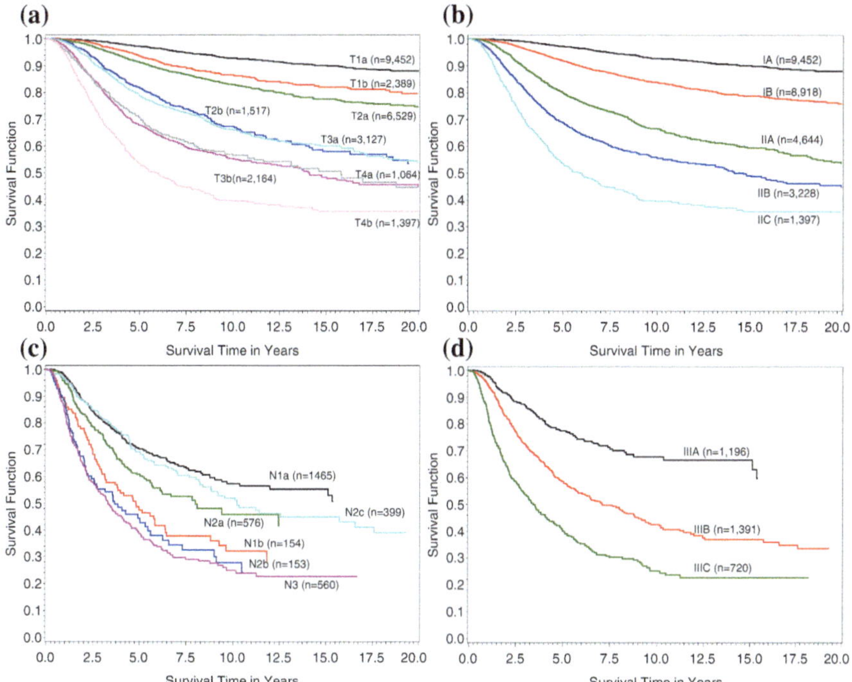

Fig. 1 Survival curves from the American Joint Committee on Cancer melanoma staging database comparing (**a**) the different T categories and (**b**) the stage groupings for stages I and II melanoma. For patients with stage III disease, survival curves are shown comparing (**c**) the different N categories and (**d**) the stage groupings. From Balch et al. [19] with permission

[19]. A subsequent expanded analysis of the 7th edition AJCC database supported this association between increasing mitotic rate (when explored as a continuous variable) and decreasing survival in patients with stage I and II disease [32].

For the remaining T categories, tumor thickness is stratified by integer cut points (T2, T3, and T4 as >1–2 mm, >2–4 mm, and >4 mm, respectively) with (b) versus (a) subclassification based on the presence or absence of primary tumor ulceration (Table 2). In the AJCC 7th edition, the 10-year survival rates for patients with T1, T2, T3, and T4 primary tumors were 92, 80, 63, and 50 %, respectively [19]. It has also been established that survival rates for patients with ulcerated primary tumors are worse than for those with non-ulcerated tumors of the same T category and actually quite similar to the survival rate of the next highest T category for non-ulcerated primaries (Fig. 1). For example, a T3a lesion (2.01–4 mm and non-ulcerated) has a 5-year survival of 79 versus 82 % for a T2b tumor (1.01–2 mm and ulcerated). Therefore, the presence of ulceration can group a T2 primary melanoma within stage IIA (rather than stage I), given the similarity of survival outcomes between thinner, ulcerated tumors and non-ulcerated tumors from the next higher T category [15].

2.2 Regional Lymph Nodes (N)

There is significant prognostic heterogeneity among patients with regional metastases. Since regional lymph nodes are the most common site of metastasis for patients who present with primary cutaneous melanoma, clinical and pathological evaluation of lymph nodes represent critical components of the melanoma staging system. Clinical staging relies upon the clinical and/or radiographic detection of metastasis-containing regional nodes, whereas pathological staging is dictated by pathological examination of the node(s) after sentinel lymph node biopsy (SLNB) or lymph node dissection (LND).

It is evident that tumor burden has a significant impact on survival outcomes and is an important prognostic factor. Several studies have shown that even limited regional node tumor burden is associated with poorer survival outcomes over time [33, 34]. Moreover, prospective randomized clinical trials, such as the Multicenter Selective Lymphadenectomy Trial-1 (MSLT-1) as well as other studies, demonstrate that patients with micrometastatic lymph node disease (i.e., detected pathologically in sentinel lymph nodes after SLNB) have significantly better survival rates than those who develop macrometastatic disease (i.e., detected clinically and confirmed by therapeutic lymphadenectomy OR when nodal metastases demonstrate gross extracapsular extension upon review of pathology) [14, 15, 19, 35–37].

Data from the AJCC melanoma staging database have demonstrated the importance of number of positive regional lymph nodes, regional node tumor burden (empirically defined in the 7th edition AJCC staging system as microscopic versus macroscopic), and the presence or absence of primary tumor ulceration as independent predictors of survival in patients with stage III melanoma (Tables 2, 3 and 4) [15, 19]. Importantly, at least some studies have reported that even small burden of nodal disease (including isolated tumor cells in sentinel nodes) can be associated with poorer melanoma-related outcomes [33, 34]. Noting their long-standing use in melanoma clinical practice, immunohistochemical analysis of regional lymph nodes was formally acknowledged in the 7th edition AJCC melanoma staging system and represents a more sensitive way of identifying melanoma cells, using melanoma-specific antibodies (e.g., HMB-45, Melan A, and MART 1), compared to use of routine hematoxylin and eosin alone. Use of this technique has been shown to increase the sensitivity of SLNB for detecting occult regional SLN metastases [38–40] and has been widely embraced for contemporary SLN pathological assessment.

The stratification of patients into the appropriate N category is primarily based upon the number of metastatic nodes, while the subclassification within the N grouping reflects the burden of disease, defined as either microscopic (a) or macroscopic (b). These categories reflect well-characterized differences in 10-year survival among these groups of patients [10, 19, 41–43]. N0 corresponds to the absence of detectable regional metastases. NX represents patients for whom the regional nodes cannot be assessed, such as those who have already had a lymphadenectomy for other reasons. N1 signifies the presence of metastasis in only 1

Table 3 AJCC 7th edition anatomic stage groupings for cutaneous melanoma

Clinical staging[a]				Pathologic staging[b]			
	T	N	M		T	N	M
0	Tis	N0	M0	0	Tis	N0	M0
IA	T1a	N0	M0	IA	T1a	N0	M0
IB	T1b	N0	M0	IB	T1b	N0	M0
	T2a	N0	M0		T2a	N0	M0
IIA	T2b	N0	M0	IIA	T2b	N0	M0
	T3a	N0	M0		T3a	N0	M0
IIB	T3b	N0	M0	IIB	T3b	N0	M0
	T4a	N0	M0		T4a	N0	M0
IIC	T4b	N0	M0	IIC	T4b	N0	M0
III	Any T	N > N0	M0	IIIA	T1–4a	N1a	M0
					T1–4a	N2a	M0
				IIIB	T1–4b	N1a	M0
					T1–4b	N2a	M0
					T1–4a	N1b	M0
					T1–4a	N2b	M0
					T1–4a	N2c	M0
				IIIC	T1–4b	N1b	M0
					T1–4b	N2b	M0
					T1–4b	N2c	M0
					Any T	N3	M0
IV	Any T	Any N	M1	IV	Any T	Any N	M1

[a]Clinical staging includes microstaging of the primary melanoma and clinical/radiologic evaluation for metastases. By convention, it should be used after complete excision of the primary melanoma with clinical assessment for regional and distant metastases

[b]Pathologic staging includes microstaging of the primary melanoma and pathologic information about the regional lymph nodes after partial (i.e., sentinel node biopsy) or complete lymphadenectomy. Pathologic stage 0 or stage IA patients are the exception; they do not require pathologic evaluation of their lymph nodes

node; N1a represents micrometastatic disease (i.e., detected upon pathological evaluation of the SLN) and N1b represents macrometastatic disease (i.e., detected clinically and confirmed by pathological review, or when nodal metastasis exhibits gross extracapsular extension) in a single node. The N2 category describes patients with 2–3 positive lymph nodes, with the same subclassification into (a) and (b) based upon the micro- versus macrometastatic disease. N2c describes patients with intransit metastases or satellites *without* regional metastatic nodes, and N3 encompasses patients with 4 or more metastatic nodes, matted nodes, or those with intransit/satellite lesions, and regional nodal disease (Table 1).

Since the publication of the 7th edition of the AJCC melanoma staging manual, several studies have examined clinicopathological factors that predict sentinel lymph node positivity and/or survival outcomes. Increasing age, often associated with

Table 4 Five-year survival rates for patients with stage III disease stratified by number of metastatic nodes, primary tumor ulceration, and nodal tumor burden (microscopic or macroscopic) ($N = 2313$)

Rates by type and no. of metastases[a]						
Primary tumor ulceration	No. of nodal micrometastases % ± SE ($n = 1872$)			No. of nodal macrometastases % ± SE ($n = 441$)		
	1	2–3	≥4	1	2–3	≥4
Absent	81.5 ± 1.9 (777[b])	73.2 ± 3.7 (246)	38.0 ± 8.5 (46)	51.6 ± 7.2 (75)	46.6 ± 7.9 (67)	45.4 ± 9.1 (50)
Present	56.6 ± 2.9 (531)	53.9 ± 4.2 (223)	34.0 ± 8.3 (49)	49.4 ± 6.2 88)	37.7 ± 6.2 (93)	29.2 ± 6.7 (68)

Note Stage III disease indicates nodal metastases
Total No. of patients = 2313
Abbreviation: *SE* standard error
[a]Overall statistical significance, $P < 0.001$
[b]Indicates the sample size for each subgroup
From Balch et al. [59] with permission

tumors containing features of more aggressive tumor biology, has been associated with a decreased incidence of a positive sentinel lymph node, but a higher melanoma-specific mortality rate compared to a younger cohort of patients [44].

The presence of non-nodal regional disease, including intransit metastases, satellites, and microsatellitosis, is clinically relevant in melanoma. The formation of these metastatic deposits reflects a spectrum of tumor biology and represents a disease entity with unique treatment options, including locoregional approaches and intralesional therapies. Intransit metastases have been classically defined as cutaneous or subcutaneous regional metastasis that are located greater than 2 cm from the primary melanoma site, between the primary melanoma site and the draining regional lymph node basin. Satellite metastases are defined as grossly visible cutaneous and/or subcutaneous metastases occurring within 2 cm of the primary melanoma. Clinically, however, satellites and intransits are generally considered to be similar manifestations of intralymphatic metastasis. Microsatellitosis is the presence of tumor nests > or at least 0.05 mm in diameter separate from the principal tumor, but separated from it by at least 0.3 mm of normal tissue and found on pathological evaluation of the primary melanoma. Importantly, while the significance of microsatellites is still not clearly defined, they have been associated with unfavorable pathological features [45]. Therefore, they are still included in N2c. In the 7th edition melanoma staging system, non-nodal regional metastasis is classified as N2c. These locoregional non-nodal melanoma metastases represent manifestations of intralymphatic disease. Survival estimates for the subset of patients with N2c disease were somewhat better than the other stage IIIB cohort [46], although they remain 90 % of stage IIIB category given their statistical fit in terms of survival outcomes [19].

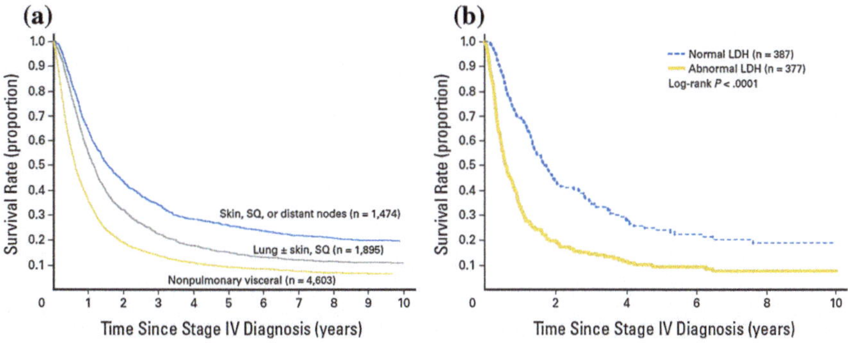

Fig. 2 Survival curves of 7635 patients with metastatic melanomas at distant sites (stage IV) subgrouped by (**a**) the site of metastatic disease and (**b**) serum lactose dehydrogenase (LDH) levels. LDH values are not used to stratify patients. *Curves* in (**a**) are based only on site of metastasis. The number of patients is shown in *parentheses*. *SQ* subcutaneous. From Balch et al. [19] with permission. Stage IV survival curves from the 7th edition of the AJCC melanoma staging database

2.3 Distant Metastases (M)

In the 7th edition AJCC staging manual, M0 represents no evidence of distant metastasis, and M1 indicates distant metastasis. M1a includes metastases to distant skin, subcutaneous tissue, or lymph nodes; M1b includes pulmonary metastases; and M1c represents metastases to all other visceral sites or distant metastases to any site in the setting of an elevated lactate dehydrogenase (LDH) level (Table 2). Based on analyses leading to the 7th edition AJCC staging system, 1-year survival rates for patients with M1a, M1b, and M1c diseases were 62, 53, and 33 %, respectively [19]. If patients have distant metastases to more than one site, they are classified according to the highest M1 category that is involved.

Although the use of a serum marker is relatively uncommon for cancer staging, the presence of an elevated LDH was included in the AJCC staging system, since the 6th edition, when it was shown to be an independent and highly significant adverse predictor of survival, regardless of the site(s) of distant disease [47–50]. The 1-year survival of patients with an elevated LDH compared to those without an elevated LDH was 32 and 65 %, respectively (Fig. 2). According to the 7th edition AJCC staging manual, it is recommended that a repeat LDH level separated by more than 24 h be performed to appropriately document an elevated serum LDH [27].

3 Stage Groupings (Table 2)

3.1 Localized Disease (Stages I and II)

The prognosis for patients with localized melanoma—i.e., without regional and/or distant metastasis and hence N0M0—is generally favorable. Stage I represents earliest-stage invasive melanoma and stage II overall represents an intermediate-risk category; there is, however, heterogeneity within these groups. Stage IA includes T1 melanomas without primary tumor ulceration and with <1 mitosis/mm^2 (i.e., Tla). Stage IB includes T1 melanomas with ulceration and/or at least 1 mitosis/mm^2 (T1b) and T2a melanomas (1.01–2 mm thick without ulceration.) Stage II patients include stage IIA (T2b and T3a), stage IIB (T3b and T4a), and stage IIC (T4b) (Tables 2 and 3).

3.2 Regional Disease (Stage III)

Stage III is defined by the presence of locoregional metastases and includes both nodal and non-nodal regional disease. Primary tumor ulceration was initially incorporated into the 6th edition AJCC stage III staging system when it was shown to be an independent adverse predictor of survival among patients with regional nodal disease [15]. This observation has been corroborated in the 7th edition AJCC analyses [19]. Similar to the adverse impact of ulceration in stages I and II disease, ulceration has also been associated with adverse survival in stage III melanoma, essentially upstaging a patient whose primary tumor is ulcerated to that of a patient with a non-ulcerated primary tumor who has a higher nodal tumor burden category (Tables 3 and 4) [51]. For these patients, pathological staging facilitates the stratification of patients according to nodal tumor burden [14, 15, 19, 36, 37].

Stage IIIA includes patients with 1–3 microscopic disease-containing regional lymph nodes (N1a and N2a), generally by sentinel node biopsy in patients with a non-ulcerated primary tumor, and is associated overall with 5-year and 10-year survival rates of 78 and 68 %, respectively [19] (Tables 2, 3, and 4 and Fig. 1). Patients with pathological stage IIIB are those with 1–3 *microscopically* involved regional lymph nodes and an ulcerated primary tumor, 1–3 *macroscopically* involved regional lymph nodes but with a non-ulcerated primary tumor, or patients with intralymphatic regional metastases (e.g., satellites, intransits) who have *no* regional lymph node metastasis (N2c). The 5-year survival rate for this group is 59 % and 10-year survival rate is 43 % [19]. Stage IIIC melanoma is comprised of patients with 1–3 macroscopically involved regional nodes and an ulcerated primary tumor, patients with N3 disease (>3 nodes) regardless of the T category, and patients who have both satellite/intransit disease *and* regional lymph node metastases. The 5-year and 10-year survival estimates for this group are 40 and 24 %, respectively (Fig. 1).

3.3 Distant Metastases (Stage IV)

Overall, the prognosis for patients with distant melanoma metastasis has historically been poor, with overall 5-year survival rates of <10 % [52–54]. Beginning with the 6th edition AJCC melanoma staging system, site of metastasis and/or presence of elevated LDH has been used to stratify M1 disease [15], with associated differences in survival outcomes (Table 2, Fig. 2) [19]. Several studies have reported that the number of distant metastases may be prognostically relevant in patients with metastatic melanoma [52, 55, 56]. While these observations are supported by the AJCC database analysis [15, 19], it has not been formally incorporated into the staging system, due at least in part to potential variability in diagnostic modalities utilized and difficulty in standardization and quantification of these data.

4 Future Directions

While the AJCC melanoma staging system offers invaluable insight into the clinical management of this disease, there are nonetheless inherent constraints to the current TNM-based staging system, such as the limited number of factors that can be included, the inability to use continuous variables, that estimates of survival are based solely at the time of diagnosis, and the inability to incorporate multiple, individual risk factors to create a truly integrated risk-assessment model [57]. The need for improved prognostication tools in melanoma is an area of great interest. Analysis of the AJCC database has yielded proof of concept tools such as a Web-based electronic prediction tool for melanoma patients with localized disease (http://www.melanomaprognosis.org/) [58].

The date and time of diagnosis is traditionally used to calculate 5-year and 10-year survival. However, these initial survival estimates may become less relevant during the course of treatment, particularly for patients with advanced disease who are alive for a period of time following diagnosis of their advanced disease [51]. Conditional probability survival analysis—defined as assessment of survival at some point in time following initial diagnosis of a particular stage of disease, can provide a more contextually relevant assessment of the clinical status of such patients. The inclusion and integration of new statistical models and contemporary analytic approaches facilitate inclusion of additional variables and/or use of continuous variables into staging and prognostic factor analyses. Such approaches will likely facilitate the inclusion of features such as molecular endpoints to better estimate melanoma-specific and disease-free survival within individual patient settings [57, 59–63].

Analysis of the 7th edition AJCC database has already identified important variables that are predictive of survival such as patient age, gender, primary tumor site, extent of microscopic burden, and number of sites of distant metastases. Improved analytic tools may allow the incorporation of these variables into refined prognostic algorithms, including extent of microscopic sentinel node tumor burden and mitotic activity (as a continuous variable) [51]. One such proof of principle tool available today developed by the AJCC provides an individual patient's 1-, 2-, 5-, and 10-year survival estimates with associated confidence intervals using a Web-based platform [63]. Further refinements to prognostic factor assessment will likely enhance clinical management and decision making in the future.

Historically, clinicopathological features have been used in the AJCC melanoma staging system to offer prognostic information and to guide patient risk stratification models. Looking forward, the integration of these variables with molecular data may allow for more detailed and biologically based staging criteria. Given the affordability and accessibility of new techniques for molecular profiling of tumors, including next-generation sequencing, there is excitement about the potential use of these techniques in tumor classification, risk stratification, and both early- and late-stage treatment decision making. While endeavors are currently focused on treatment options for patients with metastatic disease, profiling data are also facilitating a deeper understanding of tumor biology. Large-scale, multi-institutional projects, such as The Cancer Genome Atlas Program (TCGA), are ongoing and have already begun to yield multiplatform datasets from tumors that will contribute to a baseline profile of the biology and heterogeneity of various tumor types, including melanoma [64]. The identification of context-specific biomarkers and molecular profiles may allow improvements in staging and prognostication in melanoma patients [65].

Molecular profiling is now routinely used in the setting of metastatic melanoma, given advances in targeted therapies, including the FDA approval of vemurafenib dabrafenib, and trametinib in the setting of *BRAF V600E* mutant melanoma [66–72]. There is also evolving data from single-institution studies that demonstrate differences in metastatic profiles and survival outcomes in patients, based upon their specific genotype. For example, patients with NRAS mutant metastatic melanomas have been shown to be associated with poorer survival outcomes, and BRAF/NRAS mutant tumors demonstrate a proclivity for brain metastases when compared to non-BRAF/NRAS mutant tumors [62]. Other studies have demonstrated that even within the BRAF gene, different mutations are associated with patient variables and differences in survival outcomes, with poorer overall survival seen in patients with BRAF V600 K mutations versus those with BRAF V600E mutations [73].

Given the availability of new techniques for tumor profiling and characterization, it is indeed an exciting time in the melanoma arena. Immune profiling and mutanome studies, molecular and sequencing analyses, proteomic characterization, and epigenetics may allow us to more robustly understand and integrate this knowledge into our existing clinical decision-making repertoire in the not too distant future.

References

1. Commission TWotC (1927) The health organization of the league of nations: the work of the cancer commission, 1923–1927. Br Med J 1157
2. Weiss L (2000) The morphologic documentation of clinical progression, invasion metastasis—staging. Cancer Metastasis Rev 19(3–4):303–313. doi:10.1023/a:1010658607570
3. Weiss L (2000) Metastasis of cancer: a conceptual history from antiquity to the 1990s. Cancer Metastasis Rev 19(3–4):I–XI, 193–383
4. International Union against Cancer, TNM history, evolution and milestones. http://www.uicc.org/resources/tnm/resources
5. Ackerman L, DRJ (1947) Cancer diagnosis, treatment and prognosis. St Louis, CV Mosby, pp 169–181
6. Macneer G, Dasgupta T (1964) Prognosis in malignant melanoma. Surgery 56:512–518
7. Smith GJ (1975) Histopathology of melanoma. Yale J Biol Med 48(5):409–416
8. Breslow A (1970) Thickness, cross-sectional areas and depth of invasion in the prognosis of cutaneous melanoma. Ann Surg 172(5):902–908

9. Breslow A, Cascinelli N, van der Esch EP et al (1978) Stage I melanoma of the limbs: assessment of prognosis by levels of invasion and maximum thickness. Tumori 64(3):273–284
10. Balch CM, Murad TM, Soong SJ et al (1978) A multifactorial analysis of melanoma: prognostic histopathological features comparing Clark's and Breslow's staging methods. Ann Surg 188(6):732–742
11. Breslow A (1975) Tumor thickness, level of invasion and node dissection in stage I cutaneous melanoma. Ann Surg 182(5):572–575
12. Leong SP, Kashani-Sabet M, Desmond RA et al (2005) Clinical significance of occult metastatic melanoma in sentinel lymph nodes and other high-risk factors based on long-term follow-up. World J Surg 29(6):683–691. doi:10.1007/s00268-005-7736-x
13. Cascinelli N, Bombardieri E, Bufalino R et al (2006) Sentinel and nonsentinel node status in stage IB and II melanoma patients: two-step prognostic indicators of survival. J Clin Oncol Official J Am Soc Clin Oncol 24(27):4464–4471. doi:10.1200/JCO.2006.06.3198 JCO.2009.27.1627 [pii]
14. Balch CM, Soong SJ, Gershenwald JE et al (2001) Prognostic factors analysis of 17,600 melanoma patients: validation of the American joint committee on cancer melanoma staging system. J Clin Oncol Official J Am Soc Clin Oncol 19(16):3622–3634
15. Balch CM, Buzaid AC, Soong SJ et al (2001) Final version of the American joint committee on cancer staging system for cutaneous melanoma. J Clin Oncol Official J Am Soc Clin Oncol 19(16):3635–3648
16. American Joint Committee for Cancer Staging and End Results Reporting (1978) Staging for malignant melanoma. Manual for staging of cancer, pp 131–140
17. Gershenwald JE, Buzaid AC, Ross MI (1998) Classification and staging of melanoma. Hematol Oncol Clin North Am 12(4):737–765
18. American Joint Committee for Cancer Staging and End Results Reporting (1977) Staging of malignant melanoma. American Joint Committee, Manual for Staging in Cancer
19. Balch CM, Gershenwald JE, Soong SJ et al (2009) Final version of 2009 AJCC melanoma staging and classification. J Clin Oncol Official J Am Soc Clin Oncol 27(36):6199–6206. doi:10.1200/JCO.2009.23.4799 JCO.2009.23.4799 [pii]
20. Gershenwald JE, Thompson W, Mansfield PF et al (1999) Multi-institutional melanoma lymphatic mapping experience: the prognostic value of sentinel lymph node status in 612 stage I or II melanoma patients. J Clin Oncol Official J Am Soc Clin Oncol 17(3):976–983
21. Morton DL, Wen DR, Wong JH et al (1992) Technical details of intraoperative lymphatic mapping for early stage melanoma. Arch Surg 127(4):392–399
22. Yee VS, Thompson JF, McKinnon JG et al (2005) Outcome in 846 cutaneous melanoma patients from a single center after a negative sentinel node biopsy. Ann Surg Oncol 12(6): 429–439. doi:10.1245/ASO.2005.03.074
23. Francken AB, Shaw HM, Thompson JF et al (2004) The prognostic importance of tumor mitotic rate confirmed in 1317 patients with primary cutaneous melanoma and long follow-up. Ann Surg Oncol 11(4):426–433. doi:10.1245/ASO.2004.07.014 ASO.2004.07.014 [pii]
24. Eigentler TK, Buettner PG, Leiter U et al (2004) Impact of ulceration in stages I to III cutaneous melanoma as staged by the American joint committee on cancer staging system: an analysis of the German central malignant melanoma registry. J Clin Oncol Official J Am Soc Clin Oncol 22(21):4376–4383. doi:10.1200/JCO.2004.03.075 22/21/4376 [pii]
25. Balch CM, Wilkerson JA, Murad TM et al (1980) The prognostic significance of ulceration of cutaneous melanoma. Cancer 45(12):3012–3017
26. Averbook BJ, Fu P, Rao JS et al. (2002) A long-term analysis of 1018 patients with melanoma by classic cox regression and tree-structured survival analysis at a major referral center: Implications on the future of cancer staging. Surgery 132(4):589–602; discussion 602–584. S003960600200137X [pii]
27. Balch CM, Gershenwald JE, Soong S et al (2009) Melanoma of the skin. In: Edge SE, Byrd DR, Compton CA, Fritz AG, Greene FL, Trotti III A (eds) AJCC cancer staging manual, 7th edn. Springer, Berlin pp 325–346

28. Gimotty PA, Elder DE, Fraker DL et al (2007) Identification of high-risk patients among those diagnosed with thin cutaneous melanomas. J Clin Oncol Official J Am Soc Clin Oncol 25 (9):1129–1134. doi:10.1200/JCO.2006.08.1463 25/9/1129 [pii]
29. Gimotty PA, Guerry D, Ming ME et al (2004) Thin primary cutaneous malignant melanoma: a prognostic tree for 10-year metastasis is more accurate than American joint committee on cancer staging. J Clin Oncol Official J Am Soc Clin Oncol 22(18):3668–3676. doi:10.1200/JCO.2004.12.015 JCO.2004.12.015 [pii]
30. Karakousis GC, Gimotty PA, Czerniecki BJ et al (2007) Regional nodal metastatic disease is the strongest predictor of survival in patients with thin vertical growth phase melanomas: a case for SLN staging biopsy in these patients. Ann Surg Oncol 14(5):1596–1603. doi:10.1245/s10434-006-9319-y
31. Kesmodel SB, Karakousis GC, Botbyl JD et al (2005) Mitotic rate as a predictor of sentinel lymph node positivity in patients with thin melanomas. Ann Surg Oncol 12(6):449–458. doi:10.1245/ASO.2005.04.027
32. Thompson JF, Soong SJ, Balch CM et al (2011) Prognostic significance of mitotic rate in localized primary cutaneous melanoma: an analysis of patients in the multi-institutional American joint committee on cancer melanoma staging database. J Clin Oncol 29(16):2199–2205. doi:10.1200/JCO.2010.31.5812
33. Scheri RP, Essner R, Turner RR et al (2007) Isolated tumor cells in the sentinel node affect long-term prognosis of patients with melanoma. Ann Surg Oncol 14(10):2861–2866. doi:10.1245/s10434-007-9472-y
34. van Akkooi AC, de Wilt JH, Verhoef C et al (2006) Clinical relevance of melanoma micrometastases (<0.1 mm) in sentinel nodes: are these nodes to be considered negative? Ann Oncol 17(10):1578–1585. doi:10.1093/annonc/mdl176 mdl176 [pii]
35. Cascinelli N, Belli F, Santinami M et al (2000) Sentinel lymph node biopsy in cutaneous melanoma: the WHO melanoma program experience. Ann Surg Oncol 7(6):469–474
36. Morton DL, Thompson JF, Cochran AJ et al (2006) Sentinel-node biopsy or nodal observation in melanoma. New Engl J Med 355(13):1307–1317. doi:10.1056/NEJMoa060992 355/13/1307 [pii]
37. Morton DL, Thompson JF, Cochran AJ et al (2014) Final trial report of sentinel-node biopsy versus nodal observation in melanoma. New Engl J Med 370(7):599–609. doi:10.1056/NEJMoa1310460
38. Yu LL, Flotte TJ, Tanabe KK et al (1999) Detection of microscopic melanoma metastases in sentinel lymph nodes. Cancer 86(4):617–627. doi:10.1002/(SICI)1097-0142(19990815)86:4<617:AID-CNCR10>3.0.CO;2-S [pii]
39. Spanknebel K, Coit DG, Bieligk SC et al (2005) Characterization of micrometastatic disease in melanoma sentinel lymph nodes by enhanced pathology: recommendations for standardizing pathologic analysis. Am J Surg Pathol 29(3):305–317. 00000478-200503000-00003 [pii]
40. Gibbs JF, Huang PP, Zhang PJ et al (1999) Accuracy of pathologic techniques for the diagnosis of metastatic melanoma in sentinel lymph nodes. Ann Surg Oncol 6(7):699–704
41. van Akkooi AC, Bouwhuis MG, van Geel AN et al (2007) Morbidity and prognosis after therapeutic lymph node dissections for malignant melanoma. Eur J Surg Oncol 33(1):102–108. doi:10.1016/j.ejso.2006.10.032 S0748-7983(06)00426-4 [pii]
42. Meyer T, Merkel S, Gohl J et al. (2002) Lymph node dissection for clinically evident lymph node metastases of malignant melanoma. Eur J Surg Oncol 28 (4):424–430. S0748798301912624 [pii]
43. Badgwell B, Xing Y, Gershenwald JE et al (2007) Pelvic lymph node dissection is beneficial in subsets of patients with node-positive melanoma. Ann Surg Oncol 14(10):2867–2875. doi:10.1245/s10434-007-9512-7
44. Balch CM, Thompson JF, Gershenwald JE et al (2014) Age as a predictor of sentinel node metastasis among patients with localized melanoma: an inverse correlation of melanoma mortality and incidence of sentinel node metastasis among young and old patients. Ann Surg Oncol 21(4):1075–1081. doi:10.1245/s10434-013-3464-x

45. Bartlett EK, Gupta M, Datta J et al (2014) Prognosis of patients with melanoma and microsatellitosis undergoing sentinel lymph node biopsy. Ann Surg Oncol 21(3):1016–1023. doi:10.1245/s10434-013-3388-5
46. Shaikh L, Sagebiel RW, Ferreira CM et al (2005) The role of microsatellites as a prognostic factor in primary malignant melanoma. Arch Dermatol 141(6):739–742. doi:10.1001/archderm.141.6.739 141/6/739 [pii]
47. Keilholz U, Martus P, Punt CJ et al (2002) Prognostic factors for survival and factors associated with long-term remission in patients with advanced melanoma receiving cytokine-based treatments: second analysis of a randomised EORTC melanoma group trial comparing interferon-alpha2a (IFNalpha) and interleukin 2 (IL-2) with or without cisplatin. Eur J Cancer 38(11):1501–1511. S0959804902001235 [pii]
48. Keilholz U, Conradt C, Legha SS et al (1998) Results of interleukin-2-based treatment in advanced melanoma: a case record-based analysis of 631 patients. J Clin Oncol Official J Am Soc Clin Oncol 16(9):2921–2929
49. Franzke A, Probst-Kepper M, Buer J et al (1998) Elevated pretreatment serum levels of soluble vascular cell adhesion molecule 1 and lactate dehydrogenase as predictors of survival in cutaneous metastatic malignant melanoma. Br J Cancer 78(1):40–45
50. Eton O, Legha SS, Moon TE et al (1998) Prognostic factors for survival of patients treated systemically for disseminated melanoma. J Clin Oncol Official J Am Soc Clin Oncol 16 (3):1103–1111
51. Dickson PV, Gershenwald JE (2011) Staging and prognosis of cutaneous melanoma. Surg Oncol Clin N Am 20(1):1–17. doi:10.1016/j.soc.2010.09.007 S1055-3207(10)00095-5 [pii]
52. Barth A, Wanek LA, Morton DL (1995) Prognostic factors in 1521 melanoma patients with distant metastases. J Am Coll Surg 181(3):193–201
53. Manola J, Atkins M, Ibrahim J et al (2000) Prognostic factors in metastatic melanoma: a pooled analysis of Eastern Cooperative Oncology Group trials. J Clin Oncol 18(22):3782–3793
54. Unger JM, Flaherty LE, Liu PY et al (2001) Gender and other survival predictors in patients with metastatic melanoma on Southwest oncology group trials. Cancer 91(6):1148–1155. doi:10.1002/1097-0142(20010315)91:6<1148:AID-CNCR1111>3.0.CO;2-# [pii]
55. Balch CM (1992) Cutaneous melanoma: prognosis and treatment results worldwide. Semin Surg Oncol 8(6):400–414
56. Staudt M, Lasithiotakis K, Leiter U et al (2010) Determinants of survival in patients with brain metastases from cutaneous melanoma. Br J Cancer 102(8):1213–1218. doi:10.1038/sj.bjc.6605622 6605622 [pii]
57. Ascierto PA, Grimaldi AM, Curti B et al (2012) Future perspectives in melanoma research. Meeting report from the "Melanoma research: a bridge from Naples to the World. Napoli, December 5th-6th 2011". J Transl Med 10:83. doi:10.1186/1479-5876-10-83 1479-5876-10-83 [pii]
58. Soong SJ, Ding S, Coit D et al (2010) Predicting survival outcome of localized melanoma: an electronic prediction tool based on the AJCC melanoma database. Ann Surg Oncol 17 (8):2006–2014. doi:10.1245/s10434-010-1050-z
59. Balch CM, Gershenwald JE, Soong SJ et al (2010) Multivariate analysis of prognostic factors among 2313 patients with stage III melanoma: comparison of nodal micrometastases versus macrometastases. J Clin Oncol Official J Am Soc Clin Oncol 28(14):2452–2459. doi:10.1200/JCO.2009.27.1627 JCO.2009.27.1627 [pii]
60. Bowles TL, Xing Y, Hu CY et al (2010) Conditional survival estimates improve over 5 years for melanoma survivors with node-positive disease. Ann Surg Oncol 17(8):2015–2023. doi:10.1245/s10434-010-1051-y
61. Gershenwald JE, Soong SJ, Balch CM (2010) 2010 TNM staging system for cutaneous melanoma and beyond. Ann Surg Oncol 17(6):1475–1477. doi:10.1245/s10434-010-0986-3
62. Jakob JA, Bassett RL Jr, Ng CS et al (2012) NRAS mutation status is an independent prognostic factor in metastatic melanoma. Cancer 118(16):4014–4023. doi:10.1002/cncr.26724

63. Soong SJ, Ding S, Coit D et al (2010) Predicting survival outcome of localized melanoma: an electronic prediction tool based on the AJCC melanoma database. Ann Surg Oncol 17 (8):2006–2014. doi:10.1245/s10434-010-1050-z
64. https://tcga-data.nci.nih.gov/tcga
65. Boland GM, Meric-Bernstam F (2014) The role of surgeons in building a personalized medicine program. J Surg Oncol. doi:10.1002/jso.23684
66. Chapman PB, Hauschild A, Robert C et al (2011) Improved survival with vemurafenib in melanoma with BRAF V600E mutation. New Engl J Med 364(26):2507–2516. doi:10.1056/NEJMoa1103782
67. Flaherty KT, Yasothan U, Kirkpatrick P (2011) Vemurafenib. Nat Rev Drug Discov 10 (11):811–812. doi:10.1038/nrd3579 nrd3579 [pii]
68. Flaherty KT, Infante JR, Daud A et al (2012) Combined BRAF and MEK inhibition in melanoma with BRAF V600 mutations. New Engl J Med 367(18):1694–1703. doi:10.1056/NEJMoa1210093
69. Flaherty KT, Robert C, Hersey P et al (2012) Improved survival with MEK inhibition in BRAF-mutated melanoma. New Engl J Med 367(2):107–114. doi:10.1056/NEJMoa1203421
70. Larkin J, Ascierto PA, Dreno B et al (2014) Combined vemurafenib and cobimetinib in BRAF-mutated melanoma. New Engl J Med 371(20):1867–1876. doi:10.1056/NEJMoa1408868
71. Long GV, Stroyakovskiy D, Gogas H et al (2014) Combined BRAF and MEK inhibition versus BRAF inhibition alone in melanoma. New Engl J Med 371(20):1877–1888. doi:10.1056/NEJMoa1406037
72. Sosman JA, Kim KB, Schuchter L et al (2012) Survival in BRAF V600-mutant advanced melanoma treated with vemurafenib. New Engl J Med 366(8):707–714. doi:10.1056/NEJMoa1112302
73. Bucheit AD, Syklawer E, Jakob JA et al (2013) Clinical characteristics and outcomes with specific BRAF and NRAS mutations in patients with metastatic melanoma. Cancer 119 (21):3821–3829. doi:10.1002/cncr.28306

Surgical Management of Melanoma

Vadim P. Koshenkov, Joe Broucek and Howard L. Kaufman

Abstract

The surgical management of melanoma has undergone considerable changes over the past several decades, as new strategies and treatments have become available. Surgeons play a pivotal role in all aspects of melanoma care: diagnostic, curative, and palliative. There is a high potential for cure in patients with early-stage melanoma and the selection of an appropriate operation is very important for this reason. Staging the nodal basin has become widespread since the adoption of sentinel lymph node biopsy (SLNB) for the management of melanoma. This operation provides the best prognostic information that is currently available for patients with melanoma. The surgeon plays a central role in the palliation of symptoms resulting from nodal disease and metastases, as melanoma has a propensity to spread to almost any site in the body.

Keywords

Melanoma · Surgery · Treatment

Abbreviations

FNA	Fine needle aspiration
SLNB	Sentinel lymph node biopsy
MSLT-1	Multicenter selective lymphadenectomy trial 1
VGP	Vertical growth phase
DM	Desmoplastic melanoma

V.P. Koshenkov (✉) · J. Broucek · H.L. Kaufman
Division of Surgical Oncology, Rutgers Cancer Institute of New Jersey,
195 Little Albany St., Suite 3001, New Brunswick, NJ 08901, USA
e-mail: vpk10@cinj.rutgers.edu

H.L. Kaufman and J.M. Mehnert (eds.), *Melanoma*,
Cancer Treatment and Research 167, DOI 10.1007/978-3-319-22539-5_6

HILP	Hyperthermic isolated limp perfusion
ILI	Isolated limb infusion
IPI	Ipilimumab
IL-2	Interleukin 2

Contents

1 Introduction

Over the last several decades, the incidence of melanoma has continued to rise at an almost exponential pace, matched only by esophageal carcinoma. It is now the fifth most common cancer in the USA. Breast, prostate, lung, and colon cancer are the only malignancies that are more common than melanoma [105]. Annually, almost 10,000 deaths are estimated to occur as a result of melanoma. Despite the far higher incidence of approximately 3.5 million annual cases of basal cell carcinoma and squamous cell carcinoma, melanoma accounts for about 50–75 % of all skin cancer deaths [72]. According to the National Cancer Database, 91.2 % of melanomas are cutaneous, 5.3 % are ocular, 2.2 % are of unknown site, and 1.3 % are mucosal [25]. A normal melanocyte resides at the dermal/epidermal junction and transforms via a stepwise progression to become melanoma. It first turns into an atypical melanocyte, which can undergo hyperplasia, and then develops a radial growth phase. Afterward, vertical growth phase (VGP) occurs, and this is when the melanocyte has metastatic potential. Epidemiologic studies have shown that men are not only more likely to be afflicted with melanoma, but to also die from it. Factors, such as a delay in seeking medical attention for suspicious skin lesions, less careful protection from sunlight, and more frequent head and neck melanomas, locations that are more difficult to treat adequately, have been implicated in the differences of incidence and mortality between men and women. In women, legs are the most common site of melanoma, as opposed to the trunk in men.

The most evident etiologic factor for melanoma is sunlight exposure. Both ultraviolet-A radiation (UVA) and ultraviolet-B radiation (UVB) have been implicated, although the latter appears to be more directly associated with acute sunburn and melanin pigment production [43, 69]. Sunburns in either childhood or adolescence have been shown to increase the rates of subsequent development of melanoma [38]. It has been estimated that 98.2 % of cutaneous melanomas occur in the Caucasian population [25]. This disproportionate distribution is explained by the more harmful effect of ultraviolet irradiation to fair-skinned individuals. Thus, it is the combination of excessive sunlight exposure and sensitive skin that burns easily that causes the development of most melanomas. Less commonly, there may be a heritable predisposition to melanoma or a presence of rare conditions, such as dysplastic nevus syndrome or xeroderma pigmentosum. Lastly, therapeutic radiation administered to children has been shown to increase the risk of melanoma development [49].

Classically, five melanoma subtypes have been described and are defined by their histologic growth patterns (Table 1). Superficial spreading melanoma is the most common subtype and is usually found on the trunk and extremities. Nodular melanoma is unique in that it skips the radial growth phase, progressing straight to the VGP. As a result, these lesions tend to be deeper than other subtypes, and because of this have a worse prognosis. However, it is important to note that the prognosis is the same for a non-nodular melanoma and a nodular melanoma when the Breslow thickness is the same. Lentigo maligna melanoma usually occurs on the face of the elderly and is most commonly a thin lesion. Acral lentiginous melanoma is found on subungual, plantar, palmar, and mucosal surfaces. Sunlight exposure

Table 1 Melanoma subtypes

	Superficial spreading	Nodular	Lentigo maligna	Acral lentiginous	Desmoplastic
Incidence	60–70 %	10–20 %	5–10 %	<5 %	<5 %
Location	Trunk Extremity	Anywhere	Face Upper Chest	Acral Mucosal	Head Neck

likely plays a lesser role with this subtype and is more common in African, Asian, and Hispanic populations [105]. A delay in diagnosis is not uncommon with this melanoma subtype as the lesions may be confused with benign conditions. Moreover, biopsy of concerning lesions of mucosal surfaces or subungual locations can be challenging. Desmoplastic melanoma (DM) is the least frequent subtype. Despite a propensity for local recurrence, prognosis is no worse than for other subtypes of melanoma [71].

2 Prognostic Factors

A broad spectrum of outcomes exists for patients diagnosed with melanoma. For those with early-stage I melanoma, 5-year survival rates approach 98 %. For those with widespread metastatic disease, 5-year survival rates are in the single digits [37]. Several features of the primary lesion determine the risk of lymph node and distant metastases. The thickness of the lesion, as measured in millimeters and classified as Breslow thickness, is the best predictor of metastatic spread. Deeper melanomas metastasize at higher rates than superficial melanomas and this is reflected in the staging system (Fig. 1). Clark's level is an alternate method to describe the thickness of the lesion. It is determined by which layers of the skin are involved by the melanoma, such as the epidermis, papillary dermis, reticular dermis, and subcutaneous tissue. In the current 7th edition of AJCC Cancer Staging Manual, Clark's level is no longer used to guide the staging of the lesion. However, several recent publications have highlighted the importance of Clark's level IV–V in the prediction of lymph node metastases, and hence prognosis, as determined by a sentinel lymph node biopsy (SLNB) in thin cutaneous melanomas [17, 53, 68].

The presence of ulceration and mitotic figures are the other features of the primary lesion that are important to consider for prognostication, as either one predicts worse survival. This is demonstrated with ulcerated melanomas that portend the same prognosis as non-ulcerated melanomas one T stage higher [8, 9]. As a result, such lesions are grouped together to define the same stages [37]. Presence of one or more mitotic figures defines a T1b melanoma, and this was one of the major changes instituted in the 7th Edition of AJCC Cancer Staging Manual [3, 45, 111]. Other variables such as gender, location of the primary lesion, and age also affect prognosis of patients with melanoma. Males have lower survival rates than females, most likely because their melanomas are usually deeper, more commonly ulcerated, and more frequently located on the head and neck [8, 9, 102]. Melanomas that are on the head and neck locations are more challenging to treat. First, adequate margins are not always possible because of proximity to vital structures. Second, higher false-negative sentinel node biopsy rates exist due to more variable lymph node drainage patterns. With respect to age, it appears that elderly patients have a worse prognosis [8, 9, 63]. This is paradoxical because younger patients have higher rates of lymph node metastases as determined by a sentinel node biopsy [92, 111]. Several theories have been proposed to explain this paradox. One argues that

AJCC Staging System for Melanoma, Seventh Edition, 2010					
STAGE	TNM Classification	Breslow Depth	Ulceration	Mitotic Rate	Nodal status, Intransit or distant metastases
IA	T1a N0 M0	≤ 1.0 mm	NO	<1/mm²	------
IB	T1b N0 M0	≤ 1.0 mm	Yes	≥1/mm²	------
	T2a N0 M0	1.01-2.0 mm	No		------
IIA	T2b N0 M0	1.01-2.0 mm	Yes		------
	T3a N0 M0	2.01-4.0 mm	No		------
IIB	T3b N0 M0	2.01-4.0 mm	Yes		------
	T4a N0 M0	> 4.0 mm	No		------
IIC	T4b N0 M0	> 4.0 mm	Yes		------
IIIA	T1a-4a N1a M0	Any	No		one node with micro. Metastasis
	T1a-4a N2a M0	Any	No		2-3 nodes, micro metastasis
IIIB	T1-4b N1a M0	Any	Yes		One node with micro metastasis
	T1-4b N2a M0	Any	Yes		2-3 nodes with micro metastasis
	T1-4a N1b M0	Any	No		one node with Macro. Metastasis
	T1-4a N2b M0	Any	No		2-3 nodes with Macro. Metastasis
	T1-4a N2c M0	Any	Any		Intransit/satellite without nodes
IIIC	T1b-4b N1b M0	Any	Yes		One node with Macro. Metastasis
	T1b-4b N2b M0	Any	Yes		2-3 nodes with macro. Metastasis
	T1-4a N2c M0	Any	Any		Intransit/satellite without nodes
	Any T N3 M0	Any	Any		≥ 4 metast/matted Nodes/ In-transit/ satellitosis
Stage IV	AnyT AnyN AnyM	Any	Any		
	M1a - distant skin, subcutaneous or nodal metastases				
	M1b - Lung metastases				
	M1c - other viscera and distant metastases				

Fig. 1 AJCC 7th edition TNM staging of melanoma. Adapted from AJCC Cancer Staging Manual, 7th edition (2010). Springer, New York

nodal metastases, especially micrometastases, worsen the survival of older patients to a greater degree than younger patients, underlying a likely role for a more robust immune system and its relation to cancer. Another possible explanation lies in the more favorable clinicopathologic profile of younger patients who tend to have thinner lesions with less ulceration [25].

3 Diagnosis and Selection of Biopsy Techniques

Abnormal cutaneous lesions that are concerning for melanoma should always be biopsied for a definitive diagnosis. Suspicious lesions may have changed over time or have certain appearance that prompts the clinician to perform a biopsy. The ABCDEs mnemonic of melanoma nicely summarizes the concerning appearance that many melanomas have asymmetry, border irregularity, color variation, diameter greater than 6 mm, and evolution of the lesion (Fig. 2). However, some melanomas are non-pigmented, while benign lesions such as seborrheic keratoses can often be confused for this malignancy. For these reasons, biopsy is critical for confirming a diagnosis.

There are multiple ways to biopsy a melanoma. Shave and punch biopsies are easily performed in an office setting, do not require anesthesia, and are well-tolerated by patients. As a result, the majority of melanomas are diagnosed via one of these methods. The upside to these diagnostic modalities is the rapidity with which they can be scheduled and performed. The downside is that neither one is as accurate as an excisional biopsy. The rates of positive deep margins, especially with shave biopsies, are considerably higher than with excisional biopsy, ranging from 22 to 37 % [113, 126]. In the presence of a positive deep margin on initial biopsy, the true thickness of melanoma is unknown. This creates uncertainty with respect to the type of operation that should be performed, as it is primarily the Breslow thickness that determines margins of excision and a need for a SLNB [68]. Governing bodies and societies such as the National Institute of Health, the National Comprehensive Cancer Network, and the American Academy of Dermatology have proclaimed the excisional biopsy to be the gold standard of diagnosing a melanoma [110]. Regrettably, adherence to these guidelines is low. The issue of a correct prebiopsy identification of a melanoma is also an important one to consider when arguing for or against a diagnostic modality. Zager and colleagues found that only 34 % of lesions that turned out to be melanoma were suspected of being one at the time of the initial evaluation. One of the authors' conclusions was that a harsh stance against shave biopsies would discourage against their use and could result in less frequent diagnoses of melanoma [126]. If early diagnosis of melanoma is the ultimate goal, then the elimination of shave and punch biopsies would certainly undermine it. It appears that the best recommendation at this time is to perform an excisional biopsy whenever the clinician is comfortable doing so, and implement alternative techniques otherwise.

Incisional biopsy and fine needle aspiration (FNA) are two other diagnostic modalities that are available to physicians in the diagnosis of melanoma. The former is performed when a large lesion is identified, with a diameter of 1.5 cm serving as a useful cutoff. These biopsies should include the deepest or darkest portions of the lesion. Further definitive management will still be necessary, but the information obtained from the incisional biopsy will allow the clinician to ascertain the need for other surgical approaches, such as lymph node mapping and biopsy, and a metastatic work-up. A FNA uses a thin needle (e.g., 22-gauge) to extract a small sample of cells for microscopic evaluation. Usually, enough tissue is obtained

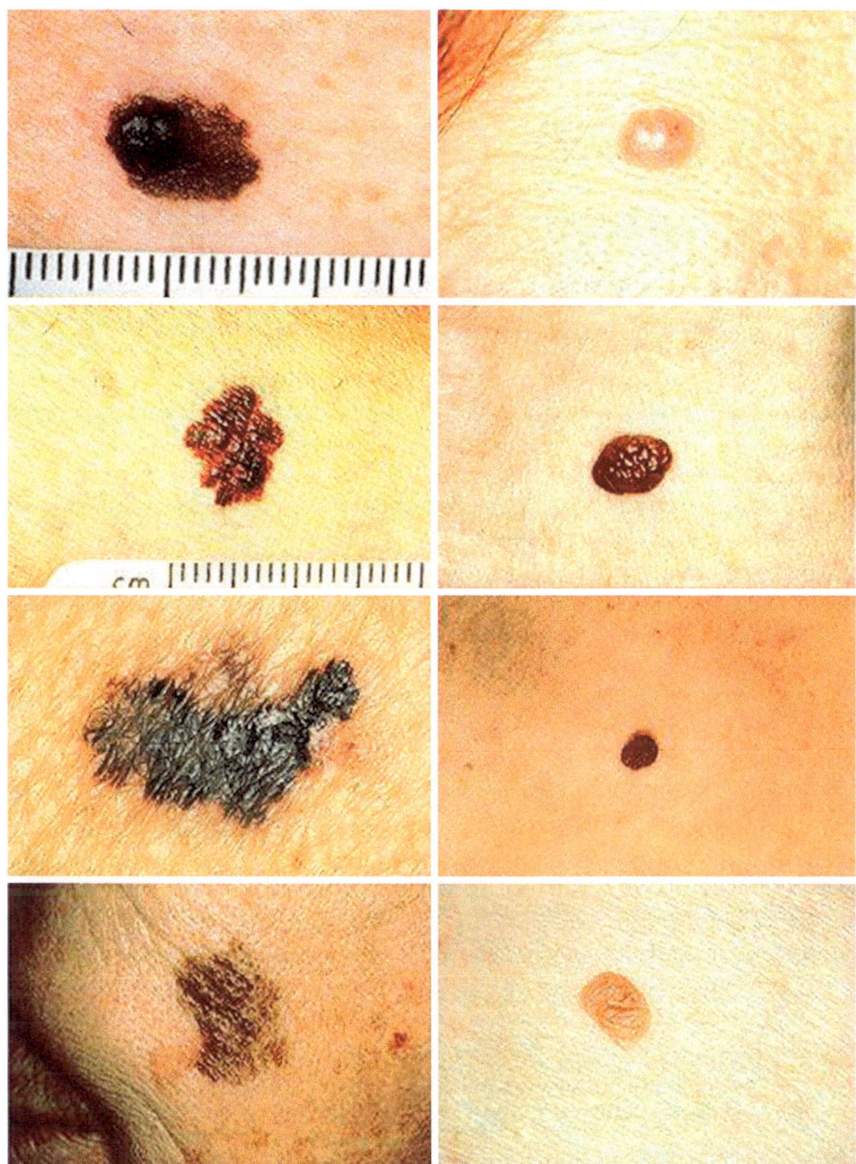

Fig. 2 The ABCDEs of melanoma are illustrated

to allow for a variety of immunohistochemical stains, such as S100, MART-1, and tyrosinase, to be performed on the specimen. A FNA is highly sensitive for detecting melanoma cells but should not be used as a method to diagnose the primary lesion, as tumor thickness along with other important histologic features cannot be determined. Its best application is for the assessment of a nodal mass.

4 Surgical Management of Primary Melanoma Lesions

Wide local excision is the definitive management of primary cutaneous melanoma and consists of resecting the entire melanoma and surrounding skin, while including the epidermis, dermis, and subcutaneous fat. During the operation, the surgeon measures the appropriate margin around the external border of visible pigmentation or prior biopsy scar and often employs an elliptical incision to allow for primary closure. If the primary melanoma diameter is small, the operation can usually be performed without intravenous anesthesia under a local anesthetic.

Surgical excision of melanoma is a fundamental step in achieving local control of the cancer. For most of the twentieth century, surgical management of cutaneous melanoma involved aggressive excisions of the primary lesion with circumferential margins of 3–5 cm [50, 103]. Wide margins of excision became the surgical dogma after an early study showed abnormal melanocytes to display a "field effect" whereby abnormal cells were isolated up to 5 cm away from the primary lesion [54]. In addition, early reports on the biological course of melanoma demonstrated dismal survival rates that were somewhat improved in patients subjected to radical excisions [91]. As a result, this led to fears that inappropriately narrow margins would promote disease recurrence. In addition, closure with placement of a split-thickness skin graft was strongly advocated and regarded as an important step in management.

It was not until the late 1970s when new data on the prognostic value of tumor depth surfaced and surgeons began to employ narrower margins with good outcomes [6, 20, 39]. Controversy ensued over optimal margins of excision as there was no sound evidence to guide surgical practice at the time. Beginning in the late 1970s with Program Trial No. 10 conducted by the World Health Organization, there have been several randomized trials carried out to evaluate the safety of performing excisions with narrower surgical margins (Table 2). The investigators of the first trial set out to compare 1-cm and 3- to 5-cm margins for patients with melanomas whose thickness measured ≤2.0 mm [118]. They found no differences in survival between the two groups and concluded that 1-cm margin was safe for thin melanomas (≤1.0 mm). There were more local recurrences in 1.01–2.0 mm melanomas and even though statistical significance was not reached, many surgeons remained hesitant to adapt the 1-cm margin for these patients. Both the Swedish Melanoma Study Group and the French Cooperative Group trials examined the same type of population as the WHO Melanoma Program Trial No. 10 trial, but treated them with a 2-cm margin or a 5-cm margin [33, 66]. The survival rates did not differ between conservative and aggressive excisions in both trials. The investigators concluded that 2-cm margins were safe in patients with melanomas up to 2.0 mm in thickness.

The Intergroup Melanoma Surgical Trial aimed to address the issue of appropriate margins of excision for patients with intermediate-thickness melanomas (1.01–4.0 mm) [8, 9]. The authors chose 2- and 4-cm margins for comparison. Neither the overall survival nor the number of local recurrences differed between

Table 2 Randomized clinical trials of excision margins

Trial	*N*	Tumor thickness (mm)	Margins (cm)	Local recurrence	Disease-free survival	Overall survival	Outcome
WHO Melanoma Group Trial #10	612	0–2.0	1 versus 3–5	8 versus 3 for 1–2 mm subgroups (NS) None in <1 mm		No difference	1-cm margin for <1 mm
Swedish Melanoma Group Trial	989	0.8–2.0	2 versus 5	3 versus 4	No difference	No difference • Corrected 5 yr survival • 90.9 % in 2 cm • 93.7 % in 5 cm	2-cm margin for ≤2 mm
French Cooperative Group Trial	337	0–2.0	2 versus 5	22 in 2 cm 33 in 5 cm	At 10 years: • 85 % in 2 cm • 83 % in 5 cm	No difference At 10 years: • 87 % versus 86 %	2-cm margin for ≤2 mm
Intergroup Melanoma Surgical Trial	486	1–4.0	2 versus 4	0.4 % versus 0.9 % as first relapse 2.1 % versus 2.6 % any time		No difference At 10 years: • 70 % versus 77 % (NS)	2-cm margin for 1–4.0 mm
UK Melanoma Study	900	≥2	1 versus 3	26 % greater rate of locoregional failure with 1 cm ($p = 0.05$)		No difference	Avoid 1-cm margins in melanomas thicker than 2 mm
European Multicenter Trial	936	≥2	2 versus 4	20 versus 9 ($p = 0.06$)	No difference	No difference • 65 % versus 65 %	2-cm margins for ≥2 mm

the two groups. Additionally, surgical morbidity, length of hospital stay, and the need for skin grafting were all lower with narrower margins, leading the investigators to make a recommendation of 2-cm margin of excision for intermediate-thickness melanomas.

The first trial to include patients with thick melanomas (>4.0 mm) was the British Cooperative Group Trial [114]. The authors compared 1- and 3-cm margins of excision for melanomas ≥2.0 mm. Despite more locoregional recurrences in the 1-cm group, the difference in overall survival did not reach statistical significance. However, patients did not have staging of the regional nodal basin and so the conclusions and the applicability of this study are limited. A more recent trial conducted across nine European centers tested 2-cm versus 4-cm margins for melanomas ≥2.0 mm [44]. Despite more local recurrences in the 2-cm group, overall survival was not different. Not surprisingly, skin grafting was more frequently utilized in the 4-cm group. The authors' recommendation was to use 2-cm margins for melanomas ≥2.0 mm.

The current recommendations for margins of excision of melanoma are listed in Table 3. There continues to be a controversy about the management of thick melanomas with some surgeons advocating for a 3-cm margin. Only two of the randomized trials included patients with thick melanomas. However, these patients were underrepresented in both trials. Thus, recommendations for deep melanomas frequently require expert assessment by a surgical oncologist trained in melanoma surgery.

Dissection to the muscular fascia is the prevailing surgical practice as there does not appear to be any benefit in excising it. While there have been several randomized trials evaluating the role of margin width in local control of primary melanomas, few studies have examined the role that dissection depth plays in rates of locoregional recurrence and survival. Grotz and colleagues performed a retrospective analysis of patients with primary melanoma undergoing resection over a 29-year period revisiting the cases of 964 patients with melanomas ≥1.0 mm [48]. The muscular fascia was left intact in 686 (71 %) of the study population and excised in the remainder. The review found no difference in the rate of local recurrence between the two groups, but did find a significant reduction in the rate of in-transit and nodal metastases when the muscular fascia was preserved. There is concern that some of the data may have been confounded by advancements in practice that made sentinel node biopsies standard of care toward the end of the study period. Nonetheless, a conclusion could be drawn that resection of the muscular fascia did not improve patient outcomes following wide local excision and may serve to increase the risks of nodal recurrences [65, 90].

Table 3 Recommendations for margins of excision for treatment of melanoma

Depth of primary tumor	Margin of excision (cm)
In situ	0.5
<1 mm	1
1–4 mm	2
>4 mm	2–3

5 Sentinel Lymph Node Biopsy

The importance that surgeons place in the management of regional nodal disease comes from an understanding that melanoma commonly spreads via a lymphatic route. The impact of nodal metastases on survival has been studied extensively over the last several decades. The single most important factor in overall survival has been shown to be the status of disease within local lymph nodes [81]. The identification of metastatic melanoma in a nodal basin is important for staging, prognostication, and making treatment decisions.

Historically, elective lymph node dissection was felt to be appropriate for intermediate-thickness melanoma. Nodal staging was not considered in the treatment of thin melanomas because of low incidence of metastases. On the other hand, nodal staging was viewed as overtreatment of thick melanomas, as these patients were thought to have a high likelihood of developing distant metastases [5]. Two large cohort studies initially showed a benefit in survival for patients with intermediate-thickness melanoma who underwent this operation [76, 96]. Upon further review with more accurate, longer follow-up, elective lymph node dissection did not improve the survival of patients with no clinically involved nodes [32, 108]. While failing to show a benefit, the frequent implementation of this operation led to many patients suffering from wound complications and lymphedema. Subsequently, several prospective randomized trials further revealed there to be no improvement in survival from elective lymph node dissection in this population group [7, 106, 117].

The concept of a SLNB was applied to melanoma in the late twentieth century. The idea was first introduced by Cabanas for the treatment of penile carcinoma in 1977 [23]. However, it was not until SLNB was studied in the arena of melanoma treatment at the John Wayne Cancer Institute by Donald Morton that it became popularized [80]. The concept behind this technique is that lymphatic drainage progresses in an organized fashion. Rather than removing all lymph nodes for evaluation, only one could be excised to determine whether the primary tumor has spread. Several methods exist for the detection of a sentinel node(s). An intradermal injection of a radionuclide around the melanoma allows for the identification of sentinel nodes in the lymph node basin with a handheld gamma probe. This is the most common method utilized to perform a SLNB, because radiocolloid alone has been shown to be very safe and to have very low false-negative rates of 2–4 %. The high accuracy of this procedure is likely due to improved technology of gamma probes and their widespread use in the last two decades [55]. Alternatively, an injection of blue dye (isosulfan blue or methylene blue) intradermally around the melanoma will lead to its migration to the lymph node basin. The surgeon will then search for "blue" nodes in the appropriate nodal basin. A combination of these techniques can also be used and has been shown to result in greater accuracy in the identification of sentinel nodes [41]. The use of blue dyes, whether alone or in combination with radiocolloid, is less common than radionuclide because of several safety concerns. These include allergic reactions, tissue necrosis, and skin graft failures. Allergic reactions at a rate of 1.5 % have mostly been reported with isosulfan blue dye [34]. The risk of an anaphylactic reaction can be considerably reduced when less than 2 ml of the dye is administered. Tissue necrosis and skin graft complications have occurred when methylene blue dye has been used, especially in certain locations such as the face, wrists, and ankles [88]. As some institutions have limited or altogether eliminated the availability of isosulfan blue dye in order to contain costs, the surgeon must be keenly aware of the problems that may be encountered with the cheaper methylene blue dye.

After studies validated the accuracy and safety of lymph node mapping and sentinel node biopsy, surgeons started to identify the many benefits of this approach. A major advantage of the SLNB is that it is less likely to result in both immediate (seroma, wound infection) and long-term (lymphedema) complications when compared to elective node dissection [82, 123]. Another clear benefit of a SLNB, particular to the radiocolloid technique, is that it allows the surgeon to preoperatively localize the draining nodal basin(s), which is especially important for lesions of the trunk and the head and neck. Finally, sentinel nodes provide limited amount of tissue for the pathologist to examine, and both sensitive (S-100) and specific (MART-1) melanoma immunohistochemical stains can be applied at high frequency. As a result, the diagnosis is not only more accurate, but more precise, as the volume of metastatic disease can be quantified in each node.

6 Multicenter Selective Lymphadenectomy Trial-1

It is now widely accepted that the status of the sentinel lymph node is the most important prognostic factor in patients with melanoma. It is most consistently predicted by Breslow thickness of the primary lesion [31]. While previous reports showed no benefit in survival with elective lymph node dissection for patients with intermediate-thickness melanomas and no clinically evident nodal disease, the impact of a SLNB was yet to be determined for this metric. This was the goal of the Multicenter Selective Lymphadenectomy Trial-1 (MSLT-1). An analysis of 1347 patients, with a 60-month median follow-up, detected no benefit to melanoma-specific survival when the combination of a SLNB and wide local excision was compared to wide local excision alone (86.6 % vs. 87.1 %, HR = 0.92, p = 0.58) [83]. The addition of a SLNB did improve the disease-free survival (73.1 % vs. 78.3 %, HR = 0.74, p = 0.009), and benefits to survival were particularly pronounced in a subgroup of patients with positive sentinel nodes. In this group of patients, a superior 5-year melanoma-specific survival was identified when immediate completion lymphadenectomy was performed rather than a delayed lymphadenectomy (72.3 % vs. 52.4 %, HR = 0.51, p = 0.007). There are several criticisms of the subgroup analysis: The trial was not adequately powered to detect differences in this subset of patients, and false negatives were not included in it. Additionally, while immediate lymphadenectomy treated patients with micrometastatic disease, delayed lymphadenectomy treated bulky recurrent disease, essentially macrometastases, that were detected during oncologic surveillance. Since the volume of metastatic disease has consistently been shown to impact survival and is reflected in the staging system [37], the comparison of such groups may not have been appropriate.

The authors of the trial designed the ongoing MSLT-2 trial specifically to address the issue that was raised by the subset analysis. If properly powered, will there be an improved disease-specific survival when an immediate lymphadenectomy is performed in the setting of a positive SLNB versus a delayed lymphadenectomy? This trial is currently accruing patients. Importantly, updated results with 10-year follow-up have recently been reported for MSLT-1 [84]. At ten years, melanoma-specific survival remained similar between the two groups (81.4 % vs. 78.3 %, HR = 0.85, $p = 0.18$). Ten-year disease-free survival continued to be higher in the combination group (71.3 % vs. 64.7 %, HR = 0.76, $p = 0.01$). The prognostic significance of the sentinel node persisted at 10 years. Additionally, the report revealed same outcomes for 290 patients with thick melanomas. The appropriate inclusion of the patients with false-negative SLNB strengthened the survival results that were presented at 10-year follow-up. Whether the subgroup analysis is deemed to be appropriate or not by the reader of the published reports, MSLT-1 did demonstrate that SLNB is the best staging tool available to surgeons treating melanoma patients and delays the time to recurrence in intermediate-thickness melanomas. The benefit in disease-free survival is a metric that should not be overlooked as patients place considerable value in it, even when it does not translate into an improvement in disease-specific survival [67]. Additionally, many clinical trials require an assessment of the nodal basin as an inclusion parameter, and the lower morbidity associated with this operation as opposed to elective lymph node dissection makes it an ideal tool to do so.

7 Sentinel Lymph Node Biopsy for Thin and Thick Melanomas

Currently, SLNB is recommended for all patients with intermediate-thickness primary melanomas. There is more controversy about the role of a SLNB in patients with thin or thick melanomas. Since the incidence of lymph node metastases is low with thin melanomas, and concurrent distant metastases are not infrequent with thick melanomas, the value of this operation continues to be questioned in these patient populations. The benefits of a SLNB, such as improved disease-free survival and the ability to most accurately predict the prognosis, likely exist for both thin and thick melanomas. However, enthusiasm for performing the SLNB needs to be tempered with several facts. First, the incidence of lymph node metastases in melanomas <1 mm without any other clinicopathologic risk factors (ulceration, mitoses, etc.) is under 5 % [16, 86, 122]. Second, since approximately 70 % of all cutaneous melanomas are thin, the number of complications that would result from a SLNB would carry a significant toll. This is despite the fact that morbidity is usually minor occurs in only 5–10 % of patients and is most commonly managed on an outpatient basis [82, 123]. Third, the issue of cost has been carefully studied in patients with thin melanomas and remains a strong deterrent to widespread use of the operation [1]. For all of these reasons, lymph node mapping and sentinel node biopsy is advocated to patients with thin melanomas selectively. With respect to thick melanomas, limited evidence exists that SLNB has clinical benefit, but some surgeons argue that the procedure provides staging and prognostic information. The risk of distant metastases is not insignificant in these patients and a metastatic work-up is often considered prior to definitive surgical management. In the event that metastatic disease is found, prevention of future symptoms via adequate locoregional control is the major goal of surgical management, not cure of the disease. Patients without evidence of distant metastases should be treated with curative intent, and SLNB may be appropriate for above-mentioned reasons. Table 4 represents a summary of current recommendations for SLNB in patients with melanoma.

Certain factors, such as ulceration or mitoses, have been shown to increase the rate of lymph node metastasis from under 5 % to 5–14.7 % in thin melanomas [53, 62]. Both are used to define T1b thin melanoma, which has a slightly worse prognosis than T1a thin melanoma [37]. Additionally, multiple reports identified a considerable difference in the rate of SLNB positivity for patients with Breslow thickness under and over 0.75 mm. For melanomas <0.75 mm, lymph node metastases occur in less than 3 % of patients [53, 94, 123]. For thin melanomas ≥0.75 mm, regional nodal metastases are found in 5–10 % of patients [53, 87]. Most surgeons agree that presence of ulceration or mitoses in an otherwise thin melanoma should prompt the performance of a SLNB, especially when tumor depth is over 0.75 mm.

Clark's level is a way to state the depth of a melanoma based on which layers of epidermis/dermis it involves. Clark's level used to define T1b melanoma as recently as in the 6th edition of the AJCC Cancer Staging Manual, but was subsequently replaced with mitotic index in the 7th Edition. This occurred because multiple institutional studies reported that when mitoses were taken into account, Clark's level no longer predicted lymph node metastases or played a role in prognosis [40, 62, 86, 94, 119, 121]. However, a recent large cohort study demonstrated that

Table 4 Indications for sentinel lymph node biopsy

Depth of primary tumor	Recommendation
In situ	Not recommended
<0.75 mm	Not recommended
0.75–1.0 mm	Selected patients with high-risk features may benefit from SLNB
1.0–4.0 mm	SLNB recommended for all patients
>4.0 mm	Selected patients only as evidence is limited of benefit for SLNB in these patients; metastatic work-up should be considered prior to surgical management

Clark's level IV–V in patients with melanomas ≥0.75 mm resulted in 8.2 % incidence of SLNB positivity [53]. Several institutional studies have also reported Clark's level to be a significant predictor of lymph node metastases in multivariate analyses [17, 68]. Until more definitive data becomes available, Clark's level IV–V may be used to recommend a SLNB.

There are other indications to perform a SLNB in thin melanomas, albeit more relative ones. The presence of a VGP has been studied most extensively by the Pigmented Lesion Group. Investigators at University of Pennsylvania found that the presence of a VGP in thin melanomas ≥0.75 mm led to a 9.7 % incidence of lymph node metastases and was also a significant variable in a multivariate analysis [12, 62]. VGP has not been widely adopted as an indication to perform a SLNB because it is somewhat subjective and is not uniformly reported by pathologists across different centers. Another relative indication is the presence of a positive deep margin on initial biopsy. In this setting, Breslow thickness is indeterminate and the surgeon may have difficulty in determining prognosis of the patient and choosing the appropriate operation, with respect to margins of excision and the need for a SLNB. In a single institutional study, patients with thin melanomas and a positive deep margin on initial biopsy had an 8.3 % incidence of SLNB positivity [68]. The true Breslow thickness could only be determined in 26 % of patients who had residual disease in the surgical specimen, with over half showing deeper lesions. At this point, there is not enough evidence to strongly support the routine use of SLNB in these patients, and so it is being used selectively at some institutions.

It is known that younger patients have higher rates of lymph node metastases. Despite this, their survival is better. Investigators at the Moffitt Cancer Center and the John Wayne Cancer Institute examined the issue of age as an indication for a SLNB. Age less than 35 or 50 years was examined at these institutions and found to be an independent predictor of lymph node metastases [40, 111]. However, this factor is not commonly used to advocate for a SLNB because the survival does not appear to be worse in this population group. Another relative indication for a SLNB in thin melanomas is male sex. Multiple reports have shown this to be an independent predictor of SLNB positivity [40, 62]. However, among all the factors that were significant, such as Breslow thickness, ulceration, mitoses, VGP, and age, male sex had the weakest predictive value. In conclusion, certain institutions use VGP, positive deep margin, age, and sex as indications for a SLNB, but the data supporting these practices are limited.

8 Local Recurrence

An inadequate initial excision with suboptimal margins may result in a local recurrence. In this situation, disease-specific survival is rarely affected. Alternatively, in the face of an appropriate initial excision, as guided by margin width, a local recurrence signifies aggressive tumor biology and often heralds metastatic disease even following successful re-excision. The definition of a local recurrence is a regrowth of cancer within 2 cm of the surgical scar following excision of the lesion [10]. Local recurrence of melanoma can occur by a number of mechanisms. The most widely accepted is that of contiguous, horizontal growth of the primary lesion. By this mechanism, recurrent melanomas arise from retained malignant melanocytes that exist beyond the boundary of excision and escape pathological detection by virtue of a sampling error [10]. This theory supports the rationale for wide local excision and highlights the importance of appropriate margins. Another theory centers on the existence of microsatellites, or tumor nests that exist independently of the main tumor body. These lesions signify lymphatic spread of the cancer and confer a greater risk of local recurrence when they are identified in primary tumor excision specimens [64]. As the depth of the tumor increases, the number of microsatellites is also believed to be increased.

Major risk factors for developing a local recurrence are Breslow thickness and ulceration. Long-term data from the Intergroup Melanoma Surgical Trial showed that the presence of ulceration was the strongest predictor of local recurrence [8, 9]. The same study reported a dismal 5-year overall survival rate of 9 % when a local recurrence was identified. Surgical excision remains the treatment of choice in patients with a local recurrence. Since common practice is to monitor patients closely after the surgical treatment of melanoma for five years or longer, majority of recurrent lesions are detected early enough to permit a second excision. No guidelines exist for this type of excision, but it appears reasonable to resect a local recurrence with a 0.5- to 1.0-cm margin to facilitate primary closure in as many patients as possible. In the presence of distant metastases, excision to a negative margin is a sensible approach. Recurrent or unresectable lesions should be considered for palliation with radiotherapy.

9 Surgical Management in Special Populations

9.1 Desmoplastic Melanoma

DM is a rare histologic subtype with certain features that make management unique. First, DM is oftentimes non-pigmented, making for a more challenging and sometimes delayed diagnosis. Second, it is not uncommon for the pathologist to identify cancer cells in the dermis, without any abnormalities in the epidermis. Third, immunohistochemical staining profile is unusual. While staining for S-100 is usually positive, the more specific melanoma stains such as MART-1, HMB-45, and tyrosinase are typically negative. Furthermore, DM can stain positive for smooth muscle markers, such as actin, desmin, and vimentin [21]. This adds complexity to correctly identifying this melanoma subtype, as it can be confused with other spindle cell neoplasms. Fourth, the most common location is on the head and neck, making the surgical management more difficult for reasons that have been previously stated.

A distinction has been made between pure and mixed DMs, as their behavior is quite different. Pure DMs usually present with greater Breslow thickness than other melanomas, but the rates of lymph node metastases are lower than expected. Moreover, pure DMs have disease-free and overall survival rates that are better than one would predict given the depth with which they present [71, 79]. In comparison, mixed DMs have higher rates of lymph node metastases and a worse disease-free and overall survival than pure DMs [28]. For thin DMs, 1-cm margin appears to be adequate for mixed lesions, but not for pure ones. Maurichi and colleagues demonstrated higher local recurrence rates and higher mortality for pure DMs that were treated with 1 cm as opposed to a 2-cm margin [75]. Taken together, DMs present multiple challenges with diagnosis and appropriate treatment and require the surgeon to have a thorough knowledge of the subject.

9.2 Pregnancy

Women who are pregnant at the time of their melanoma diagnosis should be treated in the same fashion as a non-pregnant patient. Worse outcomes were identified in older poorly designed studies that examined pregnant patients with melanoma. More recent literature has refuted those findings [73]. Similarly, there is no prognostic relevance to estrogen replacement therapy or birth control pills. Since most resections of the primary lesion can be performed under local anesthesia with or without light sedation, the operation can take place in any trimester. Recent reports have demonstrated the safety of a SLNB during pregnancy with either the use of blue dye, radiocolloid, or a combination of the two [2, 46]. If general anesthesia is anticipated, as would be the case with a therapeutic or a completion lymphadenectomy, a consultation with an obstetrician could help alleviate the anxiety of the parents, and sometimes the physician. In general, an operation in any trimester should be safe, although the second trimester is preferred. Ultimately, melanoma in a pregnant patient is not a reason to seek non-surgical treatment options and must be treated promptly with the full armamentarium that is available to surgeons.

9.3 Children

Melanoma is a rare cancer of childhood. Early studies suggested worse outcomes for children with melanoma in comparison with adults. Fortunately, more recent data demonstrated no differences between these two groups when all prognostic variables were taken into account [42]. Importantly, SLNB has been successfully used in this population and seems to provide the same benefits and prognostic information as it does in adults. The Sydney Melanoma Unit group reported that despite higher than expected incidence of lymph node metastases as detected by a SLNB, few patients had positive non-sentinel nodes in the completion lymphadenectomy specimen, and melanoma-specific death rates were low [59]. The reverse relationship between SLNB positivity and survival has been shown in young adult populations, making these findings consistent.

There are several aspects of treatment that are unique to children with melanoma. One is the issue of a giant congenital nevus, which occurs at a rate of 1 in 20,000 newborns and measures greater than 20 cm in diameter by adulthood [74]. These carry a lifetime risk of 4–7 % of melanoma development, which typically develops by the age of five, but may occur later in life. Different ways of treating these lesions have been proposed, ranging from early resection, partial ablation, close observation until adolescence, or observation throughout lifetime. Another is the issue of Spitz nevi, which usually have benign behavior, but are frequently difficult to distinguish from melanomas because of cellular atypia and structural asymmetry. These lesions are so ambiguous that several investigators treat them as they would be a melanoma, including the use of a SLNB. However, recent data determined that a positive SLNB in the setting of Spitz nevi does not convey the same negative prognosis as it does in adults or children with unambiguous melanoma, making its implementation questionable [22]. Lastly, surgical interventions, both diagnostic and therapeutic, require a form of sedation in children. Even an otherwise straightforward procedure like a shave biopsy cannot be easily performed in a conscious child. This may lead to delays in diagnostic procedures for children with suspicious cutaneous lesions. Excisional biopsy or wide local excision would certainly necessitate deep sedation, oftentimes requiring general anesthesia. All of these issues make the care of a child with the diagnosis of melanoma a specialized field that mandates a thorough understanding of all the relevant facts.

9.4 Geriatrics

Elderly patients represent a significant proportion of all those who are diagnosed with melanoma. Several variables that are inherent to this group of patients present challenges to the treating surgeon. It has been well established that older age portends a worse prognosis [8, 9, 63]. The reasons for this remain elusive. It is possible that immune surveillance plays a role, especially in the presence of nodal metastases, or that comorbidities combined with the presence of cancer result in higher mortality. Furthermore, there appears to be a lower tolerance to reconstructions that are sometimes needed after a resection of a melanoma. Longer times may sometimes be needed to recover from skin grafting or tissue advancement/rotational flaps. Additionally, fewer adjuvant therapies are available to the elderly. The ability to come for daily radiotherapy may preclude from this treatment being administered to its fullest effect. Certain age or presence of comorbidities may prevent enrollment of an elderly patient in clinical trials. Toxicities or the duration of some therapies, such as the year-long interferon treatment, may preclude from their implementation. Ultimately, the surgeon must keep in mind that for an elderly patient quality of life is frequently more important than quantity of life, and several features of melanoma treatment may adversely impact this metric.

10 Wound Closure

10.1 Primary Closure

The adoption of narrower margins of excision has not liberated melanoma patients from complex surgeries with important functional, cosmetic, and psychological implications. As research has demonstrated, appropriate margins are necessary for disease control and must not be sacrificed in favor of less complex wound closure. Melanomas of the trunk and proximal extremities are often managed with elliptical excision and primary closure. Excisions at sites such as distal extremities, head, and neck may also be amenable to primary closure, but reconstructive techniques are more likely to be needed. Sometimes, adjacent tissue has to be undermined with dissection of the skin and subcutaneous tissue from the fascial layer which will allow the skin to be advanced over the defect. Unless there is significant skin laxity, the defect is usually closed in two or more layers to lessen tension. Absorbable deep dermal sutures will maximize the integrity of the closure and allow for approximation of the epidermal layers with minimal tension. The skin can then be closed with a running subcuticular suture, interrupted stitches or staples based on surgeon preference and wound characteristics.

10.2 Reconstruction

Lower costs, better cosmetic outcomes, and less surgical morbidity all favor primary closure. However, this is not always practical when excessive tension will be placed on the wound or derangement of neighboring structures occurs. In such cases, advanced reconstructive techniques will be necessary to close the acquired defect. In increasing complexity, these are skin grafts, local flaps, regional flaps, and free tissue transfer. For many of these closures, a surgeon trained in reconstruction will be a critical member of the oncologic team.

The transfer of skin from one site to repair a defect in another is known as skin grafting. Grafts are usually obtained from the patient as opposed to a cadaver and can be either split-thickness or full-thickness. The harvesting technique employed in split-thickness grafting allows for division of the dermal layer such that the deepest layers remain to permit re-epithelialization of the donor site. This differs from full-thickness grafting where the entire dermal layer is included in the graft and independent closure of the donor site by local advancement or secondary flaps is necessary. Wound contraction is less pronounced with full-thickness grafts making them appropriate for closure of defects in critical and sensitive locations [56]. A frequently encountered problem with skin grafting arises when there is a significant difference in color between the donor and recipient tissues and is particularly relevant with reconstructions of the face. Split-thickness grafts are commonly harvested from the thigh, but can also be harvested from the trunk, back, buttocks, or neck depending on the need for a color match [116].

Rearrangement of soft tissues adjacent to a defect is another option for wound closure when the wound cannot be closed primarily. Indications for flap coverage are similar to those for skin grafts, but also include poor vascularization of the recipient bed and regional aesthetics that do not favor grafts. Local flaps have the added benefit of allowing the surgeon to maintain the normal contour of the skin and repair the defect without color matching problems [60]. These advantages make local flaps a good option for closing defects on the face. The donor site must have sufficient laxity to permit repair of the oncologic defect and for primary closure of the donor site.

Regional flaps are another method for reconstruction of complex wounds [4]. Regional flaps utilize tissue within the vicinity of the defect, but not necessarily adjacent to it. Each flap has a territorial arc of rotation and remains attached to the donor site by a vascular pedicle [10]. The flap is transposed to the donor site by moving it over or tunneling it under normal tissue. They are mainly indicated for closure of large defects or those which contain important structures such as bone, tendons, or nerves. Well-recognized regional flaps include the latissimus dorsi flap, which is frequently employed in breast reconstruction and other defects of the chest wall [78, 101], and the pectoralis flap that can be used for reconstruction of the head, neck, and axilla [70].

Free flaps are temporarily severed from their blood supply to allow transfer to the donor site [99, 104]. The feeding vessels are then anastamosed to a new artery and vein near the recipient site to reestablish perfusion to the transplanted tissue. The general indications for a free flap are for reconstruction of large soft tissue defects following major procedures, protection of exposed vital organs and restoration of function or appearance. These procedures are very complex and require a large amount of preoperative planning before they are attempted because flap loss can be a highly morbid and devastating complication.

10.3 Head and Neck

Of all areas of oncologic reconstruction, the head and neck presents one of the greatest challenges to surgeons as the slightest degree of asymmetry may produce cosmetically disappointing outcomes for the patient. The scalp is inelastic because of the galea aponeurotica and frequently requires advanced reconstructive efforts. In general, defects greater than 2 cm are difficult to approximate primarily. The scalp is very vascular and this allows for a number of reconstructive approaches to be used. Skin grafting is usually successful as long as the defect does not extend down to the bone. However, local flap coverage is a cosmetically superior method as it does not lead to alopecia and contour mismatch. Large defects of the scalp, especially when exceeding 8 cm, or situations where the cranium or dura are exposed, benefit from free tissue flaps [116]. Melanoma on the forehead, cheek, eyelids, nose, lips, and ears present similar challenges as does the scalp location. Local flaps are the most common method of defect reconstruction at these sites. Wide undermining may be necessary, and attention should be paid to the normal tension lines of the face to conceal scarring and lessen distortion. Special considerations should be made for some of these sites, such as care with facial nerve branches at medial cheek, full-thickness grafting from lower eyelid to cover upper eyelid defects but not the reverse, and the greater difficulty with upper lip reconstruction as opposed to the lower lip due to less elasticity.

10.4 Distal Extremities

Primary closure after an excision of a forearm or a leg melanoma is more challenging than in the proximal extremities because of less skin laxity, presence of a thick investing fascia, the subcutaneous location of the long bones and the tapering anatomy of the forearm and the leg. Additionally, there is a greater risk of accidental trauma to the repair postoperatively. Local flap coverage may be a better option for managing defects of the distal extremities than skin grafting because they allow for preservation of the natural contour and color matching. Nonetheless, flap coverage in these regions can be challenging because vascular supply is less robust and less reliable, necessitating a thorough knowledge of the constant points of vascular supply to the skin.

11 Surgical Management of Regional Metastases

11.1 Management of Clinically Positive Lymph Nodes

Clinically palpable lymph nodes in the presence of a melanoma near the draining nodal basin are concerning for metastatic disease. Fine needle aspiration is the best way to confirm nodal spread. Once this is established, therapeutic lymph node dissection should be offered to patients. There are several reasons for this recommendation. First, unresected nodal metastases can continue to grow and invade adjacent structures, leading to considerable morbidity. Second, despite a high rate of concurrent distant metastases, up to a third of patients can still be cured [107, 108, 124]. When a melanoma is located on the head, neck, or trunk, multiple draining nodal basins can be involved with metastases. A careful physical examination is of paramount importance to detect macroscopic nodal disease. A SLNB may be helpful in ruling out the presence of metastases in other neighboring nodal basins even in the presence of palpable disease.

11.2 Therapeutic Lymphadenectomy

Melanoma patients with macroscopic nodal disease should undergo a therapeutic lymph node dissection, essentially a complete lymphadenectomy. In contrast to breast cancer where nodal sampling with a SLNB or a limited axillary lymphadenectomy (level 1 and partial level 2) may be sufficient for clinical management, melanoma patients require complete dissection to clear all potential nodal disease. For axillary lymph node dissection, level 1, 2, and 3 nodes should be excised. With respect to inguinal lymphadenectomy, few surgeons offer both superficial and deep dissections. Most would limit the lymphadenectomy to the superficial compartment unless there was bulky nodal disease, the presence of disease in Cloquet's node (located at the junction to the deep compartment), 3 or more involved inguinal nodes, or an inguinal node ratio >0.20 [29]. The reason for this is the very high rates of distant metastases in the presence of deep iliac, obturator, or pelvic nodal involvement. Additionally, synchronous pelvic disease is rare, with some reports citing the incidence to be around 12 % [29]. Another point to make about inguinal lymphadenectomy is the attendant high rates of morbidity that accompany this operation. The rates of wound complications approach 50 % in contemporary studies, with a significant proportion of these representing dehiscences [35, 93, 99]. These high rates of serious complications have deterred many surgeons from performing this operation despite the current recommendations [15]. Others have adopted a routine transposition of the sartorius muscle during the operation in order to protect the femoral vessels in case a dehiscence develops. Moreover, several centers have developed a minimally invasive laparoscopic technique to superficial inguinal lymphadenectomy, with early results showing lower rates of wound infections and dehiscences [36, 47]. A modified radical neck dissection should be performed in the presence of cervical nodal disease. Modified radical neck dissection removes all lymph nodes in cervical levels 1–5, while preserving the internal jugular vein, the sternocleidomastoid muscle, and the spinal accessory nerve. Melanomas of the anterior scalp and face usually drain to parotid nodes, and a superficial parotidectomy is commonly performed at the time of the neck dissection.

Lymphadenectomy is a procedure that typically requires hospitalization and general anesthesia. The operation is associated with considerable potential morbidity, including lymphedema reported in up to 44 % of patients, seroma, hematoma, wound complications, and nerve damage [13, 61, 115]. Several authors have attempted to come up with standards for the various types of lymph node dissections, in terms of lymph node yield. Investigators at the Sydney Melanoma Unit have proposed the 90th percentile benchmark as a minimum acceptable lymph node count. According to their report, lymph node yield for axillary, superficial inguinal, selective neck, and modified radical neck dissection should be greater than or equal to 10, 7, 6, and 20 nodes, respectively [112].

11.3 Recurrent Regional Metastases and Isolated Limb Therapies

Prognosis is poor when melanoma recurs regionally, but a meaningful disease-free interval is possible and so is cure. Recurrent regional melanoma can present as satellite lesions, in-transit disease, or nodal metastases. Satellite lesions are within 2–5 cm of the primary melanoma location, while in-transit lesions are more than

5 cm away, but proximal to the lymph node basin. Satellite and in-transit disease both represent intralymphatic spread, and for this reason portend similar prognosis. This is reflected in the staging system [37]. These lesions should be excised to clear margins. Currently, no effective systemic therapy is available for recurrent regional disease. When multiple recurrent lesions are identified in an extremity and there are no distant metastases, isolated limb therapies can accomplish superior regional control than multiple simple excisions. Hyperthermic isolated limb perfusion (HILP) was developed in 1950s, while isolated limb infusion (ILI) is a more recent technique that has been available since 1990s. With both operations, a cytotoxic agent, commonly melphalan, is delivered to an upper or a lower extremity for the purpose of controlling diffuse, overwhelming regional disease [85]. With the older approach, a nodal lymphadenectomy is performed followed by the direct cannulation of blood vessels. In the setting of the newer operation, catheters are placed percutaneously, usually by interventionalists. The regional toxicity is higher with HILP, but so are the response rates. It appears that disease-specific survival does not vary between patients treated with either one of these therapies, making ILI more attractive in the initial setting because of lower complication rates and easier reproducibility. However, several reports have shown that with repeat operations for regional disease control, HILP has higher response rates than ILI and appears to be more appropriate [24, 95].

12 Surgical Management of Metastatic Disease

Long-term survival rates are around 10 % for patients with systemic metastatic disease [37]. However, with the advent of multiple new targeted drugs and immunotherapies, there is hope that cure rates for stage IV melanoma will improve in the near future. Even though systemic therapies are the main modality of treatment for stage IV disease, patients with isolated and resectable metastases may benefit from a surgical resection. Metastasectomy for melanoma is most commonly employed in a palliative setting, such as small bowel resection for hemorrhage or a bowel obstruction, lymphadenectomy for present or impending neurologic symptoms, and cutaneous excision for pain control. Surgical resection can also be used for curative purposes, although such events are rare. Gastrointestinal tract metastases commonly limited to small intestine, when resected completely can result in improved survival. A review of such a cohort of patients demonstrated 23.5-month survival time in patients whose disease was completely resected as opposed to patients who underwent a partial resection (8.9 months) or were not resected (4.1 months) ($p < 0.0001$) [14]. There was a selection bias in favor of patients who were selected to undergo a surgical exploration as 14 patients were deemed to be too sick to undergo an operation because of multiple comorbidities. Several other reports also determined that a complete resection of gastrointestinal metastases leads to a benefit in survival in comparison with incomplete resection, while symptomatic relief is commonly accomplished [51, 89, 100].

Distant cutaneous, nodal, and pulmonary metastases can also be surgically resected. Considerable selection bias is present in these reports because the data are retrospective, but certain trends have emerged and are helpful in the identification of patients who may benefit the most from an operation. A low number of metastases, a long disease-free interval between the time of initial diagnosis and the detection of metastatic disease, and an operation with a goal for a metastasectomy have been found to be associated with an improved survival [87, 120]. The authors of the MSLT-1 studied patients who were enrolled in the trial and subsequently developed metastases. The 4-year survival rate was superior for the 161 patients who underwent an operative approach as opposed to the 130 patients who did not (20.8 % vs. 7.0 %, HR = 0.41, $p < 0.0001$) [58]. Patients with distant skin, subcutaneous and nodal metastases (M1a disease) seemed to derive the greatest benefit from a surgical resection with or without an addition of systemic therapy. Another interesting finding was that repeat operations did not result in a worse survival in 67 patients.

Other visceral sites of melanoma metastases, such as the liver and adrenal glands, have been studied in the setting of a metastasectomy, with 5-year survival rates reaching 20.5 % [77, 98]. Patients who underwent resection demonstrated an improved survival. In the presence of brain metastases, median survival ranges from 3 to 6 months. Oftentimes, major clinical symptoms are observed and resection of such lesions may provide clinical benefits. A retrospective report studied 147 patients who underwent a craniotomy for 1–3 accessible metastases [125]. The mortality was 2 %, while the median survival reached 8.5 months, an improvement over historical cohorts treated non-operatively. Long-term cures were very rare, with only 5 % of patients surviving to 5 years. In line with other published data, this report identified an improved survival in patients with fewer lesions and complete resections. In conclusion, despite the considerable selection bias present in all reports for metastasectomy, it is clear that when the operation can be safely performed, carefully selected patients may derive a clinical benefit.

13 Surgical Management of Systemic Therapy Complications

13.1 Gastrointestinal Perforation

Since 2011, a number of new targeted therapies have become available for patients with metastatic melanoma. These include ipilimumab (IPI), an anti-CTLA-4 antibody, BRAF inhibitor, programmed death-1 inhibitor, and programmed death ligand-1 inhibitor. Some of these have been used alone, while others have been combined with other established therapies, such as interleukin-2 (IL-2). Enterocolitis is a known side effect of treatment with IPI, occurring in about 21 % of patients and is frequently reported as the most common major toxicity [11]. While most patients respond to high-dose steroids or infliximab, about 2 % develop bowel perforation requiring a colectomy. This was higher than the rate of bowel perforations in patients treated with IL-2 (0.45 %) [57]. The Surgery Branch at the National Cancer Institute reported an even higher incidence of gastrointestinal perforation (13.6 %) in patients who were first treated with IPI and then high-dose IL-2 [109]. The authors recommended patients undergo a diagnostic colonoscopy prior to initiation of IL-2 therapy to rule out the presence of chronic active colitis. Severe gastrointestinal toxicity has not been reported with the newer agents [52], but as combination therapies become more widespread, it is safe to assume that rates of severe enterocolitis leading to bowel perforation will increase, and the surgeon must remain vigilant and knowledgeable about these possibilities.

13.2 Squamous Cell Carcinoma of the Skin

Serine/threonine kinase BRAF is a component of the RAS–RAF–MEK–ERK signaling pathway that affects several cellular processes. It can be mutated in melanoma, commonly at codon 600 (V600E) [18]. A BRAF inhibitor has been approved for the treatment of metastatic melanoma [27]. Patients who are treated with this agent frequently develop a variety of cutaneous lesions. Most of these are benign, but squamous cell carcinomas can occur [30]. These can arise as early as 1 week into treatment, but usually occur 3–4 months after the start of therapy. The incidence can be as high as 26 % [19]. Given this high potential for malignant lesions to develop as a result of treatment with a BRAF inhibitor, a low threshold for a biopsy of new lesions is recommended.

14 Conclusions

Melanoma is a rare form of skin cancer that has continued to increase in incidence and accounts for a large proportion of skin cancer deaths. Surgical management can result in high cure rates for patients with early- and intermediate-stage disease. Proper treatment begins with a prompt biopsy of concerning cutaneous lesions, with a preference for an excisional biopsy as it is more accurate than other diagnostic modalities. Appropriate margins of excision are based on the thickness of the primary lesion. Nodal staging is performed with a SLNB. While this operation holds a clear clinical benefit to patients with intermediate-thickness melanomas, certain subsets of thin melanomas and thick melanomas may derive benefits as well. SLNB has not shown a survival benefit, but provides the best prognostic information available to patients with melanoma. Complete lymph node dissection remains the standard of care for patients with a positive sentinel node biopsy or clinically involved nodes. Indications for metastasectomy have continued to expand since this can lead to improved outcomes in carefully selected patients. These will likely become more prevalent as newer therapies with better outcomes continue to emerge onto the field of melanoma care.

References

1. Agnese DM, Abdessalam SF, Burak WE Jr et al (2003) Cost-effectiveness of sentinel lymph node biopsy in thin melanomas. Surgery 134:542–547
2. Andtbacka RH, Donaldson MR, Bowles TL et al (2013) Sentinel lymph node biopsy for melanoma in pregnant women. Ann Surg Oncol 20:689–696
3. Azzola MF, Shaw HM, Thompson JF et al (2003) Tumor mitotic rate is a more powerful prognostic indicator than ulceration in patients with primary cutaneous melanoma: an analysis of 3661 patients from a single center. Cancer 97:1488–1498
4. Baker SR (1990) Regional flaps in facial reconstruction. Otolaryngol Clin North Am 23:925–946
5. Balch CM (1988) The role of elective lymph node dissection in melanoma: rationale, results, and controversies. J Clin Oncol 6:163–172
6. Balch CM, Murad TM, Soong SJ et al (1979) Tumor thickness as a guide to surgical management of clinical stage I melanoma patients. Cancer 43:883–888
7. Balch CM, Soong S, Ross MI et al (2000) Long-term results of a multi-institutional randomized trial comparing prognostic factors and surgical results for intermediate thickness melanomas (1.0 to 4.0 mm). Intergroup Melanoma Surgical Trial. Ann Surg Oncol 7:87–97
8. Balch CM, Soong SJ, Gershenwald JE et al (2001) Prognostic factors analysis of 17600 melanoma patients: validation of the American Joint Committee on Cancer melanoma staging system. J Clin Oncol 200119:3622–3634
9. Balch CM, Soong SJ, Smith T et al (2001) Long-term results of a prospective surgical trial comparing 2 cm vs. 4 cm excision margins for 740 patients with 1-4 mm melanomas. Ann Surg Oncol 8:101–108
10. Balch CM, Houghton AN, Sober AJ (2003) Cutaneous melanoma. Quality Medical Publishing, St. Louis
11. Beck KE, Blansfield JA, Tran KQ et al (2006) Enterocolitis in patients with cancer after antibody blockade of cytotoxic T-lymphocyte-associated antigen 4. J Clin Oncol 24:2283–2289
12. Bedrosian I, Faries MB, Guerry D 4th et al (2000) Incidence of sentinel node metastasis in patients with thin primary melanoma (≤1 mm) with vertical growth phase. Ann Surg Oncol 7:262–267
13. Beitsch P, Balch CM (1992) Operative morbidity and risk factor assessment in melanoma patients undergoing inguinal lymph node dissection. Am J Surg 164:462–465
14. Berger AC, Buell JF, Venzon D et al (1999) Management of symptomatic malignant melanoma of the gastrointestinal tract. Ann Surg Oncol 6:155–160
15. Bilimoria KY, Balch CM, Bentrem DJ et al (2008) Complete lymph node dissection for sentinel node-positive melanoma: assessment of practice patterns in the United States. Ann Surg Oncol 15:1566–1576
16. Bleicher RJ, Essner R, Foshag LJ et al (2003) Role of sentinel lymphadenectomy in thin invasive cutaneous melanomas. J Clin Oncol 21:1326–1331
17. Boland G, Caudle A, Warneke C et al (2014) Predictors of survival in contemporary era patients with thin melanoma who underwent sentinel node biopsy. Presented at parallel melanoma session at the 67th annual society of surgical oncology cancer symposium in Phoenix, AZ
18. Bollag G, Hirth P, Tsai J et al (2010) Clinical efficacy of a RAF inhibitor needs broad target blockade in BRAF-mutant melanoma. Nature 467:596–599
19. Boussemart L, Routier E, Mateus C et al (2013) Prospective study of cutaneous side-effects associated with the BRAF inhibitor vemurafenib: a study of 42 patients. Ann Oncol 24:1691–1697
20. Breslow A (1970) Thickness, cross-sectional areas and depth of invasion in the prognosis of cutaneous melanoma. Ann Surg 172:902–908
21. Busam KJ (2011) Desmoplastic melanoma. Clin Lab Med 31:321–330

22. Busam KJ, Murali R, Pulitzer M et al (2009) Atypical spitzoid melanocytic tumors with positive sentinel lymph nodes in children and teenagers, and comparison with histologically unambiguous and lethal melanomas. Am J Surg Pathol 33:1386–1395
23. Cabanas RM (1977) An approach for the treatment of penile carcinoma. Cancer 39:456–466
24. Chai CY, Deneve JL, Beasley GM et al (2012) A multi-institutional experience of repeat regional chemotherapy for recurrent melanoma of extremities. Ann Surg Oncol 19:1637–1643
25. Chang AE, Karnell LH, Menck HR (1998) The National Cancer Data Base report on cutaneous and noncutaneous melanoma: a summary of 84836 cases from the past decade. The American College of Surgeons Commission on Cancer and the American Cancer Society. Cancer 83:1664–1678
26. Chapgar RB, Ross MI, Roentgen DS et al (2007) Factors associated with improved survival among young adult melanoma patients despite a greater incidence of sentinel lymph node metastasis. J Surg Res 143:164–168
27. Chapman PB, Hauschild A, Robert C et al (2011) Improved survival with vemurafenib in melanoma with BRAF V600E mutation. N Engl J Med 364:2507–2516
28. Chen LL, Jaimes N, Barker CA et al (2013) Desmoplastic melanoma: a review. J Am Acad Dermatol 68:825–833
29. Chu CK, Delman KA, Carlson GW et al (2011) Inguinopelvic lymphadenectomy following positive inguinal sentinel lymph node biopsy in melanoma: true frequency of synchronous pelvic metastases. Ann Surg Oncol 18:3309–3315
30. Chu EY, Wanat KA, Miller CJ et al (2012) Diverse cutaneous side effects associated with BRAF inhibitor therapy: a clinicopathologic study. J Am Acad Dermatol 67:1265–1272
31. Clary BM, Brady MS, Lewis JJ et al (2001) Sentinel lymph node biopsy in the management of patients with primary cutaneous melanoma: review of a large single-institutional experience with an emphasis on recurrence. Ann Surg 233:250–258
32. Coates AS, Ingvar CI, Petersen-Schaefer K et al (1995) Elective lymph node dissection in patients with primary melanoma of the trunk and limbs treated at the Sydney Melanoma unit from 1960 to 1991. J Am Coll Surg 180:402–409
33. Cohn-Cedermark G, Rutqvist LE, Andersson R et al (2000) Long term results of a randomized study by the Swedish Melanoma Study Group on 2-cm versus 5-cm resection margins for patients with cutaneous melanoma with a tumor thickness of 0.8–2.0 mm. Cancer 89:1495–1501
34. Daley MD, Norman PH, Leak JA et al (2004) Adverse events associated with the intraoperative injection of isosulfan blue. J Clin Anesth 16:332–341
35. de Vries M, Hoekstra HJ, Hoekstra-Weebers JE (2009) Quality of life after axillary or groin sentinel lymph node biopsy, with or without completion lymph node dissection, in patients with cutaneous melanoma. Ann Surg Oncol 16:2840–2847
36. Delman KA, Kooby DA, Ogan K et al (2010) Feasibility of a novel approach to inguinal lymphadenectomy: minimally invasive groin dissection for melanoma. Ann Surg Oncol 17:731–737
37. Edge SB, Byrd DR, Compton CC et al (2010) AJCC Cancer Staging Manual, 7th edn. Springer, New York
38. Elwood JM, Jopson J (1997) Melanoma and sun exposure: an overview of published studies. Int J Cancer 73:198–203
39. Everall JD, Dowd PM (1977) Diagnosis, prognosis, and treatment of melanoma. Lancet 2:286–289
40. Faries MB, Wanek LA, Elashoff D et al (2010) Predictors of occult nodal metastasis in patients with thin melanoma. Arch Surg 145:137–142
41. Gershenwald JE, Colome MI, Lee JE et al (1998) Patterns of recurrence following a negative sentinel lymph node biopsy in 243 patients with stage I or II melanoma. J Clin Oncol 16:2253–2260

42. Gibbs P, Moore A, Robinson W et al (2000) Pediatric melanoma: are recent advances in management of adult melanoma relevant to the pediatric population. J Pediatr Hematol Oncol 22:428–432
43. Gilchrest BA, Eller MS, Geller AC et al (1999) The pathogenesis of melanoma induced by ultraviolet radiation. N Engl J Med 340:1341–1348
44. Gillgren P, Drzewiecki KT, Niin M et al (2011) 2-cm versus 4-cm surgical excision margins for primary cutaneous melanoma thicker than 2 mm: a randomized, multicentre trial. Lancet 378:1635–1642
45. Gimotty PA, Elder DE, Fraker DL et al (2007) Identification of high-risk patients among those diagnosed with thin cutaneous melanomas. J Clin Oncol 25:1129–1134
46. Gropper AB, Calvillo KZ, Dominici L et al (2014) Sentinel lymph node biopsy in pregnant women with breast cancer. Ann Surg Oncol. 23 Apr 2014 (Epub ahead of print)
47. Grotz TE, Jakub JW (2014) Comparison of tissue sealing devices for minimally invasive inguinal lymphadenectomy. Presented at the poster session at the 67th annual society of surgical oncology cancer symposium in Phoenix, AZ
48. Grotz TE, Glorioso JM, Pockaj BA et al (2013) Preservation of the deep muscular fascia and locoregional control in melanoma. Surgery 153:535–541
49. Guerin S, Dupuy A, Anderson H et al (2003) Radiation dose as a risk factor for malignant melanoma following childhood cancer. Eur J Cancer 39:2379–2386
50. Gupta TK (1977) Results of treatment of 269 patients with primary cutaneous melanoma: a five-year prospective study. Ann Surg 186:201–209
51. Gutman H, Hess KR, Kokotsakis JA et al (2001) Surgery for abdominal metastases of cutaneous melanoma. World J Surg 25:750–758
52. Hamid O, Robert C, Daud A et al (2013) Safety and tumor responses with lambrolizumab (anti-PD-1) in melanoma. N Engl J Med 369:134–144
53. Han D, Zager JS, Shyr Y et al (2013) Clinicopathologic predictors of sentinel lymph node metastasis in thin melanoma. J Clin Oncol 31:4387–4393
54. Handley WS (1907) The pathology of melanotic growths in relation to their operative treatment. Lancet 1:927–933
55. Harlow SP, Krag DN, Ashikaga T et al (2001) Gamma probe guided biopsy of the sentinel node in malignant melanoma: a multicenter study. Melanoma Res 11:45–55
56. Harrison CA, MacNeil S (2008) The mechanism of skin graft contraction: an update on current research and potential future therapies. Burns 34:153–163
57. Heimann DM, Schwartzentruber DJ (2004) Gastrointestinal perforations associated with interleukin-2 administration. J Immunother 27:254–258
58. Howard JH, Thompson JF, Mozzillo N et al (2012) Metastasectomy for distant metastatic melanoma: analysis of data from the first multicenter selective lymphadenectomy trial (MSLT-I). Ann Surg Oncol 19:2547–2555
59. Howman-Giles R, Shaw HM, Scolyer RM et al (2010) Sentinel lymph node biopsy in pediatric and adolescent cutaneous melanoma patients. Ann Surg Oncol 17:138–143
60. Jackson IT (1985) Local flaps in head and neck reconstruction. Mosby, St. Louis
61. Karakousis CP, Driscoll DL (1994) Groin dissection in malignant melanoma. Br J Surg 81:1771–1774
62. Karakousis GC, Gimotty PA, Botbyl JD et al (2006) Predictors of regional nodal disease in patients with thin melanomas. Ann Surg Oncol 13:533–541
63. Karakousis GC, Gimotty PA, Czerniecki BJ et al (2007) Regional nodal metastatic disease is the strongest predictor of survival in patients with thin vertical growth phase melanomas: a case of SLN Staging biopsy in these patients. Ann Surg Oncol 14:1596–1603
64. Kelly JW, Sagebiel RW, Calderon W et al (1984) The frequency of local recurrence and microsatellites as a guide to reexcision margins for cutaneous malignant melanoma. Ann Surg 200:759–763
65. Kenady DE, Brown BW, McBride CM (1982) Excision of underlying fascia with a primary malignant melanoma: effect on recurrence and survival rates. Surgery 92:615–618

66. Khayat D, Rixe O, Martin G et al (2003) Surgical margins in cutaneous melanoma (2 cm versus 5 cm for lesions measuring less than 2.1-mm thick). Cancer 97:1941–1946
67. Kilbridge KL, Weeks JC, Sober AJ et al (2001) Patient preferences for adjuvant interferon alfa-2b treatment. J Clin Oncol 19:812–823
68. Koshenkov VP, Shulkin D, Bustami R et al (2012) Role of sentinel lymphadenectomy in thin cutaneous melanomas with positive deep margins on initial biopsy. J Surg Oncol 106:363–368
69. Lea CS, Scotto JA, Buffler PA et al (2007) Ambient UVB and melanoma risk in the United States: a case-control analysis. Ann Epidemiol 17:447–453
70. Liu R, Gullane P, Brown D et al (2001) Pectoralis major myocutaneous pedicled flap in head and neck reconstruction: retrospective review of indications and results in 244 consecutive cases at the Toronto General Hospital. J Otolaryngol 30:34–40
71. Livestro DP, Muzikansky A, Kaine EM et al (2005) Biology of desmoplastic melanoma: a case-control comparison with other melanomas. J Clin Oncol 23:6739–6746
72. Lomas A, Leonardi-Bee J, Bath-Hextall F (2012) A systematic review of worldwide incidence of nonmelanoma skin cancer. Br J Dermatol 166:1069–1080
73. MacKie RM (1999) Pregnancy and exogenous hormones in patients with cutaneous malignant melanoma. Curr Opin Oncol 11:129–131
74. Marghoob AA, Schoenbach SP, Kopf AW et al (1996) Large congenital melanocytic nevi and the risk for the development of malignant melanoma. A prospective study. Arch Dermatol 132:170–175
75. Maurichi A, Miceli R, Camerini T et al (2010) Pure desmoplastic melanoma: a melanoma with distinctive clinical behavior. Ann Surg 252:1052–1057
76. Milton GW, Shaw HM, McCarthy WH et al (1982) Prophylactic lymph node dissection in clinical stage I cutaneous malignant melanoma: results of surgical treatment in 1319 patients. Br J Surg 69:108–111
77. Mittendorf EA, Lim SJ, Schacherer CW et al (2008) Melanoma adrenal metastasis: natural history and surgical management. Am J Surg 195:363–368
78. Moelleken BR, Mathes SA, Chang N (1989) Latissimus dorsi muscle-musculocutaneous flap in chest-wall reconstruction. Surg Clin North Am 69:977–990
79. Mohebati A, Ganly I, Busam KJ et al (2012) The role of sentinel lymph node biopsy in the management of head and neck desmoplastic melanoma. Ann Surg Oncol 19:4307–4313
80. Morton DL, Wen DR, Wong JH et al (1992) Technical details of intraoperative lymphatic mapping for early stage melanoma. Arch Surg 127:392–399
81. Morton DL, Thompson JF, Essner R et al (1999) Validation of the accuracy of intraoperative lymphatic mapping and sentinel lymphadenectomy for early-stage melanoma: a multicenter trial. Multicenter Selective Lymphadenectomy Trial Group. Ann Surg 230:453–463
82. Morton DL, Cochran AJ, Thompson JF et al (2005) Sentinel node biopsy for early-stage melanoma: accuracy and morbidity in MSLT-I, an international multicenter trial. Ann Surg 242:302–311
83. Morton DL, Thompson JF, Cochran AJ et al (2006) Sentinel-node biopsy or nodal observation in melanoma. N Engl J Med 355:1307–1317
84. Morton DL, Thompson JF, Cochran AJ et al (2014) Final trial report of sentinel-node biopsy versus nodal observation in melanoma. N Engl J Med 370:599–609
85. Muchmore JH, Wanebo HJ (2008) Regional chemotherapy: overview. Surg Oncol Clin N Am 17:709–730
86. Murali R, Haydu LE, Quinn MJ et al (2012) Sentinel lymph node biopsy in patients with thin primary cutaneous melanomas. Ann Surg 255:128–133
87. Neuman HB, Patel A, Hanlon C et al (2007) Stage-IV melanoma and pulmonary metastases: factors predictive of survival. Ann Surg Oncol 14:2847–2853
88. Nieves RI, Reynolds BQ, Hazard SW et al (2011) Increased post-operative complications with methylene blue versus lymphazurin in sentinel lymph node biopsies for skin cancers. J Surg Oncol 103:421–425

89. Ollila DW, Essner R, Wanek LA et al (1996) Surgical resection for melanoma metastatic to the gastrointestinal tract. Arch Surg 131:975–979
90. Olsen G (1964) Removal of fascia—cause of more frequent metastases of malignant melanomas of the skin to regional lymph nodes? Cancer 17:1159–1164
91. Pack GT, Gerber DM, Scharnagel IM (1952) End results in the treatment of malignant melanoma; a report of 1190 cases. Ann Surg 136:905–911
92. Paek SC, Griffith KA, Johnson TM et al (2007) The impact of factors beyond Breslow depth on predicting sentinel lymph node positivity in melanoma. Cancer 109:100–108
93. Poos HP, Kruijff S, Bastiaannet E et al (2009) Therapeutic groin dissection for melanoma: risk factors for short term morbidity. Eur J Surg Oncol 35:877–883
94. Ranieri JM, Wagner JD, Wenck S et al (2006) The prognostic importance of sentinel lymph node biopsy in thin melanomas. Ann Surg Oncol 13:927–932
95. Raymond AK, Beasley GM, Broadwater G et al (2011) Current trends in regional therapy for melanoma: lessons learned from 225 regional chemotherapy treatments between 1995 and 2010 at a single institution. J Am Coll Surg 213:306–316
96. Reintgen DS, Cox EB, McCarthy KS Jr et al (1983) Efficacy of elective lymph node dissection in patients with intermediate thickness primary melanoma. Ann Surg 198:379–385
97. Roehl KR, Mahabir RC (2013) A practical guide to free tissue transfer. Plast Reconstr Surg 132:147e–158e
98. Ryu SW, Saw R, Scolyer RA et al (2013) Liver resection for metastatic melanoma: equivalent survival for cutaneous and ocular primaries. J Surg Oncol 108:129–135
99. Sabel MS, Griffth KA, Arora A et al (2007) Inguinal node dissection for melanoma in the era of sentinel lymph node biopsy. Surgery 141:728–735
100. Sanki A, Ra Scolyer, Thompson JF (2009) Surgery for melanoma metastases of the gastrointestinal tract: indications and results. Eur J Surg Oncol 35:313–319
101. Schneider WJ, Hill HL Jr, Brown RG (1977) Latissimus dorsi myocutaneous flap for breast reconstruction. Br J Plast Surg 30:277–281
102. Scoggins CR, Ross MI, Reintgen DS et al (2006) Gender-related differences in outcome for melanoma patients. Ann Surg 243:693–698
103. Seigler HF, Fetter BF (1977) Current management of melanoma. Ann Surg 186:1–12
104. Shestak KC, Myers EN, Ramasastry SS et al (1993) Vascularized free-tissue transfer in head and neck surgery. Am J Otolaryngol 14:148–154
105. Siegel R, Ma J, Zou Z et al (2014) Cancer Statistics, 2014. CA Cancer J Clin 64:9–29
106. Sim FH, Taylor WF, Pritchard DJ et al (1986) Lymphadenectomy in the management of stage I malignant melanoma: a prospective randomized study. Mayo Clin Proc 61:697–705
107. Slingluff CL Jr, Vollmer R, Seigler HF (1988) Stage II malignant melanoma: presentation of a prognostic model and an assessment of specific active immunotherapy in 1,273 patients. J Surg Oncol 39:139–147
108. Slingluff CL Jr, Stidham KR, Ricci WM et al (1994) Surgical management of regional lymph nodes in patients with melanoma. Experience with 4682 patients. Ann Surg 219:120–130
109. Smith FO, Goff SL, Klapper JA et al (2007) Risk of bowel perforation in patients receiving interleukin-2 after therapy with anti-CTLA 4 monoclonal antibody. J Immunother 30:130
110. Sober AJ, Chuang TY, Duvic M et al (2001) Guidelines of care for primary cutaneous melanoma. J Am Acad Dermatol 45:579–586
111. Sondak VK, Taylor JM, Sabel MS et al (2004) Mitotic rate and younger age are predictors of sentinel lymph node positivity: lessons learned from the generation of a probabilistic model. Ann Surg Oncol 11:247–258
112. Spillane AJ, Cheung BL, Stretch JR et al (2009) Proposed quality standards for regional lymph node dissections in patients with melanoma. Ann Surg 249:473–480
113. Stell VH, Norton HJ, Smith KS et al (2007) Method of biopsy and incidence of positive margins in primary melanoma. Ann Surg Oncol 14:893–898
114. Thomas JM, Newton-Bishop J, A'Hern R et al (2004) Excision margins in high-risk malignant melanoma. N Engl J Med 350:757–766

115. Urist MM, Maddox WA, Kennedy JE et al (1983) Patient risk factors and surgical morbidity after regional lymphadenectomy in 204 melanoma patients. Cancer 51:212–216
116. van Aalst JA, McCurry T, Wagner J (2003) Reconstructive considerations in the surgical management of melanoma. Surg Clin North Am 83:187–230
117. Veronesi U, Adamus J, Bandiera DC et al (1977) Inefficacy of immediate node dissection in stage 1 melanoma of the limbs. N Engl J Med 297:627–30
118. Veronesi U, Cascinelli N, Adamus J et al (1988) Thin stage I primary cutaneous malignant melanoma. Comparison of excision with margins of 1 or 3 cm. N Engl J Med 318:1159–1162
119. Warycha MA, Zakrzewski J, Ni Q et al (2009) Meta-analysis of sentinel lymph node positivity in thin melanomas (≤1 mm). Cancer 115:869–879
120. Wasif N, Bagaria SP, Ray P et al (2011) Does metastasectomy improve survival in patients with stage IV melanoma? A cancer registry analysis of outcomes. J Surg Oncol 104:111–115
121. Wong SL, Brady MS, Busam KJ et al (2006) Results of sentinel lymph node biopsy in patients with thin melanoma. Ann Surg Oncol 13:302–309
122. Woods JE, Soule EH, Creagan ET (1983) Metastasis and death in patients with thin melanomas (less than 0.76 mm). Ann Surg 198:63–64
123. Wrightson WR, Wong SL, Edwards MJ et al (2003) Complications associated with sentinel lymph node biopsy for melanoma. Ann Surg Oncol 10:676–680
124. Young SE, Martinez SR, Faries MB et al (2006) Can surgical therapy alone achieve long-term cure of melanoma metastatic to regional nodes? Cancer J 12:207–211
125. Zacest AC, Basser M, Stevens G et al (2002) Surgical management of cerebral metastases from melanoma: outcome in 147 patients treated at a single institution over two decades. J Neurosurg 96:552–558
126. Zager JS, Hochwald SN, Marzban SS et al (2011) Shave biopsy is a safe and accurate method for the initial evaluation of melanoma. J Am Coll Surg 212:454–460

Adjuvant Therapy of Melanoma

Diwakar Davar and John M. Kirkwood

Abstract

The incidence of melanoma is rapidly increasing, especially in younger female and older male patients. Recent fundamental advances in our knowledge of melanoma tumorigenesis have established roles for inhibitors of the MAPK pathway and regulatory immune checkpoints CTLA-4 and PD-1/PD-L1. However, the majority of patients continue to present with non-metastatic disease—typically managed with surgical resection and adjuvant therapy. High-dose IFN-α2b (HDI) is the main adjuvant therapeutic mainstay in high-risk disease following definitive resection. In this chapter, we review the evidence supporting the use of adjuvant HDI in high-risk melanoma. We also discuss some of the other treatment modalities that have been evaluated including vaccines, chemotherapy, and radiotherapy.

Keywords

Melanoma · Adjuvant · High-dose IFN-α2b · HDI · Pegylated IFN · Vaccines · Chemotherapy · Radiotherapy · PD-1 · PD-L1 · CTLA-4 · Ipilimumab · Nivolumab · Pembrolizumab

D. Davar · J.M. Kirkwood (✉)
Division of Hematology-Oncology, Department of Medicine,
University of Pittsburgh Medical Center, 5150 Centre Avenue, Pittsburgh,
PA 15232, USA
e-mail: kirkwoodjm@upmc.edu

D. Davar
e-mail: davard@upmc.edu

H.L. Kaufman and J.M. Mehnert (eds.), *Melanoma*,
Cancer Treatment and Research 167, DOI 10.1007/978-3-319-22539-5_7

Contents

1 Introduction

Data from the US Surveillance, Epidemiology, and End Results (SEER) program indicate that melanoma is rapidly increasing in incidence. In 2014 there were 76,100 new cases of melanoma and 9,710 deaths—an incidence that has quadrupled over the past 4 decades, increasing by 2.6 % annually over the last 10 years [1].

Patients with early-stage (T1-2) disease have generally excellent outcomes following surgery. However, patients with thicker (≥T3) or ulcerated tumors, or with regional lymph node involvement, have a higher risk of relapse and death, underscoring the interest in effective adjuvant therapy for resected high-risk disease.

Early studies of interferons demonstrated a broad range of direct antitumor activities as well as immunomodulatory functions in a range of preclinical disease models. Clinical activity in the advanced disease setting was modest and attention turned to evaluating interferons in the adjuvant setting. The pivotal Eastern Cooperative Oncology Group trial (E1684) randomized high-risk patients defined as those with T4 primary lesions or any nodal involvement either at presentation or at regional recurrence to high-dose IFN-α2b (HDI) versus observation and demonstrated substantial improvements in relapse-free survival (RFS) and overall survival (OS) and led the first Food and Drug Administration (FDA) approval for an adjuvant therapy of resected high-risk melanoma [2]. HDI and the more recently approved pegylated IFN (pegIFN) remain the only approved adjuvant treatments for resected high-risk melanoma (primary tumor thickness ≥T4 mm and/or regional lymph node metastases) [2].

Although approved in the USA, Australia, and Europe, substantial treatment-related constitutional, hematologic, hepatic, and psychiatric toxicities have impeded the adoption of this regimen in parts of Europe and the USA, as well as in Australia. Subsequent trials have evaluated various dosages, schedules, and routes of administration in an attempt to improve the therapeutic index while assessing which treatment component was most critical to efficacy. These studies have not offered substantial evidence that any alternative schedule or dose has benefits that would rival those observed with HDI. Retrospective studies evaluating a variety of predictive biomarkers have suggested several promising candidates, none of which have been prospectively evaluated.

In this chapter, we first discuss the clinical factors associated with recurrence risk. We outline the development of IFN-α in the adjuvant setting, focusing on the various clinical studies that led HDI to becoming the standard of adjuvant therapy, and discuss emerging options including pegylated IFN, vaccines, CTLA-4 blockade, chemotherapy, and radiotherapy.

2 Indications for Adjuvant Therapy

Adjuvant therapy is typically considered for patients whose risk of recurrence is higher than 30–40 % at 5 years, following the surgical extirpation of detectable disease, for the purposes of preventing the likelihood of recurrence and ultimately toward the goal of improving the overall long-term disease-specific survival.

Of the various clinicopathologic factors important in melanoma, 5 factors with independent predictive value in relation to relapse and mortality have been identified based on relapse and survival data from patients in the American Joint Committee on Cancer (AJCC) Melanoma Staging Database [3]. These factors were included in the revised 2009 classification on the staging and prognosis of cutaneous melanoma copublished by the AJCC and the International Union Against Cancer (UICC):

- Primary tumor depth or Breslow thickness.
  - Measured in millimeters [<1.00 mm (T1), 1.01–2.00 mm (T2), 2.01–4.00 mm (T3), and >4.00 mm (T4)], and this is the most important prognostic factor, with survival decreasing commensurately to increasing thickness.
- Ulceration.
  - Adversely increases the prognosis of melanoma of any thickness—ulcerated melanoma of any T depth is associated with a risk of relapse and/or death of the next higher non-ulcerated T depth.
- Mitotic rate.
  - Defined as the number of mitoses per square millimeter (mm^2) in the primary tumor, and this discriminates between aggressive lesions (>1 mitoses/mm^2) and less aggressive lesions (<1 mitoses/mm^2) especially in T1 melanomas. Besides ulceration, the mitotic index separates T1a from T1b lesions.
- Regional metastatic burden.
  - Absolute risk of lymph node involvement increases proportionally to tumor thickness—2–5 % for T1 and up to 34 % for T4 lesions [4]. Both macroscopic tumor burden (1, 2–3 and ≥4) and microscopic tumor burden have prognostic implications—latter subdividing N1 and N2 classifications into N1a/N2a (micro-metastatic) and N1b/N2b (macro-metastases). Survival decreases with increasing lymph node involvement—5-year survival ranges

from 78 % (stage IIIA) to 59 % (stage IIIB) down to 40 % (stage IIIC). Prognostic implication of sub-micro-metastases (<0.1 mm) is contentious: Some authors deem sentinel lymph node (SLN) involvement of any degree significant, while others argue that patients with melanoma micro-metastases have similar rates of relapse and/or death as patients with SLN-negative disease [4, 5].

- Location and extent of distant metastatic disease.
  - Location and extent of distant metastases and serum lactate dehydrogenase (LDH) enzyme level predict survival. Of the former, distant skin, subcutaneous, and/or lymph node metastases (M1a) have the best prognosis, while non-lung visceral metastases and tumors with LDH elevation (M1c) have the worst. Pulmonary metastases (M1b) have an intermediate prognosis. The extent of tumor, and particularly whether the disease is solitary or not, has been shown to be important both in the regional lymph node and in the distant visceral sites including the brain [6].

Several authors have developed prediction tools that use proprietary nomograms to estimate the risk of nodal metastases (Memorial Sloan Kettering Sentinel Node Metastasis prediction tool) and 5-/10-year survival (AJCC Individualized Melanoma Patient Outcome Prediction Tool) [7, 8].

Current practice standards advocate either clinical trial enrollment or adjuvant therapy with interferon [either high-dose interferon for 1 year or pegylated interferon (pegIFN) for 2 years] in patients with high-risk resected melanoma whose estimated risk of recurrence exceeds 30 %, i.e., high-risk node-negative disease (T3b or T4 a/b) and node-positive melanoma.

3 Evolution of HDI and PegIFN in Adjuvant Therapy of High-Risk Resected Melanoma

Melanoma is an immunogenic solid tumor, as first suggested by reports of spontaneous regressions in advanced disease; and by the subsequent documentation of melanoma-specific immune responses to cancer germ line antigens (MAGE and NY-ESO-1), melanoma differentiation antigens, and presence of tumor-infiltrating lymphocytes (TILs). These observations paralleled our early forays into understanding the cellular and humoral basis of immunity.

Evidence of the antineoplastic effects of a variety of cytokines including IFN-α, IL-2, IL-7, and IL-21 heralded the dawn of cancer immunotherapy. These early results yielded in a series of trials in an array of preclinical disease models and in human melanoma. Early studies of IFN-α in metastatic melanoma were promising, with several durable responses and occasional complete responses, although overall response rates were low ($\sim$15 %)—a response pattern that came to characterize the antitumor efficacy of early immunomodulatory agents in this setting. Encouraged by observed activity in the setting of advanced disease, investigators turned to evaluating IFN-α in the adjuvant postoperative high-risk setting. Following initial dose-finding trials, US, European, and Australian investigators conducted multiple adjuvant phase III trials evaluating different subtypes (IFN-α2a, IFN-α2b, and IFN-α2c), dosages (low dose, ≤ 3 MU/dose; intermediate dose, 5–10 MU/dose; and high dose ≥10 MU/dose), routes [intravenous (IV), intra-muscular (IM), subcutaneous (SC)], and schedules (induction, maintenance, combination) to refine the therapeutic index. These trials are summarized in Table 1 [9–28].

The first two prospective randomized phase III trials of high-dose IFN-α2b (HDI) in stage II/III melanoma were the North Central Cancer Treatment Group (NCCTG) 83-0752 and the Eastern Cooperative Group (ECOG) E1684 trials. NCCTG 83-0752 randomized 262 patients (61 % lymph node positive) to either IFN-α2a (20 MU/m^2 thrice weekly IM for 12 weeks) or observation and reported non-significant trends towards reduced recurrence and improved survival with IFN-α2a [9, 10]. ECOG E1684 utilized IFN-α2b and tested a longer regimen comprising induction (IV 20 MU/m^2 daily for 5 days for 4 weeks) and maintenance (SC 10 MU/m^2 thrice weekly for 48 weeks) phases in 287 stage II/III patients, 89 % of whom had regional lymph node metastases. When initially reported at 6.9 years median follow-up, HDI significantly improved both disease-free survival (DFS) and OS compared to observation. Subset analysis suggested that node-positive patients benefited disproportionately though node-negative patients only represented 11 % of the cohort. Toxicity consisted of near-universal constitutional and flu-like symptoms that were readily supported by properly trained allied health professional teams, and hematologic, and hepatic laboratory findings which were the basis of dose-modification along with the constitutional toxicities, and psychiatric and depressive symptoms that were encountered in <10%. In overview, the toxicities of this therapy resulted in treatment delay and/or dose reduction in ~50 % of patients although the toxicities were nearly all reversible. Based on these statistically significant RFS and OS results at nearly 7 years of median follow-up, the FDA approved HDI for the indication of adjuvant therapy in 1995. When the 7 year survival data were re-analyzed at 12.6 years median follow-up, RFS improvement favored treatment although at this horizon, the originally noted significant benefit in terms of OS were no longer nominally statistically significant. This may have reflected competing causes of death in an elderly cohort.

Subsequent trials seeking to develop less difficult regimens that might show efficacy have evaluated lower doses of IFN-α in an attempt to extend the OS/RFS benefits [11–27]. Alternative regimens have evaluated *very low-dose regimens* (1 MU SC every other day) in the European Organization for Research and Treatment of Cancer (EORTC) 18871; *low-dose regimen* (3 MU SC thrice weekly) tested in WHO Melanoma Program Trials 16, ECOG E1690 (T4N1), UKCCCR AIM-High trial, Scottish trial, German DeCOG 2008, and DeCOG 2010 studies; and *intermediate-dose regimen* tested in EORTC 18952/18991 and Nordic Melanoma Cooperative Group's Nordic IFN trial. Although several of these reported improvements in RFS, only the German DeCOG 2008 study reported an OS benefit although this trial was only powered to assess the combined regimen of low-dose IFN-α (LDI) with dacarbazine (DTIC), rather than LDI alone, and has never been replicated.

Efforts to add chemotherapeutic agents to HDI to augment the benefits seen with HDI have been generally disappointing with high toxicity rates given the relative duration and toxicity of the HDI regimen itself. Southwest Oncology Group's (SWOG) S0008 was an attempt to evaluate how a shorter (but more intensive) biochemotherapy regimen consisting of IL-2, IFN, cisplatin, vinblastine, and dacarbazine would compare to standard HDI [28]. 402 patients with stage III (24 % IIIC) cutaneous melanoma were randomized to either HDI or biochemotherapy. At a median follow-up of 7.2 years, biochemotherapy was associated with fewer relapse events and improved overall survival; albeit with 40 % incidence of grade 4 toxicity (7 % for HDI) though grade 3/4 toxicity rates and treatment discontinuation rates were similar in both cohorts. Further evaluation of this regimen is not planned with future use being restricted to highly selected patients at experienced centers.

Nineteen phase III trials have evaluated the role of IFN-α2b in reducing risk of relapse and improving overall survival in high-risk melanoma. Two systematic reviews [29, 30], a pooled individual patient data analysis [31], and two meta-analyses of the literature [32, 33] have analyzed the collective data with the singular conclusion that IFN-α-based adjuvant therapy reliably improves RFS by 17 % (HR 0.83, 95 % confidence interval 0.78–0.87, *p* value significant), with a lesser improvement in OS of 9 % (HR 0.91, 95 % confidence interval 0.85–0.97, *p* value significant) based on the most recent Cochrane database review by Mocellin et al. [30].

Post-hoc analyses in E1684 indicated that the greatest reduction in risk of relapse occurred early with this therapy—raising the possibility that the value of the HDI regimen's induction phase was both necessary and perhaps sufficient for this treatment benefit. Three prospective randomized trials have evaluated the efficacy of a truncated treatment course in relation to the full year of treatment or observation: Hellenic He13A/98 (modified induction only versus modified induction and maintenance) [14], E1697 (HDI induction only versus observation) [16], and a recently reported Oxford UK phase II study (HDI induction only vs. HDI induction and maintenance) [34]. Hellenic He13A/98 study authors chose a non-inferiority design and elected to use modified induction/maintenance doses: 25 % dose-reduced induction (IV 15 MU/m^2 rather than 20 MU/m^2) and a flat maintenance (SC 10 MU rather than 10 MU/m^2) with an otherwise unchanged administration schedule. Although Hellenic He13A/98 authors concluded that the modified induction-only regimen was non-inferior to the extended induction/maintenance therapy, the relatively lower percentage of stage III patients enrolled (58 %) and lack of an observation control arm and lower doses of IFN-α used are noteworthy. E1697 was terminated early for futility at interim analysis of 1150 patients of a planned enrollment of 1420. At ASCO 2011, authors reported not noting any significant improvement in either recurrence-free or 5-year survival for the truncated treatment schedule. A recently published British randomized phase II study of HDI induction versus HDI induction/maintenance in 194 patients (77 % lymph node positive) reached similar conclusions with borderline statistical superiority of the 1-year versus the 1-month treatment in terms of the OS of patients in this study.

Other authors have sought to answer the alternative question of whether prolonged duration of therapy might confer greater treatment benefit. Given the toxicity and frequency of treatment with HDI, studies of longer than one year of this regimen have not been undertaken; however, the greater potential facility of treatment with pegylated species and the familiarity of lower dosage regimens with recombinant IFN are used for hepatitis C, studies evaluating longer durations of treatment have utilized PegIFN or lower dosages of IFN-α: E1690 [11], WHO 16 [27], EORTC 18952 [17], 18991 [18] and the Nordic IFN trial [19]. Neither ECOG E1690 nor the European WHO trial 16 demonstrated any RFS/OS benefit with 2–3 years of lower dose IFN (3 MU TIW). Although EORTC 18952 concluded that adjuvant intermediate-dose IFN-α2b given for an extended duration failed to improve distant metastasis-free interval (DMFI), distant metastasis-free survival (DMFS), or OS, post hoc analysis noted a survival benefit for patients with stage IIB/C disease suggesting that lower tumor burdens predicted for IFN response. However, both the Nordic IFN trial and EORTC 18991 concluded that adjuvant IFN (IFN-α2b and PegIFN, respectively) improved RFS but not OS after 1 year of therapy with no incremental benefit from additional treatment. A separate finding from subgroup analysis in EORTC 18991 of RFS/DMFS/OS benefit in patients with ulcerated primaries and/or microscopic nodal metastases is being prospectively evaluated in EORTC 18081 (adjuvant PegIFN for 2 years compared to observation in ulcerated node-negative patients).

HDI and PegIFN are approved by American, European (HDI only, not PegIFN) and Australian health authorities for the adjuvant treatment of high-risk resected melanoma conventionally accepted to comprise either node-positive disease or node-negative disease with a primary of Breslow thickness T2b or greater. Both HDI (given for 1 year) and PegIFN (given for 2 years) improve the RFS from 30 % (HDI) to 13 % (PegIFN). Treatment related toxicity is considerable with both regimens—leading to delays or discontinuation in ~50 % of treated patients.

4 Other Adjuvant Therapeutic Options—Vaccines, Chemotherapy, and Radiotherapy

Other adjuvant immunotherapy modalities that have been evaluated include other cytokines and nonspecific immune stimulants (BCG, Corynebacterium parvum, levamisole including combinations with DTIC). Other than isolated, non-reproducible results in early phase studies, these trials have been largely negative. These data are reviewed in detail elsewhere [35].

Cancer vaccines are subdivided based on the nature of the antigen(s) or cell(s) incorporated—whole cell/cell lysate (autologous, allogeneic), dendritic cell (DC), peptide, ganglioside, and DNA vaccines. Of the randomized trials of allogeneic cell-based vaccines evaluated in the adjuvant setting, most have yielded negative results and this approach is no longer being pursued [36]. Peptide vaccines typically utilize melanocyte lineage antigens (MART-1, gp100, tyrosinase) or cancer–testis antigens (NY-ESO-1, MAGE-A3) and include adjuvants or Toll-like receptor

(TLR) ligands without which tolerance would result. Promising leads in early phase studies have not increased RFS compared to placebo in randomized trials. A large phase III trial of a MAGE-A3 vaccine is underway in patients with stage III B/C melanoma whose tumors are positive for the MAGE-A3 germ line lineage antigen. This vaccine contains a proprietary immune-stimulant AS15 and elicits robust CD8 + cytotoxic T-cell responses. However, recent reports indicate that the trial failed to meet its DFS end point at interim analysis though the trial will continue until the second coprimary end point (DFS in gene signature-positive subpopulation) is assessed [37]. Other cancer vaccines currently in phase III trials for melanoma include Vical's Allovectin-7® (NCT00395070), Amgen's Talimogene laherparepvec, and OncoVEXGM-CSF® (NCT00769704). Although final data have not been released, interim reports indicate that Vical's Allovectin-7® failed to improve either primary (24 week overall response rate) or secondary (overall survival) efficacy end points compared to chemotherapy [38].

Three phase III trials have reviewed the role of adjuvant chemotherapy after surgical resection. Neither RFS nor OS benefits have been obtained with this approach. In the most recent of these (E1673), neither BCG alone nor the DTIC/BCG combination improved RFS/OS over observation in stage I–III patients [39–41]. Combinations of chemotherapy with immunotherapy (biochemotherapy, BCT) are associated with higher response rates when compared to DTIC, although no survival advantage has been demonstrated and toxicity is greater [42]. Adjuvant BCT was evaluated before the negative data from the use of BCT versus chemotherapy in metastatic melanoma was available. In S008, a randomized phase III trial by South West Oncology Group (SWOG), the reference one-year HDI was compared to three cycles of cisplatin, vinblastine, DTIC, IL-2, and IFN-α2b in patients with high-risk resected melanoma (stage IIIA-C, 100 % node positive). At ASCO 2012, the authors reported that compared to standard HDI in this high-risk cohort, biochemotherapy improved RFS (HR 0.77) with no discernible influence upon OS at a median follow-up of 6 years. Grade 3 constitutional toxicity was higher in the HDI arm, but grade 4 toxicity was noted in 40 % of patients receiving BCT [43].

Acral/mucosal melanoma is a distinct clinical entity associated with mutations in KIT at a higher frequency [15–20 % (mucosal) and 10–20 % (acral)] than present in cutaneous melanomas (2 %) [44–46]. Given the relative rarity of acral/mucosal melanoma outside Asia, prior US/European adjuvant trials have neither selectively evaluated the role of adjuvant therapy in this population nor have mucosal melanoma been separately delineated in previously reported trials. A Chinese phase II study compared HDI versus temozolomide/cisplatin chemotherapy to observation in high-risk resected mucosal melanoma and noted that although both HDI and chemotherapy improved RFS/OS compared to surgery alone, HDI appeared less effective than chemotherapy in RFS terms [47]. Although yet to be validated in a phase III trial, this observation underscores the different biology of acral/mucosal melanoma and may drive differential responses to adjuvant HDI.

Melanoma has long thought to be a radiotherapy (RT) resistant tumor—largely since the 1970s when cell survival curves for human cancer cell lines were first published which showed a broad shoulder for melanoma cell lines and implied high

Table 1 Phase III studies of IFN-α for advanced melanoma

Study reference	Patients eligible for analysis	Stage	IFN type	Dose and schedule—treatment arm	Median follow-up at reporting (years)	DFS/RFS	OS	% node positive
High dose								
NCCTG 83-7052 [9]	262	II–III (T2-4N0M0 or TanyN+M0)	IFN-α2a versus observation	IM 20 MU/m^2 thrice weekly for 4 months	6.1	HR: 1.20 (HDI vs. observation) (NS)	HR: 1.11 (HDI vs. observation) (NS)	61
ECOG E1684 [10]	287	II–III (T4N0M0 or TanyN+M0)	IFN-α2b versus observation	IV 20 MU/m^2 5 days a week for 4 weeks → then → SC 10 MU/m^2 3 days a week for 48 weeks	12.6	HR: 1.38 (HDI vs. observation) (S)	HR: 1.22 (HDI vs. observation) (S at 6.9 years but NS at 12.6 years)	89
ECOG E1690 [11]	642	II–III (T4N0M0 or TanyN+M0)	IFN-α2b—high dose versus low dose versus observation	High dose: IV 20 MU/m^2 5 days a week for 4 weeks → then → SC 10 MU/m^2 3 days a week for 48 weeks Low dose: SC 3 MU/m^2 2 days a week for 2 years	4.3	HR: 1.28 (HDI vs. observation) (S) 1.19 (LDI vs. observation) (NS) RFS: 44 % (HDI) versus 40 % (LDI) versus 35 % (observation)	HR: 1.0 (HDI vs. observation) (NS) 1.04 (LDI vs. observation) (NS) OS: 52 % (HDI) versus 53 % (LDI) versus 55 % (observation)	74
ECOG E1694 [12]	774	II–III (T4N0M0 or TanyN+M0)	IFN-α2b versus GMK vaccine	IV 20 MU/m^2 5 days a week for 4 weeks → then → SC 10 MU/m^2 2 days a week for 48 weeks	2.1	HR: 1.49 (HDI vs. GMK) (S) RFS: 25 % (HDI) versus 39 % (GMK)	HR: 1.38 (HDI vs. GMK) (S) OS: 78 % (HDI) versus 73 % (GMK)	77

(continued)

Table 1 (continued)

Study reference	Patients eligible for analysis	Stage	IFN type	Dose and schedule—treatment arm	Median follow-up at reporting (years)	DFS/RFS	OS	% node positive
ECOG E2696 [13]	107	II–IV	GMK vaccination with concurrent HDI (Arm A) versus GMK vaccination with HDI beginning D28 (Arm B) versus GMK vaccination alone (Arm C)	HDI: IV 20 MU/m^2 5 days a week for 4 weeks → then → SC 10 MU/m^2 3 days a week for 48 weeks GMK vaccination: GM2-KLH/QS-21 on D1, 8, 15, 22 then weeks 12, 24,36	2.4	HR: 1.75 (C vs. A) (S) 1.96 (C vs. B) (S) RFS: Not reached (A) versus 30.72 months (B) versus 14.85 months (C)	HR: not reported OS: not reached (A, B or C)	Not reported
Hellenic He13A/98 [14]	364	IIB-C/III (T3/4N0M0 or TanyN+M0)	Modified IFN-α2b induction-only (Arm A) versus modified IFN-α2b induction and maintenance (Arm B)	Non-inferiority design. Modified induction: IV 15 MU/m^2 5 days a week for 4 weeks Modified maintenance: SC 10 MU 3 days a week for 48 weeks	5.3	Median RFS: 24.1 months (Arm A) versus 27.9 (Arm B) (NS, primary non-inferiority endpoint met)	Median OS: 64.4 months (Arm A) versus 65.3 (Arm B) (NS)	58
Italian Melanoma Intergroup [15]	330	III (TanyN1-3M0)	Intensified IFN-α2b (IHDI) every other month versus IFN-α2b for 1 year	IHDI: IV 20 MU/m^2 5 days a week for 4 weeks every other month for 4 cycles	5.0	Median RFS: 47.9 months (IHDI) versus 35.6 months (HDI) (NS)	Median OS: 88.7 months 5 year OS: 60.1 % (IHDI) versus 82.6 % (HDI) (NS)	100

(continued)

Table 1 (continued)

Study reference	Patients eligible for analysis	Stage	IFN type	Dose and schedule—treatment arm	Median follow-up at reporting (years)	DFS/RFS	OS	% node positive
				Standard HDI: IV 20 MU/m^2 5 days a week for 4 weeks → then → SC 10 MU/m^2 3 days a week for 48 weeks		5 year RFS: 45.8 % (IHDI) versus 44.3 % (HDI)		
E1697 [16]	1150 (1420 planned enrollment)	IIB-C/III (T2-4N0M0 or TanyN1a/2aM0)	Induction HDI versus observation	HDI induction: IV 20 MU/m^2 5 days a week for 4 weeks	Not reported	Median RFS: 6.8 years (HDI induction) versus 7.3 years (observation) (NS)	5 year OS: 82 % (HDI induction) vs. 85 % (observation) (NS)	19
S0008 [28]	402	IIIA-IIIC	HDI vs. biochemotherapy (IL-2, IFN, cisplatin, vinblastine, and dacarbazine)	HDI: IV 20MU/m2 5 days a week for 4 weeks→then→SC 10MU/m2 3 days a week for 48 weeks Biochemotherapy: Dacarbazine 800 mg/m^2 (day 1); Cisplatin 20 mg/m^2, Vinblastine 1.2 mg/m^2, IL-2 at 9 MU/m^2 continuous IV infusion (days 1-4); IFN 5MU/m2 (day 1-5, 8, 10, 12). Repeated every 21 days for 3 cycles.	7.2	Median RFS: 4.0 years (biochemotherapy) vs. 1.9 years (HDI) (S) 5 year RFS: 39 % (biochemotherapy) vs. 48 % (HDI) (S)	Median OS: 9.9 years (biochemotherapy) vs. 6.7 years (HDI) (S) 5 year OS: 56 % (biochemotherapy) vs. 56 % (HDI) (NS)	24

(continued)

Table 1 (continued)

Study reference	Patients eligible for analysis	Stage	IFN type	Dose and schedule—treatment arm	Median follow-up at reporting (years)	DFS/RFS	OS	% node positive
Intermediate dose								
EORTC 18952 [17]	1388	II–III (T4N0M0 or TanyN+M0)	IFN-α2b for 1 year versus 2 years versus observation	Induction: IV 10 MU 5 days a week for 4 weeks Maintenance: SC 10 MU 3 days a week for 1 year *OR* SC 5 MU 3 days a week for 2 years	4.7	DMFI: HR: 0.93 (13 month versus observation) (NS) 0.83 (25 month versus observation) (S)	DMFS: HR: 0.95 (13 month versus observation) (NS) 0.85 (25 month versus observation) (NS)	74
EORTC 18991 [18]	1256	III (TanyN+M0)	PegIFN versus observation	Induction: SC 6 μg/kg/week for 8 weeks Maintenance: SC 3 μg/kg/week for 5 years	7.6	34.8 months (IFN) versus 25.6 months (observation); S	Not reported	100
Nordic IFN [19]	855	IIB-IIIB (T4N0M0 or TanyN1-2M0)	IFN-α2b for 1 year versus 2 years versus observation	Observation (A) versus SC 10 MU 5 days a week for 4 weeks then SC 10 MU 3 days a week for 1 year	6.0	23.2 months (A) versus 37.8 months (B) versus 28.6 months (C)	56.1 months (A) versus 72.1 months (B) versus 64.3 months (C) (NS)	81

(continued)

Table 1 (continued)

Study reference	Patients eligible for analysis	Stage	IFN type	Dose and schedule—treatment arm	Median follow-up at reporting (years)	DFS/RFS	OS	% node positive
				(B) versus SC 10 MU 5 days a week for 4 weeks then SC 10 MU 3 days a week for 2 years (C)		IFN versus observation and IFN 1 year versus observation (S); IFN 2 year versus observation (NS)		
Low dose								
Austrian Melanoma Cooperative Group (AMCG) [20]	311	II (T2-4N0M0)	IFN-α2a versus observation	SC 3 MU 7 days a week for 3 weeks → then → SC 3 MU 3 days a week for 1 year	3.4	RFS/DMFS not reported Rate of relapse: (24.0 % LDI vs. 36.3 % obs)	Not reported	0
French Melanoma Cooperative Group (FCGM) [21]	499	II (T2-4N0M0)	IFN-α2a versus observation	SC 3 MU 3 days a week for 18 months	>3	HR: 0.74 (LDI versus observation) (S)	HR: 0.70 (LDI versus observation) (S)	0
WHO Melanoma Program Trial 16 [22]	444	III (TanyN+M0)	IFN-α2a versus observation	SC 3 MU 3 days a week for 36 months	7.3	NS	NS	100
Scottish Melanoma Cooperative Group [23]	96	II–III (T3-4N0M0 or TanyN+M0)	IFN-α2a versus observation	SC 3 MU 3 days a week for 6 months	>6	NS	NS	Not reported

(continued)

Table 1 (continued)

Study reference	Patients eligible for analysis	Stage	IFN type	Dose and schedule—treatment arm	Median follow-up at reporting (years)	DFS/RFS	OS	% node positive
EORTC 18871/DKG 80-1 [24]	728	II–III (T3-4N0M0 or TanyN+M0)	IFN-α2b versus IFN-γ versus ISCADOR M® versus. observation	IFN-α2b: SC 1 MU every other day for 12 months IFN-γ: SC 0.2 mg every other day for 12 months	8.2	NS	NS	58
UKCCCR/AIM HIGH [25]	674	II–III (T3-4N0M0 or TanyN+M0)	IFN-α2a versus observation	SC 3 MU 3 days a week for 24 months	3.1	NS	NS	Not reported
DeCOG [26]	840	III (T3anyN +M0)	IFN-α2a	SC 3 MU 3 days a week for 18 months (A) versus 5 years (B)	4.3	5 year DMFS 81.9 % (A) versus 79.7 % (B) (NS)	5 year OS 85.9 % (A) versus 84.9 % (B) (NS)	Not reported
DeCOG [27]	444	III (TanyN+M0)	IFN-α2a	SC 3 MU 3 days a week for 24 months (A) versus SC 3 MU 3 days a week for 24 months + DTIC 850 mg/m^2 every 4–8 weeks for 24 months (B) versus observation (C)	3.9	HR: 0.69 (A) versus 1.01 (B) versus 1.0 (C)	HR: 0.62 (A) versus 0.96 (B) versus 1.0 (C)	100 %

Key: *NS* not significant; *S* significant; *HR* hazard ratio; *DFS* disease free survival; *OS* overall survival level of damage repair. Investigators assumed that melanoma was less likely to respond to conventionally fractionated radiation (2–2.5 Gy/fraction) and that hyperfractionation (≥4 Gy/fraction) was required to result in equivalent outcomes. RTOG 83-05 prospectively randomized 126 patients with measurable disease to either hyperfractionated or conventionally fractionated radiation schedules [48]. However, the study was closed prematurely for futility as complete and partial remission rates were similar in both arms indicating that not only is melanoma a radio-responsive disease, but conventional fractionation schedules may be equivalent to hyperfractionated schedules for treatment of the disease. RT has been shown to reduce the risk of loco-regional relapse. The ANZMTG trial was a prospective multicenter phase III study in which 250 patients with high-risk disease were randomized to either observation or regional nodal basin RT (48 Gy in 20 fractions). RT significantly reduced risk of loco-regional recurrence although survival was reduced, albeit in a non-statistically significant fashion—a result that is poorly understood at this time [49].

Currently, given HDI's role in reducing local and systemic recurrence risk, RT is primarily indicated to reduce the risk and morbidity of local recurrence in patients who either decline or are unsuitable for HDI. Based on several studies including the ANZMTG trial, clinicopathologic features that predispose to local recurrence despite adequate surgical margins have been identified and include:

- Extra-capsular lymph node extension.
- Involvement of four or more nodes.
- Bulky disease (exceeding 3 cm in size).
- Cervical lymph node location.
- Recurrent disease.

5 Ongoing Adjuvant Trials

The current spectrum of adjuvant clinical trials spans several classes of agents including standard (HDI and pegIFN) and novel immunotherapeutic agents including checkpoint inhibitors (anti-CTLA-4, anti-PD1, and anti-PDL1); new targeted molecular signaling inhibitor therapies (BRAF, MEK); and novel vaccine approaches. These are summarized in Table 2.

Based on observations in EORTC 18952/18991 of selective OS/RFS benefits in patients with node-negative ulcerated primary melanomas who received adjuvant IFN (IFN-α2b and PegIFN), the EORTC has designed a prospective randomized trial—EORTC 18081—to compare 2 years of PegIFN to observation in 1200 patients with node-negative melanoma and ulcerated primaries greater than 1 mm thickness (T2-4bN0M0). Accrual has commenced.

The discovery of the critical role of oncogenic driver mutations has profoundly altered the therapeutic landscape of many malignancies including melanoma. Prior histopathologic nomenclature (superficial spreading, nodular, lentigo maligna, acral

Table 2 Phase III studies of Ipilimumab for advanced melanoma

Study reference	Patients eligible for analysis	Study design	Endpoints	Dose and schedule—treatment arm	Median Follow-up at Reporting (years)	RFS and OS	Grade 3/4 Toxicity (ipilimumab vs. placebo)
IImmunotherapies							
EORTC 18071 (NCT00636168)	951	Phase III, randomized, open-label study in T2b-4bN1-3M0 melanoma following resection Stage breakdown (% in ipilimumab and placebo arms) •IIIA (restricted to ≥1 mm LN involvement): 21 %/18 % •IIIB: 45 %/43 % •IIIC: 35 %/38 %	Primary—RFS Secondary—OS, DMFS, quality of life, quality-of-life-adjusted survival	Ipilimumab vs. placebo Ipilimumab:*Induction*—10 mg/kg q3weeks for 4 doses *Maintenance*—10 mg/kg q3 months for a maximum of 36 months	2.7	RFS (ipilimumab vs. placebo): •Median 26.1 months vs. 17.1 months •HR: 0.75 (0.64-0.90) (S) •1-year: 63.5 % vs. 56.1 %. •2-year: 51.5 % vs. 43.8 %. •3-year: 46.5 % vs. 34.8 %.	Grade 5 AE: 1 % (in both groups) Grade 4 AE: 8 % vs. 3 % All Grade 3/4 irAE: 41 % vs. 2.5 % Cutaneous: 4.5 % vs. 0.0 % Gastrointestinal: 16 % vs. 0.8 % •Colitis: 7.6 % vs. 0.2 % •Hepatic: 10.7 % vs. 0.2 % Endocrine: 8.5 % vs. 0.0 % •Hypophysitis: 5.1 % vs. 0.0 % •Hypothyroidism: 0.2 % vs. 0.0 %

(continued)

Table 2 (continued)

Study reference	Patients eligible for analysis	Study design	Endpoints	Dose and schedule—treatment arm	Median Follow-up at Reporting (years)	RFS and OS	Grade 3/4 Toxicity (ipilimumab vs. placebo)
							Resolution: •Cutaneous: 89.1 % vs. 92.9 % •Gastrointestinal: 93.8 % vs. 94.4 % •Hepatic: 94.8 % vs. 80.0 % •Endocrine: 56.0 % vs. 80.0 %
E1609 (NCT01274338)	1500	Phase III, randomized, open-label study in high-risk (IIIB-C or resected IVA) resected melanoma *Biomarker evaluation: •Ipilimumab—MDSC, Treg, IL-17 •HDI—S100B	Primary—RFS and OS Secondary—Toxicity, global quality of life	Ipilimumab in 2 dose levels vs. HDI Ipilimumab: *Induction*–3 or 10 mg/kg q3weeks for 4 doses *Maintenance*—3 or 10 mg/kg q6weeks until week 48 then q12weeks afterwards HDI: *Induction*—I.V. 20MU/m^2 5 days a week for 4 weeks *Maintenance*—S.C. 10MU/m^2 3 days a week for 48 weeks	N/A	N/A	N/A

Key: *NS* not significant; *S* significant; *HR* hazard ratio; *DFS* disease free survival; *RFS* relapse free survival; *OS* overall survival; *irAE* immune-related adverse events lentiginous) is increasingly being replaced by genetically defined subgroups (BRAF, NRAS, KIT, and for uveal melanoma, GNAQ/GNA11). Somatic mutations in BRAF have been described in approximately 40–60 % of malignant melanomas, especially those that arise from intermittent sun-exposed skin [50–53]. Most prevalent are missense mutations in valine 600. These single base alterations most often substitute glutamine for valine (V600E, 80–90 %), with other substitutions being less common—lysine for valine (V600K, 5–12 %) and arginine/aspartic acid for valine (V600 R/D, respectively, <5 %). Regardless of type, these mutations result in enhanced BRAF kinase activity and increased activity of downstream targets such as MEK [54, 55].

Inhibitors of BRAF (vemurafenib and dabrafenib) and MEK kinases (trametinib) have significantly improved survival in patients with advanced disease, although acquired resistance is common and tumor progression occurs in most patients [56–58]. Proven activity in the former setting has led to interest in the adjuvant arena; currently, there are several studies evaluating RAF/MEK inhibitors either singly or in combination for adjuvant treatment of melanoma. COMBI-AD (NCT01682083) and BRIM-8 (NCT01667419) are randomized, double-blind phase III studies enrolling high-risk stage III patients to placebo versus combined RAF/MEK inhibition with dabrafenib and trametinib (COMBI-AD) or RAF inhibition alone with vemurafenib (BRIM-8). Primary end points are RFS (COMBI-AD) and disease-free survival (BRIM-8) with the proposed duration of treatment in both studies being 12 months. Investigators from Memorial Sloan Kettering Cancer Center are performing a phase II adjuvant study of 4 cycles of monthly dabrafenib in resected stage IIIC BRAF-mutated patients with RFS as a primary end point (NCT01682213). Chinese investigators are comparing imatinib to a modified IFN-α2b schedule in KIT-mutated patients (NCT01782508). These trials are slated to open in 2013 with estimated completion between 2014 and 2016.

T-cell responses to antigen presentation are modulated by a system of positive and negative feedback loops following initial antigen presentation. Following binding of cognate ligands to CD4+ T-cell receptors, T cells are primed but require a second "costimulatory" signal between B7-1/B7-2 (CD80/86) on antigen presenting cells (APCs) and T-cell CD28 for full activation. CD28 transmits a stimulatory signal, while CTLA-4 transmits an inhibitory signal—with the functional outcome depending on the relative engagement of APC with CD28 versus CTLA-4. PD-L1 is ubiquitously expressed on tumors and engages with T-cell PD-1 to downregulate CD8+ T-cell responses possibly through suppression of PI3K/AKT activation [59]. CTLA-4 and PD-1 are negative regulators of T-cell responses that function in initiator and effector phases of the T-cell response, respectively. By blocking negative regulators of the immune response, CTLA-4 (and PD-1) inhibitors enhance CD8+ T-cell proliferation and response.

Ipilimumab (Yervoy™, Medarex Inc/Bristol-Myers Squibb) is a humanized $IgG1_K$ monoclonal antibody that competitively inhibits CTLA-4 negative regulatory checkpoint. Ipilimumab has been evaluated in two randomized trials in metastatic melanoma patients: against a gp100 peptide vaccine in the second line (3 mg/kg) and against dacarbazine in the first line (10 mg/kg) [60, 61]. Of these, both trials demonstrated improved OS and PFS with durable responses in a minority of treated patients. Use is associated with a novel pattern of side effects involving skin, liver, bowel, and/or endocrine system—collectively termed immune-related adverse events (irAEs). Ipilimumab use is also associated with a variety of radiographic response patterns, distinct from those observed with traditional cytotoxic chemotherapy [62].

Evaluation in the adjuvant setting is proceeding in both Europe and the USA. EORTC 18071 evaluated ipilimumab 10 mg/kg against placebo in 951 high-risk stage IIIA-C melanoma patients post-resection, and interim results were presented at ASCO 2014 [63, 64]. Specifically in the IIIA cohort, investigators only enrolled patients with >1 mm lymph node involvement. Accrual commenced June 2008 and completed July 2011, and as at June 2014, a median of 2.7 years (and 56 % of events) had elapsed. Ipilimumab use was associated with a 25 % reduction in risk of relapse (HR 0.74, 0.64–0.90). This translated into a 9.0-month (26.1 vs. 17.1 months) improvement in RFS over placebo and a difference in absolute risk of 8 % at 2 years and 12 % at 3 years, respectively. This is similar although three years less mature than the initial report of adjuvant efficacy for high-dose IFN. RFS improvement was noted in all subgroups but was greatest in patients with stage IIIC disease, ulcerated primaries, or microscopic nodal involvement which may be due to the greater relative maturity of the data in this subset. Toxicity profile was consistent with studies of ipilimumab in advanced melanoma though somewhat higher (42 % grade 3/4 events including 7.6 % grade 3/4 colitis, 5.1 % grade 3/4 hypophysitis) and included 5 treatment-related deaths. Although most patients discontinued therapy secondary to intolerance or progression, benefit was seen after a median of 4–5 doses suggesting that the first four induction doses accounted for majority of RFS benefit. Data regarding secondary end points (DMFS and OS) are immature and will be reported later.

ECOG has led an intergroup trial E1609 that is an open-label randomized phase III trial comparing ipilimumab at both the approved dosage level (3 mg/kg) and the higher potentially more active dosage of 10 mg/kg versus HDI in 1600 patients with high-risk melanoma (stages IIIB-C/IV) following resection. Unlike EORTC 18071, E1609 was powered with RFS and OS as coprimary end points and will answer whether ipilimumab 10 mg/kg has RFS (or OS) benefit over IFN, and if so, whether 3 mg/kg is efficacious. Accrual is near complete, and initial results are expected in 2016. These data are awaited due to the fact that the primary end points of this trial were both OS and RFS, and it has tested the lower and already US FDA-approved dosage of 3 mg/kg of ipilimumab, where the fatal and grade ¾ toxicity rate is anticipated to be substantially lower than for the 10 mg/kg studied in EORTC 18071. Moreover, the comparator IFN therapy is more relevant to the worldwide community where IFN has been adopted as the approved reference standard.

Table 3 Ongoing adjuvant studies in high-risk resected melanoma

Study reference	Estimated enrollment	Study design	Primary endpoint	Secondary endpoint(s)	Dose and schedule—treatment arm	Start date	Estimated completion
Immunotherapies							
Ipilimumab vs. HDI (E1609; NCT01274338)	1500	Phase III, randomized, open-label study in high-risk (IIIB-C or resected IVA) resected melanoma *Biomarker evaluation: •Ipilimumab—MDSC, Treg, IL-17 •HDI—S100B	RFS, OS	Toxicity, global quality of life	Ipilimumab in 2 dose levels vs. HDI Ipilimumab: *Induction*—3/10 mg/kg q3weeks for 4 doses *Maintenance*—3/10 mg/kg q6weeks until week 48 then q12weeks afterwards HDI: *Induction*—I.V. 20MU/m^2 5 days a week for 4 weeks *Maintenance*—S.C. 10MU/m2 3 days a week for 48 weeks	June 2008	September 2014
E1609 (NCT01274338)	1500	Phase III, randomized, open-label study in high-risk (IIIB-C or resected IVA) resected melanoma *Biomarker evaluation: • Ipilimumab – MDSC, Treg, IL-17 • HDI—S100B	RFS, OS	Toxicity, global quality of life	Ipilimumab in 2 dose levels versus HDI Ipilimumab: *Induction*—3/10 mg/kg q3 weeks for 4 doses *Maintenance*—3/10 mg/kg q6 weeks until week 48 then q12 weeks afterward HDI: *Induction*—I.V. 20 MU/m^2 5 days a week for 4 weeks *Maintenance*—S.C. 10 MU/m^2 3 days a week for 48 weeks	May 2011	May 2018

(continued)

Table 3 (continued)

Study reference	Estimated enrollment	Study design	Primary endpoint	Secondary endpoint(s)	Dose and schedule—treatment arm	Start date	Estimated completion
Pegylated IFN-α2b (EORTC 18081; NCT01502696)	1200	Phase III, randomized, open-label study in ulcerated node-negative (T2b-4bN0M0) melanoma	RFS	OS, DMFS, quality of life	Pegylated IFN-α2b 3 μg/kg weekly injections for 2 years	April 2012	April 2020
Nivolumab vs. Ipilimumab (CheckMate 23; NCT02388906)	800	Phase III, randomized, double-blind placebo-controlled study in resected stage III B/C melanoma	RFS	OS	Nivolumab 3 mg/kg q2 weeks + Ipilimumab matched placebo q3 weeks for 1 year Ipilimumab 3 mg/kg q3 weeks + Nivolumab matched placebo q2 weeks for 1 year	March 2015	June 2020
Pembrolizumab (KEYNOTE 054; NCT02362594)	900	Phase III, randomized, double-blind placebo-controlled study in resected stage III melanoma *Biomarker evaluation: •Pembrolizumab—PD-L1 expression	RFS and RFS in PD-L1 positive tumors	DMFS (and DMFS in PD-L1 positive tumors); OS (and OS in PD-L1 positive tumors)	Pembrolizumab 200 mg q3 weeks for 1 year Matched placebo in same schedule	July 2015	September 2023
Vaccines							
MAGE-A3 vaccine (NCT00796445)	1349	Phase III, randomized, open-label study in T2b-4bN0M0 melanoma *Biomarker evaluation: •Expression of MAGE-A3 Antigen-specific cancer immunotherapeutic (ASCI) gene signature	DFS	OS, DMFS, anti-MAGE-A3 and antiprotein D seropositivity status, quality of life	MAGE-A3 vaccine with 2 adjuvants including QS-21 (Stimulon™, Agenus) and a proprietary Toll-like receptor 9 agonist (VaxImmune™, Coley Pharmaceuticals)	December 2008	October 2016

(continued)

Table 3 (continued)

Study reference	Estimated enrollment	Study design	Primary endpoint	Secondary endpoint(s)	Dose and schedule—treatment arm	Start date	Estimated completion
Molecularly targeted agents							
Dabrafenib (NCT01682213)	23	Non-randomized open label phase II study in high-risk (IIIC) resected BRAF V600E/K mutant melanoma	RFS	OS, safety, toxicity	Dabrafenib 150 mg B.I.D. per cycle (28 days) for 4 cycles	September 2012	September 2014
Imatinib (NCT01782508)	40	Non-randomized open label phase II study in high-risk (IIB-IIIC) resected CKIT mutant melanoma	RFS	OS	Imatinib 400 mg daily versus modified IFN-α2b	August 2012	December 2014
Vemurafenib (BRIM8, NCT01667419)	725	Phase III, randomized, double-blinded study in high-risk (IIC or IIIA-C) resected BRAF V600E mutant melanoma	DFS	OS, DMFS, quality of life, pharmacokinetics, safety, toxicity	Vemurafenib 960 mg B.I.D. vs. placebo for 12 months	September 2012	June 2016
Dabrafenib and Trametinib (COMBI-AD, NCT01682083)	850	Phase III, randomized, double-blinded study in high-risk (IIIA-C) resected BRAF V600E/K mutant melanoma	RFS	OS, DMFS, FFR, safety, toxicity	Dabrafenib 150 mg B.I.D. ANDTrametinib 2 mg once daily vs. placebos for 12 months	November 2012	July 2015
Crizotinib (NCT02223819)	30	Open label phase II study in high-risk uveal melanoma as determined by gene expression profiling (Castle Biosciences, class II)	RFS	OS, disease specific survival, toxicity	Crizotinib 250 mg B.I.D. per 4 week cycle for 12 cycles	August 2014	August 2016

(continued)

Table 3 (continued)

Study reference	Estimated enrollment	Study design	Primary endpoint	Secondary endpoint(s)	Dose and schedule—treatment arm	Start date	Estimated completion
Dabrafenib and Trametinib (COMBI-NEO, NCT02231775)	84	Randomized open-label phase II study of neoadjuvant and adjuvant Dabrafenib /Trametinib and surgery compared to surgery alone in clinical stage IIIB–C or oligometastatic stage IV melanoma	1 year RFS	N/A	Dabrafenib 150 mg B.I.D. and Trametinib 2 mg daily for 8 weeks prior to surgery; then surgery; then Dabrafenib/Trametinib in patients with stable/responding disease for an additional 44 weeks	October 2014	October 2017

Key: *NS* not significant; *S* significant; *HR* hazard ratio; *DFS* disease free survival; *RFS* relapse free survival; *OS* overall survival; *irAE* immune-related adverse events

6 Conclusions

Prior efforts in developing an adjuvant option in high-risk resected melanoma have centered on the use of non-selective cytokines. Approaches based on vaccines, cytotoxic chemotherapy, and BCT have largely failed to yield reproducible benefits in randomized studies. RT has a role in selecting patients as delineated above.

HDI (for 1 year) and PegIFN (for 2 years) have reproducibly demonstrated improved RFS and OS resulting in regulatory approval. Treatment-related morbidity is significant with both agents, and $\sim$50 % of patients experience treatment delays, discontinuations, and/or dose adjustments. Efforts to improve the risk/benefit ratio have evaluated lower dose regimens and longer durations of therapy with negative results. EORTC's E18081 will prospectively evaluate whether PegIFN will selectively benefit patients with ulcerated node-negative melanoma.

Advances over the preceding decade have elucidated several molecular driver (BRAF, MEK) and immune tolerogenic mechanisms (CTLA-4, PD-1/PD-L1) important in the growth and proliferation of melanoma. Agents developed based on these approaches (BRAF/MEK/KIT inhibitors, CTLA-4/PD-1/PD-L1 inhibitors) have improved survival in the advanced disease setting and are pending evaluation in the adjuvant setting—COMBI-AD (dabrafenib and trametinib combination vs. placebo in BRAF-mutated patients), BRIM-8 (vemurafenib vs. placebo in BRAF-mutated patients), and NCT01782508 (imatinib vs. modified IFN-α2b schedule in KIT-mutated patients).

Data from EORTC 18071 (ipilimumab 10 mg/kg vs. placebo) reported clinically significant improvement in RFS over placebo with adjuvant ipilimumab compared to placebo in stage III resected melanoma. Data regarding OS is immature at this time. E1609 (ipilimumab 3 mg/kg vs. ipilimumab 10 mg/kg vs. HDI) has nearly completed accrual and results are expected in 2016. Collectively results from these two studies will inform if ipilimumab has a role in the management of high-resected melanoma. These two trials are summarized in Table 3.

Recent work suggests that BRAF-mutated melanomas have greater tumor immunogenicity but paradoxically decreased antitumor immunity suggesting that combinations of targeted and immunomodulatory therapies may have additive, or synergistic, benefits. This approach is being evaluated in the advanced disease setting and if successful may be transposed to the adjuvant setting.

Acknowledgments This work was supported by Award Number P50 CA121973 from the National Cancer Institute. The content is solely the responsibility of the authors and does not necessarily represent the official views of the National Cancer Institute or the National Institutes of Health.

References

1. Surveillance, Epidemiology, and End Results Program. Turning Cancer Data into Discovery. Melanoma of the Skin. Date last modified not known. Available at: http://seer.cancer.gov/statfacts/html/melan.html. Accessed 01 Mar 2014
2. National Cancer Institute: PDQ® Melanoma Treatment. Bethesda, MD: National Cancer Institute. Date last modified 16 May 2013. Available at: http://cancer.gov/cancertopics/pdq/treatment/melanoma/HealthProfessional. Accessed 01 Mar 2014
3. Balch CM, Gershenwald JE, Soong SJ et al (2009) Final version of 2009 AJCC melanoma staging and classification. J Clin Oncol 27(36):6199–6206
4. Kettlewell S, Moyes C, Bray C et al (2006) Value of sentinel node status as a prognostic factor in melanoma: prospective observational study. BMJ 332:1423
5. van Akkooi AC, de Wilt JH, Verhoef C, Eggermont AM (2008) Isolated tumor cells and long-term prognosis of patients with melanoma. Ann Surg Oncol 15(5):1547–1548
6. Liew DN, Kano H, Kondziolka D et al (2011) Outcome predictors of gamma knife surgery for melanoma brain metastases: Clinical article. J Neurosurg 114(3):769–779
7. Melanoma Nomogram: Sentinel Node Metastasis. Date last modified unknown. Available at: http://www.mskcc.org/cancer-care/adult/melanoma/prediction-tools. Accessed 01 Mar 2014
8. Individualized Melanoma Patient Outcome Prediction Tools—developed based on the AJCC Melanoma Database. Date last modified unknown. Available at: http://www.melanomaprognosis.org/. Accessed 01 Mar 2014
9. Creagan ET, Dalton RJ, Ahmann DL et al (1995) Randomized, surgical adjuvant clinical trial of recombinant interferon alfa-2a in selected patients with malignant melanoma. J Clin Oncol 13(11):2776–2783
10. Kirkwood JM, Strawderman MH, Ernstoff MS et al (1996) Interferon alfa-2b adjuvant therapy of high-risk resected cutaneous melanoma: the Eastern Cooperative Oncology Group Trial EST 1684. J Clin Oncol 14(1):7–17
11. Kirkwood JM, Ibrahim JG, Sondak VK et al (2000) High- and low-dose interferon alfa-2b in high-risk melanoma: first analysis of intergroup trial E1690/S9111/C9190. J Clin Oncol 18 (12):2444–2458
12. Kirkwood JM, Ibrahim JG, Sosman JA et al (2001) High-dose interferon alfa-2b significantly prolongs relapse-free and overall survival compared with the GM2-KLH/QS-21 vaccine in patients with resected stage IIB-III melanoma: results of intergroup trial E1694/S9512/C509801. J Clin Oncol 19(9):2370–2380
13. Kirkwood JM, Ibrahim J, Lawson DH et al (2001) High-dose interferon alfa-2b does not diminish antibody response to GM2 vaccination in patients with resected melanoma: results of the Multicenter Eastern Cooperative Oncology Group Phase II Trial E2696. J Clin Oncol 19 (5):1430–1436
14. Pectasides D, Dafni U, Bafaloukos D et al (2009) Randomized phase III study of 1 month versus 1 year of adjuvant high-dose interferon alfa-2b in patients with resected high-risk melanoma. J Clin Oncol 27(6):939–944
15. Chiarion-Sileni V, Guida M, Romanini A et al (2011) Intensified high-dose intravenous interferon alpha 2b (IFNa2b) for adjuvant treatment of stage III melanoma: a randomized phase III Italian Melanoma Intergroup (IMI) trial [ISRCTN75125874]. J Clin Oncol 29 (suppl; abstr 8506)
16. Agarwala SS,Lee SJ, Flaherty LE et al (2011) Randomized phase III trial of high-dose interferon alfa-2b for 4weeks induction only in patients with intermediate- and high-risk melanoma (Intergroup trial E1697). J Clin Oncol 29(suppl; abstr 8505)
17. Eggermont AM, Suciu S, MacKie R et al (2005) Post-surgery adjuvant therapy with intermediate doses of interferon alfa 2b versus observation in patients with stage IIb/III melanoma (EORTC 18952): randomised controlled trial. Lancet 366(9492):1189–1196

18. Eggermont AM, Suciu S, Testori A et al (2012) Long-term results of the randomized phase III trial EORTC 18991 of adjuvant therapy with pegylated interferon alfa-2b versus observation in resected stage III melanoma. J Clin Oncol 30(31):3810–3818
19. Hansson J, Aamdal S, Bastholt L et al (2011) Two different durations of adjuvant therapy with intermediate-dose interferon alfa-2b in patients with high-risk melanoma (Nordic IFN trial): a randomised phase 3 trial. Lancet Oncol 12(2):144–152
20. Pehamberger H, Soyer HP, Steiner A et al (1998) Adjuvant interferon alfa-2a treatment in resected primary stage II cutaneous melanoma. Austrian Malignant Melanoma Cooperative Group. J Clin Oncol 16(4):1425–1429
21. Grob JJ, Dreno B, de la Salmonière P et al (1998) Randomised trial of interferon alpha-2a as adjuvant therapy in resected primary melanoma thicker than 1.5 mm without clinically detectable node metastases. French Cooperative Group on Melanoma. Lancet 351 (9120):1905–1910
22. Cascinelli N, Belli F, MacKie RM et al (2001) Effect of long-term adjuvant therapy with interferon alpha-2a in patients with regional node metastases from cutaneous melanoma: a randomised trial. Lancet 358(9285):866–869
23. Cameron DA, Cornbleet MC, Mackie RM et al (2001) Adjuvant interferon alpha 2b in high risk melanoma—the Scottish study. Br J Cancer 84(9):1146–1149
24. Kleeberg UR, Suciu S, Bröcker EB et al (2004) Final results of the EORTC 18871/DKG 80-1 randomised phase III trial. rIFN-α2b versus rIFN-gamma versus ISCADOR M versus observation after surgery in melanoma patients with either high-risk primary (thickness >3 mm) or regional lymph node metastasis. Eur J Cancer 40(3):390–402
25. Hancock BW, Wheatley K, Harris S et al (2004) Adjuvant interferon in high-risk melanoma: the AIM HIGH Study-United Kingdom Coordinating Committee on Cancer Research randomized study of adjuvant low-dose extended-duration interferon Alfa-2a in high-risk resected malignant melanoma. J Clin Oncol 22(1):53–61
26. Garbe C, Radny P, Linse R et al (2008) Adjuvant low-dose interferon α2a with or without dacarbazine compared with surgery alone: a prospective-randomized phase III DeCOG trial in melanoma patients with regional lymph node metastasis. Ann Oncol 19(6):1195–1201
27. Hauschild A, Weichenthal M, Rass K et al (2010) Efficacy of low-dose interferon α2a 18 versus 60 months of treatment in patients with primary melanoma of ≥1.5 mm tumor thickness: results of a randomized phase III DeCOG trial. J Clin Oncol 28(5):841–846
28. Flaherty LE, Othus M, Atkins MB, et al (2014) Southwest Oncology Group S0008: a phase IIItrial of high-dose interferon Alfa-2b versus cisplatin, vinblastine, and dacarbazine, plusinterleukin-2 and interferon in patients with high-risk melanoma–an intergroup study ofcancer and leukemia Group B, Children's Oncology Group, Eastern Cooperative OncologyGroup, and Southwest Oncology Group. J Clin Oncol 32(33):3771–3778
29. Lens MB, Dawes M (2002) Interferon alfa therapy for malignant melanoma: a systematic review of randomized controlled trials. J Clin Oncol 20:1818–1825
30. Mocellin S, Lens MB, Pasquali S et al (2013) Interferon alpha for the adjuvant treatment of cutaneous melanoma. Cochrane Database Syst Rev 6:CD008955
31. Wheatley K, Hancock B, Gore M et al (2007) Interferon-α as adjuvant therapy for melanoma: an individual patient data meta-analysis of randomised trials. J Clin Oncol 25(suppl 18): Abstract 8526
32. Wheatley K, Ives N, Hancock B et al (2003) Does adjuvant interferon-alpha for high-risk melanoma provide a worthwhile benefit? A meta-analysis of the randomised trials. Cancer Treat Rev 29:241–252
33. Mocellin S, Pasquali S, Rossi CR et al (2010) Interferon alpha adjuvant therapy in patients with high-risk melanoma: a systematic review and meta analysis. J Natl Cancer Inst 102: 493–501
34. Payne MJ, Argyropoulou K, Lorigan P et al (2014) Phase II pilot study of intravenous high-dose interferon with or without maintenance treatment in melanoma at high risk of recurrence. J Clin Oncol 32(3):185–190

35. Garbe C, Eigentler TK, Keilholz U et al (2011) Systematic review of medical treatment in melanoma: current status and future prospects. Oncologist 16(1):5–24
36. Blanchard T, Srivastava PK, Duan F (2013) Vaccines against advanced melanoma. Clin Dermatol 31(2):179–190
37. The Investigational MAGE-A3 Antigen-specific Cancer Immunotherapeutic Does Not Meet First Co-primary Endpoint in Phase III Melanoma Clinical Trial. N.p., 5 Sept 2013. Web. 3 Apr 2014
38. Vical Phase 3 Trial of Allovectin® Fails to Meet Efficacy Endpoints. N.p., 12 Aug 2013. Web. 3 Apr 2014
39. Hill GJ II, Moss SE, Golomb FM et al (1981) DTIC and combination therapy for melanoma: III. DTIC (NSC 45388) Surgical Adjuvant Study COG PROTOCOL 7040. Cancer 47 (11):2556–2562
40. Veronesi U, Adamus J, Aubert C et al (1982) A randomized trial of adjuvant chemotherapy and immunotherapy in cutaneous melanoma. N Engl J Med 307(15):913–916
41. Agarwala SS, Neuberg D, Park Y, Kirkwood JM (2004) Mature results of a phase III randomized trial of bacillus Calmette-Guerin (BCG) versus observation and BCG plus dacarbazine versus BCG in the adjuvant therapy of American Joint Committee on Cancer Stage I-III melanoma (E1673): a trial of the Eastern Oncology Group. Cancer 100(8): 1692–1698
42. Atkins MB, Hsu J, Lee S et al (2008) Phase III trial comparing concurrent biochemotherapy with cisplatin, vinblastine, dacarbazine, interleukin-2, and interferon α-2b with cisplatin, vinblastine, and dacarbazine alone in patients with metastatic malignant melanoma (E3695): a trial coordinated by the Eastern Cooperative Oncology Group. J Clin Oncol 26(35):5748–5754
43. Flaherty LE, Moon J, Atkins MB et al (2012) Phase III trial of high-dose interferon α-2b versus cisplatin, vinblastine, DTIC plus IL-2 and interferon in patients with high-risk melanoma (SWOG S0008): an intergroup study of CALGB, COG, ECOG, and SWOG. J Clin Oncol 30(suppl; abstr 8504)
44. Curtin JA, Busam K, Pinkel D, Bastian BC (2006) Somatic activation of KIT in distinct subtypes of melanoma. J Clin Oncol 24(26):4340–4346
45. Handolias D, Salemi R, Murray W et al (2010) Mutations in KIT occur at low frequency in melanomas arising from anatomical sites associated with chronic and intermittent sun exposure. Pigm Cell Melanoma Res 23(2):210–215
46. Kong Y, Si L, Zhu Y et al (2011) Large-scale analysis of KIT aberrations in Chinese patients with melanoma. Clin Cancer Res 17(7):1684–1691
47. Lian B, Si L, Cui C et al (2013) Phase II randomized trial comparing high-dose IFN-α2b with temozolomide plus cisplatin as systemic adjuvant therapy for resected mucosal melanoma. Clin Cancer Res 19(16):4488–4498
48. Sause WT, Cooper JS, Rush S et al (1991) Fraction size in external beam radiation therapy in the treatment of melanoma. Int J Radiat Oncol Biol Phys 20(3):429–432
49. Henderson MA, Burmeister B, Ainslie J et al (2013) Adjuvant radiotherapy after lymphadenectomy in melanoma patients: final results of an intergroup randomized trial (ANZMTG 0.1.02/TROG 02.01). J Clin Oncol 31 (suppl; abstr 9001)
50. Davies H, Bignell GR, Cox C et al (2002) Mutations of the BRAF gene in human cancer. Nature 417(6892):949–954
51. Maldonado JL, Fridlyand J, Patel H et al (2003) Determinants of BRAF mutations in primary melanomas. J Natl Cancer Inst 95(24):1878–1890
52. Wan PT, Garnett MJ, Roe SM et al (2004) Mechanism of activation of the RAF-ERK signaling pathway by oncogenic mutations of B-RAF. Cell 116(6):855–867
53. Curtin JA, Fridlyand J, Kageshita T et al (2005) Distinct sets of genetic alterations in melanoma. N Engl J Med 353(20):2135–2147
54. Rubinstein JC, Sznol M, Pavlick AC et al (2010) Incidence of the V600 K mutation among melanoma patients with BRAF mutations, and potential therapeutic response to the specific BRAF inhibitor PLX4032. J Transl Med 14(8):67

55. Lovly CM, Dahlman KB, Fohn LE et al (2012) Routine multiplex mutational profiling of melanomas enables enrollment in genotype-driven therapeutic trials. PLoS ONE 7(4):e35309
56. Chapman PB, Hauschild A, Robert C et al (2011) Improved survival with vemurafenib in melanoma with BRAF V600E mutation. N Engl J Med 364(26):2507–2516
57. Sosman JA, Kim KB, Schuchter L et al (2012) Survival in BRAF V600-mutant advanced melanoma treated with vemurafenib. N Engl J Med 366(8):707–714
58. Flaherty KT, Infante JR, Daud A et al (2012) Combined BRAF and MEK inhibition in melanoma with BRAF V600 mutations. N Engl J Med 367(18):1694–1703
59. Parry RV, Chemnitz JM, Frauwirth KA et al (2005) CTLA-4 and PD-1 receptors inhibit T-cell activation by distinct mechanisms. Mol Cell Biol 25(21):9543–9553
60. Hodi FS, O'Day SJ, McDermott DF et al (2010) Improved survival with ipilimumab in patients with metastatic melanoma. N Engl J Med 363:711–723
61. Robert C, Thomas L, Bondarenko I et al (2011) Ipilimumab plus dacarbazine for previously untreated metastatic melanoma. N Engl J Med 364:2517–2526
62. Wolchok JD, Hoos A, O'Day S et al (2009) Guidelines for the evaluation of immune therapy activity in solid tumors: immune-related response criteria. Clin Cancer Res 15:7412–7420
63. Eggermont AM, Chiarion-Sileni V, Grob JJ et al (2014) Ipilimumab versus placebo after complete resection of stage III melanoma: initial efficacy and safety results from the EORTC 18071 phase III trial. J Clin Oncol 32:5 s(suppl; abstr LBA9008)
64. Eggermont AM, Chiarion-Sileni V, Grob JJ et al (2015) Adjuvant ipilimumab versus placebo after complete resection of highriskstage III melanoma (EORTC 18071): a randomised, double-blind, phase 3 trial. LancetOncol 16(5):522–30

Chemotherapy for Melanoma

Melissa A. Wilson and Lynn M. Schuchter

Abstract

Prior to the recent therapeutic advances, chemotherapy was the mainstay of treatment options for advanced-stage melanoma. A number of studies have investigated various chemotherapy combinations in order to expand on the clinical responses achieved with single-agent dacarbazine, but these have not demonstrated an improvement in overall survival. Similar objective responses were observed with the combination of carboplatin and paclitaxel as were seen with single-agent dacarbazine. The combination of chemotherapy and immunotherapy, known as biochemotherapy, has shown high clinical responses; however, biochemotherapy has not been shown to improve overall survival and resulted in increased toxicities. In contrast, palliation and long-term responses have been observed with localized treatment with isolated limb perfusion or infusion in limb-isolated disease. Although new, improved therapeutic options exist for first-line management of advanced-stage melanoma, chemotherapy may still be important in the palliative treatment of refractory,

M.A. Wilson
Division of Hematology/Oncology, Department of Medicine, Hospital of the University of Pennsylvania, 3400 Civic Center Blvd, 16 Penn Tower, Philadelphia, PA 19104, USA
e-mail: Melissa.Wilson@nyumc.org

M.A. Wilson
Division of Hematology and Medical Oncology, Perlmutter Cancer Center, NYU School of Medicine, 160 E. 34th Street, Rm 915, New York, NY 10016, USA

L.M. Schuchter (✉)
Division of Hematology/Oncology, Department of Medicine, Abramson Cancer Center of the University of Pennsylvania, 3400 Civic Center Blvd, 1218 Penn Tower, Philadelphia, PA 19104, USA
e-mail: lynn.schuchter@uphs.upenn.edu

H.L. Kaufman and J.M. Mehnert (eds.), *Melanoma*,
Cancer Treatment and Research 167, DOI 10.1007/978-3-319-22539-5_8

progressive, and relapsed melanoma. We review the various chemotherapy options available for use in the treatment and palliation of advanced-stage melanoma, discuss the important clinical trials supporting the treatment recommendations, and focus on the clinical circumstances in which treatment with chemotherapy is useful.

Keywords
Biochemotherapy · Chemotherapy · Dacarbazine · Melanoma · Temozolomide

Contents

1 Introduction

Melanoma is the most aggressive form of skin cancer. Its incidence continues to increase yearly, with 77,000 new cases and 9500 deaths related to melanoma in 2013 [47]. In 2011, the Food and Drug Administration (FDA) approved two new drugs for the treatment of advanced-stage melanoma, the cytotoxic T-lymphocyte antigen-4 (CTLA-4)-blocking antibody, ipilimumab, and the targeted *BRAF* V600E kinase inhibitor, vemurafenib. In 2013, two additional drugs were approved which target mutant *BRAF* V600, the BRAF inhibitor, dabrafenib, and the MEK inhibitor, trametinib. These treatment advances have demonstrated improved clinical outcomes in patients with advanced-stage melanoma, with ipilimumab and vemurafenib demonstrating improved overall survival [16, 43, 83, 89], and dabrafenib and trametinib, both as single agents and in combination, demonstrating improved progression-free survival [28, 31, 33, 39, 51]. Moreover, new treatment advances, including new combinations, are being tested in clinical trials to improve treatment options for patients with melanoma, a field that had not seen new advances in a number of years. Prior to these advances in treatment options, chemotherapy, along with high-dose interleukin-2 (IL-2), remained a mainstay in the treatment of advanced-stage melanoma.

While chemotherapy no longer is frontline therapy in advanced-stage melanoma, it represents a common salvage regimen, confirming its role in the treatment paradigm of melanoma. Moreover, chemotherapy will have a more prominent role in those melanomas which do not harbor somatic mutations that can be targeted with specific inhibitors. With disease progression after receiving immunotherapy, chemotherapy is the next option, given the current lack of targeted therapies for melanomas lacking *BRAF*, *NRAS*, or *KIT* mutations. In this review, we discuss the chemotherapy regimens that have been used in the treatment of advanced-stage melanoma and the role of these agents in current treatment paradigms with the development of improved treatment options.

2 Single Chemotherapeutic Agents

2.1 Dacarbazine/Temozolomide

Dacarbazine has been a longstanding chemotherapy drug that has been used in the treatment of advanced-stage melanoma. Dacarbazine is an alkylating agent which results in DNA adducts and is cytotoxic to cells [5, 65]. Dacarbazine is metabolized by the liver into its intermediate metabolite, 3-methyl-(trianzen-1-yl)imidazole-4-carboxamide (MTIC) [74]. Dacarbazine is an intravenous infusion, and its main side effects include nausea and vomiting and myelosuppression. Dacarbazine gained FDA approval for the treatment of melanoma in 1975. In total, a number of phase I and phase II clinical trials demonstrated partial response (PR) rates of approximately 15–28 %, complete response (CR) rates of approximately 3–5 %, and very few durable responses of <2 % (reviewed in [20]). Randomized placebo-controlled trials of dacarbazine have not been performed [20]. Since its FDA approval, dacarbazine has become the standard regimen that all others have been compared, including recent clinical trials of new targeted therapies and immunotherapies with dacarbazine as the control arm [39, 83]. A number of studies have been performed that involved addition of agents in order to try to increase the efficacy of dacarbazine, including chemotherapies, immunotherapies (IFN and IL-2), and anti-estrogens, with no improvement in overall survival, and at the cost of increased side effects and decreased quality of life (reviewed in [24]). The overall outcome from these studies demonstrated that dacarbazine remained the standard chemotherapy treatment option for patients with metastatic melanoma, as had been previously suggested [16, 24].

Dose and schedules of dacarbazine vary widely, with no data to suggest that response rates are influenced by these variables. The most commonly used regimen is 800 to 1000 mg/m^2 intravenously repeated every 3–4 weeks, or 200 mg/m^2 intravenously for 5 days every 3–4 weeks. Dacarbazine is generally well tolerated. The most frequent side effects are nausea and vomiting, which can be severe. Mild to moderate myelosuppression is a common dose-related side effect.

Another chemotherapeutic agent that is used in the treatment of advanced-stage melanoma is temozolomide. Similar to dacarbazine, temozolomide is an alkylating agent, which is FDA-approved in the treatment of glioblastoma [98, 99]. Temozolomide undergoes conversion to MTIC under physiologic conditions [74]. It is an oral chemotherapeutic drug, with CNS activity as it crosses the blood–brain barrier [98], and its main side effects include headache, nausea and vomiting, and myelosuppression, including lymphopenia and thrombocytopenia [2].

A number of studies have investigated the efficacy of temozolomide versus dacarbazine. Overall, these studies demonstrated no differences between these two agents, and dacarbazine and temozolomide are generally believed to be similar agents which are interchangeable. Of note, temozolomide has demonstrated better CNS activity, as has been seen in the treatment of glioblastoma and glioma [13, 98, 99], so it is often considered in the setting of melanoma brain metastases [12]. A randomized phase III trial of temozolomide versus dacarbazine in patients with metastatic melanoma demonstrated an equivalent median overall survival (OS) (7.7 months for temozolomide-treated patients and 6.4 months for dacarbazine-treated patients, $p = 0.20$), and similar response rates between the two cohorts were observed (13.5 % for temozolomide-treated patients and 12.1 % for dacarbazine-treated patients) [73]. As has been standard practice in clinical trials, patients with brain metastases were excluded from this trial. Another trial, which also excluded brain metastases, investigated an escalated dose of temozolomide versus dacarbazine with similar results, such that no difference was observed between the two treatment arms and that escalated temozolomide dosing does not have better efficacy or outcomes than dacarbazine. Median OS was 9.1 months in the temozolomide arm and 9.4 months in the dacarbazine arms ($p = 0.99$), and overall response rate was 14.5 % in the temozolomide arm versus 9.8 % in the dacarbazine arm [77].

A retrospective case–control study investigated the effect of temozolomide in reducing CNS metastases in melanoma. Patients with metastatic melanoma were evaluated if they had responded to systemic treatment. In the 21 patients who responded to dacarbazine and the 20 patients who responded to temozolomide, nine dacarbazine-treated and two temozolomide-treated patients were found to have CNS relapse, which was statistically significant ($p = 0.03$) [78], suggesting that temozolomide may be involved in reducing development of new brain metastases. In addition, two phase II trials specifically looked at the use of temozolomide in the treatment of melanoma CNS metastases. In the first study, patients with measurable CNS disease were treated with whole-brain irradiation and temozolomide at 75 mg/m^2 daily for six weeks, with temozolomide treatment repeated every 10 weeks. A limited number of toxicities occurred, although one included a fatal episode of sepsis. Of the 31 patients treated, one patient experienced a complete CNS response for 4.5 months and two patients experienced partial CNS responses for two months and seven months [68]. While temozolomide and whole-brain irradiation demonstrated limited activity, this study demonstrated the safety of the combination. A multicenter, international study evaluated temozolomide in the treatment of CNS metastases. Temozolomide was used at 150 mg/m^2 in previously treated patients and 200 mg/m^2 in treatment-naïve patients, and treatment was on days one to five every 28 days. Of the 151 patients enrolled on study, 42 (36 %) derived some sort of clinical benefit, including one complete and seven partial responses and stable disease [2]. Brain metastases occur frequently in melanoma patients and are associated with significant mortality.

Though not FDA-approved for melanoma, temozolomide is used to treat patients with advanced melanoma based upon its ease of administration, CNS penetration, and favorable toxicity profile. Two different schedules have been evaluated. First is a 5-day regimen with a daily dose of 150–200 mg/m^2 on days 1–5. Courses are repeated every 3–4 weeks. The major side effect is mild to moderate myelosuppression. Mild nausea and vomiting also are common but can be readily controlled with standard antiemetic therapy. A second regimen, known as extended dosing of temozolomide, has been investigated, which comprises a lower daily dose for prolonged periods (75 mg/m^2 daily for 6 weeks on, 2 weeks off). This dosing regimen of temozolomide is associated with more lymphopenia, and opportunistic infections, specifically pneumocystis pneumonia, have been reported.

A recent meta-analysis reported aggregate data from five clinical trials investigating temozolomide versus temozolomide containing regimens. Results from this meta-analysis demonstrated a relative risk of 1.44 (95 % confidence interval (CI), 1.06–1.95) for temozolomide combinations compared to temozolomide alone [50]. However, there was not a significant difference between the treatment arms for the one-year survival rate. Similarly, no differences in adverse events were noted. Although limited in its analysis, this study demonstrates the safe combination of temozolomide and additional chemotherapeutic agents and, despite the lack of difference in longer term survival, the potential for short-term responses, which are sometimes desirable in rapidly progressing disease which is refractory to previous immunotherapy and targeted agents.

In an attempt to improve on previous therapies and capitalize on the improved response rates observed with the use of immune checkpoint inhibitors, clinical trials have investigated the combination of DTIC with ipilimumab. In a randomized phase II multicenter clinical trial, chemotherapy-naïve advanced-stage melanoma patients were randomized to receive ipilimumab alone at 3 mg/kg every four weeks for four doses (ipi), or ipilimumab in combination with DTIC at 250 mg/m^2 daily for up to six 5-day courses (ipi + DTIC). Overall response rate was increased in the ipi + DTIC arm compared to ipi alone, 14.3 versus 5.4 %, and median OS was 14.3 months and 11.4 months, respectively [40]. Durable responses were identified in over 50 % of patients responding to treatment, including patients on both arms of the study. Although clinical trial results did not reach statistical significance, the study demonstrated the feasibility of combining treatments with different mechanisms of action in the attempt to increase responses [40]. Concurrent with this trial, a dose-finding trial of ipilimumab identified increased response rates with ipilimumab at 10 mg/kg [96]. As such, another clinical trial investigating the combination of ipilimumab with DTIC was performed. In a randomized phase III clinical trial, treatment-naïve patients with advanced-stage melanoma were randomized to receive ipilimumab (10 mg/kg) plus DTIC (850 mg/m^2)(ipi + DTIC) or

DTIC plus placebo (DTIC) every three weeks for four treatments followed by DTIC alone every three weeks for total of 22 weeks; in addition, patients without progressive disease or dose-limiting toxicity received maintenance ipi or placebo every 12 weeks [83]. Results of this clinical trial demonstrated median OS of 11.2 months in the ipi + DTIC arm and 9.1 months in the DTIC arm (HR = 0.72, $P < 0.001$) [83]. No unexpected adverse events were identified, although toxicity was increased in the ipi + DTIC arm compared to DTIC alone, with a notable increase in liver enzymes and decrease in gastrointestinal side effects in the ipi + DTIC arm [83]. Moreover, improved responses associated with ipilimumab in combination with DTIC compared to DTIC alone were observed in all patient subsets that were analyzed, including well-known poor prognostic factors including elevated LDH and M1c disease [83].

2.2 Nitrosoureas

In addition to DTIC and temozolomide, the nitrosoureas—carmustine (BCNU) and lomustine (CCNU)—are also alkylating agents that have been used in the treatment of advanced-stage melanoma, rarely alone and usually in combination. BCNU is administered intravenously, while CCNU is taken orally. Initial studies of single-agent BCNU and CCNU date back to the late 1960s. Reports describe the use of DTIC, BCNU, and CCNU as single agents or in combination in the treatment of metastatic melanoma. In a report describing treatment of 80 patients, DTIC was given more frequently in 62 patients, but BCNU was given to 18 patients and CCNU was given to six patients; in addition, patients received sequential treatments with these agents, as well as combinations of therapy. Objective responses (complete responses and partial responses) were observed in 29 % of patients treated with DTIC, 17 % of patients treated with BCNU, and 33 % of patients treated with CCNU [42]. It is believed that treatment with BCNU or CCNU provides benefit to those patients with brain metastases, as symptomatic response was observed in a patient treated with BCNU and a patient treated with CCNU, while patients treated with DTIC relapsed with brain metastases [42], though with increased side effects. In general, carmustine and lomustine are mainly used in combination chemotherapy regimens, carmustine in the Dartmouth regimen and lomustine in BOLD, in the treatment of advanced-stage melanoma which will be discussed.

2.3 Carboplatin/Taxanes

In addition to dacarbazine and temozolomide, other chemotherapies have been examined in the treatment of advanced-stage melanoma in order to try to identify agents resulting in improved outcomes. Carboplatin has been used to treat a number of solid tumors. Treatment with carboplatin is cytotoxic to cells, resulting from DNA crosslink formation and inhibition of both replication and transcription. It has been tested in melanoma as a single agent and in combination with other chemotherapies. Taxanes, both paclitaxel and docetaxel, have also been tested in melanoma. This class of chemotherapy agents functions as microtubule inhibitors, and they function to stabilize tubulin polymerization and microtubule formation, thereby resulting in dysfunctional mitotic spindle complexes and cell death. The taxanes have also been tested alone as single agents and in combination with other agents.

A phase II trial investigated the use of carboplatin in advanced-stage melanoma. Chemotherapy-naïve metastatic melanoma patients were treated with carboplatin. Five out of 26 patients achieved PRs, resulting in a 19 % response rate (95 % CI, 8–38 %) [27]. Dose-limiting thrombocytopenia was observed, as well as moderate nausea and vomiting. The response rates observed with the treatment of carboplatin are comparable to those observed with dacarbazine [20, 27], the standard chemotherapy regimen for advanced-stage melanoma, and therefore represented a potential chemotherapy option, alone or in combination, to be further explored in melanoma patients.

The use of paclitaxel in the treatment of melanoma was explored in two phase II clinical trials. In the one study, three out of 25 chemotherapy-naïve patients treated with paclitaxel demonstrated a PR (12 %; CI, 3–13 %) [63]. In addition to these PRs, 4 out of 25 (16 %) demonstrated objective responses not qualifying as PR with durable responses between six to 17 months, and 4 out of 25 (16 %) demonstrated stable disease (SD) [63]. Side effects that were observed included neutropenia, requiring dose reduction of paclitaxel, alopecia, lower extremity bone pain, and peripheral neuropathy. An additional 34 patients were treated with paclitaxel in another study. In the 28 evaluable patients, four (14, 95 % CI, 4–33 %) demonstrated an objective response, with three patients experiencing a CR and one patient with a PR, with two patients who had continued responses at 25 and 38 months at the time of the study [25]. Five additional patients demonstrated minor responses to paclitaxel treatment [25]. Significant side effects were observed in this study. Anaphylactic reactions were observed in four patients, resulting in treatment discontinuation, as well as significant neutropenia and peripheral neuropathy [25]. These trials demonstrated that paclitaxel had activity in melanoma which was comparable to activity seen with dacarbazine [20, 25, 63] that warranted other studies, particularly in combination studies.

Similar activity was seen in clinical trials investigating activity of docetaxel in patients with advanced-stage melanoma. Docetaxel exhibited a more favorable safety profile and is more potent when compared to paclitaxel [11]. A 17 % response rate was observed in 30 patients (5/30) treated with docetaxel who were evaluable for response (but 14 % for those evaluable for response and toxicity (5/36)) [1]. A second phase II clinical trial evaluating the activity of docetaxel in melanoma patients demonstrated an overall response rate of 12.5 % (5/40 patients) (95 % CI, 6–30 %) [9], which consisted of one CR and four PRs; stable disease was also observed in 22 patients. Median OS was 13 months for patients treated with docetaxel with the median response duration being more than seven months on the study [9]. Similar side effects from docetaxel were observed in both studies which included neutropenia, alopecia, skin toxicities, and peripheral edema/fluid retention [9, 11]. Response rates for docetaxel were similar to those observed in studies for paclitaxel [25, 63] and dacarbazine [20] and suggest that docetaxel could be used in the treatment of advanced-stage melanoma.

Given the toxicities of paclitaxel and docetaxel, *nab*-paclitaxel has also been tested in the treatment of melanoma. A phase II study evaluated *nab*-paclitaxel in previously treated and chemotherapy-naïve patients with advanced-stage melanoma. Results demonstrated a 2.7 % response rate in previously treated patients and a 21.6 % response rate in treatment-naïve patients; the combination of response rate and stable disease was 37.8 % in previously treated patients and 48.6 % in chemotherapy-naïve groups [41]. Median progression-free survival (PFS) was 3.5 months and 4.5 months in treated versus naïve patients, respectively, and median OS was 12.1 months and 9.6 months in treated and naïve patients, respectively [41]. Duration of response was increased and was 12.9 months in previously treated patients and 24.0 months in chemotherapy-naïve patients, as well as a one-year survival of 49 and 41 % in previously treated and chemotherapy-naïve patients, respectively [41]. These results were similar, if not improved, compared to responses with dacarbazine [20] and demonstrated activity of *nab*-paclitaxel in the treatment of melanoma.

Combinations of platinums and taxanes have also been examined in the treatment of advanced-stage melanoma, in the attempt to identify better chemotherapy regimens with effectiveness in patients. A phase II clinical trial looked at the combination of carboplatin and paclitaxel in patients with advanced-stage melanoma. Patients were either previously untreated or treated with one prior regiment (that did not include a platinum or taxane). In this study, 15 patients were available for evaluations, as two patients developed anaphylactic reactions to paclitaxel, and demonstrated a 20 % (3/15) PR, 47 % (7/15) SD, and 33 % (5/15) with progressive disease [44]. This study demonstrated activity of the combination of carboplatin and paclitaxel in melanoma. Similarly, a retrospective analysis of past reports of patients treated with carboplatin and paclitaxel demonstrated the clinical benefit of this chemotherapy doublet as second-line treatment for melanoma patients who were previously treated. Of the twenty-nine patients who were identified to have received this treatment combination, eight patients (26 %) had a PR and six patients (19 %) had SD, resulting in an overall clinical benefit of 45 % [82]. Median OS was 7.8 months, but in the 14 patients who derived the clinical benefit, the median duration of clinical benefit was 5.7 months [82]. These results also support the use of this chemotherapy combination in advanced-stage melanoma patients. A prospective phase II trial investigated the combination of carboplatin and paclitaxel compared to paclitaxel alone in previously treated advanced-stage melanoma patients. This study was stopped early, as overall response was <10 % [100]. Indeed, no CR or PRs were observed in either treatment arm, and best response was stable disease in eight patients [100]. In all, results of these clinical trials and observations suggest the potential for activity of the combination of carboplatin and paclitaxel in the treatment of patients with advanced-stage melanoma.

The MAP kinase pathway plays an essential role in the pathogenesis of melanoma [21, 29, 30, 49], and early attempts at targeting this pathway involved the combination of targeted therapy with chemotherapy. Notably, two randomized, placebo-controlled phase III clinical trials used the carboplatin and paclitaxel chemotherapy backbone to study the addition of the multi-kinase inhibitor, sorafenib [81, 95], in treatment response rates. One clinical trial investigated the effect of sorafenib added to chemotherapy, carboplatin and paclitaxel, in patients who had progressed on dacarbazine- or temozolomide-based regimens. The addition of sorafenib did not result in improved PFS or response rate; however, median PFS of patients treated on the control arm of carboplatin and paclitaxel was 17.9 weeks and response rate was 11 % [38]. Another trial investigated the effect of sorafenib added to chemotherapy, carboplatin, and paclitaxel, in patients who were chemotherapy naïve. Results from this study demonstrated that the addition of sorafenib did not improve OS; however, median OS was 11.3 months for patients treated on the control arm of carboplatin and paclitaxel and response rate was 18 % [32]. Prior to these clinical trials, no definitive clinical trials had established evidence supporting the use of carboplatin and paclitaxel in the treatment of advanced-stage melanoma. These randomized phase III clinical trials provide survival endpoints to establish the use of carboplatin and paclitaxel in the treatment of patients with advanced-stage melanoma in both the second-line and chemotherapy-naive setting, as results are comparable to those observed with dacarbazine [20].

In addition to intracellular signaling pathways, angiogenesis, particularly vascular endothelial growth factor (VEGF), has been associated with melanoma and disease progression [10, 37, 58, 67, 93]. A randomized, placebo-controlled phase II clinical trial investigated the addition of the VEGF inhibitor, bevacizumab, or placebo to carboplatin and paclitaxel in patients with advanced melanoma (BEAM) [53]. This multi-institute phase II clinical trial enrolled 214 patients with metastatic disease (stage IV) who were treatment naïve. Although responses seemed to favor the addition of bevacizumab, results were not statistically significant. Median PFS, the primary endpoint, in the carboplatin/paclitaxel/placebo (CP) arm was 4.2 months and was 5.6 months in the carboplatin/paclitaxel/bevacizumab (CPB) (HR = 0.78, P = 0.1414), with overall response of 16.4 and 25.5 %, respectively (P = 0.1577) [53]. Initial evaluation of OS at 13 months demonstrated a benefit to the addition of bevacizumab to chemotherapy; median OS was 8.6 months in the CP arm and 12.3 months in the CPB arm (HR = 0.67, P = 0.0366). However, this benefit was not supported upon further analysis four months later; median OS was 9.2 months and 12.3 months in the CP and CPB arms, respectively (HR = 0.79, P = 0.1916) [53]. Overall, the study did not demonstrate a difference in PFS between the two treatment arms, CP and CPB, there was an increased in toxicity on the CPB arm, and duration of response was shorter on the CPB versus CP arms. In addition, survival and response rates for CP were similar to those observed in the two clinical trials combining carboplatin, paclitaxel, and sorafenib [32, 38], again demonstrating a role for combination of carboplatin/paclitaxel in the treatment of patients with metastatic melanoma. However, important observations reached in exploratory analyses of the data suggested patient cohorts possessing factors associated with poor prognosis, including M1c disease and elevated LDH, tended toward improved responses with CPB treatment [53], highlighting the importance that certain subsets of melanoma patients may respond to anti-angiogenesis therapy and the need for biomarkers of response to specific therapies in order to stratify patients for treatment.

3 Combination Chemotherapy

Given the low response rates to single chemotherapy agents, combinations of three to four chemotherapy agents have been investigated in the treatment of advanced-stage melanoma. A number of regimens have been investigated including combinations of cisplatin, vinblastine or vindesine, and dacarbazine (CVD) and what is known as the Dartmouth regimen (carmustine (BCNU), dacarbazine, cisplatin, and tamoxifen). Initial excitement for these regimens was primarily due to the observed increased response rates; however, follow-up studies incorporating multiple treatment centers demonstrated response rates similar to those seen with single-agent dacarbazine. Initial responses with CVD treatment demonstrated an overall response rate of 40 %, almost double that seen with dacarbazine treatment [62]. A multicenter phase III trial of CVD versus CVD plus interleukin-2 and interferon-α2b demonstrated a more modest response rate for CVD of 21 % [6]. And, in a study evaluating the CVD regimen setting as second-line chemotherapy, response rate in patients treated with CVD was 9.6 % with the best responses being PRs [46].

The Dartmouth regimen was investigated in a number of clinical trials. Initial trials included tamoxifen (TAM), but there was some concern of its side effects, specifically increased incidence of deep venous thrombosis and PEs, despite the increased overall response rates [70]. Further studies then compared the chemotherapy regimen alone contained within the Dartmouth regimen (carmustine (BCNU), vindesine, and dacarbazine) versus chemotherapy plus TAM. McClay et al. [70] demonstrated decreases in response rate in the absence of TAM, while two phase III trials demonstrated no differences in response rates, PFS, and OS with or without TAM added to chemotherapy [18, 86]. Margolin et al. [69] demonstrated similar objective response rates for the Dartmouth regimen, 15 % (12/79; 95 % CI, 8–25 %) as seen with single-agent treatment with dacarbazine. Chapman et al. [15] investigated the Dartmouth regimen versus the standard chemotherapy treatment, dacarbazine, in a multicenter phase III clinical trial which demonstrated that there were no differences in overall survival, although a nonsignificant increased tumor response was noted in patients treated with the Dartmouth regimen. In total, no long-term or survival benefits were observed with the Dartmouth regimen, and there were significant, increased toxicities with this regimen, suggesting that it should not replace dacarbazine as a standard chemotherapy regimen.

The combination chemotherapy regimen of bleomycin, vincristine, lomustine (CCNU), and dacarbazine (BOLD) has also been investigated in the treatment of advanced-stage melanoma. A multicenter phase II clinical trial investigated the use of BOLD plus IFN-α, evaluating the use of combination chemotherapy plus immunotherapy. Forty-three patients with stage IV disease were enrolled on the clinical trial with diverse disease characteristics, including nine patients with brain metastases, and a 27 % response rate was observed, including one complete response and ten partial responses [79]. Subset analysis in treatment-naïve patients with brain metastases demonstrated a 40 % response rate [79]. A previous study had demonstrated response rates of 62 % using BOLD plus IFN-α [80], which included patients with both stage III and stage IV disease. Additionally, there was some variations between studies using natural, leukocyte-derived IFN-α and recombinant IFN-α. As such, Vuoristo et al. [94] investigated these two forms of IFN-α with both DTIC and BOLD in a randomized phase III clinical trial. In this trial, no significant differences in responses were observed between the four treatment arms with response rates ranging from 8–24 % and median OS ranging 7.5 months–11.1 months, with six complete responses observed with BOLD [94]. Although not statistically significant, a trend toward increased responses with BOLD plus recombinant IFN-α was observed and the BOLD regimen may have improved responses in soft tissue and lung metastases [94]. However, BOLD regimen was associated with increased toxicity.

Combinations of chemotherapy have been tested in patients with the intent of identifying active agents which increase response rates. Combination therapies do not appear to offer significant increases in response rates, PFS, or OS and have increased side effects and toxicities, thereby leading to the lack of recommendations for their use. Currently, the optimal chemotherapy regimen has not been identified, although oncologists will have their own treatment preferences. Dacarbazine remains the standard chemotherapy regimen approved for the treatment of metastatic melanoma, although the combination of carboplatin and paclitaxel may also be used in the treatment of advanced-stage melanoma in current practice.

3.1 Biochemotherapy

In addition to combinations of chemotherapeutic agents, much interest surrounded the combination of chemotherapeutic agents with immunotherapy, referred to as biochemotherapy. Interferon-α (IFN-α) and interleukin-2 (IL-2) had been widely tested in advanced-stage melanoma with response rates ranging between 10–20 % [59] and 15–20 % [22, 76], respectively, with complete responses observed in approximately 5 % of patients treated with IL-2 [84]. As such, biochemotherapy was tested in the treatment of melanoma, in the metastatic setting and as neoadjuvant and adjuvant therapy in stage III disease. Initial studies demonstrated the improved response rate of sequential biochemotherapy with CVD followed by administration of IFN-α and IL-2 compared to alternating administration of CVD or IFN-α and IL-2 every six weeks [60]. In patients treated sequentially, response rate was 60 % compared to response rate of 33 % in patients treated in an alternating regimen, and there was a trend toward increased survival ($p = 0.06$) [60]. Moreover, increases in CRs and PRs were noted, with the sequential treatment resulting in 22.5 % CR and 37 % PR, while the alternating regimen resulted in 5 % CR and 27.5 % PR [60]. An increase in toxicities was observed, and although severe, they were manageable. A phase III clinical trial of sequential biochemotherapy versus chemotherapy confirmed this increase in response rate, although not to the same degree, 48 % compared to 25 % (p = 0.001) in patients treated with biochemotherapy versus CVD, respectively, with a similar non-statistically significant trend toward increased median OS [26]. However, a CR was only observed in 7 % of patients.

Given the severe toxicities associated with biochemotherapy and need for specialized care, this regimen is given in a hospital setting and sequential therapy ends up being around nine days, which is repeated every three weeks. Therefore, different regimens and dosing modifications were explored in order to deliver biochemotherapy concurrently and to try to reduce the length of hospital stays. Uncontrolled and non-randomized phase I/II and phase II clinical trials of concurrent biochemotherapy demonstrated high objective response rates, with one study demonstrating 64 % response rate and another demonstrating 48 % response rate, with CR rates of 21 and 20 %, and median OS 11.8 months and 11 months, respectively [61, 71]. Two multicenter randomized phase III clinical trials investigated the use of biochemotherapy compared to chemotherapy alone. In these studies with increased number of patients, response rates with biochemotherapy were more modest in comparison with the earlier studies. Bajetta et al. [6] demonstrated a 33 % objective response rate, 4% CR, and median OS of 11 months in patients treated with biochemotherapy compared to a 21 % objective response rate, no CRs, and median OS of 12 months in patients treated with chemotherapy alone. Similarly, Atkins et al. [4] reported a 19.5 and 13.5 % objective response rate (p = 0.140) for patients treated with biochemotherapy and chemotherapy alone, respectively. Differences in PFS, 4.8 months in the biochemotherapy arm and 2.9 months in the chemotherapy alone arm (p = 0.015) did not translate into increases in overall survival with no differences observed in the two arms, nine months and 8.7 months, respectively [4]. Other trials have been performed substituting temozolomide for dacarbazine and altered forms and dosing of IL-2 and IFN-α with no differences in responses and an approximately 20 % response rate [36].

While initial trials of biochemotherapy were thought to be promising with increased response rates, larger randomized clinical trials did not recapitulate these responses and results. A meta-analysis attempted to evaluate results from eighteen clinical trials evaluating biochemotherapy compared to chemotherapy alone, with one major criteria being that they were randomized clinical trials [48]. The analysis combined a number of trials, which had different chemotherapy backbones and with either IFN-α alone or both IFN-α and IL-2 as the added immunotherapy agent. Despite these differences, overall results demonstrated an improvement in responses rates for patients treated with any type of biochemotherapy, compared to chemotherapy alone. Increases in PR (odds ratio (OR) = 0.66; 95 % CI, 0.53–0.82, $P = 0.0001$), CR (OR = 0.50; 95 % CI, 0.35–0.73, $P = 0.003$), and overall response

(OR = 0.59; 95 % CI, 0.49–0.72, $P < 0.00001$) were observed in all biochemotherapy arms, including those receiving chemotherapy plus IFN alone and chemotherapy plus IFN and IL-2 [48]. Despite these responses, the benefits of biochemotherapy did not translate into an overall survival benefit [48]. Overall, biochemotherapy is associated with considerable toxicity including myelosuppression, nausea, vomiting, rash, hypotension, and fluid retention. Given the lack of survival benefit which has been evaluated in a randomized clinical trial, along with the toxicity, biochemotherapy is not the standard of care for patients with stage IV melanoma.

3.2 Biochemotherapy in the Adjuvant Setting

In addition to treatment for advanced-stage disease, the use of biochemotherapy has been evaluated in the neoadjuvant and adjuvant settings. Buzaid et al. [14] investigated the use of biochemotherapy in the neoadjuvant setting, for two to four cycles, in a phase II trial in melanoma patients with local regional disease, stage III. Overall pathological response in patients undergoing surgery was 50, 6.5 % pathological complete remission and 43.5 % with partial pathological response, with 44 % of patients demonstrating a partial clinical response to treatment with biochemotherapy in the adjuvant setting [14]. A multicenter phase II trial of treatment with neoadjuvant biochemotherapy demonstrated a relapse-free survival (RFS) of 64 % and an OS of 78 %, with an overall response rate of 26 % [64]. Lewis et al. [64] demonstrated a trend toward improved survival and decreased relapse in patients who had a positive sentinel lymph node, as opposed to patients who presented with clinically involved, palpable lymph nodes. In these studies, side effects were increased, but manageable.

The only FDA-approved adjuvant therapy for melanoma is high-dose interferon-α (IFN-α) [52, 54]. One randomized phase III study evaluated the use of biochemotherapy versus the standard adjuvant therapy IFN-α. A planned enrollment of 200 patients was stopped at 138 patients after a futility analysis was performed. There was no difference in RFS or OS in patients treated with either of two different IFN doses or with biochemotherapy [52]. A large cooperative group study also sought to evaluate the use of biochemotherapy in the adjuvant setting in patients with high-risk melanoma (defined as stage III disease, excluding N1a disease). Four hundred and thirty-two patients were enrolled over a seven-year period (2000–2007) and randomized to receive high-dose IFN for the standard treatment length of one year versus biochemotherapy which is given once every three weeks for three cycles (a total of nine weeks). Of the 402 evaluable patients who had at least six years of follow-up, patients who received biochemotherapy had an improved RFS (HR = 0.77; 90 % CI 0.62–0.96, $P = 0.02$) [34]. A median RFS of 4 years (90 % CI, 1.9–5.9) versus 1.9 years (90 % CI, 1.4–2.5) was observed for biochemotherapy and high-dose IFN, respectively [34]. The 5-year RFS was 47 versus 39 % in the biochemotherapy arm and high-dose IFN arm, respectively, and the 5-year OS was 56 % for both arms [34]. Moreover, increased toxicity was observed in the biochemotherapy arm compared to high-dose IFN. Despite these notable responses, these did not translate into an overall survival benefit with no differences being observed in OS between the two treatment arms [34]. However, this shorter treatment course with biochemotherapy may be an alternative treatment option to consider, compared to the standard year long course with high-dose IFN in select patients.

4 Localized Use of Chemotherapy

Until this point, the discussion has focused on the use of systemic chemotherapy in the treatment of advanced-stage melanoma. Under certain circumstances, administration of localized chemotherapy is desirable, in order to deliver high doses of chemotherapy, which would otherwise be toxic if given in the systemic setting. Indeed, in settings of disease recurrence that is unresectable and isolated to one particular limb or with limb only in-transit disease, treating the affected limb allows for the delivery of high doses of chemotherapy in order to treat local disease. Some patients can achieve long-term remissions or prevent disease progression with these approaches and should be considered when determining treatment options for patients, in particular those with local regional disease and recurrences.

Isolated limb perfusion (ILP) was developed in the 1950s [19, 75, 90] to deliver regional high-dose chemotherapy, but it is an invasive procedure. With ILP, the major vessels (artery and vein) of the specified limb are isolated and cannulated, and perfusion occurs using a bypass pump, and the application of a tourniquet completes the limb isolation from the systemic circulation. Overall response rates for ILP have been as high as 80 % with a CR rate of 54 % [75]. Hoekstra et al. [45] evaluated melphalan ILP (M-ILP) versus melphalan plus TNF-α (TM-ILP) in patients with low and high volume of disease. In 57 patients who underwent ILP, the overall response rate was 90, 84 % in the M-ILP group, and 93 % in the TM-ILP group, which included 45 % CR and 45 % PR [45]. The overall CR rate was not different between the two chemotherapy arms; however, when burden of disease was considered, low-volume disease treated with M-ILP demonstrated a 75 % CR, while high-volume disease treated with TM-ILP demonstrated a 41 % CR ($p = 0.038$) [45]. In addition, younger patients were more likely to obtain CR than older patients, 69 % CR in patients <65 years old versus 29 % CR in patients ≥65 years old ($p = 0.003$) [45]. Long-term local control has been observed with ILP and development of metastatic disease ranged from two to 135 months [45]. Moreover, the absence of CR and stage IIIC disease was demonstrated to be independent predictors for progression to systemic disease [45].

Isolated limb infusion (ILI) is a less invasive alternative to ILP, allowing for delivery of high-dose chemotherapy to the limb but with a simpler procedure. ILI was developed at the Sydney Melanoma Unit (now known as the Melanoma Institute Australia) [35, 92] and involves percutaneous access to the major artery and vein of the affected limb. This makes this procedure more tolerable and more easily repeated, if necessary. ILI is a less morbid procedure and has been shown to have response rates similar to ILP. Kroon et al. [56] performed a review of literature to ascertain experiences with ILI using melphalan plus actinomycin-D. In total, seven studies were included for a total number of 576 patients. The collective overall response rates for treatment with ILI with melphalan plus actinomycin-D was 73 %, with 33 % CR, and 40 % PR [8, 17, 23, 56, 72, 97], which are similar to responses seen with ILP [45, 75]. A prospective trial was conducted by Steinman et al. which assessed tumor burden and response to ILI with melphalan and actinomycin-D in melanoma patients, along with Merkel cell carcinoma and soft tissue sarcoma patients. In melanoma patients, low tumor burden (defined as <10 lesions and no lesion >3 cm) was correlated with increased response rates, 48 % CR, versus 9 % CR in patients with high tumor burden (defined as ≥10 lesions or a lesion >3 cm) ($p < 0.001$), in addition to increased survival, with 5-year survival 69 versus 29 %, respectively [91]. Patients with CR had increased 5-year overall survival of 91 % compared to 53 % in patients with PR ($p = 0.042$) [91], which is similar to response rates observed in other ILI studies [7, 8, 57, 88]. A recent review of an individual site experience reports similar response rates, overall response rate of 70 % with 35 % CR and 35 % PR in patients undergoing ILI with melphalan and actinomycin-D for limb localized melanoma, with some long-term responses of eight and 10 years [35]. Overall, studies have demonstrated the decreased morbidity of ILI along with tolerability of the procedure. Moreover, long-term responses and delayed progression have been observed in the setting of palliative treatment.

For ILP or ILI, melphalan is the standard chemotherapy agent used, either alone or in combination with agents such as actinomycin-D [75, 87] or tumor necrosis factor α (TNF-α) [3, 45, 66, 75, 85]. Both procedures are performed in centers highly trained in these procedures. Complications of the two procedures are similar including redness and swelling, lymphedema, compartment syndrome, infection, and thromboses, but ILI is generally associated with decreased limb complications [90]. Furthermore, fibrosis of major blood vessels and surrounding tissue following dissection and cannulization can be seen after ILP, making repeat procedures difficult, although these still occur [55]. Similar response rates have been observed with both procedures and therefore suggest that ILI is an acceptable alternative, as it is a less invasive procedure, especially in a situation where patients would otherwise not be able to tolerate an ILP procedure. These procedures are applicable to a limited number of patients and provide disease palliation and stabilization, with some long-term results. As such, ILP and ILI should be considered as treatment options for select patients.

5 Conclusions

The progress made in treatment options for advanced-stage melanoma over the recent years has transformed patient outcomes. However, despite the increased overall survival observed with treatment with ipilimumab and BRAF inhibitors, some patients have treatment refractory disease, develop treatment resistant disease, or experience disease relapse. Although new treatment options continue to be developed, it is sometimes necessary to rely on second- or third-line treatment options, including chemotherapy. Although no longer considered first-line therapy, chemotherapy still has a role in the treatment of melanoma, certainly in the palliative setting.

For a long time, dacarbazine had been the standard chemotherapy agent used in the treatment of melanoma. Temozolomide, an oral equivalent of dacarbazine, is frequently used as an alternative, particularly in the setting of CNS disease involvement, as temozolomide is able to cross the blood–brain barrier. More recently, the chemotherapy doublet carboplatin and paclitaxel has also demonstrated activity in the treatment of advanced-stage melanoma. Investigation of different chemotherapy combinations, alone or in combination with a variety of immunotherapies, has not provided improved therapeutic options. In addition, some clinical trials have also demonstrated the potential use of biochemotherapy in the adjuvant setting. Since biochemotherapy has increased side effects, this should only be considered in certain high-risk patients. Furthermore, localized therapy with ILP or ILI has produced long-term palliation of localized disease. Though no overall survival benefit has been demonstrated with chemotherapy, chemotherapy offers palliative treatment options for patients, especially if rapid tumor responses are needed, and provides patients with additional alternative treatment options.

References

1. Aamdal S, Wolff I et al (1994) Docetaxel (Taxotere) in advanced malignant melanoma: a phase II study of the EORTC early clinical trials group. Eur J Cancer 30A(8):1061–1064
2. Agarwala SS, Kirkwood JM et al (2004) Temozolomide for the treatment of brain metastases associated with metastatic melanoma: a phase II study. J Clin Oncol 22(11):2101–2107
3. Alexander HR Jr, Fraker DL et al (2010) Analysis of factors influencing outcome in patients with in-transit malignant melanoma undergoing isolated limb perfusion using modern treatment parameters. J Clin Oncol 28(1):114–118
4. Atkins MB, Hsu J et al (2008) Phase III trial comparing concurrent biochemotherapy with cisplatin, vinblastine, dacarbazine, interleukin-2, and interferon alfa-2b with cisplatin, vinblastine, and dacarbazine alone in patients with metastatic malignant melanoma (E3695): a trial coordinated by the eastern cooperative oncology group. J Clin Oncol 26(35): 5748–5754
5. Bajetta E, Del Vecchio M et al (2002) Metastatic melanoma: chemotherapy. Semin Oncol 29 (5):427–445
6. Bajetta E, Del Vecchio M et al (2006) Multicenter phase III randomized trial of polychemotherapy (CVD regimen) versus the same chemotherapy (CT) plus subcutaneous interleukin-2 and interferon-alpha2b in metastatic melanoma. Ann Oncol 17(4):571–577
7. Barbour AP, Thomas J et al (2009) Isolated limb infusion for malignant melanoma: predictors of response and outcome. Ann Surg Oncol 16(12):3463–3472
8. Beasley GM, Caudle A et al (2009) A multi-institutional experience of isolated limb infusion: defining response and toxicity in the US. J Am Coll Surg **208**(5):706–715, discussion 715–707

9. Bedikian AY, Weiss GR et al (1995) Phase II trial of docetaxel in patients with advanced cutaneous malignant melanoma previously untreated with chemotherapy. J Clin Oncol 13 (12):2895–2899
10. Birck A, Kirkin AF et al (1999) Expression of basic fibroblast growth factor and vascular endothelial growth factor in primary and metastatic melanoma from the same patients. Melanoma Res 9(4):375–381
11. Bissery MC, Guenard D et al (1991) Experimental antitumor activity of taxotere (RP 56976, NSC 628503), a taxol analogue. Cancer Res 51(18):4845–4852
12. Bleehen NM, Newlands ES et al (1995) Cancer research campaign phase II trial of temozolomide in metastatic melanoma. J Clin Oncol 13(4):910–913
13. Bower M, Newlands ES et al (1997) Multicentre CRC phase II trial of temozolomide in recurrent or progressive high-grade glioma. Cancer Chemother Pharmacol 40(6):484–488
14. Buzaid AC, Colome M et al (1998) Phase II study of neoadjuvant concurrent biochemotherapy in melanoma patients with local-regional metastases. Melanoma Res 8 (6):549–556
15. Chapman PB, Einhorn LH et al (1999) Phase III multicenter randomized trial of the Dartmouth regimen versus dacarbazine in patients with metastatic melanoma. J Clin Oncol 17(9):2745–2751
16. Chapman PB, Hauschild A et al (2011) Improved survival with vemurafenib in melanoma with BRAF V600E mutation. N Engl J Med 364(26):2507–2516
17. Coventry BJ, Kroon HM et al (2014) Australian multi-center experience outside of the Sydney melanoma unit of isolated limb infusion chemotherapy for melanoma. J Surg Oncol
18. Creagan ET, Suman VJ et al (1999) Phase III clinical trial of the combination of cisplatin, dacarbazine, and carmustine with or without tamoxifen in patients with advanced malignant melanoma. J Clin Oncol 17(6):1884–1890
19. Creech O Jr, Krementz ET et al (1958) Chemotherapy of cancer: regional perfusion utilizing an extracorporeal circuit. Ann Surg 148(4):616–632
20. Crosby T, Fish R et al (2000) Systemic treatments for metastatic cutaneous melanoma. Cochrane Database Syst Rev 2:CD001215
21. Dhomen N, Marais R (2009) BRAF signaling and targeted therapies in melanoma. Hematol Oncol Clin North Am 23(3):529–545, ix
22. Dillman RO, Church C et al (1993) Inpatient continuous-infusion interleukin-2 in 788 patients with cancer. The national biotherapy study group experience. Cancer 71(7): 2358–2370
23. Duprat Neto JP, Mauro AC et al (2012) Isolated limb infusion with hyperthermia and chemotherapy for advanced limb malignancy: factors influencing toxicity. ANZ J Surg
24. Eggermont AM, Kirkwood JM (2004) Re-evaluating the role of dacarbazine in metastatic melanoma: what have we learned in 30 years? Eur J Cancer 40(12):1825–1836
25. Einzig AI, Hochster H et al (1991) A phase II study of taxol in patients with malignant melanoma. Invest New Drugs 9(1):59–64
26. Eton O, Legha SS et al (2002) Sequential biochemotherapy versus chemotherapy for metastatic melanoma: results from a phase III randomized trial. J Clin Oncol 20(8): 2045–2052
27. Evans LM, Casper ES et al (1987) Phase II trial of carboplatin in advanced malignant melanoma. Cancer Treat Rep 71(2):171–172
28. Falchook GS, Lewis KD et al (2012) Activity of the oral MEK inhibitor trametinib in patients with advanced melanoma: a phase 1 dose-escalation trial. Lancet Oncol 13(8):782–789
29. Fecher LA, Amaravadi R et al (2008) Effectively targeting BRAF in melanoma: a formidable challenge. Pigm Cell Melanoma Res 21(4):410–411
30. Fecher LA, Amaravadi RK et al (2008) The MAPK pathway in melanoma. Curr Opin Oncol 20(2):183–189
31. Flaherty KT, Infante JR et al (2012) Combined BRAF and MEK inhibition in melanoma with BRAF V600 mutations. N Engl J Med 367(18):1694–1703

32. Flaherty KT, Lee SJ et al (2013) Phase III trial of carboplatin and paclitaxel with or without sorafenib in metastatic melanoma. J Clin Oncol 31(3):373–379
33. Flaherty KT, Robert C et al (2012) Improved survival with MEK inhibition in BRAF-mutated melanoma. N Engl J Med 367(2):107–114
34. Flaherty LE, Moon J et al (2012) Phase III trial of high-dose interferon alpha-2b versus cisplatin, vinblastine, DTIC plus IL-2 and interferon in patients with high-risk melanoma (SWOG S0008): an intergroup study of CALGB, COG, ECOG, and SWOG. J Clin Oncol (suppl)
35. Giles MH, Coventry BJ (2013) Isolated limb infusion chemotherapy for melanoma: an overview of early experience at the Adelaide melanoma unit. Cancer Manag Res 5:243–249
36. Gonzalez Cao M, Malvehy J et al (2006) Biochemotherapy with temozolomide, cisplatin, vinblastine, subcutaneous interleukin-2 and interferon-alpha in patients with metastatic melanoma. Melanoma Res 16(1):59–64
37. Gorski DH, Leal AD et al (2003) Differential expression of vascular endothelial growth factor-A isoforms at different stages of melanoma progression. J Am Coll Surg 197(3): 408–418
38. Hauschild A, Agarwala SS et al (2009) Results of a phase III, randomized, placebo-controlled study of sorafenib in combination with carboplatin and paclitaxel as second-line treatment in patients with unresectable stage III or stage IV melanoma. J Clin Oncol 27(17):2823–2830
39. Hauschild A, Grob JJ et al (2012) Dabrafenib in BRAF-mutated metastatic melanoma: a multicentre, open-label, phase 3 randomised controlled trial. Lancet 380(9839):358–365
40. Hersh EM, O'Day SJ et al (2011) A phase II multicenter study of ipilimumab with or without dacarbazine in chemotherapy-naive patients with advanced melanoma. Invest New Drugs 29 (3):489–498
41. Hersh EM, O'Day SJ et al (2010) A phase 2 clinical trial of nab-paclitaxel in previously treated and chemotherapy-naive patients with metastatic melanoma. Cancer 116(1):155–163
42. Hill GJ 2nd, Ruess R et al (1974) Chemotherapy of malignant melanoma with dimethyl traizeno imidazole carboxamide (DITC) and nitrosourea derivatives (BCNU, CCNU). Ann Surg 180(2):167–174
43. Hodi FS, O'Day SJ et al (2010) Improved survival with ipilimumab in patients with metastatic melanoma. N Engl J Med 363(8):711–723
44. Hodi FS, Soiffer RJ et al (2002) Phase II study of paclitaxel and carboplatin for malignant melanoma. Am J Clin Oncol 25(3):283–286
45. Hoekstra HJ, Veerman K et al (2014) Isolated limb perfusion for in-transit melanoma metastases: melphalan or TNF-melphalan perfusion? J Surg Oncol 109(4):338–347
46. Hofmann MA, Hauschild A et al (2011) Prospective evaluation of supportive care with or without CVD chemotherapy as a second-line treatment in advanced melanoma by patient's choice: a multicentre dermatologic cooperative oncology group trial. Melanoma Res 21 (6):516–523
47. Howlader NNA, Krapcho M, Garshell J, Neyman N, Altekruse SF, Kosary CL, Yu M, Ruhl J, Tatalovich Z, Cho H, Mariotto A, Lewis DR, Chen HS, Feuer EJ, Cronin KA (eds) (2013) SEER cancer statistics review, 1975–2010. National Cancer Institute. Bethesda, MD, http://seer.cancer.gov/csr/1975_2010/, based on November 2012 SEER data submission, posted to the SEER web site, 2013
48. Ives NJ, Stowe RL et al (2007) Chemotherapy compared with biochemotherapy for the treatment of metastatic melanoma: a meta-analysis of 18 trials involving 2621 patients. J Clin Oncol 25(34):5426–5434
49. Ji Z, Flaherty KT et al (2010) Molecular therapeutic approaches to melanoma. Mol Aspects Med 31(2):194–204
50. Jiang G, Li RH et al (2014) Efficacy and safety between temozolomide alone and temozolomide-based double therapy for malignant melanoma: a meta-analysis. Tumour Biol 35(1):315–322

51. Kim KB, Kefford R et al (2013) Phase II study of the MEK1/MEK2 inhibitor trametinib in patients with metastatic BRAF-mutant cutaneous melanoma previously treated with or without a BRAF inhibitor. J Clin Oncol 31(4):482–489
52. Kim KB, Legha SS et al (2009) A randomized phase III trial of biochemotherapy versus interferon-alpha-2b for adjuvant therapy in patients at high risk for melanoma recurrence. Melanoma Res 19(1):42–49
53. Kim KB, Sosman JA et al (2012) BEAM: a randomized phase II study evaluating the activity of bevacizumab in combination with carboplatin plus paclitaxel in patients with previously untreated advanced melanoma. J Clin Oncol 30(1):34–41
54. Kirkwood JM, Strawderman MH et al (1996) Interferon alfa-2b adjuvant therapy of high-risk resected cutaneous melanoma: the eastern cooperative oncology group trial EST 1684. J Clin Oncol 14(1):7–17
55. Klop WM, Vrouenraets BC et al (1996) Repeat isolated limb perfusion with melphalan for recurrent melanoma of the limbs. J Am Coll Surg 182(6):467–472
56. Kroon HM, Huismans AM et al (2014) Isolated limb infusion with melphalan and actinomycin D for melanoma: a systematic review. J Surg Oncol 109(4):348–351
57. Kroon HM, Moncrieff M et al (2008) Outcomes following isolated limb infusion for melanoma. A 14-year experience. Ann Surg Oncol 15(11):3003–3013
58. Lacal PM, Failla CM et al (2000) Human melanoma cells secrete and respond to placenta growth factor and vascular endothelial growth factor. J Invest Dermatol 115(6):1000–1007
59. Legha SS, Papadopoulos NE et al (1987) Clinical evaluation of recombinant interferon alfa-2a (Roferon-A) in metastatic melanoma using two different schedules. J Clin Oncol 5 (8):1240–1246
60. Legha SS, Ring S et al (1996) Treatment of metastatic melanoma with combined chemotherapy containing cisplatin, vinblastine and dacarbazine (CVD) and biotherapy using interleukin-2 and interferon-alpha. Ann Oncol 7(8):827–835
61. Legha SS, Ring S et al (1998) Development of a biochemotherapy regimen with concurrent administration of cisplatin, vinblastine, dacarbazine, interferon alfa, and interleukin-2 for patients with metastatic melanoma. J Clin Oncol 16(5):1752–1759
62. Legha SS, Ring S et al (1989) A prospective evaluation of a triple-drug regimen containing cisplatin, vinblastine, and dacarbazine (CVD) for metastatic melanoma. Cancer 64(10): 2024–2029
63. Legha SS, Ring S et al (1990) A phase II trial of taxol in metastatic melanoma. Cancer 65 (11):2478–2481
64. Lewis KD, Robinson WA et al (2006) Phase II multicenter study of neoadjuvant biochemotherapy for patients with stage III malignant melanoma. J Clin Oncol 24 (19):3157–3163
65. Li Y, McClay EF (2002) Systemic chemotherapy for the treatment of metastatic melanoma. Semin Oncol 29(5):413–426
66. Lienard D, Ewalenko P et al (1992) High-dose recombinant tumor necrosis factor alpha in combination with interferon gamma and melphalan in isolation perfusion of the limbs for melanoma and sarcoma. J Clin Oncol 10(1):52–60
67. Marcoval J, Moreno A et al (1997) Angiogenesis and malignant melanoma. Angiogenesis is related to the development of vertical (tumorigenic) growth phase. J Cutan Pathol 24(4): 212–218
68. Margolin K, Atkins B et al (2002) Temozolomide and whole brain irradiation in melanoma metastatic to the brain: a phase II trial of the cytokine working group. J Cancer Res Clin Oncol 128(4):214–218
69. Margolin KA, Liu PY et al (1998) Phase II study of carmustine, dacarbazine, cisplatin, and tamoxifen in advanced melanoma: a Southwest Oncology Group study. J Clin Oncol 16 (2):664–669
70. McClay EF, Mastrangelo MJ et al (1992) Effective combination chemo/hormonal therapy for malignant melanoma: experience with three consecutive trials. Int J Cancer 50(4):553–556

71. McDermott DF, Mier JW et al (2000) A phase II pilot trial of concurrent biochemotherapy with cisplatin, vinblastine, dacarbazine, interleukin 2, and interferon alpha-2B in patients with metastatic melanoma. Clin Cancer Res 6(6):2201–2208
72. Mian R, Henderson MA et al (2001) Isolated limb infusion for melanoma: a simple alternative to isolated limb perfusion. Can J Surg 44(3):189–192
73. Middleton MR, Grob JJ et al (2000) Randomized phase III study of temozolomide versus dacarbazine in the treatment of patients with advanced metastatic malignant melanoma. J Clin Oncol 18(1):158–166
74. Newlands ES, Stevens MF et al (1997) Temozolomide: a review of its discovery, chemical properties, pre-clinical development and clinical trials. Cancer Treat Rev 23(1):35–61
75. Nieweg OE, Kroon BB (2014) Isolated limb perfusion with melphalan for melanoma. J Surg Oncol 109(4):332–337
76. Parkinson DR, Abrams JS et al (1990) Interleukin-2 therapy in patients with metastatic malignant melanoma: a phase II study. J Clin Oncol 8(10):1650–1656
77. Patel PM, Suciu S et al (2011) Extended schedule, escalated dose temozolomide versus dacarbazine in stage IV melanoma: final results of a randomised phase III study (EORTC 18032). Eur J Cancer 47(10):1476–1483
78. Paul MJ, Summers Y et al (2002) Effect of temozolomide on central nervous system relapse in patients with advanced melanoma. Melanoma Res 12(2):175–178
79. Punt CJ, van Herpen CM et al (1997) Chemoimmunotherapy with bleomycin, vincristine, lomustine, dacarbazine (BOLD) plus interferon alpha for metastatic melanoma: a multicentre phase II study. Br J Cancer 76(2):266–269
80. Pyrhonen S, Hahka-Kemppinen M et al (1992) A promising interferon plus four-drug chemotherapy regimen for metastatic melanoma. J Clin Oncol 10(12):1919–1926
81. Qi RQ, He L et al (2011) BRAF exon 15 T1799A mutation is common in melanocytic nevi, but less prevalent in cutaneous malignant melanoma, in Chinese Han. J Invest Dermatol 131 (5):1129–1138
82. Rao GG, Rogers P et al (2005) Phase I clinical trial of weekly paclitaxel, weekly carboplatin, and concurrent radiotherapy for primary cervical cancer. Gynecol Oncol 96(1):168–172
83. Robert C, Thomas L et al (2011) Ipilimumab plus dacarbazine for previously untreated metastatic melanoma. N Engl J Med 364(26):2517–2526
84. Rosenberg SA, Yang JC et al (1994) Treatment of 283 consecutive patients with metastatic melanoma or renal cell cancer using high-dose bolus interleukin 2. JAMA 271(12):907–913
85. Rossi CR, Russano F et al (2008) TNF-based isolated limb perfusion followed by consolidation biotherapy with systemic low-dose interferon alpha 2b in patients with in-transit melanoma metastases: a pilot trial. Ann Surg Oncol 15(4):1218–1223
86. Rusthoven JJ, Quirt IC et al (1996) Randomized, double-blind, placebo-controlled trial comparing the response rates of carmustine, dacarbazine, and cisplatin with and without tamoxifen in patients with metastatic melanoma. National Cancer Institute of Canada Clinical Trials Group. J Clin Oncol 14(7):2083–2090
87. Sanki A, Kam PC et al (2007) Long-term results of hyperthermic, isolated limb perfusion for melanoma: a reflection of tumor biology. Ann Surg 245(4):591–596
88. Shetty G, Beasley GM et al (2013) Plasma cytokine analysis in patients with advanced extremity melanoma undergoing isolated limb infusion. Ann Surg Oncol 20(4):1128–1135
89. Sosman JA, Kim KB et al (2012) Survival in BRAF V600-mutant advanced melanoma treated with vemurafenib. N Engl J Med 366(8):707–714
90. Squires MH 3rd, Delman KA (2013) Current treatment of locoregional recurrence of melanoma. Curr Oncol Rep 15(5):465–472
91. Steinman J, Ariyan C et al (2014) Factors associated with response, survival, and limb salvage in patients undergoing isolated limb infusion. J Surg Oncol 109(5):405–409
92. Thompson JF, Kam PC et al (1998) Isolated limb infusion with cytotoxic agents: a simple alternative to isolated limb perfusion. Semin Surg Oncol 14(3):238–247

93. Ugurel S, Rappl G et al (2001) Increased serum concentration of angiogenic factors in malignant melanoma patients correlates with tumor progression and survival. J Clin Oncol 19 (2):577–583
94. Vuoristo MS, Hahka-Kemppinen M et al (2005) Randomized trial of dacarbazine versus bleomycin, vincristine, lomustine and dacarbazine (BOLD) chemotherapy combined with natural or recombinant interferon-alpha in patients with advanced melanoma. Melanoma Res 15(4):291–296
95. Wilhelm SM, Adnane L et al (2008) Preclinical overview of sorafenib, a multikinase inhibitor that targets both Raf and VEGF and PDGF receptor tyrosine kinase signaling. Mol Cancer Ther 7(10):3129–3140
96. Wolchok JD, Neyns B et al (2010) Ipilimumab monotherapy in patients with pretreated advanced melanoma: a randomised, double-blind, multicentre, phase 2, dose-ranging study. Lancet Oncol 11(2):155–164
97. Wong J, Chen YA et al (2013) Isolated limb infusion in a series of over 100 infusions: a single-center experience. Ann Surg Oncol 20(4):1121–1127
98. Yung WK (2000) Temozolomide in malignant gliomas. Semin Oncol 27(3 Suppl 6):27–34
99. Yung WK, Albright RE et al (2000) A phase II study of temozolomide vs. procarbazine in patients with glioblastoma multiforme at first relapse. Br J Cancer 83(5):588–593
100. Zimpfer-Rechner C, Hofmann U et al (2003) Randomized phase II study of weekly paclitaxel versus paclitaxel and carboplatin as second-line therapy in disseminated melanoma: a multicentre trial of the dermatologic co-operative oncology group (DeCOG). Melanoma Res 13(5):531–536

Checkpoint Blockade for the Treatment of Advanced Melanoma

Margaret K. Callahan, Catherine R. Flaherty and Michael A. Postow

Abstract

Immunotherapy with immune checkpoint inhibition has been improving the outcomes of patients with many different types of malignancies. Immune checkpoint inhibition has been most extensively studied in patients with advanced melanoma and there are three FDA approved antibodies already widely used in clinical practice (ipilimumab, nivolumab, and pembrolizumab). In this chapter, we review the mechanistic basis behind the development of immune checkpoint blocking antibodies. We then discuss specifics regarding each agent, unique clinical considerations in treating patients with this approach, and future directions, including combination strategies. This chapter is focused on melanoma, but the principles related to this immunotherapy approach are applicable to patients with many types of malignancies.

Keyword

Immune checkpoint · Immunotherapy · Melanoma · Immune-related response criteria · Immune-related adverse events

M.K. Callahan · C.R. Flaherty · M.A. Postow (✉)
Melanoma and Immunotherapeutics Service, Department of Medicine, Memorial Sloan Kettering Cancer Center, New York, NY, USA
e-mail: PostowM@mskcc.org

M.K. Callahan · M.A. Postow
Weill Medical College of Cornell University, New York, NY, USA

H.L. Kaufman and J.M. Mehnert (eds.), *Melanoma*,
Cancer Treatment and Research 167, DOI 10.1007/978-3-319-22539-5_9

Contents

1 Introduction

Melanoma is a challenging malignancy due to the associated high risk of recurrence after treatment of the primary tumor and often aggressive disease course in advanced stages. Chemotherapy regimens can benefit some patients with melanoma, but none have led to an improvement in overall survival. For this reason, additional treatment modalities have been of interest. Among the various systemic treatments for melanoma, immunotherapy remains an essential component.

This chapter is focused on the utilization of checkpoint blockading antibodies, a novel immunotherapeutic approach, to treat unresectable and metastatic melanoma. We discuss the preclinical rationale that led to the development of these antibodies and then review clinical experiences involving cytotoxic T lymphocyte-associated antigen (CTLA-4) and programmed cell death 1 (PD-1) receptor antibodies. We conclude with comments on promising new combination approaches.

2 Cytotoxic T Lymphocyte-Associated Antigen (CTLA-4) Blockade—Basic Biology and Pre-clinical Activity

Cytotoxic T lymphocyte-associated antigen (CTLA-4) is an important negative regulator or "checkpoint" in T cell activation [1–4]. CTLA-4 is expressed on activated T cells and binds to its ligands B7-1 and B7-2, which are expressed on antigen presenting cells [5]. CTLA-4 appears to compete with the co-stimulatory molecule, CD28, for binding to B7-1 and B7-2 [2, 6]. In addition, CTLA-4 engagement inhibits T cell cytokine production and proliferation [2, 4, 7–9]. The phenotype of CTLA-4$^{-/-}$ knockout mice supports the negative regulatory function for CTLA-4 in vivo. These mice develop a lethal hyperproliferative lymphocyte expansion and fail to live past 3 weeks [10–12].

Given the role the CTLA-4 plays as a negative regulator of T cell activation, it was hypothesized that blocking CTLA-4 could enhance immune responses against tumors by inhibiting this "checkpoint" [13]. This idea was initially tested using transplantable murine tumor lines of colon carcinoma and fibrosarcoma, where it was demonstrated that established tumors could be rejected by administration of a CTLA-4 blocking antibody [14–18]. This observation has since been validated in a variety of pre-clinical mouse models including models of melanoma [14–18]. In addition to being expressed on activated T cells, CTLA-4 is also highly expressed on regulatory T cells. It has been hypothesized that CTLA-4 blockade may also work, in part, via its effects on regulatory T cells [19–21]. CTLA-4 blockade has also shown activity in pre-clinical models in combination with established cancer therapies including radiation therapy, chemotherapy, surgery, cryoablation, and radiofrequency ablation [22–26]. In mouse models, this approach has also been combined successfully with a number of potential immunotherapies, including notable preclinical activity for the combination of CTLA-4 and PD-1 pathway blockade [27–37].

3 CTLA-4 Blocking Antibodies

Two antibodies that block human CTLA-4 have been developed and tested in patients: ipilimumab (Bristol Myers-Squibb, Princeton, NJ, USA) and tremelimumab (previously Pfizer, New York, NY and now Medimmune, Inc, Gaithersburg, MD). Ipilimumab is a fully human monoclonal IgG1 kappa antibody with a half-life of 12–14 days. Tremelimumab is a fully human monoclonal IgG2 antibody with a half-life of approximately 22 days. Ipilimumab has been approved by the FDA for the treatment of advanced melanoma. Tremelimumab is still in clinical development.

4 Ipilimumab—Clinical Development and FDA Approval

In March 2011, ipilimumab was approved for the treatment of unresectable or metastatic melanoma by the United States Food and Drug Administration (FDA). The clinical journey to FDA approval was just beginning in 2002, when some of the first evidence for clinical activity for ipilimumab in melanoma was published beginning with a phase I, single-dose study reporting two partial responses (PR) out of 17 patients with advanced melanoma [38]. The next several studies explored questions of schedule and dosing for this new agent. In several of these studies, ipilimumab was dosed once every three weeks for up to four doses. In these multi-dose studies, clinical investigators reported their first experiences with a unique toxicity profile for this new class of agents. Toxicities appeared to reflect a pattern of drug-induced, tissue-specific inflammation and were labeled immune-related adverse events (irAE). In a double-blind phase II study comparing ipilimumab at doses of 0.3, 3, and 10 mg/kg, a dose–response relationship was observed [39]. The highest dose level, 10 mg/kg, had the highest response rate (11 %), compared to 3 mg/kg (4.2 %), and 0.3 mg/kg (0 %). As might be anticipated, the rate of irAEs was also higher with the higher ipilimumab dose.

Finally, a randomized phase III trial for patients with previously treated, unresectable stage III or stage IV melanoma was reported by Hodi et al. [40]. This study demonstrated a benefit in overall survival and ipilimumab was subsequently granted FDA approval [40]. In this study, patients were randomized in a 3:1:1 ratio to be treated with ipilimumab with a peptide vaccine, ipilimumab alone, or the peptide vaccine alone as the control arm. The peptide vaccine consisted of two HLA-A*0201-restricted peptides from gp100 (a melanosomal antigen) emulsified in Montanide. Ipilimumab was dosed at 3 mg/kg. Overall survival was the primary endpoint of the study which reported that patients treated with ipilimumab plus vaccine (10.0 months) or ipilimumab alone (10.1 months) had a longer median survival than patients who received peptide vaccine alone (6.4 months). Furthermore, landmark survival at 1 or 2 years was higher in the ipilimumab-treated group versus the vaccine-treated group (45.6 % vs. 25.3 % at one year, 23.8 % vs. 16.3 % at 2 years), a finding that is especially notable since most patients completed treatment with ipilimumab within the first 3 months on study. A second phase III trial reported by Robert et al. confirmed this survival benefit. This randomized, placebo-controlled study compared ipilimumab at a dose of 10 mg/kg combined with dacarbazine chemotherapy to dacarbazine alone in patients with advanced melanoma [41]. Highlighting the long-term survival benefit to receiving ipilimumab in this population, a survival advantage was observed at 1 year (47.3 % vs. 36.3 %), 2 years (28.5 % vs. 17.9 %), and 3 years (20.8 % vs. 12.2 %) after initial treatment.

5 Kinetics of Tumor Response and Re-evaluation of Traditional Radiographic Response Endpoints

Early studies of CTLA-4 blockade suggested that patterns of radiographic response to this immunotherapy may differ from those previously described for standard chemotherapy. Patients who responded to ipilimumab after initial development of a new lesion or after progression of all measurable disease challenged the notions of what had previously been observed and expected for other types of cancer therapies. According to standard radiographic criteria such as RECIST or mWHO, increase in tumor size and/or development of new lesions is defined as progressive disease, typically suggesting that a change in therapy should be considered.

A retrospective review of radiographic responses in 487 patients enrolled in one of three multicenter phase II clinical trials of ipilimumab was undertaken to further investigate these observations [42]. In this analysis, four unique radiographic patterns associated with favorable clinical outcomes were observed and captured: (1) decrease in baseline lesions without new lesions (classical response); (2) durable stable disease; (3) initial increase in total tumor burden with later response (flare); and (4) reduction in size of baseline lesions concurrent with the growth of new lesions (mixed pattern). Importantly, each of these patterns correlated with survival —i.e., patients who had a survival benefit and would have been overlooked by traditional criteria (patterns 3 and 4) were detected by the criteria developed in this analysis. Thus, the immune-related response criteria (irRC) were proposed as novel radiographic criteria to evaluate the clinical benefit of checkpoint blockade. At present, we await prospective validation of this approach.

6 Dosing and Schedule

The FDA-approved schedule for ipilimumab is one dose every three weeks for up to four doses. Some studies of ipilimumab permitted repeating treatment with ipilimumab (reinduction) in patients who progressed after an initial response according to the original four-dose schedule. The phase III study of ipilimumab led by Hodi et al. provided modest data to suggest that reinduction benefits selected patients [43]. Of the 504 randomized to receive ipilimumab or ipilimumab plus vaccine, there were 31 patients who developed disease progression after an initial confirmed PR, complete response (CR), or at least 3 months of stable disease (SD) and then were offered reinduction. Of these selected patients who received reinduction during this time of disease progression, 21 appeared to subsequently benefit with 1 CR, 5 PRs, and 15 with SD. In other trials, additional (maintenance) doses of ipilimumab were administered every three months after the initial four doses. The benefit of continued (maintenance) dosing is unknown.

A maximum tolerated dose for ipilimumab was not identified in the original phase I studies. In a randomized, double-blinded phase II study comparing ipilimumab at three dose levels, 0.3, 3, and 10 mg/kg, the highest dose level achieved the highest response rate. Importantly, this higher response rate (0 % vs. 4.2 % vs. 11.1 %) must be considered in light of the increased rate of Grade 3/4 irAEs (0 % vs. 7 % vs. 25 %). A phase III study evaluating ipilimumab dosed at 10 mg/kg versus 3 mg/kg is expected to be reported soon.

7 Side Effects Associated with CTLA-4 Blocking Antibodies

With the exploration of the clinical activity for CTLA-4 blocking antibody came the discovery of a novel pattern of side effects not previously seen with chemotherapies, specifically a unique distribution of tissue-specific inflammation. The term immune-related adverse events (irAEs) has been employed to describe these toxicities which are thought to reflect the activation of the immune system consistent with the proposed mechanism of activity of ipilimumab. The tissues that are most often affected are the bowel (diarrhea, colitis), the liver (hepatitis, elevated liver enzymes), and the pituitary and other endocrine glands (hypophysitis, hypothyroidism, thyroiditis, adrenal insufficiency) and skin (rash, pruritus, vitiligo) [43]. Uncommon, but reported irAEs include uveitis, conjunctivitis, pancreatitis, cytopenias, neuropathy, myopathy, pneumonitis, and nephritis [44–48]. IrAEs are usually ameliorated with interruption or discontinuation of CTLA-4 blockade in combination with immunosuppressive drugs. Drugs that have been most helpful for the treatment of irAEs are corticosteroids; more rarely, TNF-blocking antibodies (for colitis) or mycophenolate mofetil (for hepatitis) or other approaches have been employed [49, 50]. For some patients that develop endocrinopathies, irreversible damage to endocrine organs during the acute period of inflammation may necessitate long-term hormone supplementation [51–53]. Guidelines for the management of individual toxicities are available [54]. Given the concern for immune-related toxicities, clinical trials of ipilimumab have generally excluded patients with pre-existing autoimmune conditions and the safety of ipilimumab in this patient population is not known. Some case reports have suggested ipilimumab has not exacerbated patients' underlying autoimmune diseases, but others have indicated this may be possible [55, 56].

8 Investigating Biomarkers for CTLA-4 Blockade

Research investigations into immunological parameters that may provide insight into the activity of checkpoint blockade have been incorporated into many of the clinical trials of ipilimumab; however, no clear biomarkers that predict response to therapy or likelihood of toxicity have been identified to date. The majority of potential biomarkers have been identified in small, retrospective analyses and have been hypothesis generating.

Several early studies of ipilimumab singled out the absolute lymphocyte count (ALC) as a marker of interest. Several subsequent retrospective analyses have linked higher ALC during treatment, either using a cutoff or measuring the rate of rise, with more favorable clinical outcomes [57, 58]. However, ALC prior to initiation of treatment has not been established as a predictive biomarker. Antigen-specific immune responses during checkpoint blockade have also been investigated for a number of cancer-related antigens. Immune responses to NY-ESO-1, a cancer-testis antigen, have been the most closely evaluated. In a single institution retrospective analysis of 15 melanoma patients treated with ipilimumab, 5/8 (62.5 %) patients with tumor reduction or stabilization had developed NY-ESO-1 antibodies [59]. This connection between tumor antigen and clinical outcome was also described in a larger, retrospective study of 144 patients with melanoma where NY-ESO-1 seropositive patients were more likely to have a CR, PR, or prolonged SD after ipilimumab treatment [60].

Inducible costimulator (ICOS) is a costimulatory molecule expressed on activated T cells. It is thought to be involved in T cell proliferation, survival, and memory [61]. ICOS expression has been hypothesized to be biomarker for clinical activity in patients treated with ipilimumab. The first studies supporting a correlation between ICOS expression and anti-tumor activity came from the analysis of tumor and peripheral blood T cells in patients with bladder cancer treated with neoadjuvant ipilimumab [62]. In a subsequent retrospective analysis of patients with advanced melanoma treated with ipilimumab, a higher frequency of peripheral blood CD4+ICOS^{high} T cells, sustained over 12 week's time, correlated positively with increased overall survival [63].

The tumor microenvironment plays in modulating anti-tumor immune responses and the tumor/tumor microenvironment may be a more relevant place to evaluate potential biomarkers. In a prospective phase II study of patients with melanoma treated with ipilimumab, utilizing gene expression profiling, expression of immune-related genes in pre-treatment tumor biopsy specimens, especially interferon gamma responsive genes, correlated positively with clinical activity [64, 65]. In a more recent retrospective study of tumor characteristics, the number and character of tumor mutations, potentially neo-antigens recognized by the immune system, correlated with the clinical outcomes in patients treated with ipilimumab [66].

9 Programmed Cell Death Protein 1 (PD-1) Pathway Blockade—Preclinical Rationale and Clinical Efficacy

Targeting CTLA-4 was the first immune checkpoint strategy that demonstrated success for patients with advanced melanoma. However, due to high clinical efficacy and excellent tolerability, much recent attention has been directed toward strategies that block another immunologic checkpoint, the programmed cell protein 1 pathway (PD-1/PD-L1). PD-1 is a negative regulator of T cell activity that limits the activity of T cells at a variety of stages of the immune response when it interacts with its two ligands PD-L1 and PD-L2 [67–69]. When engaged by ligand, through phosphatase activity, PD-1 inhibits kinase signaling pathways that normally lead to T cell activation [68]. This T cell proliferation activates the immune system. It is interesting to note that PD-1, like CTLA-4, is also expressed on Tregs and may enhance their immunosuppressive function as well [70]. The phenotype of PD-1-deficient mice characterized by autoimmune features such as dilated cardiomyopathy and arthritis differs from mice deficient in CTLA-4 [71, 72]. While the specific reasons for this are not known, it is possible that this is because PD-1 is primarily believed to inhibit effector T cell activity in the effector phase within tissue and tumors as opposed to the predominantly earlier role CTLA-4 plays in limiting T cell activation [73]. Since PD-1 is expressed on B cells and natural killer cells, therapeutic blockade of the PD-1 pathway may also affect the biology of these cell types [73, 74].

Antibodies that block the PD-1 axis are undergoing extensive clinical evaluation. Antibodies include those that target PD-1 (Nivolumab, Bristol-Myers Squibb; Pembrolizumab, Merck; Pidilizumab, CureTech) and those that target PD-L1 (MPDL3280A, Genentech; MEDI4736, MedImmune/AstraZeneca; BMS-936559, Bristol-Myers Squibb; MSB0010718C, EMD Serono). AMP-224 (Amplimmune/GlaxoSmithKline) is a PD-L2 fusion protein that does not directly target PD-1 or PD-L1, but instead is believed to deplete PD-1+ T cells [75]. While these immunotherapeutic approaches are being investigated in many diseases, data are most mature for patients with advanced melanoma, and two agents, pembrolizumab and nivolumab, are already approved by the United States Food and Drug Administration (US FDA).

Large phase I studies of nivolumab and pembrolizumab have demonstrated highly durable objective response rates (~30–40 %) with minimal toxicity involving patients with advanced melanoma [76–78]. The durability of PD-1 responses is also impressive with a median duration of response of nivolumab lasting approximately 2 years [78]. Randomized phase III data have demonstrated a superior response rate for nivolumab compared to dacarbazine and also found an overall survival benefit in favor of nivolumab in a population of patients with BRAF wild-type melanoma [79].

Pembrolizumab is believed to have similar efficacy to nivolumab, demonstrating impressive tumor responses. In September 2014, pembrolizumab was approved by the US FDA for patients with melanoma previously treated with ipilimumab and if relevant, a BRAF inhibitor [80]. This approval was based upon favorable results in a phase I randomized dose finding study [80]. No difference in efficacy or safety was seen in patients with melanoma treated with pembrolizumab 2 mg/kg every 3 weeks versus 10 mg/kg every 3 weeks, leading the FDA to approve pembrolizumab at the dose of 2 mg/kg every 3 weeks. Though the FDA has approved pembrolizumab for patients previously treated with ipilimumab and if relevant, a BRAF inhibitor, efficacy of pembrolizumab appears similar for patients with melanoma who have not had prior ipilimumab or RAF inhibition [77]. Large randomized studies comparing pembrolizumab to ipilimumab in the frontline setting and to chemotherapy in the second line setting after ipilimumab are ongoing.

While nivolumab and pembrolizumab have been most extensively evaluated, other PD-1/PD-L1 blockade approaches have included patients with melanoma. The PD-1 blocking antibody, pidilizumab was evaluated in a phase II study involving patients with melanoma. The response rate was low, but the overall survival in this study was favorable compared to historical data [81]. The discrepancy between the low response rate and improved overall survival compared to historical controls may have been due to patients with SD, but this remains speculative. Patients treated with pidilizumab in this trial had 75 % M1c disease, 16 % had brain metastases, 30 % had an elevated LDH, and 77 % had received prior systemic treatment for melanoma. It appears unlikely that selection bias alone accounted for the favorable overall survival seen in this study. Due to the overall low response rate of pidilizumab monotherapy, future studies will likely investigate this agent in combination with other approaches.

While targeting PD-L1 is a similarly promising approach, fewer patients with melanoma have been treated with antibodies that block PD-L1. In concept, targeting PD-L1 may result in different immunologic effects than targeting PD-1. PD-L1 also exerts negative signals on T cells by interacting with B7; in addition to the negative signals, PD-L1 creates by interacting with PD-1 [82]. While PD-L1 blocking antibodies prevent the interaction of PD-L1 with B7, PD-1 blocking antibodies, such as the previously described nivolumab, pembrolizumab, and pidilizumab, do not. Antibodies that block PD-L1 also do not prevent PD-1 from interacting with PD-L2. The importance of the PD-L2 and PD-1 interaction in antitumor activity remains unknown.

BMS-956559 was the first PD-L1 antibody to show objective tumor responses in patients with melanoma [83]. MPDL3280A, MEDI4736, and MSB0010718C are also undergoing clinical evaluation are similarly promising approaches [84–87]. It is possible that the role of these PD-L1 blocking antibodies in patients with melanoma may ultimately be as a component of combination strategies such as in partnership with dabrafenib and trametinib or vemurafenib and cobimetinib for patients with BRAF mutant melanoma.

10 Re-evaluating the Immune-Related Response Criteria (irRC) in the PD-1 Era

As described previously in this chapter, responses to CTLA-4 antibody blockade can often be delayed [88]. This has led to the development of the alternative response criteria termed the “immune-related response criteria (irRC)” [89, 90].

Most of the presented and published trials of PD-1/PD-L1 blockade in melanoma have reported data using traditional response criteria such as the Response Evaluation Criteria in Solid Tumors (RECIST) methodology. The use of the irRC has been more limited. Nevertheless, some patients that were treated with PD-1 agents have similarly shown "immune-related" patterns of response [76, 77]. In the phase III nivolumab versus dacarbazine study, there was an increased survival benefit with nivolumab, a PD1 blocking agent, compared to dacarbazine chemotherapy. Also, some patients appeared to benefit in unconventional ways such as 54 patients that were treated with nivolumab after progression of disease and 17 had an immune-related response pattern [79].

Though these delayed or atypical responses to PD-1/PD-L1 can be seen, they are less common and most patients with increasing tumor burdens while on PD-1 unfortunately continue to progress. Out of 192 patients treated with pembrolizumab, approximately 10 % of patients who had progressed by RECIST at week 12 subsequently achieved some benefit from pembrolizumab therapy (response or SD) [91]. In phase III evaluation of nivolumab versus chemotherapy, 10 out of 120 patients (8 %) who received nivolumab had atypical irRC responses [92].

The irRC will likely continue to be modified as additional data accumulate. Since irRC had initially developed from the bidirectional modified World Health Organization (mWHO) criteria, efforts have proposed a unidimensional irRC to be more consistent with the commonly used RECIST unidimensional measurements [93]. Randomized trials evaluating the irRC in both PD-1/PD-L1 experimental arms and chemotherapy control arms will ultimately be necessary to determine whether irRC is more effective at capturing efficacy of immunotherapy compared to the standard mWHO and RECIST.

11 Side Effects (irAEs) of PD-1

Despite the profound benefits of PD-1/PD-L1 blocking antibodies, unfortunately side effects can occur. The spectrum and frequency of side effects with PD-1/PD-L1 is somewhat distinct from that of CTLA-4, but early recognition and treatment are believed to be equally important in optimal outcomes. The most common irAE is skin toxicity. Perhaps more specific to the PD-1 experience, mucositis and/or complaints of dry mouth have been reported [78]. Treatment for skin irAEs from PD-1/PD-L1 antibodies is similar to that blocking CTLA-4 consisting of topical corticosteroids and antipruritics (i.e., hydroxyzine and diphenhydramine). Occasionally, oral corticosteroid rinses and lidocaine have helped patients with mucositis. Severe diarrhea and transaminitis are fortunately less common with antibodies that block PD-1/PD-L1 compared to those that block CTLA-4. Yet, grade 3/4 toxicity can still occur and merits treatment with steroids [76, 77]. It is essential to note that infliximab can be helpful for steroid refractory cases of diarrhea, but it should not be used in patients with steroid refractory hepatitis out of concern infliximab itself could result in hepatic toxicity. Mycophenolate mofetil (500 mg twice daily) can sometimes help cases of steroid refractory hepatitis.

The rate of less common irAEs such as endocrinopathy after PD-1 blockade is not completely known but has been reported to affect a small proportion of patients with melanoma in some of the reported trials. The treatment of endocrinopathy from PD-1 blockade is similar to the treatment of endocrinopathy arising from CTLA-4 blockade. Often a short course of steroids is needed to palliate symptoms. Then, replacement hormones are administered, depending on the deficient hormone (levothyroxine for hypothyroidism; hydrocortisone for adrenal insufficiency; gonadal hormone replacement for sex hormone deficiency). Other rare irAEs such as pneumonitis have been described. Pneumonitis is notable since treatment-related deaths have been unfortunately experienced [76].

12 PD-L1 as a Biomarker for PD-1/PD-L1 Outcomes in Patients with Melanoma

PD-1/PD-L1 treatment would ideally be matched to patients with melanoma who are most likely to benefit and least likely to experience side effects. The majority of biomarker efforts have investigated immunohistochemical expression of PD-L1 and its association with response. Though patients whose tumors express PD-L1 have numerically higher response rates to PD-1/PD-L1 blockade than patients who do not express PD-L1 [76, 94, 95], patients who do not express PD-L1 can still have great responses to PD-1 blockade. No difference in overall survival between PD-L1 positive versus PD-L1 negative patients was seen in a randomized phase III study of nivolumab compared to chemotherapy. PD-L1 negative patients also had improved overall survival compared to chemotherapy, indicating PD-L1 is not a predictive biomarker of PD-1 benefit. We therefore do not believe PD-L1 should be used to exclude a patient from the opportunity to benefit from a PD-1/PD-L1 antibody. Infiltrating immune cells as well as possibly genetic changes within the tumor can also affect PD-L1 expression, and additional research into the mechanisms involved in PD-L1 expression is warranted [96–98].

13 Combination Immunotherapy Approaches

The concurrent combination of ipilimumab and nivolumab was tested in a phase I dose-escalation study which was notable for objective response rate averaging 40 % (ranging from 21 to 53 %, $n = 52$) across all dose levels tested [99]. While cross-study comparisons should be approached with caution, previously reported response rates for monotherapy treatment with either ipilimumab or nivolumab were 11 and 31 %, respectively [43, 76, 100]. Furthermore, patients responding to the combination of ipilimumab and nivolumab appeared to have a relatively rapid response and a greater magnitude in reduction of tumor burden than typically expected for checkpoint blockade. Among responding patients, there was a very high rate of CRs or near CRs with 31 % of the patients showing a reduction in disease burden of 80 % or greater. As might be expected, the frequency of irAEs and the number of patients with multiple irAEs was higher than previously described for either monotherapy. Among all patients who received the concurrent combination, 93 % had a treatment-related toxicity of any grade and 53 % had a grade 3/4 toxicity attributed to treatment. At present, a phase II study comparing the combination to ipilimumab alone and a phase III study comparing the combination to either ipilimumab or nivolumab monotherapy are ongoing.

Many other potential immunotherapy combination approaches are presently under investigation including combinations of CTLA-4 or PD-1 pathway blockade with IL-2 as well as other novel immunotherapy agents in development. A randomized phase 2 study of ipilimumab combined with GM-CSF compared to ipilimumab alone suggested a longer overall survival and lower toxicity with the combination, meriting further investigation [101].

14 Combination Approaches with Chemotherapy

While a randomized 72-patient phase II study comparing ipilimumab (3 mg/kg) combined with dacarbazine to ipilimumab alone reported a higher objective response rate for the combination (14.3 % vs. 5.4 %), this finding has not been formally tested in larger studies. The phase III trial comparing ipilimumab (10 mg/kg) combined with dacarbazine compared to dacarbazine alone did not include an arm with ipilimumab alone and used the higher 10 mg/kg dose of ipilimumab [41]. In this study, the response rate in the combination arm was 15.2 %. In both of these studies, response rates for the combination were very close to the range of response rates previously reported for ipilimumab monotherapy. Additionally, the combination of ipilimumab at a dose of 10 mg/kg and dacarbazine had a rate of grade 3/4 irAEs of >40 % which appears to be significantly higher than previously reported for ipilimumab (10 mg/kg) alone (~25 %) [39]. As a consequence, ipilimumab combined with dacarbazine chemotherapy has not been adopted in clinical practice.

15 Combination Approaches with Targeted Inhibitors

For patients with BRAF mutant melanoma, targeted inhibitors of BRAF (vemurafenib, dabrafenib) and MEK (trametinib) have been approved by the FDA and incorporated into standard clinical practice. The potential for combining these targeted inhibitors with ipilimumab appeared attractive given their unique mechanisms of action. The first study testing the concomitant combination of ipilimumab and vemurafenib unfortunately encountered dose-limiting hepatotoxicity, limiting the clinical potential for this combination at the dose/schedule explored thus far [102]. However, a recent report at ASCO describing a phase 1 study combining the BRAF inhibitor dabrafenib with ipilimumab did not find hepatic DLTs in the 12 patients evaluated on study and only 1 case of grade 3 transaminitis that responded after 1 week of treatment with steroids [103]. Additionally, studies combining BRAF inhibition with PD-1 pathway blockade are ongoing. The potential for combined checkpoint blockade and targeted BRAF inhibition is as of yet unclear.

16 Combination Approaches with Radiotherapy

As described in a comprehensive review by Formenti and Demaria, radiotherapy may lead to a number of potentially favorable immunologic effects [104]. In murine models, radiotherapy has been shown to enhance the efficacy of CTLA-4 and PD-1 blockade [24, 105, 106]. Though a variety of trials are ongoing, no randomized prospective data have yet shown that radiotherapy adds to the clinical efficacy of immunotherapy for patients with melanoma. Nevertheless, anecdotal reports in patients treated with CTLA-4 blockade and radiotherapy show that intriguing responses have been seen and the approach is generally safe [107–110]. In a phase I study involving patients with melanoma, IL-2 was administered in combination with radiotherapy, and a high response rate was seen, justifying further study in randomized trials [111]. No clinical data for PD-1 in combination with radiotherapy are yet available but the combination similarly remains an area of active research (Tables 1 and 2).

Table 1 Checkpoint blocking antibodies in clinical development

Antibody [a]fusion protein	Target	Isotype	Clinical development
Ipilimumab (BMS)	CTLA-4	IgG1	FDA approved
Tremelimumab (Pfizer, Medimmune)	CTLA-4	IgG2	Phase 3 completed
Nivolumab/BMS-936558/MDX1106 (BMS)	PD-1	IgG4	Phase 3 completed
Pidilizumab (CureTech)	PD-1	IgG1	Phase 2 completed
Pembrolizumab (Merck)	PD-1	IgG4	FDA approved
AMP-225[a] (Amplimmune)	PD-1	NA	Phase 1
BMS-936559/MDX-1105 (BMS)	PD-L1	IgG4	Phase 1
MEDI4736 (MedImmune/AstraZeneca)	PD-L1	IgG1	Phase 1 completed
MPDL3280A/RG7446 (Genentech/Roche)	PD-L1	IgG1	Phase 1 completed

Modified from Callahan et al. [107]
[a]Fusion protein

Table 2 Immune-related adverse events (irAEs) associated with checkpoint blockade

Toxicity	Any grade	Grade 3/4
Ipilimumab[a] *(data from phase 3 study, Hodi et al.)*		
Rash	18 % (93/511)	1 % (6/511)
Pruritus	19 % (99/511)	<1 % (1/511)
Diarrhea	30 % (151/511)	4 % (20/511)
Hepatitis	1 % (5/511)	<1 % (2/511)
Hypophysitis	<1 % (4/511)	<1 % (4/511)
Hypothyroidism	2 % (8/511)	<1 % (1/511)
Pneumonitis	None reported	None reported
Nivolumab[b] *(data from phase 3 study, Larkin et al.)*		
Rash	26 % (81/313)	<1 % (2/313)
Pruritus	19 % (59/313)	None reported
Diarrhea	19 % (60/313)	2 % (7/313)
Hepatitis (increased ALT)	4 % (12/313)	1 % (4/313)
Hypophysitis	<1 % (2/313)	<1 % (1/313)
Hypothyroidism	9 % (27/313)	None reported
Pneumonitis	1 % (4/313)	<1 % (1/313)

[a]Ipilimumab monotherapy or ipilimumab plus peptide vaccine at a dose of 3 mg/kg, patients with advanced melanoma
[b]Nivolumab monotherapy at 3 mg/kg

References

1. Brunet JF, Denizot F, Luciani MF et al (1987) A new member of the immunoglobulin superfamily–CTLA-4. Nature 328(6127):267–270
2. Krummel MF, Allison JP (1995) CD28 and CTLA-4 have opposing effects on the response of T cells to stimulation. J Exp Med 182(2):459–465
3. Thompson CB, Allison JP (1997) The emerging role of CTLA-4 as an immune attenuator. Immunity 7(4):445–450
4. Walunas TL, Lenschow DJ, Bakker CY et al (1994) CTLA-4 can function as a negative regulator of T cell activation. Immunity 1(5):405–413
5. Linsley PS, Brady W, Urnes M, Grosmaire LS, Damle NK, Ledbetter JA (1991) CTLA-4 is a second receptor for the B cell activation antigen B7. J Exp Med 174(3):561–569
6. Krummel MF, Allison JP (1996) CTLA-4 engagement inhibits IL-2 accumulation and cell cycle progression upon activation of resting T cells. J Exp Med 183(6):2533–2540
7. Walunas TL, Bakker CY, Bluestone JA (1996) CTLA-4 ligation blocks CD28-dependent T cell activation. J Exp Med 183(6):2541–2550
8. Brunner MC, Chambers CA, Chan FK, Hanke J, Winoto A, Allison JP (1999) CTLA-4-Mediated inhibition of early events of T cell proliferation. J Immunol 162(10):5813–5820
9. Greenwald RJ, Boussiotis VA, Lorsbach RB, Abbas AK, Sharpe AH (2001) CTLA-4 regulates induction of anergy in vivo. Immunity 14(2):145–155
10. Waterhouse P, Penninger JM, Timms E et al (1995) Lymphoproliferative disorders with early lethality in mice deficient in Ctla-4. Science 270(5238):985–988

11. Tivol EA, Borriello F, Schweitzer AN, Lynch WP, Bluestone JA, Sharpe AH (1995) Loss of CTLA-4 leads to massive lymphoproliferation and fatal multiorgan tissue destruction, revealing a critical negative regulatory role of CTLA-4. Immunity 3(5):541–547
12. Chambers CA, Sullivan TJ, Allison JP (1997) Lymphoproliferation in CTLA-4-deficient mice is mediated by costimulation-dependent activation of CD4+ T cells. Immunity 7 (6):885–895
13. Allison JP, Hurwitz AA, Leach DR (1995) Manipulation of costimulatory signals to enhance antitumor T-cell responses. Curr Opin Immunol 7(5):682–686
14. Leach DR, Krummel MF, Allison JP (1996) Enhancement of antitumor immunity by CTLA-4 blockade. Science 271(5256):1734–1736
15. Kwon ED, Hurwitz AA, Foster BA et al (1997) Manipulation of T cell costimulatory and inhibitory signals for immunotherapy of prostate cancer. Proc Natl Acad Sci USA 94 (15):8099–8103
16. Yang YF, Zou JP, Mu J et al (1997) Enhanced induction of antitumor T-cell responses by cytotoxic T lymphocyte-associated molecule-4 blockade: the effect is manifested only at the restricted tumor-bearing stages. Cancer Res 57(18):4036–4041
17. Shrikant P, Khoruts A, Mescher MF (1999) CTLA-4 blockade reverses CD8+ T cell tolerance to tumor by a CD4+ T cell- and IL-2-dependent mechanism. Immunity 11(4):483–493
18. Sotomayor EM, Borrello I, Tubb E, Allison JP, Levitsky HI (1999) In vivo blockade of CTLA-4 enhances the priming of responsive T cells but fails to prevent the induction of tumor antigen-specific tolerance. Proc Natl Acad Sci USA 96(20):11476–11481
19. Selby MJ, Engelhardt JJ, Quigley M et al (2013) Anti-CTLA-4 antibodies of IgG2a isotype enhance antitumor activity through reduction of intratumoral regulatory T cells. Cancer immunology research 1(1):32–42
20. Simpson TR, Li F, Montalvo-Ortiz W et al (2013) Fc-dependent depletion of tumor-infiltrating regulatory T cells co-defines the efficacy of anti-CTLA-4 therapy against melanoma. J Exp Med 210(9):1695–1710
21. Peggs KS, Quezada SA, Chambers CA, Korman AJ, Allison JP (2009) Blockade of CTLA-4 on both effector and regulatory T cell compartments contributes to the antitumor activity of anti-CTLA-4 antibodies. J Exp Med 206(8):1717–1725
22. Kwon ED, Foster BA, Hurwitz AA et al (1999) Elimination of residual metastatic prostate cancer after surgery and adjunctive cytotoxic T lymphocyte-associated antigen 4 (CTLA-4) blockade immunotherapy. Proc Natl Acad Sci USA 96(26):15074–15079
23. Dewan MZ, Galloway AE, Kawashima N et al (2009) Fractionated but not single-dose radiotherapy induces an immune-mediated abscopal effect when combined with anti-CTLA-4 antibody. Clin Cancer Res 15(17):5379–5388
24. Demaria S, Kawashima N, Yang AM et al (2005) Immune-mediated inhibition of metastases after treatment with local radiation and CTLA-4 blockade in a mouse model of breast cancer. Clin Cancer Res 11(2 Pt 1):728–734
25. Mokyr MB, Kalinichenko T, Gorelik L, Bluestone JA (1998) Realization of the therapeutic potential of CTLA-4 blockade in low-dose chemotherapy-treated tumor-bearing mice. Cancer Res 58(23):5301–5304
26. den Brok MH, Sutmuller RP, Nierkens S et al (2006) Efficient loading of dendritic cells following cryo and radiofrequency ablation in combination with immune modulation induces anti-tumour immunity. Br J Cancer 95(7):896–905
27. Gregor PD, Wolchok JD, Ferrone CR et al (2004) CTLA-4 blockade in combination with xenogeneic DNA vaccines enhances T-cell responses, tumor immunity and autoimmunity to self antigens in animal and cellular model systems. Vaccine 22(13–14):1700–1708
28. Hurwitz AA, Yu TF, Leach DR, Allison JP (1998) CTLA-4 blockade synergizes with tumor-derived granulocyte-macrophage colony-stimulating factor for treatment of an experimental mammary carcinoma. Proc Natl Acad Sci USA 95(17):10067–10071

29. van Elsas A, Hurwitz AA, Allison JP (1999) Combination immunotherapy of B16 melanoma using anti-cytotoxic T lymphocyte-associated antigen 4 (CTLA-4) and granulocyte/macrophage colony-stimulating factor (GM-CSF)-producing vaccines induces rejection of subcutaneous and metastatic tumors accompanied by autoimmune depigmentation. J Exp Med 190(3):355–366
30. van Elsas A, Sutmuller RP, Hurwitz AA et al (2001) Elucidating the autoimmune and antitumor effector mechanisms of a treatment based on cytotoxic T lymphocyte antigen-4 blockade in combination with a B16 melanoma vaccine: comparison of prophylaxis and therapy. J Exp Med 194(4):481–489
31. Hurwitz AA, Foster BA, Kwon ED et al (2000) Combination immunotherapy of primary prostate cancer in a transgenic mouse model using CTLA-4 blockade. Cancer Res 60 (9):2444–2448
32. Mangsbo SM, Sandin LC, Anger K, Korman AJ, Loskog A, Totterman TH (2010) Enhanced tumor eradication by combining CTLA-4 or PD-1 blockade with CpG therapy. J Immunother 33(3):225–235
33. Curran MA, Allison JP (2009) Tumor vaccines expressing flt3 ligand synergize with ctla-4 blockade to reject preimplanted tumors. Cancer Res 69(19):7747–7755
34. Met O, Wang M, Pedersen AE, Nissen MH, Buus S, Claesson MH (2006) The effect of a therapeutic dendritic cell-based cancer vaccination depends on the blockage of CTLA-4 signaling. Cancer Lett 231(2):247–256
35. Daftarian P, Song GY, Ali S et al (2004) Two distinct pathways of immuno-modulation improve potency of p53 immunization in rejecting established tumors. Cancer Res 64 (15):5407–5414
36. Davila E, Kennedy R, Celis E (2003) Generation of antitumor immunity by cytotoxic T lymphocyte epitope peptide vaccination, CpG-oligodeoxynucleotide adjuvant, and CTLA-4 blockade. Cancer Res 63(12):3281–3288
37. Gao Y, Whitaker-Dowling P, Griffin JA, Barmada MA, Bergman I (2009) Recombinant vesicular stomatitis virus targeted to Her2/neu combined with anti-CTLA4 antibody eliminates implanted mammary tumors. Cancer Gene Ther 16(1):44–52
38. Tchekmedyian S et al (2002) MDX-010 (human anti-CTLA4): a phase I trial in malignant melanoma. Proc Am Soc Clin Oncol 21(abstr 56)
39. Wolchok JD, Neyns B, Linette G et al (2010) Ipilimumab monotherapy in patients with pretreated advanced melanoma: a randomised, double-blind, multicentre, phase 2, dose-ranging study. Lancet Oncol 11(2):155–164
40. Hodi FS, O'Day SJ, McDermott DF et al (2010) Improved survival with ipilimumab in patients with metastatic melanoma. N Engl J Med 363(8):711–723
41. Robert C, Thomas L, Bondarenko I et al (2011) Ipilimumab plus dacarbazine for previously untreated metastatic melanoma. N Engl J Med 364(26):2517–2526
42. Wolchok JD, Hoos A, O'Day S et al (2009) Guidelines for the evaluation of immune therapy activity in solid tumors: immune-related response criteria. Clin Cancer Res 15(23):7412–7420
43. Hodi FS, O'Day SJ, McDermott DF et al (2010) Improved survival with ipilimumab in patients with metastatic melanoma. N Engl J Med 363(8):711–723
44. Weber J (2009) Ipilimumab: controversies in its development, utility and autoimmune adverse events. Cancer Immunol Immunother 58(5):823–830
45. Di Giacomo AM, Biagioli M, Maio M (2010) The emerging toxicity profiles of anti-CTLA-4 antibodies across clinical indications. Semin Oncol 37(5):499–507
46. Forde PM, Rock K, Wilson G, O'Byrne KJ (2012) Ipilimumab-induced Immune-related renal failure—A case report. Anticancer Res 32(10):4607–4608
47. Maur M, Tomasello C, Frassoldati A, Dieci MV, Barbieri E, Conte P (2012) Posterior reversible encephalopathy syndrome during ipilimumab therapy for malignant melanoma. J Clin Oncol 30(6):e76–e78

48. Andrews S, Holden R (2012) Characteristics and management of immunerelated adverse effects associated with ipilimumab, a new immunotherapy for metastatic melanoma. Cancer Manage Res 4:299–307
49. Beck KE, Blansfield JA, Tran KQ et al (2006) Enterocolitis in patients with cancer after antibody blockade of cytotoxic T-lymphocyte-associated antigen 4. J Clin Oncol 24 (15):2283–2289
50. Wolchok J (2012) How recent advances in immunotherapy are changing the standard of care for patients with metastatic melanoma. Ann Oncol 23(Suppl 8): viii15–21
51. Juszczak A, Gupta A, Karavitaki N, Middleton MR, Grossman AB (2012) Ipilimumab: a novel immunomodulating therapy causing autoimmune hypophysitis: a case report and review. Eur J Endocrinol Eur Fed Endocrine Soc 167(1):1–5
52. Dillard T, Yedinak CG, Alumkal J, Fleseriu M (2010) Anti-CTLA-4 antibody therapy associated autoimmune hypophysitis: serious immune related adverse events across a spectrum of cancer subtypes. Pituitary 13(1):29–38
53. Kaehler KC, Egberts F, Lorigan P, Hauschild A (2009) Anti-CTLA-4 therapy-related autoimmune hypophysitis in a melanoma patient. Melanoma Res 19(5):333–334
54. https://www.hcp.yervoy.com/pages/rems.aspx
55. Kyi C, Carvajal RD, Wolchok JD, Postow MA (2014) Ipilimumab in patients with melanoma and autoimmune disease. J Immunother Cancer 2(1):35
56. Gettings EJ, Hackett CT, Scott TF (2014) Severe relapse in a multiple sclerosis patient associated with ipilimumab treatment of melanoma. Multiple Sclerosis
57. Berman D et al (2009) Association of peripheral blood absolute lymphocyte count (ALC) and clinical activity in patients (pts) with advanced melanoma treated with ipilimumab [abstract]. J Clin Oncol 27:3020
58. Ku GY, Yuan J, Page DB et al (2010) Single-institution experience with ipilimumab in advanced melanoma patients in the compassionate use setting: lymphocyte count after 2 doses correlates with survival. Cancer 116(7):1767–1775
59. Yuan J, Gnjatic S, Li H et al (2008) CTLA-4 blockade enhances polyfunctional NY-ESO-1 specific T cell responses in metastatic melanoma patients with clinical benefit. Proc Natl Acad Sci USA 105(51):20410–20415
60. Yuan J, Adamow M, Ginsberg BA et al (2011) Integrated NY-ESO-1 antibody and CD8 + T-cell responses correlate with clinical benefit in advanced melanoma patients treated with ipilimumab. Proc Natl Acad Sci USA 108:16723–16728
61. Burmeister Y, Lischke T, Dahler AC et al (2008) ICOS controls the pool size of effector-memory and regulatory T cells. J Immunol 180(2):774–782
62. Liakou CI, Kamat A, Tang DN et al (2008) CTLA-4 blockade increases IFNgamma-producing CD4+ ICOShi cells to shift the ratio of effector to regulatory T cells in cancer patients. Proc Natl Acad Sci USA 105(39):14987–14992
63. Carthon BC, Wolchok JD, Yuan J et al (2010) Preoperative CTLA-4 blockade: tolerability and immune monitoring in the setting of a presurgical clinical trial. Clin Cancer Res 16 (10):2861–2871
64. Hamid O, Schmidt H, Nissan A et al (2011) A prospective phase II trial exploring the association between tumor microenvironment biomarkers and clinical activity of ipilimumab in advanced melanoma. J Transl Med 9:204
65. Ji RR, Chasalow SD, Wang L et al (2012) An immune-active tumor microenvironment favors clinical response to ipilimumab. Cancer Immunol Immunother 61(7):1019–1031
66. Snyder A, Makarov V, Merghoub T et al (2014) Genetic basis for clinical response to CTLA-4 blockade in melanoma. N Engl J Med 371(23):2189–2199
67. Ishida Y, Agata Y, Shibahara K, Honjo T (1992) Induced expression of PD-1, a novel member of the immunoglobulin gene superfamily, upon programmed cell death. EMBO J 11 (11):3887–3895

68. Freeman GJ, Long AJ, Iwai Y et al (2000) Engagement of the PD-1 immunoinhibitory receptor by a novel B7 family member leads to negative regulation of lymphocyte activation. J Exp Med 192(7):1027–1034
69. Keir ME, Liang SC, Guleria I et al (2006) Tissue expression of PD-L1 mediates peripheral T cell tolerance. J Exp Med 203(4):883–895
70. Francisco LM, Salinas VH, Brown KE et al (2009) PD-L1 regulates the development, maintenance, and function of induced regulatory T cells. J Exp Med 206(13):3015–3029
71. Nishimura H, Nose M, Hiai H, Minato N, Honjo T (1999) Development of lupus-like autoimmune diseases by disruption of the PD-1 gene encoding an ITIM motif-carrying immunoreceptor. Immunity 11(2):141–151
72. Nishimura H, Okazaki T, Tanaka Y et al (2001) Autoimmune dilated cardiomyopathy in PD-1 receptor-deficient mice. Science 291(5502):319–322
73. Dong H, Strome SE, Salomao DR et al (2002) Tumor-associated B7-H1 promotes T-cell apoptosis: a potential mechanism of immune evasion. Nature Med 8(8):793–800
74. Fanoni D, Tavecchio S, Recalcati S et al (2011) New monoclonal antibodies against B-cell antigens: possible new strategies for diagnosis of primary cutaneous B-cell lymphomas. Immunol Lett 134(2):157–160
75. Jeffrey R, Infante JDP, Burris HA et al (2013) Clinical and pharmacodynamic (PD) results of a phase I trial with AMP-224 (B7-DC Fc) that binds to the PD-1 receptor. J Clin Oncol 31 (suppl; abstr 3044)
76. Topalian SL, Hodi FS, Brahmer JR et al (2012) Safety, activity, and immune correlates of anti-PD-1 antibody in cancer. N Engl J Med 366(26):2443–2454
77. Hamid O, Robert C, Daud A et al (2013) Safety and tumor responses with lambrolizumab (anti-PD-1) in melanoma. N Engl J Med 369(2):134–144
78. Topalian SL, Sznol M, McDermott DF et al (2014) Survival, durable tumor remission, and long-term safety in patients with advanced melanoma receiving nivolumab. J Clin Oncol Official J Am Soc Clin Oncol 32(10):1020–1030
79. Robert C, Long GV, Brady B et al (2014) Nivolumab in previously untreated melanoma without BRAF mutation. N Engl J Med 372:320–330
80. Robert C, Ribas A, Wolchok JD et al (2014) Anti-programmed-death-receptor-1 treatment with pembrolizumab in ipilimumab-refractory advanced melanoma: a randomised dose-comparison cohort of a phase 1 trial. Lancet
81. Atkins MB, Kudchadkar R, Sznol M et al (2014) Phase 2, multicenter, safety and efficacy study of pidilizumab in patients with metastatic melanoma. J Clin Oncol 32(5 s) (suppl; abstr 9001)
82. Butte MJ, Keir ME, Phamduy TB, Sharpe AH, Freeman GJ (2007) Programmed death-1 ligand 1 interacts specifically with the B7-1 costimulatory molecule to inhibit T cell responses. Immunity 27(1):111–122
83. Brahmer JR, Tykodi SS, Chow LQ et al (2012) Safety and activity of anti-PD-L1 antibody in patients with advanced cancer. N Engl J Med 366(26):2455–2465
84. Powles T, Vogelzang NJ, Fine GD et al (2014) Inhibition of PD-L1 by MPDL3280A and clinical activity in pts with metastatic urothelial bladder cancer (UBC). J Clin Oncol 32(5 s) (suppl; abstr 5011)
85. Segal NH, Anto SJ, Brahmer JR et al (2014) Preliminary data from a multi-arm expansion study of MEDI4736, an anti-PD-L1 antibody. J Clin Oncol 32(5 s) (suppl; abstr 3002)
86. Herbst RS, Gordon MS, Fine GD et al (2013) A study of MPDL3280A, an engineered PD-L1 antibody in patients with locally advanced or metastatic tumors. J Clin Oncol 31 (suppl; abstr 3000)
87. Heery CR, O'Sullivan Coyne GH, Madan RA et al (2014) Phase I open-label, multiple ascending dose trial of MSB0010718C, an anti-PD-L1 monoclonal antibody, in advanced solid malignancies. J Clin Oncol 32(5 s) (suppl; abstr 3064)
88. Saenger YM, Wolchok JD (2008) The heterogeneity of the kinetics of response to ipilimumab in metastatic melanoma: patient cases. Cancer Immun 8:1

89. Wolchok JD, Hoos A, O'Day S et al (2009) Guidelines for the evaluation of immune therapy activity in solid tumors: immune-related response criteria. Clin Cancer Res Official J Am Assoc Cancer Res 15(23):7412–7420
90. Hoos A, Eggermont AM, Janetzki S et al (2010) Improved endpoints for cancer immunotherapy trials. J Natl Cancer Inst 102(18):1388–1397
91. Hodi FS, Ribas, A., Daud A et al (2014) Evaluation of immune-related response criteria (irRC) in patients (pts) with advanced melanoma (MEL) treated with the anti-PD-1 monoclonal antibody MK-3475. J Clin Oncol 32(5 s) (suppl; abstr 3006)
92. Weber J, Minor D, D'Angelo S et al (2014) A phase 3 randomized, open-label study of nivolumab (anti-PD-1; BMS-936558; ONO-4538) versus investigator's choice chemotherapy (ICC) in patients with advanced melanoma after prior anti-CTLA-4 therapy. Eur Soc Med Oncol
93. Nishino M, Giobbie-Hurder A, Gargano M, Suda M, Ramaiya NH, Hodi FS (2013) Developing a common language for tumor response to immunotherapy: immune-related response criteria using unidimensional measurements. Clin Cancer Res Official J Am Assoc Cancer Res 19(14):3936–3943
94. Weber JS, Kudchadkar RR, Yu B et al (2013) Safety, efficacy, and biomarkers of nivolumab with vaccine in ipilimumab-refractory or -naive melanoma. J Clin Oncol 31(34):4311–4318
95. Grosso J HC, Inzunza D et al (2013) Association of tumor PD-L1 expression and immune biomarkers with clinical activity in patients (pts) with advanced solid tumors treated with nivolumab (anti-PD-1; BMS-936558; ONO-4538). J Clin Oncol 31 (suppl; abstr 3016)
96. Taube JM, Klein A, Brahmer JR et al (2014) Association of PD-1, PD-1 ligands, and other features of the tumor immune microenvironment with response to anti-PD-1 therapy. Clin Cancer Res Official J Am Assoc Cancer Res 20:5064–5074
97. Atefi M, Avramis E, Lassen A et al (2014) Effects of MAPK and PI3 K pathways on PD-L1 expression in melanoma. Clin Cancer Res Official J Am Assoc Cancer Res 20(13):3446–3457
98. Parsa AT, Waldron JS, Panner A et al (2007) Loss of tumor suppressor PTEN function increases B7-H1 expression and immunoresistance in glioma. Nature Med 13(1):84–88
99. Wolchok JD, Kluger H, Callahan MK et al (2013) Nivolumab plus ipilimumab in advanced melanoma. N Engl J Med 369(2):122–133
100. Sznol M, Kluger H, Hodi F, David F. McDermott RDC, Lawrence DP, Topalian SL, Atkins MB, Powderly JD, Sharfman WH, Puzanov I, Smith DC, Wigginton JM, Kollia G, Gupta AK, Sosman JA (2013) Survival and long-term follow-up of safety and response in patients (pts) with advanced melanoma (MEL) in a phase I trial of nivolumab (anti-PD-1; BMS-936558; ONO-4538). J Clin Oncol 31 (suppl; abstr CRA9006) (ASCO Annual Meeting 2013)
101. Hodi FS, Lee S, McDermott DF et al (2014) Ipilimumab plus sargramostim vs ipilimumab alone for treatment of metastatic melanoma: a randomized clinical trial. JAMA 312 (17):1744–1753
102. Ribas A, Hodi FS, Callahan M, Konto C, Wolchok J (2013) Hepatotoxicity with combination of vemurafenib and ipilimumab. N Engl J Med 368(14):1365–1366
103. Puzanov I, Callahan M, Linette G, Patel S, Luke JJ, Sosman JA, Jedd DW, Omid H, Minor DR, Orford KW, Hug BA, Ma B, Matthys GM, Hoos A (2014) Phase 1 study of the BRAF inhibitor dabrafenib (D) with or without the MEK inhibitor trametinib (T) in combination with ipilimumab (Ipi) for V600E/K mutation–positive unresectable or metastatic melanoma (MM). ASCO J Clin Oncol 32(5 s) (suppl; abstr 2511)
104. Formenti SC, Demaria S (2013) Combining radiotherapy and cancer immunotherapy: a paradigm shift. J Natl Cancer Inst 105(4):256–265
105. Deng L, Liang H, Burnette B et al (2014) Irradiation and anti-PD-L1 treatment synergistically promote antitumor immunity in mice. J Clin Invest 124(2):687–695

106. Belcaid Z, Phallen JA, Zeng J et al (2014) Focal radiation therapy combined with 4-1BB activation and CTLA-4 blockade yields long-term survival and a protective antigen-specific memory response in a murine glioma model. PLoS ONE 9(7):e101764
107. Postow MA, Callahan MK, Barker CA et al (2012) Immunologic correlates of the abscopal effect in a patient with melanoma. N Engl J Med 366(10):925–931
108. Sullivan RJ, Lawrence DP, Wargo JA, Oh KS, Gonzalez RG, Piris A (2013) Case records of the Massachusetts general hospital. Case 21-2013. A 68-year-old man with metastatic melanoma. N Engl J Med 369(2):173–183
109. Grimaldi AM, Simeone E, Giannarelli D et al (2014) Abscopal effects of radiotherapy on advanced melanoma patients who progressed after ipilimumab immunotherapy. Oncoimmunology 3:e28780
110. Barker CA, Postow MA, Khan SA et al (2013) Concurrent radiotherapy and ipilimumab immunotherapy for patients with melanoma. Cancer Immunol Res 1(2):92–98
111. Seung SK, Curti BD, Crittenden M et al (2012) Phase 1 study of stereotactic body radiotherapy and interleukin-2—tumor and immunological responses. Sci Trans Med 4 (137):137ra74
112. Larkin et al (2015) Combined nivolumab and ipilimumab or monotherapy in untreated melanoma. N Engl J Med 373(1):23–24

Targeted Therapy for Melanoma

Deborah J.L. Wong and Antoni Ribas

Abstract

Vemurafenib and dabrafenib, two potent tyrosine kinase inhibitors (TKIs) of the $\mathrm{BRAF}^{\mathrm{V600E}}$ kinase, are highly effective in the treatment of a $BRAF^{V600}$-mutant metastatic melanoma. These are selective type I inhibitors (functional against the active conformation of the kinase) of the RAF kinases, which are key players in the mitogen-activated protein kinase (MAPK) pathway. $BRAF^{V600}$ mutations are present in approximately 7 % of all cancers, including high frequencies of mutations reported in 50 % of advanced melanomas and 100 % of hairy cell leukemias. As with most targeted therapies, resistance to BRAF inhibitors is an issue, and mechanisms of resistance are varied. Combining BRAF inhibitors with MEK inhibitors such as trametinib delays the development of resistance. Rationally combining targeted therapies to address the mechanism of resistance or combining BRAF inhibitors with other effective therapies such as immunotherapy may result in further improvement in outcomes for patients.

Keywords

Melanoma · BRAF · Vemurafenib · Dabrafenib · MEK · Trametinib

D.J.L. Wong · A. Ribas (✉)
Department of Medicine, Division of Hematology/Oncology, University of California
Los Angeles (UCLA), Le Conte Avenue, Los Angeles, CA 10833, USA
e-mail: aribas@mednet.ucla.edu

A. Ribas
Jonsson Comprehensive Cancer Center, UCLA, Los Angeles, CA, USA

H.L. Kaufman and J.M. Mehnert (eds.), *Melanoma*,
Cancer Treatment and Research 167, DOI 10.1007/978-3-319-22539-5_10

Contents

1 Current Treatment Options for Advanced or Metastatic Melanoma

Until recently, there was a dearth of effective treatments for surgically unresectable or metastatic melanoma. At best, cytotoxic chemotherapy such as dacarbazine yields a response rate of approximately ten percent. Similar response rates are seen with immunotherapies, such as interleukin-2 (IL-2), but these responses may be extremely durable. Neither chemotherapy nor IL-2 clearly results in improved overall survival (OS), however [1–3].

The outlook for patients with advanced melanoma significantly brightened with the identification of specific BRAF and MEK inhibitors and immune modulating antibodies as effective therapies for this disease. Ipilimumab, a cytotoxic T-lymphocyte antigen (CTLA4) blocking antibody, was approved for the treatment of metastatic melanoma. Responses to ipilimumab are on the approximately 10–15 %. Unlike the aforementioned agents, ipilimumab does improve median OS compared to the control arms in randomized clinical trials [4, 5]. In September 2014, the programmed death-1 (PD-1) blocking antibody pembrolizumab (MK-3475, Merck) was FDA-approved for metastatic melanoma that has progressed on ipilimumab and BRAF inhibitors (if *BRAF* mutated). Pembrolizumab has an overall response rate (ORR) of 24 % with many of these responses ongoing for six months or longer [6]. In all, there have been 6 FDA-approved therapies for the treatment of patients with metastatic melanoma since 2011.

High response rates for $BRAF^{V600}$-mutant metastatic melanoma are seen with the type 1 BRAF inhibitors vemurafenib (formerly PLX4032) and dabrafenib (formerly GSK2118436) [7–11]. Unfortunately, though initial responses to these agents are impressive, progression free survival (PFS) is approximately 6–7 months. Combining BRAF inhibition with MEK inhibition results in improved PFS compared to BRAF inhibition alone [12–14]. However, not all melanomas express the mutated BRAF protein, and not all melanomas with mutant *BRAF* are responsive to these targeted therapies. Thus, effective therapies that address both de novo and acquired resistance to BRAF and MEK inhibitors remain a subject of active research. Understanding the biology of melanoma will be the key in identifying strategies to address resistance to therapy.

2 Targeting the MAPK Pathway in Melanoma

BRAF is a serine–threonine protein kinase belonging to the RAF family of kinases, which is part of the MAPK signaling pathway. Under normal signaling conditions, binding of a growth factor to a RTK such as c-KIT activates RAS which then activates the RAF kinases. There are 3 identified RAF kinases: ARAF, BRAF, and CRAF. RAF activation in turn phosphorylates MEK, leading to activation of ERK and subsequent phosphorylation of various targets that result in cell proliferation and other key biologic processes (Fig. 1). Dysregulation of the MAPK pathway is a key feature in the majority of melanomas. Indeed, about 20 % of melanomas contain activating mutations in *NRAS* [15, 16]. Mutations in *KIT* and *KRAS* have also been identified. Approximately 50 % of all melanomas contain a mutation in the *BRAF* gene, most commonly resulting in substitution of glutamic acid for valine at position 600 (V600E) [17]. The *BRAF*^{V600E} substitution leads to constitutive activation of this kinase, and consequently, constitutive ERK signaling. Mutations in *BRAF* are, in general, mutually exclusive with other mutations of other proteins in the MAPK pathway [18, 19], though recently, exceptions have been reported [20].

Inhibitors of RAF include type I inhibitors which selectively inhibit the activated RAF kinase, and type II inhibitors which inhibit the resting RAF. Type II inhibitors such as sorafenib do not have potent activity in *BRAF*^{V600E}-mutated cancers [21, 22]. In contrast, two clinically relevant type I TKIs that target BRAF$^{\mathrm{V600E}}$ are vemurafenib and dabrafenib. As published in phases I, II, and III studies, treatment

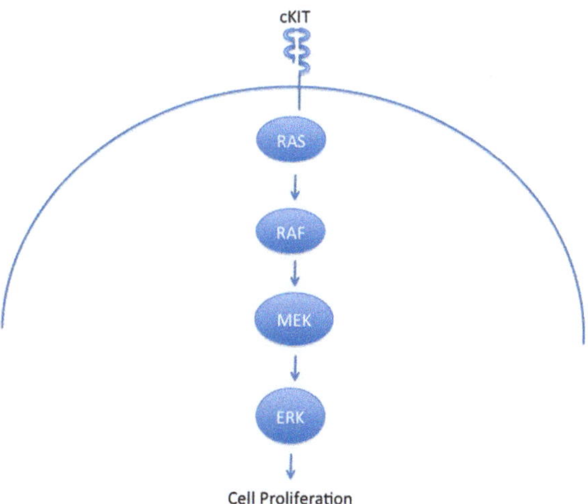

Fig. 1 Overview of the MAPK pathway. Activation of a cell surface RTK such as cKIT leads to sequential phosphorylation and activation of proteins in the MAPK pathway: RAS, RAF, MEK, and ERK. ERK activation then mediates phosphorylation of key proteins involved in cellular proliferation and other events

of patients with $BRAF^{V600E}$ advanced melanoma with vemurafenib resulted in response rates exceeding 50 % by RECIST criteria, with some degree of tumor response in over 80 % of patients, resulting in improvements in PFS and OS [7, 9, 23]. Data from the BRIM-3 phase 3 trial demonstrated that treatment with vemurafenib confers an overall response rate of 48 % compared to 5 % in dacarbazine, the only FDA-approved chemotherapy for metastatic melanoma [7]. The duration of response ranged from 2 to >18 months, with a mean duration of response of 6.7 months [9], though there are a few patients who have ongoing durable responses. Estimated OS at 6 months was 84 % for vemurafenib, compared to 64 % for dacarbazine. In the published updated analysis of BRIM-3, median OS was significantly longer in the vemurafenib group than in the dacarbazine group (13.6 months [95 % CI 12.0–15.2] vs. 9.7 months [7.9–12.8]; hazard ratio [HR] 0.70 [95 % CI 0.57–0.87]; $p = 0.0008$). Similarly, median PFS was improved (6.9 months [95 % CI 6.1–7.0] vs. 1.6 months [1.6–2.1]; HR 0.38 [95 % CI 0.32–0.46]; $p < 0.0001$) [24].

The phase I study of dabrafenib demonstrated 18/30 (60 %) of patients with a > 20 % tumor decrease by RECIST at first restaging [11]. Similarly, the open-label phase II study of dabrafenib for $BRAF^{V600E/K}$-mutant melanoma, BREAK-2, demonstrated 45/76 (59, 95 % CI 48.2–70.3) objective responses,with 7 % complete responses. For those with $BRAF^{V600E}$, median PFS was 6.3 months and median OS was 13.1 months, while it was 4.5 and 12.9 months, respectively, for those with $BRAF^{V600K}$ [25]. Furthermore, BREAK-3, the phase III study comparing dabrafenib with dacarbazine for first-line treatment of advanced melanoma, randomized 250 patients 3:1 to receive either dabrafenib or dacarbazine. The primary end point was investigator-assessed PFS. Consistent with the phase I data, the response rate was 52 %, (95 % CI 45–59) for the dabrafenib arm and 17 % (95 % CI 9–29) for the dacarbazine arm. There was a 3 % complete response rate among patients who received dabrafenib. The median PFS was 5.1 months for dabrafenib and 2.7 months for dacarbazine, with a hazard ratio (HR) of 0.30 (95 % CI 0.18–0.51; $p < 0.0001$) [26]. Given these positive data for BRAF inhibitors, vemurafenib received FDA approval in August 2011 for the treatment of patients with advanced or metastatic $BRAF^{V600E}$-mutant melanoma and dabrafenib was FDA-approved in May 2013.

Both vemurafenib and dabrafenib are generally well tolerated. With vemurafenib, adverse events were mainly grade 2 or 3 in severity and included 18 % incidence of cutaneous events (squamous cell carcinoma-SCC-, keratoacanthoma, or both) managed by excision, arthralgia (21 %), fatigue (13 %), and 12 % incidence of photosensitivity skin reactions, the most severe of which could be prevented by the use of sunblock. Adverse reactions requiring dose modifications or interruptions occurred in 38 % of patients [9]. For dabrafenib, adverse events reported in the phase I study included skin changes, low-grade cutaneous SCC, headache, nausea, fatigue, and vomiting [11]. In BREAK-2, rates of the most common AEs were as follows: arthralgia (33 %), hyperkeratosis (27 %), and pyrexia (24 %). Twenty-five patients (27 %) had a serious AE, and nine (10 %) had squamous cell carcinoma [25]. In the phase III study, 53 % of patients developed adverse events compared to 44 % in the dacarbazine arm. These include hyperkeratosis, palmar-plantar erythrodysesthesia syndrome, headache, pyrexia, arthralgia, papilloma, and alopecia. Grade 3 or 4 adverse events were uncommon in either group [26].

3 Limitations of BRAF Inhibitors

Only melanoma cells with mutated *BRAF* are susceptible to inhibition by type I Raf inhibitors. This is hypothesized to be because mutant *BRAF* is locked in an activated conformational state, which selectively allows inhibitor binding at lower concentrations than needed for inhibition of wild-type BRAF [27]. Constitutive activation of BRAF V600E may also obviate the need for binding of cofactors normally required for MAPK activation, again leading to enhanced accessibility of inhibitors to mutant BRAF. In addition, in melanoma cells with wild-type BRAF, treatment with selective RAF inhibitors leads to a paradoxical increase in MAPK signaling and activation of ERK. Similarly, in mouse models of melanoma driven by RTKs or bearing mutations of RAS (upstream of RAF in the MAPK pathway), treatment with selective RAF inhibitors stimulated tumor growth and led to development of secondary malignancies [27, 28]. This is because inhibition of BRAF in these wild-type BRAF cells allows increased signaling through CRAF, thereby allowing continued activation of the pathway. Of note, the development of cutaneous squamous cell carcinomas, most frequently of keratoacanthoma subtype, as a side effect of treatment with vemurafenib [8, 9], is a result of MAPK signaling through CRAF in cells with a pre-exiting upstream *RAS* mutation [29].

Not all patients with $BRAF^{V600\mathrm{E}}$ melanoma respond to selective inhibition with vemurafenib or dabrafenib [7, 11]. Even in patients with $BRAF^{V600E}$, development of resistance to single agent vemurafenib or dabrafenib occurs in most patients within months. Several mechanisms of acquired resistance to vemurafenib and other selective RAF inhibitors have been identified to date (Fig. 2). Some result in reactivation of the MAPK pathway, but to date, no secondary mutations (i.e. gatekeeper mutations) in the $BRAF^{V600}$ kinase, have been identified [20, 30]. Instead, mechanisms of MAPK reactivation result from gene amplification of the mutant $BRAF^{V600}$ [31], splice variants of BRAF resulting in a smaller protein with increased ability to signal [32], secondary mutations in *NRAS* such as Q61 K [20, 33], and development of mutations or deletions in *MEK1* [30, 33]. In addition, some resistant cell lines upregulate cancer Osaka thyroid (COT or MAP3K8) signaling [34]. Other mechanisms of resistance lead to enhanced cell signaling through pathways other than the MAPK. Examples include upregulation of RTKs such as the platelet-derived growth factor beta (PDGFRβ), or the insulin growth factor receptor 1 (IGF1R), or deletions of PTEN or mutations in PIK3CA or AKT [20, 35, 36]. These all lead to enhanced PI3K/AKT/mTOR signaling rather than reactivation of the MAPK pathway. These mechanisms of acquired resistance appear to develop mostly in a mutually exclusive manner. These resistance mechanisms have been

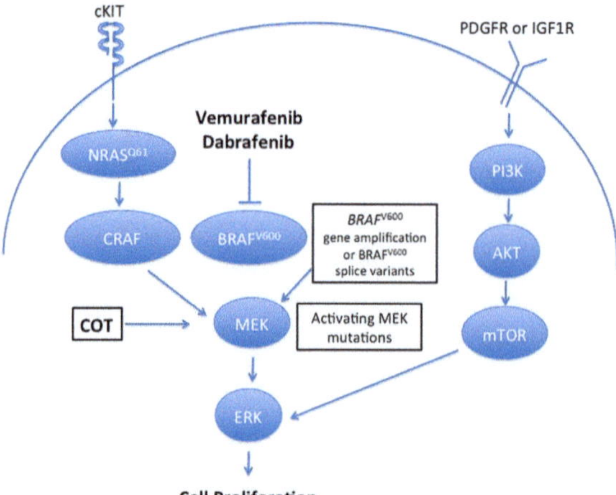

Fig. 2 Mechanisms of resistance to RAF inhibitors. Resistance to BRAF inhibitors by $BRAF^{V600}$ melanoma may occur via mechanisms that reactivate the MAPK pathway (mutations in NRAS or MEK, upregulation of COT pathway, upregulation of $BRAF^{V600}$ gene expression, or generation of BRAF splice variants) or upregulation of RTKs that signal via pathways such as AKT/PI3K/mTOR

corroborated clinically, in which these mutations or phenotypes have been identified in samples derived from patients treated with BRAF inhibitors.

4 Beyond Inhibition of Mutated BRAF

Knowledge of the mechanisms underlying resistance to vemurafenib, its analogs, or dabrafenib provides an important basis for developing rational strategies to treat patients who do not have $BRAF^{V600}$-mutated melanoma, patients with $BRAF^{V600}$-mutated melanoma who do not respond to BRAF inhibitors, or to treat patients who progress on these therapies. Data evaluating the susceptibility of cell lines derived from melanomas with acquired resistance to vemurafenib demonstrated that susceptibility to a MEK inhibitor was dependent on the mechanism of resistance [37, 38]. While initial $BRAF^{V600}$ melanoma cell lines were sensitive to both vemurafenib and the MEK inhibitor, many developed cross-resistance to both inhibitors. However, cell lines with the acquired $NRAS^{Q61}$ mutations remained sensitive to MEK inhibitor, demonstrating the continued dependence on the MAPK pathway for driver oncogenic signaling. The cell lines with RTK upregulation as the mechanism of acquired resistance did not respond to the addition of the MEK inhibitor because they use an alternative survival pathway through PI3K/AKT/mTOR. These RTK-mediated acquired resistance cell lines were indeed sensitive to the addition of an AKT inhibitor or rapamycin in combination with vemurafenib. Thus, these data demonstrate that acquired resistance to BRAF inhibitors may be overcome or partially overcome in vitro by addition of either a MEK inhibitor or an inhibitor of the AKT/mTOR pathway, depending on the mechanism of resistance. Similarly, cell lines resistant to dabrafenib remain sensitive to an inhibitor of PI3K/AKT/mTOR [33].

5 Combining Inhibition of RAF with Other MAPK Inhibitors

Given that MAPK dependence often persists even after resistance to BRAF inhibitors develops, several clinical trials evaluated MEK inhibitors, alone or in combination with type I RAF inhibitors.

In a phase I dose-escalation study of the MEK inhibitor, trametinib, Infante et al. reported a maximum tolerated dose of 2 mg daily. Dose-limiting toxicities included rash, diarrhea, and central serous retinopathy; 80 % (165/206) of patients developed rash or acneiform dermatitis and diarrhea was seen in 42 % of patients [39]. Trametinib was evaluated in a multicenter, international phase III study in V600E- or V600 K-mutant melanoma patients who were BRAF or MEK inhibitor naïve. Patients were randomized 2:1 to trametinib or chemotherapy (dacarbazine or paclitaxel), and a statistically significant improvement in investigator-assessed PFS [HR 0.47 (95 % CI: 0.34, 0.65); $p < 0.0001$] for trametinib was seen compared to chemotherapy. Objective response rate was 22 % (95 % CI, 17–28) for trametinib compared to 8 % (95 % CI, 4–15). Median PFS was 4.8 months for trametinib and 1.5 months for chemotherapy, and the 6-month overall survival rate was 81 % for trametinib, versus 67 % for chemotherapy [40]. Given these findings, the FDA approved trametinib for $BRAF^{V600E/K}$-mutant melanoma in May 2013.

In patients who had previously progressed on BRAF inhibitors, no responses to trametinib monotherapy were observed among 40 enrolled patients [40]. However, addition of the MEK inhibitor cobimetinib to vemurafenib in patients who progressed on BRAF inhibitors resulted in modest responses: 10 of 66 patients (15 %) who progressed on a BRAF inhibitor responded when cobimetinib was added. Median PFS was 2.8 months. In contrast to the modest responses in BRAF-inhibitor-pretreated patients, among the 63 BRAF-inhibitor-naïve patients evaluated, confirmed objective responses were seen in 87 % (55/63), with 10 % complete responders. The median overall survival was 13.7 months [41]. Furthermore, the combination of vemurafenib and cobimetinib resulted in a statistically significant increase in PFS compared to vemurafenib plus placebo (9.9 vs. 6.2 months, HR 0.51; 95 % CI 0.39–0.68, $p < 0.001$) [12].

Similar results have been observed for the combination of dabrafenib and trametinib. A phase I/phase II clinical trial of dabrafenib with trametinib as first-line therapy for mutant BRAF tumors demonstrated that the combination was tolerated at the full doses used in monotherapy, though rates of pyrexia were significantly higher (71 % for the combination vs. 26 % for dabrafenib alone) [12]. Furthermore, in the seminal phase III study by Robert et al. [13], the median PFS for dabrafenib and trametinib was 11.3 months, compared to 7.3 months for vemurafenib. 12-month OS rate was also improved: 72 % (95 % CI, 67–77) for the combination versus 65 % (95 % CI 59–70). Interestingly, because MEK inhibition blocks paradoxical MAPK inhibition by BRAF inhibitors [29], the incidence of squamous cell carcinomas with the combination therapy was markedly reduced. Cutaneous SCC was reported in 7 % of patients treated with dabrafenib and trametinib, compared to 19 % for dabrafenib [41, 42]. Robert et al. reported 1 % for the combination compared to 18 % for vemurafenib monotherapy [13], indicating that dual inhibition of the MAPK pathway circumvents a common adverse event seen with monotherapy with BRAF inhibitors [43]. With the statistically significant improvement in durable objective responses afforded by combination MAPK therapy, in 2014, the FDA granted accelerated approval to dabrafenib and trametinib for combination therapy for $BRAF^{V600E/K}$ metastatic melanoma.

Inhibition of MEK or ERK may also be an effective strategy for tumors that are MAPK-driven in a BRAF-independent fashion. Preclinical work in melanoma cell lines with mutant NRAS demonstrated that while these were relatively insensitive to vemurafenib, treatment with a MEK inhibitor potently inhibited growth of tumor cells and resulted in decreased phospho ERK [44]. Falchook et al. [45] reported a 10 % response rate for trametinib in BRAF wild-type melanoma. Furthermore, a phase II study of the MEK 1/2 inhibitor binimetinib reported six of 30 (20 %) with NRAS-mutated melanoma had a partial response to treatment. Among BRAF-mutant melanoma, eight of 41 (20 %) of patients responded [46]. The possibility that binimetinib may be effective in NRAS-mutant melanoma is being further explored in a randomized phase III clinical trial with dacarbazine as the control arm (NCT01763164). Other MEK inhibitors that have been or are currently under clinical investigation as single agents or combinations include TAK733 (NCT00948467) and selumetinib (NCT01974752). ERK inhibitors demonstrated promising preclinical activity in both BRAF-mutant and BRAF wild-type melanomas [47–49], and early-phase clinical trials in BRAF-, NRAS-, and MEK-mutated cancers are ongoing (NCT01781429).

6 Combining Inhibition of BRAF with PI3K/AKT/MTOR Inhibitors

As described above, PI3K/AKT/mTOR pathway activation is another important pathway driving pathogenesis in BRAF wild-type melanomas as well as in acquired resistance in BRAF-mutant melanoma. Preclinically, several published studies demonstrate the utility of inhibition of PI3K/AKT/mTOR in melanomas with acquired resistance to vemurafenib or dabrafenib [33, 37, 50]. Thus, several clinical trials of combining PI3K/AKT/mTOR inhibitors with MAPK pathway inhibitors such as BRAF or MEK inhibitors are currently ongoing or planned (NCT 1941927, NCT01902173, NCT01021748, NCT01519427, NCT01363232). One key question is whether inhibiting two key cell signaling pathways simultaneously will be tolerable at doses necessary for antitumor effect.

7 Targeted Therapy in Combination with Immunotherapy

Melanoma has long been considered an immunosensitive tumor. Data include the finding that melanomas may undergo spontaneous regression and prolonged, durable responses may be seen after treatment of metastatic melanoma with high dose IL-2, interferon, anti-CTLA4, or anti-PD1/l1. The impressive initial responses seen with BRAF inhibitors and the prolonged duration of responses that can be achieved with immunotherapy give rise to an intriguing hypothesis that combining BRAF inhibitors with immunotherapy could augment the sensitization of immune cells to the cancer cells and result in long-lasting disease control [51]. Preclinical data demonstrate that this approach may be feasible and effective. In two distinct mouse models of adoptive cell therapy for melanoma, preliminary results demonstrate that addition of vemurafenib yielded statistically significant improvements in tumor regression. Furthermore, at clinically relevant concentrations, vemurafenib neither affects the viability of lymphocytes from human peripheral blood mononuclear cells (PBMCs) nor does it significantly impair lymphocyte antigen recognition or cytotoxic activity [52], indicating that addition of vemurafenib should not adversely affect the efficacy of immunotherapy. Several clinical trials of PDL1/PD1 antibodies combined with BRAF and/or MEK inhibitors are currently accruing (NCT02130466 and NCT02027961) [51].

8 Conclusions

The recognition of the key role of the MAPK pathway, and of $BRAF^{V600}$ in particular, in driving oncogenesis in melanoma was a pivotal breakthrough allowing identification of the type I RAF inhibitors such as vemurafenib or dabrafenib as effective therapy. While initially effective, however, primary resistance or development of acquired resistance to these targeted therapies remains a significant issue. Several mechanisms of resistance have been identified, and clinical trials are ongoing to evaluate the efficacy of other MAPK inhibitors or inhibitors targeting other key signaling pathways that are altered in melanoma. Combining targeted therapies or using targeted therapies in conjunction with immunotherapy may provide additional treatment options for this disease.

Author Disclosures Deborah Wong has no conflict of interests to declare.Antoni Ribas has served as consultant for Amgen, Genentech-Roche, GSK, Merck, and Novartis with the honoraria paid to UCLA.

References

1. Comis RL (1976) DTIC (NSC-45388) in malignant melanoma: a perspective. Cancer Treat Rep 60(2):165–176
2. Tsao H, Atkins MB, Sober AJ (2004) Management of cutaneous melanoma. N Engl J Med 351(10):998–1012
3. Atkins MB et al (1999) High-dose recombinant interleukin 2 therapy for patients with metastatic melanoma: analysis of 270 patients treated between 1985 and 1993. J Clin Oncol Off J Am Soc Clin Oncol 17(7):2105–2116
4. Hodi FS et al (2010) Improved survival with ipilimumab in patients with metastatic melanoma. N Engl J Med 363(8):711–723
5. Robert C et al (2011) Ipilimumab plus dacarbazine for previously untreated metastatic melanoma. N Engl J Med 364(26):2517–2526
6. Robert C et al (2014) Anti-programmed-death-receptor-1 treatment with pembrolizumab in ipilimumab-refractory advanced melanoma: a randomised dose-comparison cohort of a phase 1 trial. Lancet 384(9948):1109–1117
7. Chapman PB et al (2011) Improved survival with vemurafenib in melanoma with BRAF V600E mutation. N Engl J Med 364(26):2507–2516
8. Flaherty KT et al (2010) Inhibition of mutated, activated BRAF in metastatic melanoma. N Engl J Med 363(9):809–819
9. Ribas A., Kim K, Schuchter L, Gonzalez R, Pavlick AC, Weber J, McArthur G, Hutson TE, Flaherty K, Moschos S, Lawrence DP, Hersey P, Kefford R, Chmielowski B, Puzanov I, Li J, Nolop K, Lee R, Joe A, Sosman J (2011) BRIM-2: An open-label, multicenter Phase II study of RG7204 (PLX4032) in previously treated patients with BRAF V600E mutation-positive metastatic melanoma. J Clin Oncol Off J Am Soc Clin Oncol 29
10. Sosman JA et al (2012) Survival in BRAF V600-mutant advanced melanoma treated with vemurafenib. N Engl J Med 366(8):707–714
11. Kefford R, Arkenau H, Brown MP, Millward M, Infante JR, Long GV, Ouellet D, Curtis M, Lebowitz PF, Falchokk GS (2010) Phase I/II study of GSK2118436, a selective inhibitor of oncogenic mutant BRAF kinase, in patients with metastatic melanoma and other solid tumors. Proc Am Soc Clin Oncol 28:611s
12. Larkin J et al (2014) Combined vemurafenib and cobimetinib in BRAF-mutated melanoma. N Engl J Med 371(20):1867–1876
13. Robert C et al (2014) Improved overall survival in melanoma with combined dabrafenib and trametinib. N Engl J Med
14. Long GV et al (2014) Combined BRAF and MEK inhibition versus BRAF inhibition alone in melanoma. N Engl J Med 371(20):1877–1888
15. Padua RA, Barrass N, Currie GA (1984) A novel transforming gene in a human malignant melanoma cell line. Nature 311(5987):671–673
16. Sekulic A et al (2008) Malignant melanoma in the 21st century: the emerging molecular landscape. In: Mayo Clinic proceedings. Mayo Clinic vol 83(7), pp 825–846
17. Brose MS et al (2002) BRAF and RAS mutations in human lung cancer and melanoma. Cancer Res 62(23):6997–7000
18. Curtin JA et al (2005) Distinct sets of genetic alterations in melanoma. N Engl J Med 353 (20):2135–2147
19. Haluska FG et al (2006) Genetic alterations in signaling pathways in melanoma. Clin Cancer Res Off J Am Assoc Cancer Res 12(7 Pt 2):2301s–2307s
20. Nazarian R et al (2010) Melanomas acquire resistance to B-RAF(V600E) inhibition by RTK or N-RAS upregulation. Nature 468(7326):973–977
21. Eisen T et al (2006) Sorafenib in advanced melanoma: a Phase II randomised discontinuation trial analysis. Br J Cancer 95(5):581–586
22. Ott PA et al (2010) A phase II trial of sorafenib in metastatic melanoma with tissue correlates. PLoS ONE 5(12):e15588

23. Bollag G et al (2010) Clinical efficacy of a RAF inhibitor needs broad target blockade in BRAF-mutant melanoma. Nature 467(7315):596–599
24. McArthur GA et al (2014) Safety and efficacy of vemurafenib in BRAF(V600E) and BRAF (V600K) mutation-positive melanoma (BRIM-3): extended follow-up of a phase 3, randomised, open-label study. Lancet Oncol 15(3):323–332
25. Ascierto PA et al (2013) Phase II trial (BREAK-2) of the BRAF inhibitor dabrafenib (GSK2118436) in patients with metastatic melanoma. J Clin Oncol Off J Am Soc Clin Oncol 31(26):3205–3211
26. Hauschild A et al (2012) Dabrafenib in BRAF-mutated metastatic melanoma: a multicentre, open-label, phase 3 randomised controlled trial. Lancet 380(9839):358–365
27. Poulikakos PI et al (2010) RAF inhibitors transactivate RAF dimers and ERK signalling in cells with wild-type BRAF. Nature 464(7287):427–430
28. Heidorn SJ et al (2010) Kinase-dead BRAF and oncogenic RAS cooperate to drive tumor progression through CRAF. Cell 140(2):209–221
29. Su F et al (2012) RAS mutations in cutaneous squamous-cell carcinomas in patients treated with BRAF inhibitors. N Engl J Med 366(3):207–215
30. Wagle N et al (2011) Dissecting therapeutic resistance to RAF inhibition in melanoma by tumor genomic profiling. J Clin Oncol Off J Am Soc Clin Oncol 29(22):3085–3096
31. Shi H et al (2012) Melanoma whole-exome sequencing identifies (V600E)B-RAF amplification-mediated acquired B-RAF inhibitor resistance. Nat Commun 3:724
32. Poulikakos PI et al (2011) RAF inhibitor resistance is mediated by dimerization of aberrantly spliced BRAF(V600E). Nature 480(7377):387–390
33. Greger JG et al (2012) Combinations of BRAF, MEK, and PI3K/mTOR inhibitors overcome acquired resistance to the BRAF inhibitor GSK2118436 dabrafenib, mediated by NRAS or MEK mutations. Mol Cancer Ther 11(4):909–920
34. Johannessen CM et al (2010) COT drives resistance to RAF inhibition through MAP kinase pathway reactivation. Nature 468(7326):968–972
35. Villanueva J et al (2010) Acquired resistance to BRAF inhibitors mediated by a RAF kinase switch in melanoma can be overcome by cotargeting MEK and IGF-1R/PI3K. Cancer Cell 18 (6):683–695
36. Shi H et al (2014) Acquired resistance and clonal evolution in melanoma during BRAF inhibitor therapy. Cancer Discov 4(1):80–93
37. Atefi M, von Euw E, Attar N, Chu C, Guo D, Nazarian R, Chmielowski B, Glaspy JA, Mischel P, Lo R, Ribas A (2011) Reversing melanoma cross-resistance to BRAF and MEK inhibitors by co-targeting the AKT/mTOR pathway. PloS one 6(12):e28973
38. Shi H et al (2011) Combinatorial treatments that overcome PDGFRbeta-driven resistance of melanoma cells to V600 EB-RAF inhibition. Cancer Res 71(15):5067–5074
39. Infante JR et al (2012) Safety, pharmacokinetic, pharmacodynamic, and efficacy data for the oral MEK inhibitor trametinib: a phase 1 dose-escalation trial. Lancet Oncol 13(8):773–781
40. Kim KB et al (2013) Phase II study of the MEK1/MEK2 inhibitor Trametinib in patients with metastatic BRAF-mutant cutaneous melanoma previously treated with or without a BRAF inhibitor. J Clin Oncol Off J Am Soc Clin Oncol 31(4):482–489
41. Ribas A et al (2014) Combination of vemurafenib and cobimetinib in patients with advanced BRAF(V600)-mutated melanoma: a phase 1b study. Lancet Oncol 15(9):954–965
42. Flaherty KT et al (2012) Combined BRAF and MEK inhibition in melanoma with BRAF V600 mutations. The New England journal of medicine 367(18):1694–1703
43. Infante JR et al (2011) Phase I/II study to assess safety, pharmacokinetics, and efficacy of the oral MEK 1/2 inhibitor GSK1120212 (GSK212) dosed in combination with the oral BRAF inhibitor GSK2118436 (GSK436). J Clin Oncol 29:p(suppl; abstr CRA8503)
44. von Euw E et al (2012) Antitumor effects of the investigational selective MEK inhibitor TAK733 against cutaneous and uveal melanoma cell lines. Mol Cancer 11(1):22
45. Falchook GS et al (2012) Activity of the oral MEK inhibitor trametinib in patients with advanced melanoma: a phase 1 dose-escalation trial. Lancet Oncol 13(8):782–789

46. Ascierto PA et al (2013) MEK162 for patients with advanced melanoma harbouring NRAS or Val600 BRAF mutations: a non-randomised, open-label phase 2 study. Lancet Oncol 14 (3):249–256
47. Hatzivassiliou G et al (2012) ERK inhibition overcomes acquired resistance to MEK inhibitors. Mol Cancer Ther
48. Wong DJ et al (2014) Antitumor activity of the ERK inhibitor SCH722984 against BRAF mutant, NRAS mutant and wild-type melanoma. Mol Cancer 13:194
49. Morris EJ et al (2013) Discovery of a novel ERK inhibitor with activity in models of acquired resistance to BRAF and MEK inhibitors. Cancer Discov 3(7):742–750
50. Lassen A et al (2014) Effects of AKT inhibitor therapy in response and resistance to BRAF inhibition in melanoma. Mol Cancer 13:83
51. Hu-Lieskovan S et al (2014) Combining targeted therapy with immunotherapy in BRAF-mutant melanoma: promise and challenges. J Clin Oncol Off J Am Soc Clin Oncol 32(21):2248–2254
52. Comin-Anduix B et al (2010) The oncogenic BRAF kinase inhibitor PLX4032/RG7204 does not affect the viability or function of human lymphocytes across a wide range of concentrations. Clin Cancer Res Off J Am Assoc Cancer Res 16(24):6040–6048

Treatment of Melanoma CNS Metastases

Sekwon Jang and Michael B. Atkins

Abstract

The discovery of the BRAFV600 mutation and the development of targeted therapies directed against this mutation as well as effective immunotherapies with durable benefits have revolutionized the treatment of patients with melanoma. Nonetheless, the frequent occurrence of brain metastases in patients with advanced melanoma represents a significant obstacle to long-term, high quality survival. The application of stereotactic radiation therapy has provided an opportunity to control brain metastases in the majority of patients with metastatic melanoma reducing the impact of these lesions on morbidity and mortality and enabling patients to receive and potentially benefit from these novel systemic treatments. Encouragingly, several of these novel new therapies have shown antitumor activity against CNS metastases that approach that seen against extracranial disease. As a consequence, several effective treatment options are now available for patients with melanoma brain metastases. With these tools in hand, it is anticipated that further investigation into the optimal sequence and/or combination of systemic therapies and local therapies along with multidisciplinary team practice will continue to improve the outcome of patients with this previously life-limiting disease complication.

S. Jang · M.B. Atkins (✉)
Georgetown Lombardi Comprehensive Cancer Center, Washington, D.C., USA
e-mail: mba41@georgetown.edu

H.L. Kaufman and J.M. Mehnert (eds.), *Melanoma*,
Cancer Treatment and Research 167, DOI 10.1007/978-3-319-22539-5_11

Keywords
Melanoma brain metastases · Stereotactic radiosurgery · Braf inhibitor therapy · Immunotherapy

Contents

Melanoma brain metastases are common, difficult to treat, and carry a poor prognosis. Local therapies such as surgery and whole-brain radiotherapy (WBRT) have historically been the only treatment approaches for patients with melanoma brain metastases. Over the past decade, stereotactic radiosurgery (SRS) has become the cornerstone of treatment for most patients. Selection and sequencing of local therapies are controversial due to lack of prospective randomized trials addressing this question. More recently, the treatment paradigm for melanoma brain metastases has begun to incorporate systemic treatments including molecularly targeted therapies such as the BRAF inhibitors dabrafenib and vemurafenib and immunotherapy with the anti-CTLA4 antibody ipilimumab. Given the expanding number of treatment options, multidisciplinary discussion is required to establish a treatment plan which balances multiple factors including reduction in symptomatic central nervous system (CNS) disease progression and the risk of neurologic death against the risk of treatment-related toxicity and competing issues related to the management of systemic disease. Further research is required to optimize the coordination of all the available therapies, both local and systemic, to improve the patient's quality of life and survival.

1 Introduction

Melanoma has high propensity to metastasize to the brain and is the third most common cause of brain metastases in the USA after lung and breast cancers [35]. Five-year cumulative incidence of brain metastases was 7 % for patients with all stages of melanoma [63]. Approximately 20 % of patients have brain metastases at first diagnosis of distant metastatic melanoma [8]. Additionally up to 45 % of patients with metastatic melanoma develop clinically documented brain metastases during their lifetime [13], and the prevalence of brain metastasis is 50–75 % in autopsy series [14, 53].

Clinicopathologic characteristics associated with the increased risk of brain metastases among patients with melanoma mirror those factors associated with metastasis and poor survival. They include male gender, melanomas arising on mucosal surfaces or on the skin of the trunk or head and neck, thick or ulcerated primary lesions, and acral lentiginous or nodular histology [61]. Also, melanoma involvement of more than three regional lymph nodes either at diagnosis or relapse was associated with the development of brain metastases [5]. Among patients with unresectable stage III or IV melanoma, elevated LDH and stage M1b or M1c were independent predictors for the risk of brain metastasis [6]. Molecular changes found in melanoma brain metastases include increased VEGF secretion, increase in phosphorylated STAT3 leading to upregulation in invasive and angiogenesis genes, and increased activity of heparanase (Chen and Davies [11]). Also, patients with melanomas containing BRAF or NRAS mutations were more likely than patients with wild-type tumors to have brain metastasis at the time they were diagnosed with distant metastatic disease [33].

Melanoma patients with brain metastases historically have had a poor prognosis with median survival of 4 months and 1-year survival rate of 10–20 % [18, 61]. An improvement in median overall survival to 8 to 10 months has been reported with SRS [39, 60]. In patients with brain metastases from melanoma, good performance status and the limited number of brain metastases were associated with a more favorable prognosis [67].

2 Treatment

2.1 Surgery

Prospective randomized studies in patients with brain metastases from largely other histologies have suggested that surgical resection followed by WBRT produced superior results to WBRT alone. For example, a randomized trial of 48 patients with a single metastasis to the brain including 3 patients with melanoma showed improvement in survival among patients who received treatment with surgical resection plus radiotherapy compared to patients treated with radiotherapy alone. Also, patients who were treated with surgery plus radiotherapy had fewer recurrences of cancer in the brain and had a better quality of life [52]. Another trial also demonstrated surgery plus radiotherapy produced superior overall and functionally independent survival compared to radiotherapy alone in patients with single brain metastasis especially those with stable extracranial disease (median survival, 12 months vs. 7 months) [70]. A systematic review also concluded that surgical resection followed by WBRT is an effective treatment for patients with a single, surgically accessible brain metastasis who have controlled extra-cranial disease and are in good general condition [21]. While this approach is an established practice for many cancers, the relevance of these findings to patients with melanoma with solitary brain metastases is uncertain as melanoma is typically less sensitive to standard low-dose fractionated WBRT approach.

Of note, a retrospective study from Australia confined to patients with melanoma showed improvement in median survival among patients with melanoma brain metastasis treated with surgery (8.9 months) or surgery and postoperative radiotherapy (9.7 months) compared to radiotherapy alone (3.4 months) or supportive care alone (2.1 months) [18]. Although the group treated with surgery likely had a significantly better pretreatment prognosis than those treated with WBRT alone or supportive care, these data are perhaps most notable for the limited benefit associated with WBRT in either the postsurgical or inoperable setting.

While surgical resection of more than one brain metastasis has been performed in cases of significant mass effect from more than one lesion, and in cases where two or more lesions are accessible through the same craniotomy approach, no robust comparative data exist to evaluate the role of surgical resection for multiple brain metastases in any cancer let alone for melanoma [36]. Retrospective review of 56 patients who underwent resection for multiple brain metastases reported improved survival in patients who had all of their brain metastases resected compared to patients who had resection of only some of the lesions (median survival, 14 months vs. 6 months) [7]. The survival was comparable to a matched control group of patients who underwent resection for a single brain metastasis. Although multiple large, symptomatic metastases can be treated with surgical resection in selected patients with favorable prognosis, SRS and/or WBRT is far more commonly employed in patients with multiple brain metastases.

2.2 Radiation Treatment

WBRT has played a central role in brain metastasis treatment and continues to be central to therapy for many tumor types with radioresponsive biology. However, melanoma cells have low responsiveness to radiation in vitro corresponding to the low efficacy of WBRT [17]. As mentioned above, patients with melanoma that had metastasized to brain who underwent WBRT alone had a median survival of only 3.4 months compared to 2.1 months for patients who received supportive care alone [18]. Given this limited benefit, WBRT in patients with melanoma has been increasingly confined to patients for whom surgery and SRS are not feasible such as those with symptomatic diffuse or leptomeningeal disease as well as inoperable large-volume brain metastatic disease.

Although prior data from patients largely with other cancers suggested a benefit for adjuvant WBRT following surgical resection [51], more recent data have called this benefit into question. A prospective randomized study conducted by the European Organisation for Research and Treatment of Cancer (EORTC) evaluated the role of adjuvant WBRT after surgery or radiosurgery in 359 patients (18 with melanoma) with one to three brain metastases and demonstrated no improvement in the duration of functional independence or overall survival despite improvement in local and distant brain control [38]. Also, adjuvant WBRT had negative impact on health-related quality of life (global health status at 9 months, physical functioning at 8 weeks, cognitive functioning at 12 months, and fatigue at 8 weeks) compared to observation [65].

In the absence of melanoma-specific data, it is difficult to estimate the benefit of WBRT as an adjuvant therapy following surgery or radiosurgery. The benefit would be expected to be greatest for patients undergoing resection or radiosurgery to large metastases (i.e., >4 cm) where the radiosurgery dose to tumor or resection cavity would need to be relatively low [56].

In contrast to the limited benefit and role of WBRT, SRS has emerged as a vital alternative local therapy for patients with melanoma brain metastases. This approach utilizes multiple convergent radiation beams to deliver a high dose of focused radiation to one or more tumor masses with rapid dose falloff beyond the tumor margin. Multiple single-institution retrospective analyses reported 1-year local control rates of 50–75 % in patients who underwent SRS for melanoma brain metastases [9, 39]. Studies identified tumor volume as an independent predictor of local tumor control [9, 42] and survival [73]. Also, patients with controlled extracranial melanoma metastases had better survival [39, 73].

Although there is substantial experience with SRS in patients with melanoma brain metastases, there is no prospective randomized melanoma-specific trial addressing the benefit of SRS to patient survival. The Radiation Therapy Oncology Group (RTOG) conducted a trial including multiple histologies (13 of 333 patients with melanoma) with up to three brain metastases and randomized patients to WBRT + SRS or WBRT alone [3]. The addition of SRS improved survival for patients with single unresectable brain metastasis but not for patients with multiple metastases. Patients who had WBRT + SRS were more likely to maintain a stable or improved performance status at 3 and 6 months compared to patients who had WBRT alone. Based on this, the authors concluded that SRS should be a standard treatment for patients with a single unresectable brain metastasis and considered for patients with two or three brain metastases.

Current radiosurgery delivery systems are capable of treating multiple (up to 10) metastases in a single session. However, the optimal treatment of patients with multiple brain metastases (4 or more) remains controversial, and only a few retrospective studies have included patients with 4 or more metastatic lesions. One study showed that patients with single brain metastasis had better survival compared with patients with multiple brain metastases after SRS (Radbill et al. [55]). Another study also showed that the number of brain metastases was an independent predictor of survival; however, long-term survival was observed in patients with up to 8 brain metastases, no prior WBRT, and good functional status [39]. Although these data once again come largely from patients with other cancer types, these data suggest that SRS is a valuable option for patients with controlled systemic disease even if they have multiple brain metastases.

The effectiveness of SRS compared to conventional surgery remains uncertain. In the absence of randomized trial, surgery is preferred if a single metastatic lesion is causing neurologic symptoms and is easily accessible. Large posterior fossa tumors or those with the large amounts of surrounding edema causing significant effacement of the fourth ventricle or cerebral aqueduct should be resected to prevent the development of obstructive hydrocephalus. SRS is preferred for smaller lesions and those in eloquent or relatively inaccessible areas of the brain.

There has been a great interest to add SRS following surgical resection of a brain metastasis. Multiple retrospective studies have demonstrated that a postoperative SRS boost in lieu of WBRT is associated with high local control rate with acceptable toxicity [33, 66]. While further studies evaluating SRS versus WBRT, or fractionated stereotactic radiotherapy, may clarify the optimal radiation modality in this setting for patients with radiosensitive malignancies, given the relative radioresistance of melanoma, adjuvant SRS is likely to be the preferred option for patients with melanoma brain metastases.

Radiation necrosis is the most common complication following SRS. It is diagnosed from radiologic evidence of increased peritumoral edema and rim enhancement at the radiosurgical site. In one series, radiation necrosis occurred in 24 % of treated lesions, being symptomatic in 10 % and asymptomatic in 14 % [46]. Predictive factors for radiation necrosis included tumor size, location, and volume of normal brain receiving 10, 12, and 16 Gy (V10, V12, and V16) especially when located in or near eloquent areas. The standard treatment for symptomatic radiation necrosis consists of corticosteroids. For patients with melanoma, steroid treatment may adversely affect the efficacy of systemic immunotherapies such as interleukin-2 or ipilimumab. In such cases, aggressive management including surgical resection of the necrotic area may be considered. Administration of low-dose bevacizumab has also been reported to be effective in the treatment of radiation-induced necrosis [2] and could be considered particularly in situations where corticosteroids are contraindicated and surgical resection is not feasible. Upfront surgical resection or fractionated stereotactic radiotherapy may be considered for metastases that would be associated with excessive risk of radiation necrosis following SRS.

2.3 Systemic Treatment

2.3.1 Chemotherapy

Cytotoxic chemotherapy has limited efficacy for patients with metastatic melanoma to the brain. Temozolomide and fotemustine can penetrate the blood–brain barrier and have produced the highest response rates among conventional chemotherapies. Temozolomide was evaluated in a phase II study in patients with melanoma brain metastases who did not require immediate radiotherapy [1]. Of 151 patients enrolled, 117 who had no prior systemic chemotherapy received temozolomide 200 mg m^2 day for 5 days every 28 days, whereas 34 who had prior chemotherapy received 150 mg m^2 day for 5 days every 28 days. Response rates were 7 % for previously untreated patients and 3 % for previously treated patients. Median overall survival was poor—3.5 and 2.2 months for previously untreated patients and for previously treated patients, respectively. Another phase II study evaluated the combination of temozolomide and thalidomide and found modest response rate of 12 % with increased toxicity such as intracranial hemorrhage, pulmonary embolism, and deep vein thrombosis [31]. Clinical activity of fotemustine was initially suggested in a phase II trial showing a response rate of 24 % in patients with melanoma brain metastases [32]. However, in a phase III trial of fotemustine compared with dacarbazine, tumor responses were observed rarely in brain (5.9 % with fotemustine vs. 0 % with dacarbazine) among patients with brain metastases at baseline.

2.3.2 Immunotherapy

Interleukin-2

Prior to 2011, high-dose interleukin-2 (IL-2) was the only approved immunotherapy in the USA for patients with advanced melanoma and has been used for patients without brain metastases with objective responses observed in 15–20 % and durable complete responses in 5–7 % of patients. Data are limited on the safety and efficacy of high-dose IL-2 in patients with untreated brain metastases. In a retrospective review from the US National Cancer Institute, IL-2 yielded objective response rate of 18 % in patients with previously irradiated brain metastases but only 6 % in patients with untreated brain metastases [23]. There were no significant differences in toxicity profiles. Given the substantial capillary leak syndrome and the associated risk for peritumoral edema, seen with high-dose IL-2 therapy, treatment of patients with large CNS metastases, even if recently irradiated, may be associated with significant CNS toxicity. Further, the CNS is a frequent site of isolated disease relapse for patients with ongoing systemic response to IL-2-based immunotherapy, suggesting that the efficacy of this treatment in controlling disease in the brain is even more limited than its modest ability to treat systemic metastatic disease [30, 47]. Finally, IL-2 therapy has been shown to be ineffective in patients taking steroids [45]. Consequently, the use of HD IL-2 in patients with extensive CNS melanoma metastases is to be discouraged.

Adoptive T-cell Therapy

Adoptive T-cell therapy is a complex treatment that is performed in few centers worldwide. It uses autologous antitumor lymphocytes plus interleukin-2 following a lymphodepleting preparative regimen used to eliminate the immunosuppressive factors within the tumor microenvironment. This approach has a high antitumor activity in patients with systemic metastases from melanoma [59]. A retrospective analysis from US National Cancer Institute Surgery Branch reported that this approach also has activity against CNS metastases [29]. Patients were eligible for treatment if they had asymptomatic oligometastases each less than 10 mm in size and unassociated with mass effect or edema. A complete response was reported in 7 of 17 evaluable patients (41 %), and 6 of these patients achieved an overall partial response. One patient developed a tumor-associated subarachnoid hemorrhage during the thrombocytopenic phase of therapy. This impressive result should be interpreted with caution given the small number of highly selected patients analyzed.

Ipilimumab

Ipilimumab is a fully human monoclonal antibody (IgG1) which inhibits the function of cytotoxic T-cell-associated antigen 4 (CTLA4) and enhances an immune response against melanoma cells. Ipilimumab 3 mg/kg intravenously every 3 weeks for up to 4 cycles was approved in 2011 for patients with metastatic melanoma based on a survival advantage over a melanoma vaccine [27]. Also, ipilimumab in combination with DTIC improved survival compared with DTIC alone [57]. Patients with active or untreated brain metastases were excluded from these trials. However, ipilimumab was observed to induce immune effector cell infiltration and tumor necrosis in brain metastases, and cases of regression or stabilization of previously progressing brain metastases in ipilimumab-treated patients have been reported [28, 62].

Activity of ipilimumab against brain metastases was specifically addressed by a phase II study including two cohorts of patients [44]. Patients in cohort A ($n = 51$) had one or more untreated brain lesions who were neurologically asymptomatic and were not receiving corticosteroid treatment at study entry. Those in cohort B ($n = 21$) were symptomatic and on a stable dose of corticosteroids. Patients were treated with ipilimumab, 10 mg/kg intravenously every 3 weeks for 4 cycles followed by same dose every 12 weeks for those who were clinically stable. Intracranial disease control (objective response or stable disease) rate was 24 % in cohort A and 10 % in cohort B using modified WHO criteria and 25 % in cohort A and 10 % in cohort B using immune-related response criteria. Extracranial disease control was mostly concordant with the intracranial disease control. The 24-month overall survival was 26 % in cohort A and 10 % in cohort B. The lower antitumor activity and worse survival in cohort B could be attributable to their less favorable prognostic characteristics as well as the inhibition of the immunostimulatory effects of CTLA4 checkpoint blockade by concomitant corticosteroid blockade. There were no unexpected toxicities, but it should be noted that one patient had a grade 4 intratumoral hemorrhage attributed to disease progression. Overall, ipilimumab has activity in melanoma brain metastases particularly when patients are asymptomatic and not receiving corticosteroids. Further study is required to determine the optimal dose (3 mg/kg vs. 10 mg/kg) and schedule (4 doses only vs. 4 doses plus every 12 weeks) of ipilimumab in this as well as other treatment settings.

Programmed Death 1 Inhibitors

Programmed death (PD) 1 is an inhibitory co-receptor on antigen-activated T cells. Inhibiting the PD-1 receptor with a blocking antibody enhances T-cell responses and antitumor activity. Early clinical trials investigating antibodies to PD-1 or PD-L1 in patients with melanoma have shown response rates ranging from 25 to 50 % [24, 69]. In addition, a study evaluating the concurrent administration of the combination of ipilimumab and the PD1 antibody nivolumab produced rapid and deep tumor responses in patients with metastatic melanoma and an overall response rate of 53 % in a small number of patients [72]. The promising results seen with various anti-PD1 and PD-L1 antibodies either alone or in combination with ipilimumab have led to multiple randomized clinical trials of comparing anti-PD-1 antibodies alone or in combination with ipilimumab to standard of care in patients with metastatic melanoma (NCT01704287, NCT01866319, NCT01844505). These new agents will likely soon be added to the therapeutic armamentarium for patients with metastatic melanoma. To date, patients with active brain metastases have been excluded from these studies; however, ongoing and future trials are anticipated to provide data on the intracranial activity of these promising agents.

2.3.3 Targeted Therapy

Activating mutations in the mitogen-activated protein kinase (MAPK) pathway, which incorporates the enzymes RAS (rat sarcoma; encoded by HRAS, NRAS, and KRAS), RAF (rapidly accelerated fibrosarcoma; encoded by ARAF, BRAF, and CRAF), MEK (MAPK/ERK kinase; encoded by MAP2K1 and MAP2K2), and ERK (extracellular signal-regulated kinase; encoded by MAPK1 and MAPK3), results in constitutive signaling leading to oncogenic cell proliferation and escape from apoptosis [22]. Approximately 40–50 % of melanomas harbor a mutation in the *BRAF*, mostly confined to a specific point mutation at nucleotide 1799 leading to a change in the V600 amino acid [12]. V600E mutation (substitution of glutamic acid for valine at position 600) is the most common *BRAF* mutation in melanoma occurring in 70–90 % of *BRAF*-mutant melanomas, with the remainder of mutations largely resulting from other amino acid substitutions at this position (V600K, V600D, or V600R) [40, 71].

In 2011, vemurafenib became the first oral BRAF inhibitor approved by US FDA for the treatment of patients with unresectable or metastatic melanoma with *BRAFV600E* mutation. A phase 3 randomized trial comparing vemurafenib to dacarbazine in 675 patients with previously untreated, metastatic melanoma with the *BRAFV600E* mutation demonstrated significantly increased overall survival (HR 0.37, 95 % confidence interval [CI], 0.26–0.55; $P < 0.001$) and progression-free survival (HR 0.26, 95 % CI, 0.20–0.33; $P < 0.001$) at the first planned interim analysis conducted after a median follow-up of only 3.7 months [10]. Response rates were 48 % for vemurafenib and 5 % for dacarbazine. Common side effects of vemurafenib were arthralgia, rash, fatigue, alopecia, photosensitivity, nausea, and diarrhea. Cutaneous squamous cell carcinomas (the majority, keratoacanthoma type) were reported in up to 26 % of patients with a significant proportion of these tumors harboring a mutation in *HRAS* [68]. These skin lesions were treated with local excision and did not require dose interruption or reduction of vemurafenib. As with many registration trials, patients with brain metastases were ineligible for the study unless the disease had been treated and was stable for at least three months and not requiring steroids.

A case report of dramatic response in a melanoma brain metastasis to vemurafenib [58] led to an open-label, single-arm trial in 24 patients with V600E *BRAF* mutation—positive melanoma and symptomatic and progressing brain metastases

[15]. These patients had a very poor prognosis at enrollment, and there was no size criteria for the brain lesions. Of 19 patients with measurable intracranial disease, seven (37 %) achieved >30 % intracranial tumor regression, and three (16 %; 95 % CI, 3.4–39.6 %) achieved a confirmed PR. Median progression-free survival was 3.9 (95 % CI, 3.0–5.5) months, and median overall survival was 5.3 (95 % CI, 3.9–6.6) months. A larger phase II study of vemurafenib in patients with *BRAF V600*-mutant melanoma and active brain metastases included patients with both symptomatic and asymptomatic brain metastases, as well as patients with untreated or previously treated CNS disease (NCT01378975). This trial has completed accrual, and the results are anticipated shortly.

Dabrafenib is a reversible, ATP-competitive inhibitor of mutant *BRAFV600* (IC50 0.5 nmol/L). Dabrafenib was approved by US FDA in 2013. In a phase 3 clinical trial, 250 patients with previously untreated, stage IV or unresectable stage III *BRAFV600E* mutant melanoma were randomized to receive either dabrafenib (187 patients) or dacarbazine (63 patients) [26]. Patients assigned to the dacarbazine arm were permitted to crossover to dabrafenib at the time of disease progression. The primary end point of this trial was progression-free survival. Dabrafenib showed a statistically significant improvement in median progression-free survival of 5.1 months compared to 2.7 months for dacarbazine. Confirmed objective response rate by independent review committee was 50 % in dabrafenib with a 3 % complete response rate. These results are similar to what was observed in the vemurafenib phase III trial indicating a likely equivalent antitumor activity for these two agents. In an updated report, the median overall survival for the dabrafenib-treated group was 18.2 months compared to 15.6 months in dacarbazine group. These survival results were confounded by crossover of the majority of patients initially assigned to dacarbazine to dabrafenib (HR 0.76, 95 % CI 0.48–1.21) [25]. The most common adverse events were cutaneous (hyperkeratosis, papillomas, palmar-plantar erythrodysaesthesia), fatigue, headache, and arthralgia, which together required dose reduction in 28 % of patients. Squamous cell carcinoma or keratoacanthomas were observed in 6 % of patients. Photosensitivity reactions were rarely seen with dabrafenib; however, grade 2 or 3 pyrexia was observed in 8 and 3 %, respectively.

The activity of dabrafenib for patients with melanoma brain metastases was first reported from the phase I expansion cohort study [16]. Among 10 patients with asymptomatic, untreated brain metastases who were treated with recommended phase II dose of 150 mg twice daily, nine patients had a reduction in the size of the brain metastases and four had a complete response in the brain. These results led to the large phase II study which enrolled 172 patients with *BRAFV600E*- or *V600K*-mutant melanoma with documented brain metastasis into one of two cohorts distinguished by whether or not they had received prior radiation therapy to brain [41]. Dabrafenib showed antitumor activity with an overall intracranial response rate of 39 and 31 % for the patients with *BRAFV600E*-mutant melanoma without and with prior brain irradiation, respectively. Median progression-free survival was 4 months, and median overall survival approximately 8 months in both cohorts. Objective responses were also seen in 5 of 33 patients (15 %) with *BRAFV600K*-

mutant melanoma. In the safety analysis, only 1 patient developed treatment-related cerebral hemorrhage.

Although a preclinical study suggests that dabrafenib may have greater brain penetration compared with vemurafenib [48], there are no data comparing the clinical intracranial activity of dabrafenib and vemurafenib. Neoadjuvant studies in patients with resectable brain metastases are planned for dabrafenib (NCT01978236) and vemurafenib (NCT 01781026) which will provide information on brain penetration of these agents.

Trametinib is an orally available, small-molecule, selective inhibitor of MEK1 and MEK2 which was approved by US FDA in 2013 for the treatment of patients with unresectable or metastatic melanoma with *BRAFV600E* or *V600K* mutations. In a phase 3 open-labeled trial, 322 patients with metastatic melanoma with *BRAFV600E* or *V600K* mutation were randomized to receive either trametinib or chemotherapy (either dacarbazine or paclitaxel) in 2:1 ratio [20]. Median progression-free survival was improved to 4.8 months in the trametinib group compared to 1.5 months in the chemotherapy group. Overall survival rate at 6 months was 81 % in the trametinib group and 67 % in the chemotherapy group even though 51 of 108 patients (47 %) in the chemotherapy group crossed over to receive trametinib (hazard ratio for death, 0.54; 95 % CI, 0.32 to 0.92; $P = 0.01$). The response rate was 22 %, and most common side effects were rash, diarrhea, and peripheral edema in the trametinib group. This trial included only a few patients with stable brain metastases (9 in trametinib and 2 in chemotherapy); therefore, the single-agent activity of trametinib against active melanoma brain metastases is currently not known.

Combination of dabrafenib and trametinib in BRAF inhibitor-naïve patients has shown improvement in response rate (76 % vs. 54 %) as well as median progression survival (9.4 months vs. 5.8 months) compared with dabrafenib alone in a randomized phase II trial which led to accelerated approval of combination therapy by US FDA in 2014 [19]. Also, the incidence of cutaneous squamous cell carcinoma was 7 % in combination group compared with 19 % for dabrafenib monotherapy, suggesting that the addition of a MEK inhibitor was able to block the paradoxical activation of MAPK pathway that contributed to these skin lesions. The intracranial activity of this combination is going to be evaluated in a planned clinical trial (NCT02039947).

2.4 Combination

2.4.1 Chemotherapy and Radiotherapy

Concurrent chemotherapy and WBRT have been evaluated in multiple clinical trials. In a phase III trial, the combination of fotemustine with whole-brain radiation delayed the time to CNS progression of melanoma brain metastases compared with fotemustine alone, but this benefit was not associated with a significant improvement in terms of objective disease control or overall survival [49]. The Cytokine

Working Group conducted phase II trials of concurrent temozolomide and whole-brain radiation [43] as well as the concurrent temozolomide, thalidomide, and whole-brain radiation [4] for patients with brain metastases from melanoma which also showed very limited antitumor activity. Once again, the addition of thalidomide was associated with an unacceptably high rate of thromboembolic disease.

2.4.2 Immunotherapy and Radiotherapy

Limited data are available investigating the use of definitive SRS and ipilimumab in patients with melanoma brain metastases. In a retrospective analysis of patients treated with radiosurgery, 27 of 77 patients received ipilimumab after radiosurgery [37]. Patients who received ipilimumab had a median survival of 21.3 months compared with 4.9 months in patients who did not receive this agent. However, these groups were not comparable. Although uni- and multivariable Cox proportional hazard analyses with data censored at 24 months demonstrated an improved hazard ratio (HR) for death in patients treated with ipilimumab compared to those who did not receive ipilimumab (HR 0.48 [95 % CI, 0.24–0.93]; $P = 0.03$), a significant role for ipilimumab could not be established in the final multivariate analysis (HR 0.61 [95 % CI, 0.33–1.10]; $P = 0.12$). Nonetheless, some groups have reported a sensitizing effect or even an abscopal effect for focused RT when used in conjunction with immunotherapy [54]. Consequently, the combination of ipilimumab and radiosurgery or whole-brain radiation is being prospectively investigated in clinical trials (NCT01703507).

2.4.3 BRAF Inhibitor and Radiotherapy

The efficacy of vemurafenib concomitant with or in patients who were previously treated with either SRS or whole-brain radiation was evaluated in a retrospective analysis in 12 patients with melanoma brain metastases [50]. Seven patients had a neurologic improvement, and radiographic responses were seen in 36 of 48 index lesions (75 %). This result suggests that BRAF inhibitor and radiotherapy-based techniques have high efficacy although they need to be validated in randomized controlled clinical trials. Of note, unusual skin reactions such as excessive acute radio-dermatitis and late skin reaction can occur during and after treatment with a combination of vemurafenib and whole-brain radiation [64]. Therefore, careful dermatologic monitoring is required for those who undergo concurrent radiation and BRAF inhibitor therapy. The safety and efficacy of dabrafenib combined with SRS are currently being investigated (NCT01721603).

3 Conclusion

The discovery of *BRAFV600* mutation and the development of targeted therapies directed against this mutation as well as effective immunotherapies with durable benefits have revolutionized the treatment of patients with melanoma. The application of stereotactic radiation therapy has provided an opportunity to control brain metastases in majority of patients with metastatic melanoma reducing the impact that these lesions have on mortality and enabling such patients to receive and potentially benefit from these novel systemic treatments. Encouragingly, several of these novel agents have shown antitumor activity against CNS metastases use approaches that are effective against extracranial disease. As a consequence, several effective treatment options are now available for patients with melanoma brain metastases. With these tools in hand, it is anticipated that further investigation into the optimal sequence and/or combination of systemic therapies and local therapies along with multidisciplinary team practice will continue to improve the outcome of patients with this previously life-limiting disease complication.

References

1. Agarwala SS, Kirkwood JM, Gore M, Dreno B, Thatcher N, Czarnetski B, Rankin EM (2004) Temozolomide for the treatment of brain metastases associated with metastatic melanoma: a phase II study. J Clin Oncol 22(11):2101–2107. doi:10.1200/jco.2004.11.044
2. Alessandretti M, Buzaid AC, Brandao R, Brandao EP (2013) Low-dose bevacizumab is effective in radiation-induced necrosis. Case Rep Oncol 6(3):598–601. doi:10.1159/000357401
3. Andrews DW, Scott CB, Sperduto PW, Flanders AE, Gaspar LE, Schell MC, Curran WJ Jr (2004) Whole brain radiation therapy with or without stereotactic radiosurgery boost for patients with one to three brain metastases: phase III results of the RTOG 9508 randomised trial. Lancet 363(9422):1665–1672. doi:10.1016/s0140 6736(04)16250-8
4. Atkins MB, Sosman JA, Agarwala S, Logan T, Clark JI, Ernstoff MS, Margolin KA (2008) Temozolomide, thalidomide, and whole brain radiation therapy for patients with brain metastasis from metastatic melanoma: a phase II Cytokine Working Group study. Cancer 113 (8):2139–2145. doi:10.1002/cncr.23805
5. Ballo MT, Ross MI, Cormier JN, Myers JN, Lee JE, Gershenwald JE, Zagars GK (2006) Combined-modality therapy for patients with regional nodal metastases from melanoma. Int J Radiat Oncol Biol Phys 64(1):106–113. doi:10.1016/j.ijrobp.2005.06.030
6. Bedikian AY, Wei C, Detry M, Kim KB, Papadopoulos NE, Hwu WJ, Hwu P (2011) Predictive factors for the development of brain metastasis in advanced unresectable metastatic melanoma. Am J Clin Oncol 34(6):603–610. doi:10.1097/COC.0b013e3181f9456a
7. Bindal RK, Sawaya R, Leavens ME, Lee JJ (1993) Surgical treatment of multiple brain metastases. J Neurosurg 79(2):210–216. doi:10.3171/jns.1993.79.2.0210
8. Carlino MS, Atkins MB, Warneke CL et al (2010) Differences between Australia (OZ) and the United States (US) in the patterns, prognosis, and treatment of melanoma CNS metastases: Analysis from the PHAMOUS (prognostic heterogeneity in patients with advanced melanoma between OZ and the US) study. Paper presented at the Melanoma Congress
9. Chang EL, Selek U, III Hassenbusch SJ, Maor MH, Allen PK, Mahajan A, Woo SY (2005). Outcome variation among "radioresistant" brain metastases treated with stereotactic radiosurgery. Neurosurgery 56(5):936–945 (discussion 936–945)
10. Chapman PB, Hauschild A, Robert C, Haanen JB, Ascierto P, Larkin J, McArthur GA (2011) Improved survival with vemurafenib in melanoma with BRAF V600E mutation. N Engl J Med 364(26):2507–2516. doi:10.1056/NEJMoa1103782
11. Chen G, Davies MA (2012) Emerging insights into the molecular biology of brain metastases. Biochem Pharmacol 83(3):305−314

12. Davies H, Bignell GR, Cox C, Stephens P, Edkins S, Clegg S, Futreal PA (2002) Mutations of the BRAF gene in human cancer. Nature 417(6892):949–954. doi:10.1038/nature00766
13. Davies MA, Liu P, McIntyre S, Kim KB, Papadopoulos N, Hwu WJ, Bedikian A (2011) Prognostic factors for survival in melanoma patients with brain metastases. Cancer 117 (8):1687–1696. doi:10.1002/cncr.25634
14. de la Monte SM, Moore GW, Hutchins GM (1983) Patterned distribution of metastases from malignant melanoma in humans. Cancer Res 43(7):3427–3433
15. Dummer R, Goldinger SM, Turtschi CP, Eggmann NB, Michielin O, Mitchell L, Rinderknecht JD (2014) Vemurafenib in patients with BRAF(V600) mutation-positive melanoma with symptomatic brain metastases: final results of an open-label pilot study. Eur J Cancer 50(3):611–621. doi:10.1016/j.ejca.2013.11.002
16. Falchook GS, Long GV, Kurzrock R, Kim KB, Arkenau TH, Brown MP, Kefford RF (2012) Dabrafenib in patients with melanoma, untreated brain metastases, and other solid tumours: a phase 1 dose-escalation trial. Lancet 379(9829):1893–1901. doi:10.1016/s0140-6736(12) 60398-5
17. Fertil B, Malaise EP (1985) Intrinsic radiosensitivity of human cell lines is correlated with radioresponsiveness of human tumors: analysis of 101 published survival curves. Int J Radiat Oncol Biol Phys 11(9):1699–1707
18. Fife KM, Colman MH, Stevens GN, Firth IC, Moon D, Shannon KF, Thompson JF (2004) Determinants of outcome in melanoma patients with cerebral metastases. J Clin Oncol 22 (7):1293–1300. doi:10.1200/jco.2004.08.140
19. Flaherty KT, Infante JR, Daud A, Gonzalez R, Kefford RF, Sosman J, Weber J (2012) Combined BRAF and MEK inhibition in melanoma with BRAF V600 mutations. N Engl J Med 367(18):1694–1703. doi:10.1056/NEJMoa1210093
20. Flaherty KT, Robert C, Hersey P, Nathan P, Garbe C, Milhem M, Schadendorf D (2012) Improved survival with MEK inhibition in BRAF-mutated melanoma. N Engl J Med 367 (2):107–114. doi:10.1056/NEJMoa1203421
21. Gaspar LE, Mehta MP, Patchell RA, Burri SH, Robinson PD, Morris RE, Kalkanis SN (2010) The role of whole brain radiation therapy in the management of newly diagnosed brain metastases: a systematic review and evidence-based clinical practice guideline. J Neurooncol 96(1):17–32. doi:10.1007/s11060-009-0060-9
22. Gray-Schopfer V, Wellbrock C, Marais R (2007) Melanoma biology and new targeted therapy. Nature 445(7130):851–857. doi:10.1038/nature05661
23. Guirguis LM, Yang JC, White DE, Steinberg SM, Liewehr DJ, Rosenberg SA, Schwartzentruber DJ (2002) Safety and efficacy of high-dose interleukin-2 therapy in patients with brain metastases. J Immunother 25(1):82–87
24. Hamid O, Robert C, Daud A, Hodi FS, Hwu WJ, Kefford R, Ribas A (2013) Safety and tumor responses with lambrolizumab (anti-PD-1) in melanoma. N Engl J Med 369(2):134–144. doi:10.1056/NEJMoa1305133
25. Hauschild A, Grob JJ, Demidov LV et al (2013) An update on BREAK-3, a phase III, randomized trial: dabrafenib (DAB) versus dacarbazine (DTIC) in patients with BRAF V600E-positive mutation metastatic melanoma (MM)
26. Hauschild A, Grob JJ, Demidov LV, Jouary T, Gutzmer R, Millward M, Chapman PB (2012) Dabrafenib in BRAF-mutated metastatic melanoma: a multicentre, open-label, phase 3 randomised controlled trial. Lancet 380(9839):358–365. doi:10.1016/s0140-6736(12)60868-x
27. Hodi FS, O'Day SJ, McDermott DF, Weber RW, Sosman JA, Haanen JB, Urba WJ (2010) Improved survival with ipilimumab in patients with metastatic melanoma. N Engl J Med 363 (8):711–723. doi:10.1056/NEJMoa1003466
28. Hodi FS, Oble DA, Drappatz J, Velazquez EF, Ramaiya N, Ramakrishna N, Mihm M (2008) CTLA-4 blockade with ipilimumab induces significant clinical benefit in a female with melanoma metastases to the CNS. Nat Clin Pract Oncol 5(9):557–561. doi:10.1038/ncponc1183

29. Hong JJ, Rosenberg SA, Dudley ME, Yang JC, White DE, Butman JA, Sherry RM (2010) Successful treatment of melanoma brain metastases with adoptive cell therapy. Clin Cancer Res 16(19):4892–4898. doi:10.1158/1078-0432.ccr-10-1507
30. Hurst R, White DE, Heiss J, Lee DS, Rosenberg SA, Schwartzentruber DJ (1999) Brain metastasis after immunotherapy in patients with metastatic melanoma or renal cell cancer: is craniotomy indicated? J Immunother 22(4):356–362
31. Hwu WJ, Lis E, Menell JH, Panageas KS, Lamb LA, Merrell J, Houghton AN (2005) Temozolomide plus thalidomide in patients with brain metastases from melanoma: a phase II study. Cancer 103(12):2590–2597. doi:10.1002/cncr.21081
32. Jacquillat C, Khayat D, Banzet P, Weil M, Fumoleau P, Avril MF et al (1990) Final report of the French multicenter phase II study of the nitrosourea fotemustine in 153 evaluable patients with disseminated malignant melanoma including patients with cerebral metastases. Cancer 66 (9):1873–1878
33. Jakob JA, Bassett RL Jr, Ng CS, Curry JL, Joseph RW, Alvarado GC, Davies MA (2012) NRAS mutation status is an independent prognostic factor in metastatic melanoma. Cancer 118(16):4014–4023. doi:10.1002/cncr.26724
34. Jensen CA, Chan MD, McCoy TP, Bourland JD, deGuzman AF, Ellis TL, Tatter SB (2011) Cavity-directed radiosurgery as adjuvant therapy after resection of a brain metastasis. J Neurosurg 114(6):1585–1591. doi:10.3171/2010.11.jns10939
35. Johnson JD, Young B (1996) Demographics of brain metastasis. Neurosurg Clin N Am 7 (3):337–344
36. Kalkanis SN, Kondziolka D, Gaspar LE, Burri SH, Asher AL, Cobbs CS, Linskey ME (2010) The role of surgical resection in the management of newly diagnosed brain metastases: a systematic review and evidence-based clinical practice guideline. J Neurooncol 96(1):33–43. doi:10.1007/s11060-009-0061-8
37. Knisely JP, Yu JB, Flanigan J, Sznol M, Kluger HM, Chiang VL (2012) Radiosurgery for melanoma brain metastases in the ipilimumab era and the possibility of longer survival. J Neurosurg 117(2):227–233. doi:10.3171/2012.5.jns111929
38. Kocher M, Soffietti R, Abacioglu U, Villa S, Fauchon F, Baumert BG, Mueller RP (2011) Adjuvant whole-brain radiotherapy versus observation after radiosurgery or surgical resection of one to three cerebral metastases: results of the EORTC 22952-26001 study. J Clin Oncol 29 (2):134–141. doi:10.1200/jco.2010.30.1655
39. Liew DN, Kano H, Kondziolka D, Mathieu D, Niranjan A, Flickinger JC, Lunsford LD (2011) Outcome predictors of Gamma Knife surgery for melanoma brain metastases. Clinical article. J Neurosurg 114(3):769–779. doi:10.3171/2010.5.jns1014
40. Long GV, Menzies AM, Nagrial AM, Haydu LE, Hamilton AL, Mann GJ, Kefford RF (2011) Prognostic and clinicopathologic associations of oncogenic BRAF in metastatic melanoma. J Clin Oncol 29(10):1239–1246. doi:10.1200/jco.2010.32.4327
41. Long GV, Trefzer U, Davies MA, Kefford RF, Ascierto PA, Chapman PB, Schadendorf D (2012) Dabrafenib in patients with Val600Glu or Val600Lys BRAF-mutant melanoma metastatic to the brain (BREAK-MB): a multicentre, open-label, phase 2 trial. Lancet Oncol 13 (11):1087–1095. doi:10.1016/s1470-2045(12)70431-x
42. Lwu S, Goetz P, Monsalves E, Aryaee M, Ebinu J, Laperriere N, Zadeh G (2013) Stereotactic radiosurgery for the treatment of melanoma and renal cell carcinoma brain metastases. Oncol Rep 29(2):407–412. doi:10.3892/or.2012.2139
43. Margolin K, Atkins B, Thompson A, Ernstoff S, Weber J, Flaherty L, Johnson D (2002) Temozolomide and whole brain irradiation in melanoma metastatic to the brain: a phase II trial of the Cytokine Working Group. J Cancer Res Clin Oncol 128(4):214–218. doi:10.1007/s00432-002-0323-8
44. Margolin K, Ernstoff MS, Hamid O, Lawrence D, McDermott D, Puzanov I, Hodi FS (2012) Ipilimumab in patients with melanoma and brain metastases: an open-label, phase 2 trial. Lancet Oncol 13(5):459–465. doi:10.1016/s1470-2045(12)70090-6

45. Mier JW, Vachino G, Klempner MS, Aronson FR, Noring R, Smith S, Atkins MB (1990) Inhibition of interleukin-2-induced tumor necrosis factor release by dexamethasone: prevention of an acquired neutrophil chemotaxis defect and differential suppression of interleukin-2-associated side effects. Blood 76(10):1933–1940
46. Minniti G, Clarke E, Lanzetta G, Osti MF, Trasimeni G, Bozzao A, Enrici RM (2011) Stereotactic radiosurgery for brain metastases: analysis of outcome and risk of brain radionecrosis. Radiat Oncol 6:48. doi:10.1186/1748-717x-6-48
47. Mitchell MS (1989) Relapse in the central nervous system in melanoma patients successfully treated with biomodulators. J Clin Oncol 7(11):1701–1709
48. Mittapalli RK, Vaidhyanathan S, Dudek AZ, Elmquist WF (2013) Mechanisms limiting distribution of the threonine-protein kinase B-RaF(V600E) inhibitor dabrafenib to the brain: implications for the treatment of melanoma brain metastases. J Pharmacol Exp Ther 344 (3):655–664. doi:10.1124/jpet.112.201475
49. Mornex F, Thomas L, Mohr P, Hauschild A, Delaunay MM, Lesimple T, Clavel M (2003) A prospective randomized multicentre phase III trial of fotemustine plus whole brain irradiation versus fotemustine alone in cerebral metastases of malignant melanoma. Melanoma Res 13 (1):97–103. doi:10.1097/01.cmr.0000043161.28051.2d
50. Narayana A, Mathew M, Tam M, Kannan R, Madden KM, Golfinos JG, Pavlick AC (2013) Vemurafenib and radiation therapy in melanoma brain metastases. J Neurooncol 113(3):411–416. doi:10.1007/s11060-013-1127-1
51. Patchell RA, Tibbs PA, Regine WF, Dempsey RJ, Mohiuddin M, Kryscio RJ, Young B (1998) Postoperative radiotherapy in the treatment of single metastases to the brain: a randomized trial. JAMA 280(17):1485–1489
52. Patchell RA, Tibbs PA, Walsh JW, Dempsey RJ, Maruyama Y, Kryscio RJ, Young B (1990) A randomized trial of surgery in the treatment of single metastases to the brain. N Engl J Med 322(8):494–500. doi:10.1056/nejm199002223220802
53. Patel JK, Didolkar MS, Pickren JW, Moore RH (1978) Metastatic pattern of malignant melanoma. A study of 216 autopsy cases. Am J Surg 135(6):807–810
54. Postow MA, Callahan MK, Barker CA, Yamada Y, Yuan J, Kitano S, Wolchok JD (2012) Immunologic correlates of the abscopal effect in a patient with melanoma. N Engl J Med 366 (10):925–931. doi:10.1056/NEJMoa1112824
55. Radbill AE1, Fiveash JF, Falkenberg ET, Guthrie BL, Young PE, Meleth S, Markert JM (2004) Initial treatment of melanoma brain metastases using gamma knife radiosurgery: an evaluation of efficacy and toxicity. Cancer 101(4):825−833
56. Ramakrishna N, Margolin KA (2013) Multidisciplinary approach to brain metastasis from melanoma; local therapies for central nervous system metastases. Am Soc Clin Oncol Educ Book 33:399–403. doi:10.1200/EdBook_AM.2013.33.399
57. Robert C, Thomas L, Bondarenko I, O'Day S, Jeffrey Weber MD, Garbe C, Wolchok JD (2011) Ipilimumab plus dacarbazine for previously untreated metastatic melanoma. N Engl J Med 364(26):2517–2526. doi:10.1056/NEJMoa1104621
58. Rochet NM, Kottschade LA, Markovic SN (2011) Vemurafenib for melanoma metastases to the brain. N Engl J Med 365(25):2439–2441. doi:10.1056/NEJMc1111672
59. Rosenberg SA, Yang JC, Sherry RM, Kammula US, Hughes MS, Phan GQ, Dudley ME (2011) Durable complete responses in heavily pretreated patients with metastatic melanoma using T-cell transfer immunotherapy. Clin Cancer Res 17(13):4550–4557. doi:10.1158/1078-0432.ccr-11-0116
60. Samlowski WE, Watson GA, Wang M, Rao G, Klimo P Jr, Boucher K, Jensen RL (2007) Multimodality treatment of melanoma brain metastases incorporating stereotactic radiosurgery (SRS). Cancer 109(9):1855–1862. doi:10.1002/cncr.22605
61. Sampson JH, Carter JH Jr, Friedman AH, Seigler HF (1998) Demographics, prognosis, and therapy in 702 patients with brain metastases from malignant melanoma. J Neurosurg 88 (1):11–20. doi:10.3171/jns.1998.88.1.0011

62. Schartz NE, Farges C, Madelaine I, Bruzzoni H, Calvo F, Hoos A, Lebbe C (2010) Complete regression of a previously untreated melanoma brain metastasis with ipilimumab. Melanoma Res 20(3):247–250. doi:10.1097/CMR.0b013e3283364a37
63. Schouten LJ, Rutten J, Huveneers HA, Twijnstra A (2002) Incidence of brain metastases in a cohort of patients with carcinoma of the breast, colon, kidney, and lung and melanoma. Cancer 94(10):2698–2705
64. Schulze B, Meissner M, Wolter M, Rodel C, Weiss C (2014) Unusual acute and delayed skin reactions during and after whole-brain radiotherapy in combination with the BRAF inhibitor vemurafenib. Two case reports. Strahlenther Onkol 190(2):229–232. doi:10.1007/s00066-013-0474-3
65. Soffietti R, Kocher M, Abacioglu UM, Villa S, Fauchon F, Baumert BG, Bottomley A (2013) A European Organisation for Research and Treatment of Cancer phase III trial of adjuvant whole-brain radiotherapy versus observation in patients with one to three brain metastases from solid tumors after surgical resection or radiosurgery: quality-of-life results. J Clin Oncol 31(1):65–72. doi:10.1200/jco.2011.41.0639
66. Soltys SG, Adler JR, Lipani JD, Jackson PS, Choi CY, Puataweepong P, Chang SD (2008) Stereotactic radiosurgery of the postoperative resection cavity for brain metastases. Int J Radiat Oncol Biol Phys 70(1):187–193. doi:10.1016/j.ijrobp.2007.06.068
67. Sperduto PW, Kased N, Roberge D, Xu Z, Shanley R, Luo X, Mehta M (2012) Summary report on the graded prognostic assessment: an accurate and facile diagnosis-specific tool to estimate survival for patients with brain metastases. J Clin Oncol 30(4):419–425. doi:10.1200/jco.2011.38.0527
68. Su F, Viros A, Milagre C, Trunzer K, Bollag G, Spleiss O, Marais R (2012) RAS mutations in cutaneous squamous-cell carcinomas in patients treated with BRAF inhibitors. N Engl J Med 366(3):207–215. doi:10.1056/NEJMoa1105358
69. Topalian SL, Hodi FS, Brahmer JR, Gettinger SN, Smith DC, McDermott DF, Sznol M (2012) Safety, activity, and immune correlates of anti-PD-1 antibody in cancer. N Engl J Med 366 (26):2443–2454. doi:10.1056/NEJMoa1200690
70. Vecht CJ, Haaxma-Reiche H, Noordijk EM, Padberg GW, Voormolen JH, Hoekstra FH et al (1993) Treatment of single brain metastasis: radiotherapy alone or combined with neurosurgery? Ann Neurol 33(6):583–590. doi:10.1002/ana.410330605
71. Wan PT, Garnett MJ, Roe SM, Lee S, Niculescu-Duvaz D, Good VM, Marais R (2004) Mechanism of activation of the RAF-ERK signaling pathway by oncogenic mutations of B-RAF. Cell 116(6):855–867
72. Wolchok JD, Kluger H, Callahan MK, Postow MA, Rizvi NA, Lesokhin AM, Sznol M (2013) Nivolumab plus ipilimumab in advanced melanoma. N Engl J Med 369(2):122–133. doi:10.1056/NEJMoa1302369
73. Yu C, Chen JC, Apuzzo ML, O'Day S, Giannotta SL, Weber JS, Petrovich Z (2002) Metastatic melanoma to the brain: prognostic factors after gamma knife radiosurgery. Int J Radiat Oncol Biol Phys 52(5):1277–1287

Treatment of Uveal Melanoma

Alexander N. Shoushtari and Richard D. Carvajal

Abstract

Uveal melanoma (UM) comprises approximately 5 % of all melanoma diagnoses in the USA each year. Approximately half of patients with UM eventually develop metastases, most commonly involving the liver. Historically, prognosis for these patients has been poor, with death occurring 6–12 months from the time of metastases. Multiple trials of cytotoxic treatments largely extrapolated from cutaneous melanoma have been ineffective in metastatic UM. Trials of regional hepatic-directed therapy have led to high response rates, but these have yet to be translated into a survival benefit. Recently, it was discovered that the majority of UMs harbor activating mutations in genes encoding one of two G-alpha protein subunits, GNAQ and GNA11. This knowledge has led to the rational development of clinical trials specifically for UM utilizing targeted inhibitors of the activated signaling pathways such as mitogen-activated protein kinase, Akt, and protein kinase C. A recent trial of the oral MEK inhibitor selumetinib was the first to show clinical benefit for any systemic therapy in a randomized fashion. This increasing understanding of the biology of UM offers hope that novel treatments will continue to benefit patients with metastatic disease.

A.N. Shoushtari (✉)
Melanoma and Immunotherapeutics Service, Memorial Sloan Kettering Cancer Center, 300 East 66th Street, New York, NY 10065, USA
e-mail: shoushta@mskcc.org

R.D. Carvajal
Melanoma and Experimental Therapeutics Services, Columbia University Medical Center, 161 Fort Washington Avenue, New York, NY 10032, USA
e-mail: rdc2150@cumc.columbia.edu

H.L. Kaufman and J.M. Mehnert (eds.), *Melanoma*,
Cancer Treatment and Research 167, DOI 10.1007/978-3-319-22539-5_12

Keywords
Uveal melanoma · MAP Kinase · MEK · Protein Kinase C · Selumetinib

Abbreviations

BAC	Best alternative care
COMS	Collaborative ocular melanoma study
GEP	Gene expression profiling
MAPK	Mitogen-activated protein kinase
mTOR	Mammalian target of rapamycin
OS	Overall survival
PFS	Progression-free survival
PKC	Protein kinase C
PI3K	Phosphatidylinositide-3 kinase
TACE	Transhepatic arterial chemoembolization
UM	Uveal melanoma
Y	Yttrium

Contents

1 Introduction

1.1 Epidemiology and Initial Presentation

Uveal melanoma (UM) arises from melanocytes of the uveal tract, which consist of the iris, ciliary body, and choroid. UM is the most common primary intraocular malignancy in adults, accounting for 5 % of all melanoma diagnoses each year. The yearly incidence is 5–6 cases per million, and it is more common in males, with a M:F ratio of 1.2:1. The median age at diagnosis is 62 years, and Caucasians comprise approximately 98 % of all reported cases [49].

Most UMs arise within the pigmented nevi, which can present with visual disturbances or as asymptomatic lesions noted on funduscopic examination. A large case series comprising 2514 choroidal nevi followed with the serial examinations noted 13 % transformed into UM by 10 years, signifying that the majority of nevi can safely be followed by ophthalmologists with serial assessments. Risk factors associated with malignant transformation included the presence of visual symptoms, thickness >2 mm, margin near the optic disk, presence of subretinal fluid or orange pigment within the nevus, absence of a surrounding amelanotic "halo," or a hollow lesion on ultrasound [48].

1.2 Staging and Prognosis

In the AJCC 7th Edition Cancer Staging Manual, stage I–III disease is determined by tumor diameter and thickness, as well as the presence of ciliary body or extraocular involvement. Stage IV disease includes disease with evidence of any spread to lymph nodes or other organs. In a large retrospective analysis of 7731 patients, this system stratified for risk of metastasis and death. For example, T1 through T4 tumors had 10-year risk of death of 8, 13, 27 and 43 %, respectively [47].

Distant metastases occur in approximately 50 % of patients within twenty years of initial diagnosis. The liver is the most common site of metastasis, representing the initial site for 60 % of patients and eventually affecting over 90 % [39, 51]. Other common sites of metastasis include the lung, soft tissue, bone, and brain [39]. Perhaps due to the historical lack of efficacious systemic treatment strategies, the prognosis of metastatic disease is dismal. Median overall survival (OS) ranges from 6 to 12 months [5, 39].

Clinical predictors of worse disease outcome include age >60, the presence of hepatic metastases (versus lung or soft tissue), and shorter metastasis-free intervals [39]. Primary tumor features that predict poorer outcomes include larger tumor diameter, thickness, and location in the ciliary body versus the rest of uveal tract [26]. Either cytogenetics or gene expression profiling (GEP) can be utilized to predict whether primary tumors have a high or low risk of metastasis. Cytogenetic markers of high-risk primary tumors include monosomy 3 and 8q24 duplication, which correspond to a worse disease-free and overall survival [8, 50]. A multivariate analysis of cytogenetic and clinicopathologic data from a retrospective series of 356 patients found that monosomy 3, basal diameter, and epithelioid cellularity could distinguish groups with varying 5-year disease-specific mortality [13]. The 5-year risk of death from UM ranged from 0 % in the lowest risk group to 66 % in the highest risk group.

A fifteen-gene GEP panel (DecisionDx-UM, Castle Biosciences) has been prospectively validated to stratify tumors into risk categories corresponding to a <5 or >70 % risk of metastasis at 5 years [34]. In this trial of 459 patients, GEP classification was superior to other clinicopathologic criteria, including chromosome 3 status, in predicting the development of metastases. The five-year risk of metastasis in patients with tumors at lowest risk, GEP "Class 1A"; low risk, GEP "Class 1B"; and high risk, GEP "Class 2" are 2, 21, and 72 %, respectively.

Recently, the genetic underpinnings of varying tumor behavior have become more clear. William Harbour's group discovered a gene on chromosome 3p, BRCA-associated protein 1 (BAP1), that was frequently mutated in UM metastases [17]. In vitro data suggest that BAP1 loss may lead to a more dedifferentiated melanocyte, providing a plausible genetic link between the presence of monosomy 3 and the more aggressive clinical phenotype of these tumors [27].

More recently, tumors with disomy 3 have been shown to have increased frequency of mutations in SF3B1 or EIF1AX that are mutually exclusive with BAP1 [16, 32]. Interestingly, a proportion of tumors with disomy 3 that had developed metastases had SF3B1 mutations in a distinct codon than those seen in tumors without metastases. Further research is ongoing to understand how these and other genetic alterations impact clinical behavior.

2 Local Therapy

Historically, enucleation has been the primary treatment for uveal melanomas. More recently, radiation therapy (RT) has been increasingly utilized in an effort to spare the globe in these patients. Retrospective studies have reported equivalent rates of local control, metastasis, and overall survival for RT and enucleation in medium-sized melanomas [1, 4, 46]. Two broad categories of RT utilize either proton beam or brachytherapy with plaque insertion. The only randomized, Phase III trial (Collaborative Ocular Melanoma Study (COMS)) comparing enucleation with RT utilized plaque Iodine-125 therapy in medium-sized tumors (apical height 2.5–10 mm or basal diameter ≤16 mm). It demonstrated no difference in overall survival at 5 and 12 years [12, 14]. A randomized COMS trial reported no mortality benefit with combined neoadjuvant RT and enucleation for large tumors [18].

Overall, local therapy choices are guided by size of the primary tumor, location relative to the macula, optic disk, or anterior segment, and comorbidities such as visual status of the fellow eye or systemic vasculopathies. Despite improvements in RT and surgical techniques, the rates of distant metastases and disease-specific mortality remain unchanged [11].

3 Regional Therapy

The vast majority of patients with metastatic UM die of sequelae of hepatic metastases. As a result, various combinations of surgery, hepatically directed embolization, chemotherapy, and radiation therapy have been utilized as regional therapy for hepatic metastasis.

Surgical resection is a potential option for a minority of patients with hepatic metastases, particularly those with small-volume disease in one lobe. Published reports suggest that patients with metastatic recurrence greater than 5 years from initial diagnosis can have prolonged recurrence-free intervals following surgical debulking [3, 20]. A French study enrolled 75 patients into a prospective study of laparotomy plus 6 months of hepatically directed intra-arterial chemotherapy with fotemustine, dacarbazine, and/or platinum agents [41]. In the roughly one-quarter of patients with curative resection, median OS improved from 9 months to 22 months. This study suggested little, if any, benefit to surgical resection with grossly positive margins [41].

Tumors in the liver are disproportionately perfused by the arterial system rather than the portal system. Another regional treatment approach, transhepatic arterial chemoembolization (TACE), utilizes microspheres to embolize the hepatic artery and release drug directly into the liver. Various Phase II studies of TACE utilizing cytotoxic agents such as cisplatin, carmustine, and mitomycin have demonstrated objective responses in a minority of patients without the evidence of survival benefit. Patients with lower hepatic tumor burden (<20–25 % involvement) appear to derive more benefit from this approach [21, 35].

To date, two Phase III trials of hepatically directed chemotherapy have been conducted: one trial randomizing 93 patients, 82 of whom had UM, to 4–6 treatments of hepatic arterial infusion of melphalan versus best alternative care per treating physician. The study was powered to detect a 4-month increase in hepatic PFS at a level of 80 %. It met its primary endpoint of increasing hepatic PFS from 49 days to 245 days, albeit with notable toxicity. Three of 40 patients died related to toxicity from hepatically directed treatment, and rates of Grade 3 or higher neutropenia and thrombocytopenia were seen in 61 and 74 %, respectively. An intent-to-treat analysis of overall survival showed no benefit, and this therapy did not receive regulatory approval by the US Food and Drug Administration [38].

The second Phase III trial of hepatically directed chemotherapy utilized intra-arterial versus intravenous of fotemustine in patients who had not received prior therapy [28]. The study was originally designed to detect a hazard ratio (HR) of 0.67 with 85 % power after 220 deaths. Due to poor accrual, an unplanned interim analysis was performed after 134 deaths to assess futility. The study demonstrated an increased response rate of 11 versus 2 %, but OS was unchanged, with HR = 1.09 and a power of 79 %.

Other regional approaches are earlier in development. Sato and colleagues reported a Phase I trial utilizing immunoembolization with granulocyte-macrophage colony-stimulating factor [42]. Despite the fact that the maximum tolerated dose was not reached, 10 of 31 patients had an objective response, and the median OS was 14.4 months. A randomized Phase II trial of immunoembolization versus bland embolization was subsequently completed, and the results are anxiously awaited. Kennedy et al. [23] reported their retrospective experience of 11 patients with UM and hepatic metastases treated with radioembolization utilizing Yttrium-90 microspheres. All 11 patients had PET/CT responses with SUVs declining to less than 2, and 8 of 10 evaluable patients survived to 1 year. A list of ongoing trials of hepatically directed therapy are listed in Table 1.

Table 1 Trials utilizing hepatically directed therapy for uveal melanoma

Intervention	Phase	Sponsor/lead center	Clinicaltrials.gov ID
90-Y microspheres	II	Thomas Jefferson	NCT01473004
Liver transplantation	II	Oslo University	NCT01311466
Isolated hepatic perfusion versus BAC	III	Sahlgrenska University	NCT01785316
Sorafenib + 90-Y microspheres	I	Centre Hospitalier Universitaire Vaudois	NCT01893099
Ipilimumab + 90-Y microspheres	0	Case Comprehensive Cancer Center	NCT01730157

Y Yttrium; *BAC* Best alternative care

4 Systemic Therapy

4.1 Cytotoxic Treatment

Conventional cytotoxic chemotherapy has been ineffective in metastatic UM. A retrospective review of 143 patients with metastatic UM treated at MD Anderson noted 1 objective response [6]. Twelve prospective trials have treated 447 patients with various systemic therapies, and the objective response rate ranged from 0 to 6 % [5, 7, 19, 25, 28, 30, 33, 37, 40, 43–45]. See Table 2 for further details of these trials. Randomized trials in particular have proven challenging, with a Phase III trial of intrahepatic versus intravenous fotemustine terminating early due to poor enrollment [28] and the Phase II trial of sunitinib versus dacarbazine terminating early following pre-planned futility analysis [30].

4.2 Immunotherapy

The immune checkpoint activator ipilimumab is approved for metastatic cutaneous melanoma, but data in uveal melanoma are more limited. Multiple retrospective analyses of heavily pretreated cohorts indicate clinical benefit for a subset of patients [22, 24, 29, 31]. The largest series consisted of 83 patients and reported a 3-month disease control rate of 35 % and a median OS of 6 months [31]. Similar results were reported in a series of 39 patients from Memorial Sloan Kettering Cancer Center, Dana-Farber Cancer Institute, and University Hospital of Lausanne, with a 3-month disease control rate of 46 % and a median OS of 9 months [29].

Thus far, no data have been presented regarding newer immune checkpoint activators that target PD1 and PDL1 in patients with UM. Further study is needed to define the role of immune checkpoint inhibitors in this disease.

Table 2 Selected clinical trials of systemic therapy in uveal melanoma

First author	Phase	Intervention	n	RR (%)	PFS/TTP (months)	OS (months)
Kivelä (2003)	II	BOLD + IFNa2b	22	0	1.9	10.6
Bedikian (2003)	II	Temozolomide	14	0	1.8	6.7
Schmidt-Hieber (2004)	II	Bendamustine	9	0	NR	NR
Schmittel (2005)	II	Cisplatin, Gemcitabine, Treosulfan	17	0	3	7.7
O'Neill (2006)	II	Dacarbazine, Treosulfan	15	0	3	6.9
Schmittel (2006)	II	Treosulfan ± Gemcitabine	48	2	2–3	NR
Penel (2008)	II	Imatinib	10	0	NR	10.8
Homsi (2010)	II	DHA-paclitaxel	22	4	3	9.8
Bhatia (2012)	II	Sorafenib + Carboplatin + Paclitaxel	25	0	4	11
Mahipal (2012)	I	Sunitinib	20	5	4.2	8.2
Leyvraz (2012)	III	Fotemustine (IV vs. HAI)	171	6	3.7–4.5	13–14.6
Sacco (2013)	II	Sunitinib versus Dacarbazine	84	4	2.8–3.9	6.4–8.7

RR response rate; *PFS* progression-free survival; *TTP* time to progression; *OS* overall survival; *BOLD* Bleomycin, Vincristine, Lomustine, Dacarbazine; *IV* intravenous; *HAI* hepatic artery infusion; *MO* months; *DHA* docosahexaenoic acid; *NR* not reported

4.3 Targeted Therapy

Recent insights into the mechanisms of UM tumor growth have provided novel rational therapeutic strategies. Van Raamsdonk and colleagues reported two mutually exclusive activating mutations in G-alpha subunits (GNAQ and GNA11) of UM cells that resulted in constitutive signaling downstream of G-protein-coupled receptors [52, 53]. Several downstream growth signaling pathways are thus upregulated, including mitogen-activated protein kinase (MAPK), protein kinase C (PKC), and phosphatidylinositol-3 kinase (PI3K)/Akt/mammalian target of rapamycin (mTOR) [36]. This discovery has led to the development of a new generation of clinical trials based upon preclinical work by our group and others demonstrating the mutation-dependent anti-tumor effects of MEK, Akt, and PKC pathway inhibition [2, 54].

We led a randomized Phase II trial of the MEK inhibitor selumetinib versus investigator's choice of chemotherapy (temozolomide or dacarbazine) that was the first study to demonstrate clinical efficacy of any agent in a randomized fashion in metastatic UM. PFS increased from 7 weeks with chemotherapy to 16 weeks with selumetinib [9]. Sustained MAPK pathway inhibition was documented on tumor samples after 14 days of selumetinib treatment. Specifically, phosphorylated ERK (pERK) and cyclinD1, downstream effectors of MEK, were decreased by a median of 48 and 76 %, respectively. Radiologic response to selumetinib was significantly correlated with pERK inhibition, and there was a trend toward correlation between

Table 3 Ongoing or recently accrued targeted therapy trials in uveal melanoma

Target(s)	Intervention	Phase	Sponsor/lead center	Clinicaltrials.gov ID
MEK	Dacarbazine ± Selumetinib	II	AstraZeneca	NCT01974752
MEK, Akt	Trametinib ± GSK2141795	II	CTEP/MSKCC	NCT01979523
MEK, PKC	AEB071 + MEK162	I/II	Novartis	NCT01801358
PKC	AEB071	I	Novartis	NCT01430416
PKC, PI3Kα	AEB071 + BYL719	I	Novartis	NCT02273219

CTEP Cancer Therapy Evaluation Program; *MSKCC* Memorial Sloan Kettering Cancer Center

pERK inhibition and clinical benefit. Notably, for the 35 patients who crossed over to selumetinib after progression with chemotherapy, no objective responses were seen, and the rate of any tumor regression dropped from 50 to 23 %. This suggests that the efficacy of MEK inhibition may be decreased in previously treated patients.

Limited results are available for another oral MEK inhibitor, trametinib, in 16 heavily pretreated patients with UM [15]. Trametinib achieved stable disease in 50 % of patients and demonstrated a clinical benefit rate of 25 % at 4 months with no objective responses. This more modest response with trametinib may be attributable to the fact that these patients had received a median of 3 prior therapies, given our data with selumetinib following crossover from chemotherapy as noted above.

Based on the progress afforded by MEK inhibition, additional clinical trials building upon MEK as a backbone are under way. See Table 3 for a list of planned or ongoing trials in UM. Several of these trials are based upon preclinical work demonstrating that multiple pathways, including PKC and PI3K/Akt/mTOR, are activated in UM and may underlie resistance to monotherapy with MEK inhibitors.

A randomized Phase II trial of dacarbazine with or without selumetinib will test the hypothesis that MEK inhibition enhances the cytotoxic effects of chemotherapy (NCT01974752). A Phase I trial of the PKC inhibitor AEB071 (NCT01430416) has demonstrated a median PFS of 15.4 weeks (cite ASCO 2014 abstract found at http://meetinglibrary.asco.org/content/128300-144; Piperno-Neumann et al).

Our group has demonstrated in preclinical models that adding an Akt inhibitor to selumetinib produces a synergistic inhibitory effect on GNAQ mutant UM [2]. Based on these data, we have recently launched a randomized, multicenter Phase II trial of the MEK inhibitor trametinib with or without the Akt inhibitor GSK2141795 for patients with previously untreated metastatic UM (NCT01979523). Boris Bastian's group has shown that combined MEK and PKC inhibition leads to synergistic inhibition of UM growth in vivo [10]. This has led to a combination trial of AEB071 plus MEK162, another oral inhibitor of MEK1/2 (NCT01801358).

Overall, the improved understanding of the molecular mechanisms underlying UM growth has accelerated the pace of developing novel therapeutic strategies. With continued preclinical insights to guide rational drug targets and these novel multicenter clinical trials, there is reason to believe that major advances will be made in treating patients with metastatic UM over the next several years.

5 Conclusion

The relative rarity of uveal melanoma has historically impeded progress in developing novel therapeutic strategies, with interventions extrapolated from cutaneous melanomas. Over the past several years, it has become clear that melanomas arising from the uveal tract are biologically distinct from cutaneous melanomas. Uveal melanomas harbor distinct mutational patterns compared to cutaneous melanomas that may underlie distinct responses to kinase inhibitors as well as cytotoxic and immunologic agents. Given our increasing understanding of relevant molecular targets for in uveal melanoma, future clinical trials promise to improve our ability to treat patients with these tumors.

References

1. Adams KS, Abramson DH, Ellsworth RM, Haik BG, Bedford M, Packer S, Seddon J, Albert D, Polivogianis L (1988) Cobalt plaque versus enucleation for uveal melanoma: comparison of survival rates. Br J Ophthalmol 72(7):494–497
2. Ambrosini G, Musi E, Ho AL, de Stanchina E, Schwartz GK (2013) Inhibition of mutant GNAQ signaling in uveal melanoma induces AMPK-dependent autophagic cell death. Mol Cancer Ther 12(5):768–776. doi:10.1158/1535-7163.mct-12-1020
3. Aoyama T, Mastrangelo MJ, Berd D, Nathan FE, Shields CL, Shields JA, Rosato EL, Rosato FE, Sato T (2000) Protracted survival after resection of metastatic uveal melanoma. Cancer 89(7):1561–1568
4. Augsburger JJ, Correa ZM, Freire J, Brady LW (1998) Long-term survival in choroidal and ciliary body melanoma after enucleation versus plaque radiation therapy. Ophthalmology 105 (9):1670–1678. doi:10.1016/s0161-6420(98)99037-6
5. Bedikian AY, Papadopoulos N, Plager C, Eton O, Ring S (2003) Phase II evaluation of temozolomide in metastatic choroidal melanoma. Melanoma Res 13(3):303–306. doi:10.1097/01.cmr.0000056231.78713.e2
6. Bedikian AY, Legha SS, Mavligit G, Carrasco CH, Khorana S, Plager C, Papadopoulos N, Benjamin RS (1995) Treatment of uveal melanoma metastatic to the liver: a review of the M. D. Anderson cancer center experience and prognostic factors. Cancer 76(9):1665–1670
7. Bhatia S, Moon J, Margolin KA, Weber JS, Lao CD, Othus M, Aparicio AM, Ribas A, Sondak VK (2012) Phase II Trial of sorafenib in combination with carboplatin and paclitaxel in patients with metastatic uveal melanoma: SWOG S0512. PLoS ONE 7(11):e48787. doi:10.1371/journal.pone.0048787
8. Bornfeld N, Prescher G, Becher R, Hirche H, Jöckel KH, Horsthemke B (1996) Prognostic implications of monosomy 3 in uveal melanoma. The Lancet 347(9010):1222–1225
9. Carvajal RD, Sosman JA, Quevedo F, Milhem MM, Joshua AM, Kudchadkar RR, Linette GP, Gajewski T, Lutzky J, Lawson DH, Lao CD, Flynn PJ, Albertini MR, Sato T, Paucar D, Panageas KS, Dickson MA, Wolchok JD, Chapman PB, Schwartz GK (2013) Phase II study

of selumetinib (sel) versus temozolomide (TMZ) in gnaq/Gna11 (Gq/11) mutant (mut) uveal melanoma (UM). J Clini Oncol Official J Am Soc Clin Oncol 31(suppl, abstr CRA9003)
10. Chen X, Wu Q, Tan L, Porter D, Jager MJ, Emery C, Bastian BC (2013) Combined PKC and MEK inhibition in uveal melanoma with GNAQ and GNA11 mutations. Oncogene 2014 Sep 25; 33(39):4724–434. doi:10.1038/onc.2013.418
11. COMS (2005) Development of metastatic disease after enrollment in the coms trials for treatment of choroidal melanoma: collaborative ocular melanoma study group report no. 26. Archives of Ophthalmology 123(12): 1639–1643. doi:10.1001/archopht.123.12.1639
12. COMS (2006) The COMS randomized trial of iodine 125 brachytherapy for choroidal melanoma: V. twelve-year mortality rates and prognostic factors: COMS report No. 28. Arch Ophthalmol 124(12):1684–1693. doi:10.1001/archopht.124.12.1684
13. Damato B, Duke C, Coupland SE, Hiscott P, Smith PA, Campbell I, Douglas A, Howard P (2007) Cytogenetics of uveal melanoma: a 7-year clinical experience. Ophthalmology 114 (10):1925–1931.e1921. doi:http://dx.doi.org/10.1016/j.ophtha.2007.06.012
14. Diener-West M, Earle JD, Fine SL, Hawkins BS, Moy CS, Reynolds SM, Schachat AP, Straatsma BR (2001) The COMS randomized trial of iodine 125 brachytherapy for choroidal melanoma, III: initial mortality findings. COMS Report No. 18. Arch Ophthalmol 119(7):969–982
15. Falchook GS, Lewis KD, Infante JR, Gordon MS, Vogelzang NJ, DeMarini DJ, Sun P, Moy C, Szabo SA, Roadcap LT, Peddareddigari VGR, Lebowitz PF, Le NT, Burris Iii HA, Messersmith WA, O'Dwyer PJ, Kim KB, Flaherty K, Bendell JC, Gonzalez R, Kurzrock R, Fecher LA (2012) Activity of the oral MEK inhibitor trametinib in patients with advanced melanoma: a phase 1 dose-escalation trial. Lancet Oncol 13(8):782–789. doi:10.1016/S1470-2045(12)70269-3
16. Harbour JW, Roberson ED, Anbunathan H, Onken MD, Worley LA, Bowcock AM (2013) Recurrent mutations at codon 625 of the splicing factor SF3B1 in uveal melanoma. Nat Genet 45(2):133–135. doi:10.1038/ng.2523
17. Harbour JW, Onken MD, Roberson EDO, Duan S, Cao L, Worley LA, Council ML, Matatall KA, Helms C, Bowcock AM (2010) Frequent mutation of BAP1 in metastasizing uveal melanomas. Science 330(6009):1410–1413. doi:10.1126/science.1194472
18. Hawkins BS (2004) The Collaborative ocular melanoma study (COMS) randomized trial of pre-enucleation radiation of large choroidal melanoma: IV. Ten-year mortality findings and prognostic factors. COMS report number 24. Am J Ophthalmol 138(6):936–951. doi:10.1016/j.ajo.2004.07.006
19. Homsi J, Bedikian AY, Papadopoulos NE, Kim KB, Hwu WJ, Mahoney SL, Hwu P (2010) Phase 2 open-label study of weekly docosahexaenoic acid-paclitaxel in patients with metastatic uveal melanoma. Melanoma Res 20(6):507–510. doi:10.1097/CMR.0b013e3283403ce9
20. Hsueh EC, Essner R, Foshag LJ, Ye X, Wang HJ, Morton DL (2004) Prolonged survival after complete resection of metastases from intraocular melanoma. Cancer 100(1):122–129. doi:10.1002/cncr.11872
21. Huppert PE, Fierlbeck G, Pereira P, Schanz S, Duda SH, Wietholtz H, Rozeik C, Claussen CD (2010) Transarterial chemoembolization of liver metastases in patients with uveal melanoma. Eur J Radiol 74(3):e38–e44. doi:10.1016/j.ejrad.2009.03.064
22. Kelderman S, van der Kooij MK, van den Eertwegh AJ, Soetekouw PM, Jansen RL, van den Brom RR, Hospers GA, Haanen JB, Kapiteijn E, Blank CU (2013) Ipilimumab in pretreated metastastic uveal melanoma patients. Results of the Dutch Working group on Immunotherapy of Oncology (WIN-O). Acta Oncologica 52(8):1786–1788 (Stockholm, Sweden). doi:10.3109/0284186x.2013.786839
23. Kennedy AS, Nutting C, Jakobs T, Cianni R, Notarianni E, Ofer A, Beny A, Dezarn WA (2009) A first report of radioembolization for hepatic metastases from ocular melanoma. Cancer Invest 27(6):682–690. doi:10.1080/07357900802620893

24. Khattak MA, Fisher R, Hughes P, Gore M, Larkin J (2013) Ipilimumab activity in advanced uveal melanoma. Melanoma Res 23(1):79–81. doi:10.1097/CMR.0b013e32835b554f
25. Kivela T, Suciu S, Hansson J, Kruit WH, Vuoristo MS, Kloke O, Gore M, Hahka-Kemppinen M, Parvinen LM, Kumpulainen E, Humblet Y, Pyrhonen S (2003) Bleomycin, vincristine, lomustine and dacarbazine (BOLD) in combination with recombinant interferon alpha-2b for metastatic uveal melanoma. Eur J Cancer 39(8):1115–1120
26. Kujala E, Damato B, Coupland SE, Desjardins L, Bechrakis NE, Grange JD, Kivela T (2013) Staging of ciliary body and choroidal melanomas based on anatomic extent. J Clin Oncol 31 (22):2825–2831. doi:10.1200/jco.2012.45.2771
27. Landreville S, Agapova OA, Matatall KA, Kneass ZT, Onken MD, Lee RS, Bowcock AM, Harbour JW (2012) Histone deacetylase inhibitors induce growth arrest and differentiation in uveal melanoma. Clin Cancer Res 18(2):408–416. doi:10.1158/1078-0432.ccr-11-0946
28. Leyvraz S, Suciu S, Piperno-Neumann S, Baurain J-F, Zdzienicki M, Testori A, Marshall E, Scheulen ME, Jouary T, Negrier S, Vermorken JB, Kaempgen E, Durando X, Schadendorf D, Gurunath RK, Polders L, de Schaetzen G, Vanderschaeghe S, Gauthier M-P, Keilholz U (2012) Randomized phase III trial of intravenous (IV) versus hepatic intra-arterial (HIA) fotemustine in patients with liver metastases from uveal melanoma: final results of the EORTC 18021 study. J Clin Oncol 30(Suppl, abstract 8532)
29. Luke JJ, Callahan MK, Postow MA, Romano E, Ramaiya N, Bluth M, Giobbie-Hurder A, Lawrence DP, Ibrahim N, Ott PA, Flaherty KT, Sullivan RJ, Harding JJ, D'Angelo S, Dickson M, Schwartz GK, Chapman PB, Wolchok JD, Hodi FS, Carvajal RD (2013) Clinical activity of ipilimumab for metastatic uveal melanoma: a retrospective review of the Dana-Farber Cancer Institute, Massachusetts General Hospital, Memorial Sloan-Kettering Cancer Center, and University Hospital of Lausanne experience. Cancer 119(20):3687–3695. doi:10.1002/cncr.28282
30. Mahipal A, Tijani L, Chan K, Laudadio M, Mastrangelo MJ, Sato T (2012) A pilot study of sunitinib malate in patients with metastatic uveal melanoma. Melanoma Res 22(6):440–446. doi:10.1097/CMR.0b013e328358b373
31. Maio M, Danielli R, Chiarion-Sileni V, Pigozzo J, Parmiani G, Ridolfi R, De Rosa F, Del Vecchio M, Di Guardo L, Queirolo P, Picasso V, Marchetti P, De Galitiis F, Mandala M, Guida M, Simeone E, Ascierto PA (2013) Efficacy and safety of ipilimumab in patients with pre-treated, uveal melanoma. Ann Oncol Official J Eur Soc Med Oncol ESMO 24(11):2911–2915. doi:10.1093/annonc/mdt376
32. Martin M, Masshofer L, Temming P, Rahmann S, Metz C, Bornfeld N, van de Nes J, Klein-Hitpass L, Hinnebusch AG, Horsthemke B, Lohmann DR, Zeschnigk M (2013) Exome sequencing identifies recurrent somatic mutations in EIF1AX and SF3B1 in uveal melanoma with disomy 3. Nat Genet 45(8):933–936. doi:10.1038/ng.2674
33. O'Neill PA, Butt M, Eswar CV, Gillis P, Marshall E (2006) A prospective single arm phase II study of dacarbazine and treosulfan as first-line therapy in metastatic uveal melanoma. Melanoma Res 16(3):245–248. doi:10.1097/01.cmr.0000205017.38859.07
34. Onken MD, Worley LA, Char DH, Augsburger JJ, Correa ZM, Nudleman E, Aaberg TM Jr, Altaweel MM, Bardenstein DS, Finger PT, Gallie BL, Harocopos GJ, Hovland PG, McGowan HD, Milman T, Mruthyunjaya P, Simpson ER, Smith ME, Wilson DJ, Wirostko WJ, Harbour JW (2012) Collaborative ocular oncology group report number 1: prospective validation of a multi-gene prognostic assay in uveal melanoma. Ophthalmology 119(8):1596–1603. doi:10.1016/j.ophtha.2012.02.017
35. Patel K, Sullivan K, Berd D, Mastrangelo MJ, Shields CL, Shields JA, Sato T (2005) Chemoembolization of the hepatic artery with BCNU for metastatic uveal melanoma: results of a phase II study. Melanoma Res 15(4):297–304
36. Patel M, Smyth E, Chapman PB, Wolchok JD, Schwartz GK, Abramson DH, Carvajal RD (2011) Therapeutic implications of the emerging molecular biology of uveal melanoma. Clin Cancer Res Official J Am Assoc Cancer Res 17(8):2087–2100. doi:10.1158/1078-0432.ccr-10-3169

37. Penel N, Delcambre C, Durando X, Clisant S, Hebbar M, Negrier S, Fournier C, Isambert N, Mascarelli F, Mouriaux F (2008) O-Mel-Inib: a Cancero-pole Nord-Ouest multicenter phase II trial of high-dose imatinib mesylate in metastatic uveal melanoma. Invest New Drugs 26 (6):561–565. doi:10.1007/s10637-008-9143-2
38. Pingpank JF HM, Alexander HR, Faries MR, Zager JS, Royal R, Whitman ED, Nutting CW, Siskin GP, Agarwala SS (2010) A phase III random assignment trial comparing percutaneous hepatic perfusion with melphalan (PHP-mel) to standard of care for patients with hepatic metastases from metastatic ocular or cutaneous melanoma. J Clin Oncol 28(18(supp)): LBA8512. Abstract
39. Rietschel P, Panageas KS, Hanlon C, Patel A, Abramson DH, Chapman PB (2005) Variates of survival in metastatic uveal melanoma. J Clin Oncol 23(31):8076–8080. doi:10.1200/jco.2005.02.6534
40. Sacco JJ, Nathan PD, Danson S et al (2013) Sunitinib versus dacarbazine as first-line treatment in patients with metastatic uveal melanoma. J Clin Oncol 31(Suppl, abstract 9031)
41. Salmon RJ, Levy C, Plancher C, Dorval T, Desjardins L, Leyvraz S, Pouillart P, Schlienger P, Servois V, Asselain B (1998) Treatment of liver metastases from uveal melanoma by combined surgery-chemotherapy. Eur J Surg Oncol J Eur Soc Surg Oncol Br Assoc Surg Oncol 24(2):127–130
42. Sato T, Eschelman DJ, Gonsalves CF, Terai M, Chervoneva I, McCue PA, Shields JA, Shields CL, Yamamoto A, Berd D, Mastrangelo MJ, Sullivan KL (2008) Immunoembolization of malignant liver tumors, including uveal melanoma, using granulocyte-macrophage colony-stimulating factor. J Clin Oncol Official J Am Soc Clin Oncol 26(33):5436–5442. doi:10.1200/jco.2008.16.0705
43. Schmidt-Hieber M, Schmittel A, Thiel E, Keilholz U (2004) A phase II study of bendamustine chemotherapy as second-line treatment in metastatic uveal melanoma. Melanoma Res 14 (6):439–442
44. Schmittel A, Scheulen ME, Bechrakis NE, Strumberg D, Baumgart J, Bornfeld N, Foerster MH, Thiel E, Keilholz U (2005) Phase II trial of cisplatin, gemcitabine and treosulfan in patients with metastatic uveal melanoma. Melanoma Res 15(3):205–207
45. Schmittel A, Schmidt-Hieber M, Martus P, Bechrakis NE, Schuster R, Siehl JM, Foerster MH, Thiel E, Keilholz U (2006) A randomized phase II trial of gemcitabine plus treosulfan versus treosulfan alone in patients with metastatic uveal melanoma. Ann Oncology Official J Eur Soc Med Oncol ESMO 17(12):1826–1829. doi:10.1093/annonc/mdl309
46. Seddon JM, Gragoudas ES, Egan KM, Glynn RJ, Howard S, Fante RG, Albert DM (1990) Relative survival rates after alternative therapies for uveal melanoma. Ophthalmology 97 (6):769–777
47. Shields CL, Kaliki S, Furuta M, Fulco E, Alarcon C, Shields JA (2013) American joint committee on cancer classification of posterior uveal melanoma (tumor size category) predicts prognosis in 7731 patients. Ophthalmology 120(10):2066–2071. doi:10.1016/j.ophtha.2013.03.012
48. Shields CL, Furuta M, Berman EL, Zahler JD, Hoberman DM, Dinh DH, Mashayekhi A, Shields JA (2009) Choroidal nevus transformation into melanoma: analysis of 2514 consecutive cases. Arch Ophthalmol 127(8):981–987. doi:10.1001/archophthalmol.2009.151
49. Singh AD, Turell ME, Topham AK (2011) Uveal melanoma: trends in incidence, treatment, and survival. Ophthalmology 118(9):1881–1885. doi:10.1016/j.ophtha.2011.01.040
50. Sisley K, Rennie IG, Parsons MA, Jacques R, Hammond DW, Bell SM, Potter AM, Rees RC (1997) Abnormalities of chromosomes 3 and 8 in posterior uveal melanoma correlate with prognosis. Genes Chromosom Cancer 19(1):22–28
51. The Collaborative Ocular Melanoma Study G (2001) Assessment of metastatic disease status at death in 435 patients with large choroidal melanoma in the collaborative ocular melanoma study (coms): Coms report no. 15. Arch Ophthalmol 119(5):670–676. doi:10.1001/archopht.119.5.670

52. Van Raamsdonk CD, Bezrookove V, Green G, Bauer J, Gaugler L, O'Brien JM, Simpson EM, Barsh GS, Bastian BC (2009) Frequent somatic mutations of GNAQ in uveal melanoma and blue naevi. Nature 457(7229):599–602. doi:10.1038/nature07586
53. Van Raamsdonk CD, Griewank KG, Crosby MB, Garrido MC, Vemula S, Wiesner T, Obenauf AC, Wackernagel W, Green G, Bouvier N, Sozen MM, Baimukanova G, Roy R, Heguy A, Dolgalev I, Khanin R, Busam K, Speicher MR, O'Brien J, Bastian BC (2010) Mutations in GNA11 in uveal melanoma. New Engl J Med 363(23):2191–2199. doi:10.1056/NEJMoa1000584
54. Wu X, Li J, Zhu M, Fletcher JA, Hodi FS (2012) Protein kinase C inhibitor AEB071 targets ocular melanoma harboring GNAQ mutations via effects on the PKC/Erk1/2 and PKC/NF-κB Pathways. Mol Cancer Ther 2012 Sep; 11(9):1905–1914. doi:10.1158/1535-7163.mct-12-0121

Mucosal Melanoma: Epidemiology, Biology and Treatment

Kristen R. Spencer and Janice M. Mehnert

Abstract

Mucosal melanoma is an exceedingly rare variant of cutaneous melanoma that, due to its rarity, is poorly described and infrequently studied. Primary sites of origin include the head and neck, anorectum and vulvovaginal regions. It is uniquely different from cutaneous melanoma with respect to epidemiology, etiology, pathogenesis and prognosis. The etiology and pathogenesis remain unclear. Unlike cutaneous melanoma, exposure to UV light is not an apparent risk factor. Furthermore, distinct molecular features including a lower incidence of *BRAF* oncogene mutations but a higher incidence of *KIT* oncogene mutations suggest divergent genetic etiologies. Mucosal melanomas generally present at a later stage, are more aggressive and carry a worse prognosis regardless of the stage at diagnosis. Establishing standardized treatment guidelines has been challenging due to the rarity of the disease. Early detection provides the best chance at survival but is often difficult due to anatomic location. Surgery remains the primary therapeutic intervention if complete resection is technically feasible given the anatomic location. Radiotherapy may be used to achieve local control when resection is not feasible, or adjuvantly to enhance locoregional control, but most studies have failed to demonstrate an improvement in overall survival.

K.R. Spencer (✉) · J.M. Mehnert
Rutgers Cancer Institute of New Jersey, 195 Little Albany Street,
New Brunswick, NJ 08901, USA
e-mail: spencekr@rwjms.rutgers.edu

J.M. Mehnert
e-mail: mehnerja@cinj.rutgers.edu

H.L. Kaufman and J.M. Mehnert (eds.), *Melanoma*,
Cancer Treatment and Research 167, DOI 10.1007/978-3-319-22539-5_13

There are no consensus guidelines on the optimal systemic therapy, and regimens are often extrapolated from data based on therapies used to treat advanced cutaneous melanoma. Clinical trials, particularly utilizing newer targeted therapies and immunotherapies, are investigating novel treatment approaches.

Keywords
KIT · Mucosal · Melanoma · Imatinib · BRAF · Immunotherapy · Targeted

Contents

1 Introduction

Mucosal melanoma is an exceedingly rare variant of cutaneous melanoma [7, 14, 24, 29, 41, 45–49, 54, 57, 63], representing approximately 0.03 % of all cancer diagnoses [38] and 1.3 % of all melanomas [3, 7, 9, 10, 14, 29, 31, 38, 41, 46, 48, 54–57]. It was first described in 1856 by Weber et al., but not classified as its own distinct disease process until 1869 by Lucke [28, 38, 57]. Unfortunately, because of its rarity, it is a poorly described and infrequently studied disease process, and as a result there is a paucity of consistent data regarding its epidemiology, etiology and pathogenesis, as well as limited data to support general recommendations regarding its proper diagnosis and treatment [14, 28, 29, 46, 57].

Mucosal melanomas can arise from any mucosal surface [9, 14, 29, 31, 41, 45, 48, 55, 57], most typically the mucosal epithelium of the respiratory, alimentary and genitourinary tracts, where melanocytes are present [3, 10, 28, 31, 41, 45, 47, 54, 57]. Primary sites of origin include the head and neck (55 %), the anorectum (24 %) and the vulvovaginal region (18 %) [3, 7, 9, 10, 14, 29, 38, 41, 45, 47, 50, 54, 56, 57]. Less frequently, mucosal melanoma has been found in the urinary tract (3 %) [3, 7, 10, 29, 46, 56, 57], as well as the tracheobronchial tree, esophagus, stomach, small and large intestine, gall bladder and cervix [9, 10, 28].

2 Etiology

Mucosal melanoma is a distinct entity from cutaneous melanoma with respect to epidemiology, etiology, pathogenesis and prognosis [24, 26, 28, 29, 41, 46, 48, 49, 54, 55, 57]. While the incidence of cutaneous melanoma is rapidly increasing in the United States, the incidence of mucosal melanoma appears stable [9, 10, 21, 25, 29, 41, 46, 48, 56, 57]. In general, patients with mucosal melanoma present at a much later age, about one to two decades later than cutaneous melanoma [14, 29, 46, 54], with a majority of cases reported between the ages of 50–80 [10, 14, 28, 29, 31, 38, 41, 45, 54, 56, 63], and a median age at diagnosis of 70 [9, 21, 46, 48]. Females are diagnosed more often than males [7, 9, 10, 14, 21, 28, 29, 31, 41, 46, 48, 56], in many reports up to twice as often [9, 14, 29, 41, 48], due to cases of vulvovaginal disease, with estimated prevalence in the United States at 2.8 cases per million women versus 1.5 cases per million men [29, 41]. Notably, a slight male predominance in cases of the head and neck mucosal melanoma subtypes has been suggested [14, 45, 46]. Overall mucosal melanoma does not seem to have a racial predilection, although it makes up a higher percentage of overall melanoma cases diagnosed in Black, Asian and Hispanic populations, likely reflecting the lower incidence of cutaneous melanoma in these populations. It has also been described that considered separately, mucosal melanoma of the oral cavity may be more common in Black and Japanese populations [9, 10, 38].

The etiology and pathogenesis of mucosal melanoma remain unclear [14, 38, 41, 46]. To date there are no clearly established risk factors for its development [7, 9, 14, 48, 57]. Unlike cutaneous melanoma, the common anatomic locations for mucosal melanoma preclude exposure to UV light as a risk factor [7, 9, 14, 21, 24, 26, 28, 29, 38, 41, 46, 48, 54, 56, 57]. There is no definitive evidence that common carcinogens such as tobacco and formaldehyde, or exposure to carcinogenic viruses such as the human papilloma viruses, human herpes viruses or polyomavirus have a role in its pathogenesis [7, 29, 38, 41, 48, 54]. Nevertheless, some studies have suggested various correlations between the mucosal melanoma subtypes and various predisposing risk factors, though strong evidence for any of these correlations is lacking [9]. Melanocytes have an established role in the sinonasal region in the metabolization of polycyclic aromatic hydrocarbons, suggesting a link between inhaled environmental and immune factors and the development of sinonasal mucosal melanoma [9, 38, 46, 57]. Because of the higher incidence of oral cavity mucosal melanoma in the Japanese population, some researchers have suggested a correlation between this particular subtype and unidentified common hereditary or environmental factors [38, 41, 46, 54, 57, 63]. In addition, up to one third of oral cavity mucosal melanomas appear to be preceded by melanosis, which has been suggested to represent the radial growth phase prior to the vertical growth phase [9, 38, 41, 43, 45, 46, 48, 54, 57, 63], a phenomenon reported in head and neck mucosal melanoma as well [43, 57]. Although no direct correlation has been established, 66 % of patients with laryngeal or pharyngeal mucosal melanoma have a history of smoking [38]. Anorectal mucosal melanoma appears to be more prevalent in patients with HIV [9, 28, 54, 63]. Finally, vulvovaginal mucosal melanoma has been suggested to be associated with chronic inflammatory conditions, viral infections and chemical irritants. Genetic factors may also play in the development of vulvovaginal disease, as 15 % of patients with vulvar mucosal melanoma provide a family history of cutaneous melanoma, and one study reported a patient with vulvar mucosal melanoma with a germline mutation in the melanocortin type I receptor [9, 46, 54].

3 Molecular Biology

Mucosal melanomas have distinct molecular features that suggest divergent genetic etiologies (see Fig. 1) [8, 29, 31, 41, 46, 49, 54]. Studies of comparative genomic hybridization have shown distinct chromosomal aberrations such as gains of 1q, 6p and 8q [29, 54], gain of function mutations such as K642E, L576P, D816H and

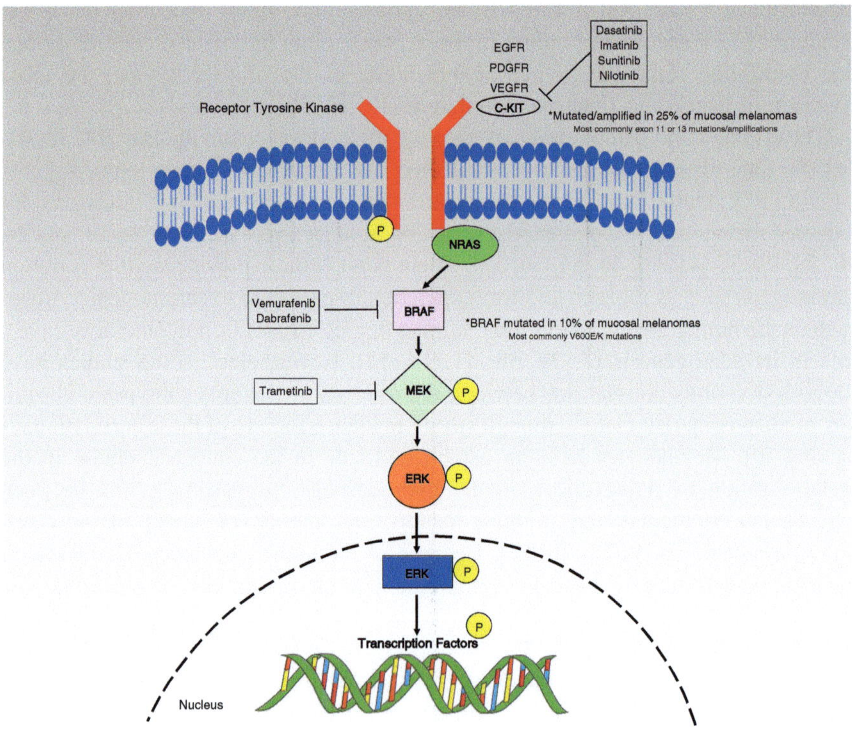

Fig. 1 Signaling pathways and therapeutic targets in mucosal melanoma

V559A [38, 54] and amplifications of the 4q12 locus [54]. While the incidence of activating mutations in the BRAF oncogene is quite common in cutaneous melanoma, it appears to be rare in mucosal melanoma, with an incidence estimated at 10 % [3, 7–9, 19, 29, 38, 41, 46, 48–50, 54, 56, 61]. More salient from a treatment perspective is that mucosal melanomas appear to have a high incidence of activating mutations and/or amplifications in the KIT oncogene. Curtin et al. first demonstrated the presence of KIT mutations in mucosal melanomas and estimated the rate of these mutations to be 39 %, while similar mutations were found in cases of non-chronic, sun damaged cutaneous melanoma cases [3, 12, 38, 41, 50, 54]. Beadling et al. found KIT mutations in 15.6 % of mucosal melanoma cases studied [4, 41, 62]. Finally, Carvajal et al. reported that of 295 tumor samples screened for the presence of KIT mutations or amplifications, abnormalities were found in 25 % [9, 48], a rate of KIT mutations and/or amplifications that has been similar across multiple reports [7–9, 19, 24, 26, 29, 31, 38, 39, 48–50, 54, 61, 62].

4 Prognosis

Mucosal melanomas are often aggressive and carry a worse prognosis, regardless of the stage at the time of diagnosis [3, 9, 14, 22, 26, 28, 29, 31, 32, 38, 41, 45, 46, 48, 54–57, 62, 63]. In contrast to cutaneous melanomas, mucosal melanomas more frequently are amelanotic and present in a multifocal fashion [2]. While different staging systems are in place for mucosal melanomas of different primary sites, a generalized staging system can be utilized as follows: Stage I, clinically localized disease; Stage II, regional nodal involvement; and Stage III, distant metastatic involvement [2]. The often concealed locations of mucosal melanoma present a challenge for routine screening and result in frequent presentations of advanced disease [3, 9, 14, 22, 26, 28, 29, 31, 32, 38, 41, 45, 46, 48, 54–57, 62, 63]. In addition, unique to these anatomic locations are vast vascular and lymphatic networks in close proximity to the primary tumor, allowing for diffuse spread [9, 14, 28, 29, 46, 54, 57], with approximately one third of patients having nodal involvement at diagnosis [10, 14, 29, 38, 45, 46]. Local treatment failure is common [48, 54, 55], with recurrences rates suggested to be as high as 50–90 % even with complete surgical resection [9]. Local recurrences are considered a harbinger for simultaneous or subsequent metastatic spread [43, 48, 54]. In all likelihood, most patients have micrometastatic disease at the time of presentation, resulting in a disease course characterized by local recurrences followed by metastatic disease, even despite aggressive surgical resection and adjuvant therapy [3, 7, 14, 29, 31, 32, 38, 46, 48, 54, 55, 57]. Thus, even for patients with presumed early-stage disease, the prognosis is poor, with 5 year survival rates of only 25 % [3, 9, 10, 22, 28, 29, 31, 32, 38, 43, 45, 46, 54, 55].

5 Treatment

Establishing guidelines for the clinical course of mucosal melanoma has been challenging due to the rarity of the disease. This renders conducting large, randomized, controlled trials to investigate various treatment modalities in this particular melanoma subtype difficult [3, 7, 14, 29, 46, 54], thus standards of care have not been formulated. As well, assumptions regarding the natural history and appropriate management of mucosal melanoma are based on retrospective case series, which are often limited by small numbers of cases and inconsistent treatment regimens [29, 43, 48]. Like most malignancies, early detection still provides the best chance at survival, but is difficult as previously discussed [14, 45, 46, 54]. Surgical considerations are often dictated by the anatomic location of the tumor, with adjuvant radiotherapy a consideration for local control. Limited data exist concerning adjuvant systemic therapy for the disease, and systemic treatments for distant disease often follow established paradigms for cutaneous melanoma [7, 14, 28, 29, 31, 41, 57], unless targets unique to mucosal melanoma are discovered within the primary or metastatic tumor.

5.1 Surgery

Surgery remains the primary therapeutic intervention for mucosal melanoma [9]. Regardless of subtype, when technically feasible, complete resection for local control provides the best chance at prolonged disease-free survival and cure, especially in light of the lack of effective systemic treatment options [9, 10, 14, 28, 46, 54, 57]. Unfortunately, complete resection is often challenging due to the anatomy of the commonly involved regions and the tendency for these tumors to have a lentiginous growth pattern [9, 14, 31, 48, 54, 55, 57]. Historically, the surgical management of mucosal melanoma involved radical procedures such as abdominoperineal resections (APR) for anorectal disease and pelvic exenteration for vulvovaginal disease [7, 9, 32, 48]. These operations resulted in significant morbidity and functional impairments [7, 9, 32]. While studies have shown improved local control with aggressive surgical resection, retrospective reports suggest they confer no overall survival benefit over more conservative techniques [7, 9, 32, 48]. Furthermore, because most patients will develop local recurrences and ultimately metastatic disease regardless of the intervention chosen, multiple additional considerations such as patient preference and quality of life often become more relevant considerations [9, 14, 32, 48, 57]. Thus, in general, conservative procedures by way of wide local excisions have replaced aggressive procedures as primary management [9, 48]. In addition, recent evidence has suggested that less-invasive endoscopic resections may be a feasible alternative for achieving aggressive local control with less morbidity for patients. This may become particularly relevant for patients with multiple local recurrences requiring repeat resections and patients with multifocal disease [9].

Lymph node status remains a controversial topic when discussed in relationship to mucosal melanoma. Unlike cutaneous melanoma, where lymph node status is a vital prognostic factor, the implications of lymph node status in cases of mucosal melanoma are less apparent. Toward that end, there is no widely accepted standard of care for the management of lymph nodes in mucosal melanoma [9]. As with other types of malignancies, evaluation of the sentinel lymph node has become routine in cases of cutaneous melanoma [9]. While this is often feasible in cases of mucosal melanoma, because of the uncertainty surrounding the prognostic importance of a positive finding, the role of sentinel lymph node biopsies remains undefined. Moreover, in light of the known course of this disease to involve frequent recurrences and distant metastases despite aggressive therapy, the question of if and how a positive sentinel lymph node should change subsequent therapy remains [9, 48]. Similarly, while most are in agreement that therapeutic lymph node dissection is reasonable to address clinically apparent, bulky or symptomatic disease, the performance of prophylactic lymphadenectomy is falling out of favor [14]. Anatomic location of a mucosal melanoma also influences surgical treatment options, as summarized below.

5.1.1 Mucosal Melanomas of the Head and Neck

Mucosal melanoma of the head and neck region constitutes 55 % of all mucosal melanomas, but <10 % of all melanomas of the head and neck region [3, 7, 9, 10, 14, 28, 29, 38, 41, 45, 47, 50, 54, 56, 57]. A majority of these tumors are found in the sinonasal regions (~55 %), while the rest are located in the oral cavity (25–40 %) [9, 28, 38, 41, 46–48, 54, 56, 57]. Among sinonasal cases, approximately 80 % are located in the nasal cavity itself, most commonly the turbinates and lateral nasal wall [9, 28, 38, 41, 43, 46, 54], while 20 % occur in the paranasal sinuses, most commonly the maxillary and ethmoid sinuses, followed by the frontal and sphenoid sinuses [9, 28, 38, 41, 46, 54]. Lesions in the oral cavity are most commonly found in the large palate and upper alveolus [9, 28, 38, 41, 46, 47, 54, 57]. Lesions within the larynx or pharynx are extremely rare, with only sixty cases reported in the literature.

Table 1 AJCC staging of melanoma of head and neck

Stage III	T3N0M0
Stage IVA	T4a*N0M0 T3* or T4a, N1, M0
	*T3 Mucosal disease *T4a Moderately advanced disease involving the deep soft tissue, bone, cartilage, or overlying skin
Stage IVB	T4b*, Any N, M0
Stage IVC	Any T, Any N, M1
	*T4b Very advanced disease involving the brain, dura, skull base, lower cranial nerves (IX, I, XI, XII), masticator space, carotid artery, prevertebral space or mediastinal structures N1 Regional nodal disease present M1 Distant disease present [9, 16, 43, 47]

*signify AJCC definition of what T3 or T4a/b means.

These tumors are most commonly located in the supraglottic region (62.2 %) followed by the vocal cords (37.8 %) [28, 38, 41, 46].

The American Joint Committee on Cancer (AJCC) staging system for head and neck mucosal melanoma is often utilized, beginning at stage III (see Table 1). The primary therapeutic modality is complete surgical resection for mostly localized stage III and IVA disease [3, 14, 41, 43, 46–48, 54, 57, 63]. The type of surgical approach used is dependent upon the location and extension of the tumor, but the goal is negative margins with minimal cosmetic or functional derangements [43, 47]. Surgery is not advised for very advanced stage IVB or metastatic stage IVC disease aside from attempting to achieve local control for symptomatic purposes [47, 48]. Unfortunately, achieving melanoma-free margins is often procedurally challenging due to the anatomical complexity of the region and the close proximity of critical anatomic structures [41, 43, 44, 48, 54, 57, 63]. The primary approach should be accompanied by appropriate surgical reconstruction for the area [14, 48, 54, 57]. However, rates of recurrence and widespread disease remain high [43, 48, 57]; it is thus difficult to justify the use of radical surgical procedures in a majority of patients, and morbidity should be a prime consideration [43]. In the setting of local recurrence, repeat surgical resections may be considered, but only after performing an extensive re-staging work-up [48]. For the multitude of reasons above, endoscopic resections are being performed more frequently to avoid the morbidity associated with open procedures [43, 48].

As discussed previously, although biopsy of the sentinel lymph node is technically feasible in head and neck mucosal melanoma, because of the uncertain prognostic implications provided by the sentinel node and the ambiguity of how it guides further management, its role in diagnosis is still under investigation [9, 27, 48, 54]. Unlike many other malignancies, the clinical significance of detecting a positive sentinel lymph node remains uncertain, as there are no clear data to suggest that outcomes are improved if management is altered to address discovered nodal disease [48]. The role of prophylactic lymph node dissection is contested as well. It is often recommended in cases of oral cavity mucosal melanoma because of the high incidence of lymph node involvement, but in cases of sinonasal disease, where the lymph nodes are less commonly involved, elective dissection is not routinely recommended [47, 54]. There is also evidence to suggest that, even in cases of oral cavity melanoma, prophylactic neck dissection does not change ultimate outcomes [48, 57]. Therapeutic neck dissection is considered in patients with clinically evident nodal disease for the purposes of local control and to address symptomatic concerns [47, 48, 57]. Much like elective lymph node dissection, there is no compelling evidence to suggest therapeutic dissection results in an overall survival benefit, even in patients without an eventual lymph node recurrence, suggesting that this procedure should be reserved for patients with clinically apparent nodal disease requiring local control, and not done empirically [48, 57].

5.1.2 Mucosal Melanomas of the Anus and Rectum

Anorectal mucosal melanoma represents 24 % of all mucosal melanomas, but <1 % of all malignant tumors of the anorectal region [3, 7, 9, 10, 14, 28, 29, 32, 38, 41, 45–47, 50, 54, 56, 57, 63]. The area known as the transitional zone of the anal canal harbors a variety of epithelial cells, including squamous-type, and the presence of melanocytes is known here, particularly beneath the dentate line [7, 28, 46, 54, 57]. The concentration of melanocytes increases distally from the dentate line toward the anoderm. For this reason, it is presumed anorectal mucosal melanoma arises within melanocytes distal to the dentate line, then has a tendency to extend proximally into the rectum [7, 28, 46, 54, 57]. There are rare cases of melanocytes present in the intestinal mucosal epithelium above the dentate line in normal patients, thus, melanoma at times can arise in the proximal anus or distal rectum [7, 54]. It is important to note, however, that only 1/3 of anorectal mucosal melanomas are pigmented, and that the presence of amelanotic melanoma is an adverse prognostic sign. Mucosal anorectal melanomas must be differentiated from anal melanomas of cutaneous origin, as the latter are more likely to behave like typical cutaneous melanomas. Approximately one third of anorectal mucosal melanoma cases are thought to originate within the anal canal, while 42 % arise from the rectum and 25 % have an indeterminate origin [9, 48]. Perineural invasion, tumor size, and thickness have also been found to be adverse prognostic factors.

Similarly to head and neck mucosal melanoma, the mainstay of treatment for anorectal melanoma is surgical resection, though there is no standard of care or agreed upon optimal approach as in colorectal carcinoma [7, 46, 50, 54, 57, 63]. Historically more aggressive surgical approaches were considered to be superior, and abdominoperineal resection (APR) was the standard of care [7, 9, 32, 48]. Once retrospective reviews of clinical outcomes data were available, and it was suggested that the extent of the surgical intervention did not significantly improve overall survival [7, 9, 14, 32, 46, 48, 54, 57], more conservative, sphincter-sparing, wide local excisions became the procedure of choice [7, 14, 32, 41, 48, 54, 57]. There has been some suggestion that performing an APR improves local control and recurrence rates over wide local excisions, but the benefit of that control appears limited. Local recurrence rates have been estimated at 8 % with APR versus 20 % with wide local excision, but as stated, this has not resulted in an improvement in overall survival [7, 14, 32, 41, 46, 48, 54, 57]. Furthermore, on multivariate analysis, type of resection was not shown to be significantly associated with prognosis [57].

The goal, of course, remains to achieve negative surgical margins if feasible, as studies have suggested a survival benefit in patients where negative margins are obtained. One study showed a 5-year survival rate of 19 % in patients with negative surgical resection margins, versus 6 % in those with positive margins [7]. APR remains an option for patients with bulky locally confined disease, and in some patients with local recurrences after conservative excision, though it still confers high morbidity and functional limitations [14, 32, 54]. As in the other subtypes of mucosal melanoma, because most patients develop recurrences and distant disease regardless of primary surgical intervention, and because of the aforementioned controversy over the impact of the extent of surgery on clinical outcomes, quality of life considerations should be a top priority [7, 32, 48].

The diagnostic and therapeutic considerations surrounding lymph nodes in cases of head and neck mucosal melanoma translate to cases of anorectal melanoma. Nodal involvement is also of uncertain prognostic significance in this mucosal melanoma subtype, as studies have suggested that regional lymph node metastases have not affected disease recurrence or survival rates. Additionally, data suggest prophylactic lymph node dissection is not associated with improved long-term prognosis. Thus, there is no established role for sentinel lymph node biopsy or indication for elective lymph node dissection [7, 9, 48, 57]. Therapeutic lymphadenectomy should be offered in cases of clinically apparent disease. It should be noted, however, that because the lymphatic drainage of the anorectum differs by tumor location, either superficial inguinal lymph nodes or hypogastric and obturator lymph nodes (and subsequently the sigmoid and peri-aortic rectal groups) may be involved [48, 57]. Thus, there may be significant morbidity associated with such lymph node dissections.

5.1.3 Mucosal Melanomas of the Vulva and Vagina

Vulvovaginal mucosal melanoma represents 18 % of all mucosal melanomas, while vulvar melanoma accounts for 10 % of all vulvar malignancies and vaginal <3 % of all vaginal malignancies [3, 7, 9, 10, 14, 21, 22, 28, 29, 38, 41, 45–47, 50, 54, 56, 57, 63]. Melanoma of the cervix and uterus are quite rare [28, 41, 46]. Vulvar melanomas vastly outnumber vaginal melanomas, with <5 % of vulvovaginal mucosal melanomas arising from the vagina [9, 21, 22, 41, 46, 48, 54]. Some reports suggest up to 20 % of cases are multi-focal, and the precise site is unidentifiable [9, 41, 54]. This is also complicated by the fact that vulvar melanomas may extend to the mucocutaneous vaginal border, obscuring the primary site of origin [46]. Of vulvar melanomas, most cases arise from the labia minora, clitoris, or inner labia majora [9, 22, 41, 46, 57, 59, 63]. The periurethral area and vaginal introitus are less commonly involved [26, 41, 57, 63]. Of vaginal melanomas, most are confined to the lower third of the vagina and the anterior wall [5, 9, 17, 28, 41, 46, 57, 63]. Bleeding, discharge, and palpation of a discernible mass are common presenting signs [5, 17, 59]. Vulvar melanomas are actually staged according to the 2002 TNM staging system for melanoma, whereas vaginal melanomas are staged by the generalized staging system discussed earlier in this chapter [5, 46, 59]. Five year survival rates for vulvar melanoma range from 24 to 77 %, and are poorer for vaginal melanoma, with rates of 5–25 % [5, 59].

Similar to anorectal melanoma, aggressive surgical approaches were the standard of care in the past, and among the options were vulvectomy, vaginectomy, urethrocystectomy, radical hysterectomy and pelvic exenteration [9, 14, 21, 22, 41, 46, 48, 54, 57]. As with anorectal melanoma, though studies have shown improved local control with these more aggressive approaches, retrospective data suggests they result in no significant improvement in overall survival as compared to more conservative, wide local excisions, thus they have fallen out of favor [9, 14, 21, 22,

41, 46, 48, 54, 57, 59]. In light of the high rates of local recurrence and metastatic spread, the benefit of improved local control is called into question, making patient preference and functional deformity important considerations [9, 14, 48, 57]. Unfortunately, obtaining negative margins without aggressive surgical procedures may be technically difficult due to the multifocality of these tumors and the anatomic constraints of the region [57]. In general, 1 cm margins should be obtained for small melanomas <1 mm; 2 cm margins can be entertained for patients with larger tumors, if possible. When wide local excision is not technically feasible, more aggressive approaches may be judiciously considered, or excision may be combined with adjuvant radiation in the setting of close or positive margins [41]. Cervical and uterine mucosal melanomas are generally still treated with radical procedures such as radical hysterectomies and vaginectomies with lymphadenectomies [28, 41].

Again, the issue of lymph node management in vulvovaginal mucosal melanoma is unclear [48]. However, sentinel lymph node mapping is feasible in patients with vulvar melanoma and recommended by some experts [35], although studies have yielded conflicting results regarding the prognostic relevance and effects on overall survival [21, 48]. While prophylactic lymph node dissection may reduce the chance of recurrence in the lymph node bed, it does not appear to impact outcomes [21, 54, 57]. Lymphadenectomy may be considered on a therapeutic basis in the setting of clinically apparent or symptomatic disease [48]. In contrast, sentinel lymph node mapping for vaginal melanomas is likely to be difficult given the complexity of lymph node drainage to the pelvic and/or inguinal basins, and cannot routinely be recommended [35].

5.1.4 Mucosal Melanomas of Other Rare Sites

Mucosal melanoma has been reported in a number of exceedingly rare sites, including the tracheobronchial tree, esophagus, stomach, small and large intestine, biliary tract, and urinary tract. Primary melanoma of the lung, specifically the tracheobronchial tree is extremely rare, with only approximately thirty cases reported in the literature [28, 41]. The treatment of choice is lobectomy and pneumonectomy in conjunction with lymph node resection. The role of adjuvant therapies, including both radiotherapy and chemotherapy, is undefined [41]. Mucosal melanoma of the esophagus is also rare, representing 0.1–0.2 % of all esophageal malignancies [28, 41, 46, 63] with just over 300 cases reported as of 2011 [63]. It is predominantly confined to the middle and lower parts of the esophagus, with only 10 % of cases located in the upper third [28, 41, 57, 63]. Radical surgical resections with nodal dissections are often the chosen primary treatment, though they have not been demonstrated to improve survival [28, 41, 46, 57]. Adjuvant therapy has been used in these cases in a palliative role [41]. Mucosal melanoma of the stomach constitutes 2.7 % of mucosal melanomas of the GI tract, with <20 cases reported in the literature [41]. Melanoma of the small intestine comprises 2.3 %, and is most commonly located in the ileum [41]. Melanoma of the biliary tract represents 1.4 % of mucosal melanomas of the GI tract, with only nine cases of bile duct and thirty cases of gallbladder melanoma reported [28, 41]. Finally, mucosal melanoma of the large intestine makes up 0.9 %, with only twelve cases reported to date [41]. Surgery is still the mainstay of therapy, and as is the trend in mucosal melanoma, has not improved overall survival [41].

Mucosal melanoma of the urinary tract includes melanomas of the urethra and bladder. Urethral melanoma represents 3 % of all mucosal melanomas, and only 4 % of all urethral malignancies, with only about 25 cases in males and 40 cases in females reported [28, 41, 46, 63]. There have only been around 20 cases of bladder melanoma reported [28, 41]. Urethral melanoma is most commonly located in the distal urethra, followed next in frequency by the meatus [41, 46, 57, 63]. Thus, treatment typically involves partial penectomy or urethrectomy with or without inguinal lymph node dissection. In the cases of more proximal urethral lesions, radical cystoprosto urethectomy or anterior exenteration may be required [46]. The optimal extent of surgery still remains undefined, and additional options have been used in female patients including radiotherapy and cryosurgery [41, 46]. Bladder melanoma is predominantly treated with surgical resection [41]. Regardless of approach used, the survival benefit is limited [46].

5.1.5 Radiotherapy

Radiotherapy may be used to achieve local control in patients with mucosal melanoma for whom surgical resection is not possible, or to enhance control after surgery particularly when resection is suboptimal, a not infrequent occurrence given the anatomic locations of these tumors. Most studies have failed to demonstrate an improvement in overall survival with adjuvant radiotherapy, although these findings are complicated by the fact that there is a tendency for radiotherapy to be favored in more advanced cases [9, 43]. Radiation is also clearly useful for most of these tumors in the palliative setting to control symptomatic local disease [41, 46, 57]. Multiple ongoing studies to investigate newer technologies that are capable of more precise delivery of radiotherapy such as protons and heavy ions that take advantage of higher linear energy transfer [9] may better define the role for radiation in the upfront management of these tumors.

With regard to mucosal melanomas of the head and neck, most clinicians agree on the use of adjuvant radiotherapy when surgery is not appropriate or feasible, and in the setting of extracapsular disease, two or more nodes involved, large nodes (3 cm or greater), positive or close margins and in the setting of residual disease or recurrence after primary surgical resection [43, 46, 47, 54, 57], and on omission of RT in clinically sensitive locations such as the eye. While several studies have accounted improved local control with the addition of radiotherapy, overall survival is not significantly affected [41, 43, 47, 48, 54, 57]. The use of prophylactic radiotherapy without clinically apparent disease post-operatively or in the above indications is contested, with some recommending post-operative radiotherapy in almost all cases because of the high risk of potentially devastating local recurrence, while others argue against its use as it has not been demonstrated to improve recurrence rates even in spite of that risk [54]. Although not an exclusive test of radiotherapy in mucosal melanoma, the Trans-Tasman randomized trial of radiotherapy or observation after lymphadenectomy for patients with high-risk melanoma can safely be extrapolated to mucosal presentations. This trial demonstrated a significant improvement in LR recurrence (HR 0.56), but without improvements in RFS or OS. The fractionation used in the RT arm was 48 Gray (Gy) in 20 fractions [6]. With respect to additional reports of optimal dosing and fractionation, a series of 28 patients reported a 49 % local control rate at 3 years using a treatment schedule of 50–55 Gy in 15–16 fractions; a similar 44 % local control rate was achieved in 25 patients treated with 8 Gy on days 7 and 21 [18, 23]. Of note, Moreno et al. reported standard fractionation at a dose greater than 54 Gy resulted in superior results as compared to a hypofractionated schedule, with locoregional failure rates of 54.6 % versus 100 % respectively [43]. Some retrospective studies noted better local control with modification of dose schedule, whereas others note both improved local control and overall survival [9, 43].

Importantly, radiotherapy has also been useful as an adjunct to sphincter-sparing local excision in anorectal melanomas, as an alternative to APR in order to preserve quality of life [32, 41, 48], although even in reports of high local control rates, 5 year survival remains low [30]. Similarly in patients with vaginal melanomas, where pelvic exenteration would be required for complete excision with unclear impact on survival, radiation may be an important tool to enhance local control when used adjuvantly and may reduce morbidity if used in the neoadjuvant setting. The fractionation schedule for radiation used for anal or vulvovaginal melanoma is based on patient and tumor anatomy with careful consideration of expected acute and chronic toxicities; with standard fractionation schedules used in the adjuvant or neoadjuvant setting and hypofractionation used primarily in the palliative or limited postoperative setting. However, no improvement in overall survival in vaginal or vulvovaginal melanoma has been reported in two recent studies, respectively [17, 33]; as such the role of radiation is largely to palliate local or metastatic disease.

5.2 Systemic Therapy

There are no consensus guidelines on the optimal systemic therapy for mucosal melanoma. Most conclusions regarding systemic therapies to date are based on case reports on a limited number of patients [3, 22, 32]. As a result, systemic therapy regimens vary widely [3, 22, 32] and are extrapolated from data based on therapies used to treat advanced cutaneous melanoma [3, 9, 50]. Contributing to the ambiguity is that many past and ongoing studies have excluded patients with mucosal melanoma [3]. Even still, with limited data available, no systemic therapy has been shown to significantly improve outcomes [9, 14, 19, 31, 57]. As it stands, the medial overall survival reported with most treatment regimens is 4.9–9.7 months [25]. Chemotherapy, targeted therapies and immunotherapies have each been examined in small studies (Table 2) and form the basis of ongoing clinical trials examining novel approaches.

Table 2 Summary of major systemic therapies impacting treatment of mucosal melanoma

Author	Study type	Agents investigated	Conditions	Major results
Lian	Phase II	Surgery alone versus high-dose IFN-α (IFN) versus temozolomide + cisplatin	Resected mucosal melanoma	• RFS surgery alone 5.4 mos; vs. 9.4 mos HDI; 20.8 mos combination chemotherapy • Median OS surgery alone 21.2 mos; vs. HDI 40.4 mos; vs. 48.7 mos combination chemotherapy
Kim	Retrospective analysis	Combinations of biochemotherapies: cisplatin, vinblastine, dacarbazine, IFA & interleukin-2 (IL-2)	Metastatic anorectal mucosal melanoma	• 8 (44 %) major responses • 2 (11 %) CR • Median PFS 6.2 mos • Median OS 12.2 mos
Harting	Retrospective analysis	Combinations of biochemotherapies: cisplatin, vinblastine, dacarbazine, IFN & IL-2 in first line setting	Advanced vulvovaginal mucosal melanoma	• 4 (36 %) PR • 0 CR • Median PFS 3 mos • Median OS 10 mos
Bartell	Retrospective analysis	Combinations of biochemotherapies: cisplatin, vinblastine, dacarbazine, IFN & IL-2	Advanced head and neck mucosal melanoma	• 3 (20 %) PR • 4 (27 %) CR • Median PFS 10 mos • Median OS 22 mos
Carvajal	Single arm Open-label Phase II	Imatinib	Advanced melanoma with KIT mutations or amplifications	• 2 (8 %) CR • 4 (16 %) PR-2 (50 %) durable, 2 (50 %) transient • 5 (20 %) SD • Median PFS 12 weeks • Median OS 46.3 weeks
Guo	Single arm Open-label Phase II	Imatinib	Metastatic melanoma with KIT mutations or amplifications	• 10 (23.3 %) PR • 13 (30.2 %) SD • Median PFS 3.5 mos • Median OS 14 mos

(continued)

Table 2 (continued)

Author	Study type	Agents investigated	Conditions	Major results
Hodi	Multi-center Phase II	Imatinib	Advanced acral, mucosal or chronically sun-damaged melanoma with KIT mutations and/or amplifications	• 7 (28 %) PR • 5 (20 %) CR • Median PFS 3.7 mos • Median OS 12.5 mos
Postow	Multi-center Retrospective analysis	Ipilimumab	Unresectable or metastatic mucosal melanoma	• By immune-mediated response criteria: 1 CR, 1 PR, 6 SD, 22 PD By WHO response criteria: 1 CR, 1 PR, 5 SD, 23 PD • Median OS 6.4 mos
Del Vecchio	Expanded access program	Ipilimumab	Metastatic mucosal melanoma	• RR 12 % • Immune-mediated disease control rate 36 % • Median PFS 4.3 mos • Median OS 6.4 mos

5.2.1 Chemotherapy

The benefit of adjuvant chemotherapy in mucosal melanoma is unclear. There has been some experience among these patients with cisplatin and interferon, but outcomes in general show limited benefit. Some studies even suggest a possible decrease in survival rates in cases where these agents have been tried [46, 57]. However, as mentioned above, systematic trials of chemotherapy regimens specifically involving mucosal melanoma patients are lacking [54]. In a single study of 189 Chinese patients with resected mucosal melanoma, chemotherapy prolonged relapse free survival versus interferon or observation (20.8 vs. 9.4 and 5.4 months) and significantly increased overall survival (49 vs. 40 and 21 months) [36].

There are limited data regarding the efficacy of additional chemotherapeutic agents in mucosal melanoma patients, and while some retrospective series suggest these therapies produce responses in these patients equivalent to those seen in cases of cutaneous melanoma, others have demonstrated mucosal melanoma patients have worse outcomes in similar dacarbazine-based regimens [9, 48]. A trial examining the combination of chemotherapy with bevacizumab in advanced patients is under way (Table 3). Small retrospective series exist reporting antitumor activity of biochemotherapy based regimens similar to those in cutaneous melanoma [3, 32]. Kim et al. reported the retrospective evaluation of cisplatin, vinblastine, dacarbazine, IFN-a 2b and/or IL-2 in patients with anorectal mucosal melanoma [3, 22, 32, 48]. Of 18 treated patients, 8 patients (44 %) had major responses, including two (11 %) with complete responses. Median time to progression of evaluated patients was 6.2 months and the median overall survival was 12.2 months. Prolonged survival was seen in a subset of treated patients ranging from 14.0 to 43.7 months, and response rates were highest in those who received treatment first line [32, 48]. Harting et al. looked at eleven patients with advanced vulvovaginal mucosal melanoma treated with biochemotherapy in the first line, with roughly a third of the patients achieving a partial response, and median follow-up at 10 months demonstrating median overall survival of 10 months [22, 48]. Finally, a third study by Bartell et al. evaluated variations of the above regimen in fifteen patients with advanced head and neck mucosal melanoma, demonstrating four patients (27 %) with complete responses and three patients (20 %) with partial responses. The median time to progression was 10 months, though again a longer time to progression (50 months) was observed among responding patients; median overall survival was 22 months [3, 48].

These studies discussed suggest response rates in advanced mucosal melanoma patients that parallel rates in cutaneous melanoma patients treated with comparable regimens [48]. Unfortunately, a phase three trial of patients with cutaneous melanoma treated with identical biochemotherapy regimens failed to confirm a survival benefit, and significant toxicity is sustained; the authors of these studies concluding that this approach could be considered in judiciously selected patients [3, 22, 48]. While this introduces doubt into the strength of evidence in favor of biochemotherapy, it also hints at the possibility that, like other alternative therapies, there is a subset of melanoma patients that may derive benefit from these regimens [3, 48].

Table 3 Mucosal melanoma trials in progress (Ongoing and Planned)

Trial name	Phase	Agent	Conditions
A phase II trial of PLX3397 in the treatment of KIT mutated advanced acral and mucosal melanoma	II	KIT inhibitor	Advanced acral melanoma Advanced mucosal melanoma
A randomized phase II study evaluating the activity of bevacizumab in combination with carboplatin plus paclitaxel in patients with previously untreated advanced mucosal melanoma	II	VEGF inhibitor	Metastatic mucosal melanoma
A phase II trial of Nilotinib in the treatment of patients with c-KIT mutated advanced acral and mucosal melanoma	II	Tyrosine kinase inhibitor	Advanced mucosal lentiginous melanoma Advanced acral lentiginous melanoma
A phase II trial of dasatinib in patients with unresectable locally advanced or stage IV mucosal, acral and vulvovaginal melanomas	II	Tyrosine kinase inhibitor	Locally advanced or metastatic mucosal melanoma Locally advanced or metastatic acral melanoma
A phase II study of imatinib in patients with mucosal or acral/lentiginous melanoma and melanomas that arise on chronically sun damaged skin	II	Tyrosine kinase inhibitor	Acral melanoma Mucosal melanoma Melanoma of chronically sun damaged skin
A phase II study of SU011248 in patients with metastatic mucosal or acral/lentiginous melanoma	II	Tyrosine kinase inhibitor	Metastatic mucosal lentiginous melanoma Acral lentiginous melanoma
Phase II study of Nilotinib in metastatic melanoma with KIT aberrations	II	Tyrosine kinase inhibitor	Metastatic melanoma with c-KIT Aberrations
A phase II study of Nilotinib (AMN107) in TKI resistant or intolerant patients with metastatic mucosal, acral or chronically sun damaged melanoma	II	Tyrosine kinase inhibitor	Metastatic acral melanoma Metastatic mucosal melanoma Melanoma of chronically sun damaged skin

Targeted Therapies

A better comprehension of the pathogenesis of mucosal melanoma, in particular its molecular aberrations, has provided important insights into targets for future therapies [9, 29, 54, 62]. As mentioned previously, a large portion of mucosal melanomas, regardless of subset, have mutations and/or amplifications in the *KIT* oncogene which encodes for a receptor tyrosine kinase protein involved in multiple processes of cell division and survival [3, 7–9, 19, 24, 26, 29, 31, 38, 39, 41, 48–50, 54, 61, 62]. Imatinib is an inhibitor of multiple tyrosine kinases, including *KIT* [8, 9, 19, 24, 26]. The initial clinical trials of imatinib showed the agent to be ineffective in a general population of patients with advanced cutaneous melanoma [8, 19, 24, 26, 61, 62]. While the early studies of the drug were coming to a close, Curtin et al. published their identification of *KIT* gene aberrations (discussed above), prompting researchers to begin examining tumors for *KIT* abnormalities and treat identified cases with tyrosine kinase inhibitors with activity against KIT [8, 12, 26, 62]. Since that time there has been anecdotal evidence that imatinib results in rapid and durable tumor responses to KIT inhibitors specifically in patients with *KIT* mutations [29, 31, 41, 48, 54, 61]. Lutzky et al. were among the first investigators to report a complete response to imatinib therapy in the case of a 69 year old woman with advanced loco-regional mucosal melanoma of the anus harboring both a mutation and an amplification of *KIT* [39, 62]. Hodi et al. then reported a patient with primary anal melanoma with a mutation of *KIT*, most specifically a seven-codon duplication in exon 11. This patient demonstrated a near-complete response as measured by PET/CT as well as a greater than 50 % reduction in tumor volume after only 2 weeks of therapy with imatinib [19, 24, 62].

After these observational reports, several clinical trials of imatinib in patients with melanoma specifically bearing *KIT* alterations have subsequently taken place [8, 19, 26, 29, 41, 48, 54, 62]. Carvajal et al. conducted a single-arm, open-label, phase two clinical trial and reported the effects of imatinib on 25 evaluable patients with melanoma harboring *KIT* mutations. Their study showed 2 complete responses and 4 partial responses, two of which were transient, and five had stable disease for 12 weeks or more. The overall durable response rate was 16 %, with the four patients with durable responses maintaining disease stability for more than a year. The median overall survival was 46.3 weeks. All six patients with responses were noted to have mutations in L576P on exon 11 or K642E on exon 13; both with complete responses had both an L576P exon 11 mutation and a concomitant *KIT* amplification [8, 26, 48, 62].

In a second single-arm, open-label phase II clinical trial of imatinib in patients with *KIT* mutations or amplifications, Guo et al. studied 43 patients, with partial responses observed in 10 (23 %) while 13 patients (30 %) had stable disease. A majority of the patients who responded had *KIT* mutations in exons 11 and 13, though one patient with a KIT amplification alone responded. The median progression free survival time was 3.5 months, and the median overall survival was 14 months [19, 26].

Finally, Hodi et al. conducted a multicenter, phase II clinical trial of imatinib in 24 patients with advanced acral, mucosal or chronically sun-damaged melanoma with *KIT* mutations and/or amplifications, including 17 patients with mucosal melanoma. There was an overall disease control rate of 50 %, again favoring patients with *KIT* aberrations. Partial responses were seen in 7 of the 13 patients with *KIT* mutations (54 %), but no responses in patients with *KIT* amplifications or without KIT deviations [26].

Patients with *KIT* anomalies have also been reported to positively respond to other *KIT* inhibitors such as sorafenib, dasatinib and sunitinib [31, 50, 54, 61, 62]. Quintas-Cardama et al. described a case of a 79 year old male with *KIT* positive metastatic anal mucosal melanoma who was treated with temozolomide and sorafenib and achieved a complete response for 5 months before eventually expiring from progressive disease [50, 61, 62]. Woodman, et al. described two cases of metastatic mucosal melanoma in patients with L576P *KIT* mutations treated with dasatinib. Both of these patients had a significant reduction in tumor burden (>50 %) and elimination of tumor by PET imaging, one of which who had previously failed therapy with imatinib. This also suggests melanoma with L576P *KIT* mutations that are resistant to imatinib may be sensitive to additional KIT inhibitors. Unfortunately, both patients developed tumor re-growth by PET imaging after 4 months of treatment [61, 62]. Finally, Zhu et al. detailed a patient with *KIT* mutated metastatic nasal melanoma who received sunitinib and had a partial response with tumors shrinking by 70 % which was maintained 5 months after the initiation of therapy at the time of publication [64].

Taken collectively, these reports demonstrate that, while genetically selected tumors with *KIT* anomalies have better response rates to *KIT* inhibitors than the general population, these responses are variable. However, there is a pattern that suggests tumors with specific *KIT* alterations may be more likely to respond to these agents than others. Multiple reports suggested aberrations in exon 11 (most commonly L576P) and exon 13 (most commonly K642E) have better and longer sustained responses over tumors with *KIT* amplifications or *KIT* alterations in other regions [8, 9, 19, 26, 48, 50, 61, 62, 64]. These findings suggest perhaps only a few *KIT* variations are truly oncogenic and are appropriate targets for therapy [8, 26]. Furthermore, they suggest not all *KIT* alterations equivocally forecast benefit from *KIT* inhibition, but that further molecular discrimination may be required to better identify patients for which these agents are appropriate [8, 9, 19, 26, 48, 62].

Unfortunately, most patients who demonstrate an initial response to *KIT* inhibiting agents will only achieve brief periods of disease response and resistance ultimately leads to progressive disease. This is in contrast to other malignancies where *KIT* inhibition is commonly used, such as chronic myelogenous leukemia (CML) and gastrointestinal stromal tumors (GIST), where durable responses commonly occur [48]. While the mechanism of resistance in GIST tumors is understood to involve the acquisition of additional, unique KIT mutations, the mechanisms behind resistance to *KIT* inhibition in mucosal melanoma are unclear [19, 26, 48]. Some have suggested it may be due to pre-existing concomitant mutations in a variety of other oncogenes, while others have implicated acquired resistance mechanisms, particularly in the case of KIT amplifications. There is limited data available for both hypotheses [26], with more investigation in this area warranted. Indeed, multiple clinical trials are ongoing to further define the activity of KIT inhibition in populations of *KIT* mutant tumors, and to examine the use of additional KIT inhibiting agents (Table 3).

Finally, some mention of the role of BRAF inhibition in the treatment of mucosal melanomas is warranted given the albeit small presence of *BRAF* V600E mutations in about 10 % of mucosal melanomas [3, 7–9, 19, 29, 38, 41, 46, 48–50, 54, 56, 61]. As covered more thoroughly in Chap. 10, vemurafenib and dabrafenib are inhibitors of *BRAF* that specifically harbor an activating mutation wherein valine is substituted for glutamic acid at position 600. These agents have been approved for the treatment of metastatic melanoma based on trials that have shown superior response rates, progression free and overall survival in melanoma compared with chemotherapy [1, 11]. As almost all tumors become resistant to single agent BRAF inhibition, combinatorial therapy with MEK inhibition was studied in two randomized phase III trials, both of which have shown superior progression free survival [34, 37] and most recently overall survival with trametnib/dabrafenib [52]. The question remains whether patients with mucosal melanoma with *BRAF* mutations will see similar response rates to BRAF or BRAF/MEK inhibition as has been seen in patients with cutaneous melanoma. This has yet to investigated [9], although BRAF and MEK inhibitor therapy in mucosal melanomas with *BRAF* V600 mutations is a reasonable scientific approach for patients not able to participate in protocols.

5.2.2 Immunotherapies

In 2011, the FDA issued approval for ipilimumab, which has been shown to improve overall survival in advanced cutaneous melanoma [8, 9, 25, 48, 49, 51]. The approval of immune checkpoint inhibitor therapies for the treatment of advanced melanoma, which have the ability to produce long term durable remissions, has revolutionized the treatment of this disease and are detailed further in Chap. 10. Ipilimumab is a fully human, IgG antibody that targets cytotoxic T lymphocyte-associated antigen 4 (CTLA-4), an inhibitor receptor on T cells. By blocking this receptor, ipilimumab enhances T cell activation and proliferation, thus enhancing anti-tumor immunity [9, 11, 25, 48, 49, 51]. Ipilimumab is the first therapy to demonstrate a survival advantage in a randomized phase III trial [9, 25]. Mucosal melanoma patients were not specifically excluded from this study, but there were few in the study population [25, 48].

To date there have been no randomized trials of ipilimumab in mucosal melanoma patients, but anecdotal cases of benefit with use of this agent have been reported [9, 48, 49]. A multicenter, retrospective analysis of 33 patients with either unresectable or advanced mucosal melanoma treated with ipilimumab described one complete response, one partial response, six cases of stable disease and twenty two with progressive disease after 12 weeks of therapy. The overall durable response rate was 6.7 %, consistent with the rates of 4.2–10.9 % reported in patients with cutaneous melanoma who underwent ipilimumab monotherapy. The median overall survival was 6.4 months with a range of 1.8–26.7 months. Although these response rates were comparatively low, this study demonstrated ipilimumab could result in antitumor effects in patients specifically with mucosal melanoma [49]. An additional analysis of 71 patients with mucosal melanoma treated as part of an expanded access program in Italy showed a 12 % response rate and immune related disease control rate of 36 %; progression free survival and overall survival were 4.3 and 6.4 months [13].

The landscape of treatment for cutaneous melanoma has been further transformed by the development of inhibitors of programmed death 1 (PD-1) receptor and programmed death receptor ligand (PDL 1). Anti PD-1 inhibitors have yielded impressive durable responses in phase I trials [20, 58], as well as improved progression free survival in melanoma compared with chemotherapy [15], and improved overall survival was observed in patients wild type for BRAF mutation compared with chemotherapy [53]. Response rates are yet higher in patients treated with anti-CTLA-4 and anti-PD-1 combinations accompanied by higher toxicity [60]. To date, one case report documents a durable response of a mucosal melanoma patient treated with the anti-PD 1 antibody pembrolizumab following treatment with ipilimumab; this patient also experienced hypothyroidism and rhabdomyolysis as a consequence of therapy [42]. Clinical trials to assess the efficacy of checkpoint inhibition in the subset of patients with mucosal melanoma will further evaluate potential therapeutic benefits of anti-PD-1 inhibitors, alone or in combination with other checkpoint inhibitors or immunomodulatory agents.

Given the ever-evolving intricacies of tumor pathogenesis as well as the complex mechanics of our own immune response, combination therapy is the next logical step in cancer research in order to broaden clinical responses and prevent the development of resistance to single agents, which has been shown to develop rapidly [40]. In addition, novel agents that have been shown to be efficacious in one setting should continue to be investigated in additional settings that make scientific sense. The aforementioned therapies are only the beginning in a promising future for mucosal melanoma patients.

References

1. Ascierto PA, Minor D, Ribas A, Lebbe C, O'Hagan A, Arya N, Guckert M, Schadendorf D, Kefford RF, Grob JJ, Hamid O, Amaravadi R, Simeone E, Wilhelm T, Kim KB, Long GV, Martin AM, Mazumdar J, Goodman VL, Trefzer U (2013) Phase II trial (BREAK-2) of the BRAF inhibitor dabrafenib (GSK2118436) in patients with metastatic melanoma. J Clin Oncol 31(26):3205–3211. doi:10.1200/JCO.2013.49.8691
2. Ballantyne AJ (1970) Malignant melanoma of the skin of the head and neck. An analysis of 405 cases. Am J Surg 120(4):425–431
3. Bartell HL, Bedikian AY, Papadopoulos NE, Dett TK, Ballo MT, Myers JN, Hwu P, Kim KB (2008) Biochemotherapy in patients with advanced head and neck mucosal melanoma. Head Neck 30(12):1592–1598. doi:10.1002/hed.20910
4. Beadling C, Jacobson-Dunlop E, Hodi FS, Le C, Warrick A, Patterson J, Town A, Harlow A, Cruz F 3rd, Azar S, Rubin BP, Muller S, West R, Heinrich MC, Corless CL (2008) KIT gene mutations and copy number in melanoma subtypes. Clin Cancer Res 14(21):6821–6828. doi:10.1158/1078-0432.CCR-08-0575
5. Borazjani G, Prem KA, Okagaki T, Twiggs LB, Adcock LL (1990) Primary malignant melanoma of the vagina: a clinicopathological analysis of 10 cases. Gynecol Oncol 37(2):264–267

6. Burmeister BH, Henderson MA, Ainslie J, Fisher R, Di Iulio J, Smithers BM, Hong A, Shannon K, Scolyer RA, Carruthers S, Coventry BJ, Babington S, Duprat J, Hoekstra HJ, Thompson JF (2012) Adjuvant radiotherapy versus observation alone for patients at risk of lymph-node field relapse after therapeutic lymphadenectomy for melanoma: a randomised trial. Lancet Oncol 13(6):589–597. doi:10.1016/S1470-2045(12)70138-9
7. Carcoforo P, Raiji MT, Palini GM, Pedriali M, Maestroni U, Soliani G, Detroia A, Zanzi MV, Manna AL, Crompton JG, Langan RC, Stojadinovic A, Avital I (2012) Primary anorectal melanoma: an update. J Cancer 3:449–453. doi:10.7150/jca.5187
8. Carvajal RD, Antonescu CR, Wolchok JD, Chapman PB, Roman RA, Teitcher J, Panageas KS, Busam KJ, Chmielowski B, Lutzky J, Pavlick AC, Fusco A, Cane L, Takebe N, Vemula S, Bouvier N, Bastian BC, Schwartz GK (2011) KIT as a therapeutic target in metastatic melanoma. JAMA 305(22):2327–2334. doi:10.1001/jama.2011.746
9. Carvajal RD, Spencer SA, Lydiatt W (2012) Mucosal melanoma: a clinically and biologically unique disease entity. J Natl Compr Cancer Netw JNCCN 10(3):345–356
10. Chang AE, Karnell LH, Menck HR (1998) The National Cancer Data Base report on cutaneous and noncutaneous melanoma: a summary of 84,836 cases from the past decade. The American College of Surgeons Commission on Cancer and the American Cancer Society. Cancer 83(8):1664–1678
11. Chapman PB, Hauschild A, Robert C, Haanen JB, Ascierto P, Larkin J, Dummer R, Garbe C, Testori A, Maio M, Hogg D, Lorigan P, Lebbe C, Jouary T, Schadendorf D, Ribas A, O'Day SJ, Sosman JA, Kirkwood JM, Eggermont AM, Dreno B, Nolop K, Li J, Nelson B, Hou J, Lee RJ, Flaherty KT, McArthur GA, Group B-S (2011) Improved survival with vemurafenib in melanoma with BRAF V600E mutation. N Engl J Med 364(26):2507–2516. doi:10.1056/NEJMoa1103782
12. Curtin JA, Busam K, Pinkel D, Bastian BC (2006) Somatic activation of KIT in distinct subtypes of melanoma. J Clin Oncol 24(26):4340–4346. doi:10.1200/JCO.2006.06.2984
13. Del Vecchio M, Di Guardo L, Ascierto PA, Grimaldi AM, Sileni VC, Pigozzo J, Ferraresi V, Nuzzo C, Rinaldi G, Testori A, Ferrucci PF, Marchetti P, De Galitiis F, Queirolo P, Tornari E, Marconcini R, Calabro L, Maio M (2014) Efficacy and safety of ipilimumab 3 mg/kg in patients with pretreated, metastatic, mucosal melanoma. Eur J Cancer 50(1):121–127. doi:10.1016/j.ejca.2013.09.007
14. DeMatos P, Tyler DS, Seigler HF (1998) Malignant melanoma of the mucous membranes: a review of 119 cases. Ann Surg Oncol 5(8):733–742
15. Dummer R, Daud A, Puzanov I, Hamid O, Schadendorf D, Robert C, Schachter J, Pavlick A, Gonzalez R, Hodi F, Cranmer L, Blank C, O'Day S, Ascierto P, Salama A, Li NX, Zhou W, Lis J, Ebbinghaus S, Kang P, Ribas A (2015) A randomized controlled comparison of pembrolizumab and chemotherapy in patients with ipilimumab-refractory melanoma. Journal of Translational Medicine 13(Suppl 1):O5
16. Edge SB, Compton CC (2010) The American Joint Committee on Cancer: the 7th edition of the AJCC cancer staging manual and the future of TNM. Ann Surg Oncol 17(6):1471–1474. doi:10.1245/s10434-010-0985-4
17. Frumovitz M, Etchepareborda M, Sun CC, Soliman PT, Eifel PJ, Levenback CF, Ramirez PT (2010) Primary malignant melanoma of the vagina. Obstet Gynecol 116(6):1358–1365. doi:10.1097/AOG.0b013e3181fb8045
18. Gilligan D, Slevin NJ (1991) Radical radiotherapy for 28 cases of mucosal melanoma in the nasal cavity and sinuses. Br J Radiol 64(768):1147–1150
19. Guo J, Si L, Kong Y, Flaherty KT, Xu X, Zhu Y, Corless CL, Li L, Li H, Sheng X, Cui C, Chi Z, Li S, Han M, Mao L, Lin X, Du N, Zhang X, Li J, Wang B, Qin S (2011) Phase II, open-label, single-arm trial of imatinib mesylate in patients with metastatic melanoma harboring c-Kit mutation or amplification. J Clin Oncol 29(21):2904–2909. doi:10.1200/JCO.2010.33.9275

20. Hamid O, Robert C, Daud A, Hodi FS, Hwu WJ, Kefford R, Wolchok JD, Hersey P, Joseph RW, Weber JS, Dronca R, Gangadhar TC, Patnaik A, Zarour H, Joshua AM, Gergich K, Elassaiss-Schaap J, Algazi A, Mateus C, Boasberg P, Tumeh PC, Chmielowski B, Ebbinghaus SW, Li XN, Kang SP, Ribas A (2013) Safety and tumor responses with lambrolizumab (anti-PD-1) in melanoma. N Engl J Med 369(2):134–144. doi:10.1056/NEJMoa1305133
21. Hardie C, Siddiqui N (2011) Primary Malignant Melanoma of the Vulva and Vagina. In: Reed N, Green JA, Gershenson DM, Siddiqui N, Connor R (eds) Rare and uncommon gynecologic cancers. Springer, New York
22. Harting MS, Kim KB (2004) Biochemotherapy in patients with advanced vulvovaginal mucosal melanoma. Melanoma Res 14(6):517–520
23. Harwood AR, Cummings BJ (1982) Radiotherapy for mucosal melanomas. Int J Radiat Oncol Biol Phys 8(7):1121–1126
24. Hodi FS, Friedlander P, Corless CL, Heinrich MC, Mac Rae S, Kruse A, Jagannathan J, Van den Abbeele AD, Velazquez EF, Demetri GD, Fisher DE (2008) Major response to imatinib mesylate in KIT-mutated melanoma. J Clin Oncol 26(12):2046–2051. doi:10.1200/JCO.2007.14.0707
25. Hodi FS, O'Day SJ, McDermott DF, Weber RW, Sosman JA, Haanen JB, Gonzalez R, Robert C, Schadendorf D, Hassel JC, Akerley W, van den Eertwegh AJ, Lutzky J, Lorigan P, Vaubel JM, Linette GP, Hogg D, Ottensmeier CH, Lebbe C, Peschel C, Quirt I, Clark JI, Wolchok JD, Weber JS, Tian J, Yellin MJ, Nichol GM, Hoos A, Urba WJ (2010) Improved survival with ipilimumab in patients with metastatic melanoma. N Engl J Med 363(8):711–723. doi:10.1056/NEJMoa1003466
26. Hodi FS, Corless CL, Giobbie-Hurder A, Fletcher JA, Zhu M, Marino-Enriquez A, Friedlander P, Gonzalez R, Weber JS, Gajewski TF, O'Day SJ, Kim KB, Lawrence D, Flaherty KT, Luke JJ, Collichio FA, Ernstoff MS, Heinrich MC, Beadling C, Zukotynski KA, Yap JT, Van den Abbeele AD, Demetri GD, Fisher DE (2013) Imatinib for melanomas harboring mutationally activated or amplified KIT arising on mucosal, acral, and chronically sun-damaged skin. J Clin Oncol 31(26):3182–3190. doi:10.1200/JCO.2012.47.7836
27. Hurria A, Dale W, Mooney M, Rowland JH, Ballman KV, Cohen HJ, Muss HB, Schilsky RL, Ferrell B, Extermann M, Schmader KE, Mohile SG, Cancer, Aging Research G (2014) Designing therapeutic clinical trials for older and frail adults with cancer: U13 conference recommendations. Journal Clin Oncol 32 (24):2587–2594. doi:10.1200/JCO.2013.55.0418
28. Hussein MR (2008) Extracutaneous malignant melanomas. Cancer Invest 26(5):516–534. doi:10.1080/07357900701781762
29. Keller DS, Thomay AA, Gaughan J, Olszanski A, Wu H, Berger AC, Farma JM (2013) Outcomes in patients with mucosal melanomas. J Surg Oncol 108(8):516–520. doi:10.1002/jso.23445
30. Kelly P, Zagars GK, Cormier JN, Ross MI, Guadagnolo BA (2011) Sphincter-sparing local excision and hypofractionated radiation therapy for anorectal melanoma: a 20-year experience. Cancer 117(20):4747–4755. doi:10.1002/cncr.26088
31. Kim HS, Kim EK, Jun HJ, Oh SY, Park KW, Lim do H, Lee SI, Kim JH, Kim KM, Lee DH, Lee J (2010) Noncutaneous malignant melanoma: a prognostic model from a retrospective multicenter study. BMC Cancer 10:167. doi:10.1186/1471-2407-10-167
32. Kim KB, Sanguino AM, Hodges C, Papadopoulos NE, Eton O, Camacho LH, Broemeling LD, Johnson MM, Ballo MT, Ross MI, Gershenwald JE, Lee JE, Mansfield PF, Prieto VG, Bedikian AY (2004) Biochemotherapy in patients with metastatic anorectal mucosal melanoma. Cancer 100(7):1478–1483. doi:10.1002/cncr.20113
33. Kirschner AN, Kidd EA, Dewees T, Perkins SM (2013) Treatment approach and outcomes of vaginal melanoma. International J Gynecol Cancer 23(8):1484–1489. doi:10.1097/IGC.0b013e3182a1ced8

34. Larkin J, Ascierto PA, Dreno B, Atkinson V, Liszkay G, Maio M, Mandala M, Demidov L, Stroyakovskiy D, Thomas L, de la Cruz-Merino L, Dutriaux C, Garbe C, Sovak MA, Chang I, Choong N, Hack SP, McArthur GA, Ribas A (2014) Combined vemurafenib and cobimetinib in BRAF-mutated melanoma. N Engl J Med 371(20):1867–1876. doi:10.1056/NEJMoa1408868
35. Leitao MM Jr (2014) Management of vulvar and vaginal melanomas: current and future strategies. American Society of Clinical Oncology educational book/ASCO American Society of Clinical Oncology Meeting e277–281. doi:10.14694/EdBook_AM.2014.34.e277
36. Lian B, Si L, Cui C, Chi Z, Sheng X, Mao L, Li S, Kong Y, Tang B, Guo J (2013) Phase II randomized trial comparing high-dose IFN-alpha2b with temozolomide plus cisplatin as systemic adjuvant therapy for resected mucosal melanoma. Clin Cancer Res 19(16):4488–4498. doi:10.1158/1078-0432.CCR-13-0739
37. Long GV, Stroyakovskiy D, Gogas H, Levchenko E, de Braud F, Larkin J, Garbe C, Jouary T, Hauschild A, Grob JJ, Chiarion Sileni V, Lebbe C, Mandala M, Millward M, Arance A, Bondarenko I, Haanen JB, Hansson J, Utikal J, Ferraresi V, Kovalenko N, Mohr P, Probachai V, Schadendorf D, Nathan P, Robert C, Ribas A, DeMarini DJ, Irani JG, Casey M, Ouellet D, Martin AM, Le N, Patel K, Flaherty K (2014) Combined BRAF and MEK inhibition versus BRAF inhibition alone in melanoma. N Engl J Med 371(20):1877–1888. doi:10.1056/NEJMoa1406037
38. Lourenco SV, Fernandes JD, Hsieh R, Coutinho-Camillo CM, Bologna S, Sangueza M, Nico MM (2014) Head and neck mucosal melanoma: a review. Am J Dermatopathol 36 (7):578–587. doi:10.1097/DAD.0000000000000035
39. Lutzky J, Bauer J, Bastian BC (2008) Dose-dependent, complete response to imatinib of a metastatic mucosal melanoma with a K642E KIT mutation. Pigm Cell Melanoma Res 21 (4):492–493. doi:10.1111/j.1755-148X.2008.00475.x
40. Mellman I, Coukos G, Dranoff G (2011) Cancer immunotherapy comes of age. Nature 480 (7378):480–489. doi:10.1038/nature10673
41. Mihajlovic M, Vlajkovic S, Jovanovic P, Stefanovic V (2012) Primary mucosal melanomas: a comprehensive review. Int J Clin Exp Pathol 5(8):739–753
42. Min L, Hodi FS (2014) Anti-PD1 following ipilimumab for mucosal melanoma: durable tumor response associated with severe hypothyroidism and rhabdomyolysis. Cancer Immunol Res 2 (1):15–18. doi:10.1158/2326-6066.CIR-13-0146
43. Moreno MA, Roberts DB, Kupferman ME, DeMonte F, El-Naggar AK, Williams M, Rosenthal DS, Hanna EY (2010) Mucosal melanoma of the nose and paranasal sinuses, a contemporary experience from the M.D. Anderson Cancer Center. Cancer 116(9):2215–2223. doi:10.1002/cncr.24976
44. Nieder C (2012) Ipilimumab in patients with melanoma and brain metastases. Lancet Oncol 13 (7):e277; author reply e277–278. doi:10.1016/S1470-2045(12)70303-0
45. Pandey M, Mathew A, Abraham EK, Ahamed IM, Nair KM (1998) Primary malignant melanoma of the mucous membranes. European J Surg Oncol 24(4):303–307
46. Patrick RJ, Fenske NA, Messina JL (2007) Primary mucosal melanoma. J Am Acad Dermatol 56(5):828–834. doi:10.1016/j.jaad.2006.06.017
47. Pfister DG, Ang KK, Brizel DM, Burtness B, Cmelak AJ, Colevas AD, Dunphy F, Eisele DW, Gilbert J, Gillison ML, Haddad RI, Haughey BH, Hicks WL Jr, Hitchcock YJ, Kies MS, Lydiatt WM, Maghami E, Martins R, McCaffrey T, Mittal BB, Pinto HA, Ridge JA, Samant S, Sanguineti G, Schuller DE, Shah JP, Spencer S, Trotti A 3rd, Weber RS, Wolf G, Worden F, National Comprehensive Cancer N (2012) Mucosal melanoma of the head and neck. J Natl Compr Cancer Network JNCCN 10(3):320–338
48. Postow MA, Hamid O, Carvajal RD (2012) Mucosal melanoma: pathogenesis, clinical behavior, and management. Curr Oncol Rep 14(5):441–448. doi:10.1007/s11912-012-0244-x
49. Postow MA, Luke JJ, Bluth MJ, Ramaiya N, Panageas KS, Lawrence DP, Ibrahim N, Flaherty KT, Sullivan RJ, Ott PA, Callahan MK, Harding JJ, D'Angelo SP, Dickson MA,

Schwartz GK, Chapman PB, Gnjatic S, Wolchok JD, Hodi FS, Carvajal RD (2013) Ipilimumab for patients with advanced mucosal melanoma. Oncologist 18(6):726–732. doi:10.1634/theoncologist.2012-0464

50. Quintas-Cardama A, Lazar AJ, Woodman SE, Kim K, Ross M, Hwu P (2008) Complete response of stage IV anal mucosal melanoma expressing KIT Val560Asp to the multikinase inhibitor sorafenib. Nat Clin Pract Oncol 5(12):737–740. doi:10.1038/ncponc1251
51. Robert C, Thomas L, Bondarenko I, O'Day S, Weber J, Garbe C, Lebbe C, Baurain JF, Testori A, Grob JJ, Davidson N, Richards J, Maio M, Hauschild A, Miller WH Jr, Gascon P, Lotem M, Harmankaya K, Ibrahim R, Francis S, Chen TT, Humphrey R, Hoos A, Wolchok JD (2011) Ipilimumab plus dacarbazine for previously untreated metastatic melanoma. N Engl J Med 364(26):2517–2526. doi:10.1056/NEJMoa1104621
52. Robert C, Karaszewska B, Schachter J, Rutkowski P, Mackiewicz A, Stroiakovski D, Lichinitser M, Dummer R, Grange F, Mortier L, Chiarion-Sileni V, Drucis K, Krajsova I, Hauschild A, Lorigan P, Wolter P, Long GV, Flaherty K, Nathan P, Ribas A, Martin AM, Sun P, Crist W, Legos J, Rubin SD, Little SM, Schadendorf D (2015) Improved overall survival in melanoma with combined dabrafenib and trametinib. N Engl J Med 372(1):30–39. doi:10.1056/NEJMoa1412690
53. Robert C, Long GV, Brady B, Dutriaux C, Maio M, Mortier L, Hassel JC, Rutkowski P, McNeil C, Kalinka-Warzocha E, Savage KJ, Hernberg MM, Lebbe C, Charles J, Mihalcioiu C, Chiarion-Sileni V, Mauch C, Cognetti F, Arance A, Schmidt H, Schadendorf D, Gogas H, Lundgren-Eriksson L, Horak C, Sharkey B, Waxman IM, Atkinson V, Ascierto PA (2015) Nivolumab in previously untreated melanoma without BRAF mutation. N Engl J Med 372(4):320–330. doi:10.1056/NEJMoa1412082
54. Seetharamu N, Ott PA, Pavlick AC (2010) Mucosal melanomas: a case-based review of the literature. Oncologist 15(7):772–781. doi:10.1634/theoncologist.2010-0067
55. Smyth EC, Flavin M, Pulitzer MP, Gardner GJ, Costantino PD, Chi DS, Bogatch K, Chapman PB, Wolchok JD, Schwartz GK, Carvajal RD (2011) Treatment of locally recurrent mucosal melanoma with topical imiquimod. J Clin Oncol 29(33):e809–811. doi:10.1200/JCO.2011.36.8829
56. Tas F, Keskin S, Karadeniz A, Dagoglu N, Sen F, Kilic L, Yildiz I (2011) Noncutaneous melanoma have distinct features from each other and cutaneous melanoma. Oncology 81(5–6):353–358. doi:10.1159/000334863
57. Tomicic J, Wanebo HJ (2003) Mucosal melanomas. Surg Clin North Am 83(2):237–252. doi:10.1016/S0039-6109(02)00100-7
58. Topalian SL, Sznol M, McDermott DF, Kluger HM, Carvajal RD, Sharfman WH, Brahmer JR, Lawrence DP, Atkins MB, Powderly JD, Leming PD, Lipson EJ, Puzanov I, Smith DC, Taube JM, Wigginton JM, Kollia GD, Gupta A, Pardoll DM, Sosman JA, Hodi FS (2014) Survival, durable tumor remission, and long-term safety in patients with advanced melanoma receiving nivolumab. J Clin Oncol 32(10):1020–1030. doi:10.1200/JCO.2013.53.0105
59. Verschraegen CF, Benjapibal M, Supakarapongkul W, Levy LB, Ross M, Atkinson EN, Bodurka-Bevers D, Kavanagh JJ, Kudelka AP, Legha SS (2001) Vulvar melanoma at the M. D. Anderson Cancer Center: 25 years later. Int J Gynecol Cancer 11(5):359–364
60. Wolchok JD, Kluger H, Callahan MK, Postow MA, Rizvi NA, Lesokhin AM, Segal NH, Ariyan CE, Gordon RA, Reed K, Burke MM, Caldwell A, Kronenberg SA, Agunwamba BU, Zhang X, Lowy I, Inzunza HD, Feely W, Horak CE, Hong Q, Korman AJ, Wigginton JM, Gupta A, Sznol M (2013) Nivolumab plus ipilimumab in advanced melanoma. New Engl J Med 369(2):122–133. doi:10.1056/NEJMoa1302369
61. Woodman SE, Trent JC, Stemke-Hale K, Lazar AJ, Pricl S, Pavan GM, Fermeglia M, Gopal YN, Yang D, Podoloff DA, Ivan D, Kim KB, Papadopoulos N, Hwu P, Mills GB, Davies MA (2009) Activity of dasatinib against L576P KIT mutant melanoma: molecular, cellular, and clinical correlates. Mol Cancer Ther 8(8):2079–2085. doi:10.1158/1535-7163.MCT-09-0459

62. Woodman SE, Davies MA (2010) Targeting KIT in melanoma: a paradigm of molecular medicine and targeted therapeutics. Biochem Pharmacol 80(5):568–574. doi:10.1016/j.bcp.2010.04.032
63. Wu E, Golitz LE (2000) Primary noncutaneous melanoma. Clinics Lab Med 20(4):731–744
64. Zhu YSL, Kong Y, Chi Z, Yuan X, Cui C, Sheng X, Guo J, Shen L (2009) Response to sunitinib in Chinese KIT-mutated metastatic mucosal melanoma. J Clin Oncol 27(15s):e20017

Acral Lentiginous Melanoma

James S. Goydos and Steven L. Shoen

Abstract

Acral lentiginous melanoma (ALM) is a rare subtype of melanoma mainly arising on the palms, soles, and nail beds. ALM is the most common subtype of melanoma found in patients of Asian or African descent and tends to more advanced at presentation due to delays in diagnosis. Surgical treatment is difficult owing to the complexity and functional importance of the hands and feet and reconstruction after resection is usually needed. The prognosis for patients with ALM depends on stage of disease and tends to be worse than with other subtypes of melanoma. Newer treatment modalities such as immunotherapies and targeted agents are being tested in patients with advanced ALM with some promising preliminary results.

Keywords

Acral · Subungual · c-Kit · Reconstruction · Delayed diagnosis

J.S. Goydos (✉)
Division of Surgical Oncology, Rutgers Robert Wood Johnson Medical School, Melanoma and Soft Tissue Oncology, Rutgers Cancer Institute of New Jersey, New Jersey, USA
e-mail: goydosjs@cinj.rutgers.edu

S.L. Shoen
Plastic and Reconstructive Surgery, Robert Wood Johnson University Hospital, New Jersey, USA
e-mail: stevenshoen@comcast.net

H.L. Kaufman and J.M. Mehnert (eds.), *Melanoma*,
Cancer Treatment and Research 167, DOI 10.1007/978-3-319-22539-5_14

Contents

1 Introduction

Acral lentiginous melanoma (ALM) is a subtype of melanoma that occurs on acral skin, which includes the palms, soles, and nail beds. ALM is an uncommon subtype of melanoma, accounting for only 4–6 % of all melanoma diagnoses in Caucasian populations [1]. However, even though still uncommon, it is the most common subtype of melanoma found in individuals with darker skin including those of Asian or African descent [2, 3]. Patients with ALM tend to have a poor prognosis, mainly caused by delays in diagnosis and advanced disease at presentation [3]. Although we are learning more about the genetic alterations found in ALM [4], factors influencing the pathogenesis of this melanoma subtype are poorly understood; however, trauma or chronic inflammation has been proposed as possible inciting factors [5]. Patients with ALM tend to be older, have fewer atypical nevi, and have a lower incidence of sun burning than patients with superficial spreading melanoma (SSM). Patients with ALM also tend to have a higher personal and family history of non-cutaneous malignancies [2].

2 Clinical Features

As with most melanomas, early ALM is asymptomatic and is usually picked up on visual inspection (Fig. 1). Many patients, but especially elderly individuals, have difficulty examining the soles of the feet, and it is common for even experienced practitioners to mistake subungual melanomas as either traumatic injuries or fungal infections [6]. This leads to delay in diagnoses and a worse prognosis for patients with this subtype of melanoma [6, 7]. It is therefore important that skin screening examinations include the soles, palms, and nail beds, including examination between the toes and fingers. As patients with ALM tend to have fewer cutaneous nevi, they are often not in follow-up with dermatology, and it is therefore important for physicians in non-dermatologic specialties to be familiar with the clinical characteristics of ALM.

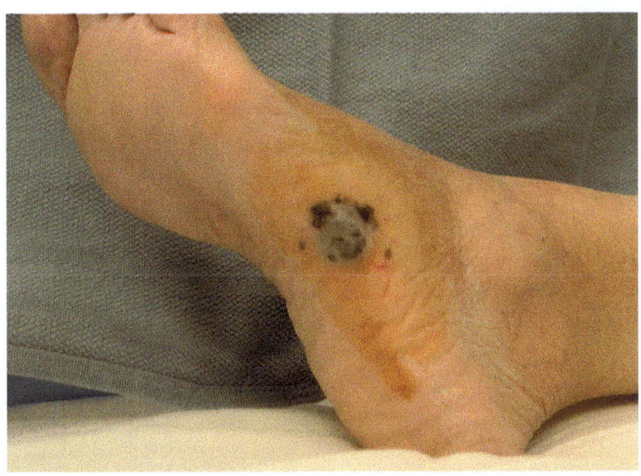

Fig. 1 Visual inspection of ALM

On gross inspection, ALM usually presents as a pigmented macule or papule on the soles or palms that has an irregular border and variegated pigment. As it advances, ALM lesions may become large, exophytic nodules containing areas of blue-black pigment. Amelanotic lesions are common and present as pink macules or nodules. ALM is often at first mistaken for other conditions including non-healing traumatic wounds, warts, fungal infections, pyogenic granulomas, or hematomas [6]. Subungual melanomas are especially hard to diagnose, particularly if amelanotic. These lesions can be treated for many years as fungal infections or non-healing traumatic wounds. It is often not until the lesion becomes exophytic or pigmented that a biopsy is performed and the diagnosis is made [6]. Subungual melanomas often first present as pigmented streaks in the nail bed and can often be confused with subungual hemorrhages. However, subungual hemorrhages will move as the nail grows while ALM lesions will remain in place [6, 7].

3 Histologic Features

Histologically, ALM usually consists of confluent dendritic or epithelioid melanocytes, both singly and in nests, found along the dermal–epidermal junction. There can be upward pagetoid migration as well as extension down adnexal structures. Dermal invasion usually presents as atypical epithelioid nests or cords, with occasional spindle cell components intermixed [7]. As with other types of melanoma, ulceration and a high mitotic rate are considered poor prognostic signs [8]. The diagnosis of ALM, especially subungual lesions, can be difficult, and it is important to obtain an adequate biopsy specimen. As one would expect, it is most difficult to obtain subungual biopsies, and as the melanocytes in normal nail matrix can have a pagetoid appearance it is especially important to get adequate biopsies of these lesions [9].

4 Genetics

The genetic factors influencing the pathogenesis and progression of the different subtypes of melanoma are becoming better understood, and we can therefore divide melanoma into different subtypes based on these genetic factors [10]. The majority of superficial spreading and nodular cutaneous melanomas (SSM/NM) contain activating mutations of either *NRAS* (17 %) or *BRAF* (50 %), and many of the tumors that contain *BRAF* mutations also have inactivation of *PTEN* [10, 11]. In contrast, ALMs have a much lower incidence of activating mutations of BRAF (17 %), rarely have mutations in *PTEN*, have approximately the same incidence of activating mutations in *NRAS* (15 %), and often have activating mutations or amplifications of wild-type *KIT* (15–40 %), a type of receptor tyrosine kinase [4, 10].

5 Treatment

The treatment of ALM is similar to that of cutaneous melanomas: wide local excision to obtain adequate negative margins and appropriate staging including sentinel lymph node mapping and selective lymphadenectomy when appropriate [12]. Wide excision of ALM of the hands and feet often requires plastic surgical reconstruction to preserve cosmesis and function [13]. Local recurrence of adequately resected ALM is no higher than for SSM, and topical agents such as imiquimod have been used successfully to treat residual disease in difficult cases [14, 15].

6 Surgical and Reconstructive Considerations When Addressing ALM of the Hand

Wide local excision of the primary lesions in patients with ALM often requires amputation of digits, especially with subungual melanoma. However, with modern reconstructive techniques, it is often possible to preserve a patient's digits while still performing an adequate excision of the primary tumor [16]. Preservation of digital length, avoiding joint stiffness, maintenance of sensation, and providing durable painless coverage must be considered when planning tumor ablation and reconstruction for tumors of the hand [17]. Achieving these goals requires a thorough knowledge of hand anatomy, meticulous surgical technique, and an understanding of the principles that govern hand function. An optimal functional result often requires the intervention of a certified hand therapist, working in concert with the hand surgeon.

While it is intuitive that preservation of digital length is important, the functional benefit of digital length depends on the ray. Thumb length should always be maximized as digital opposition of the first ray correlates directly with thumb length.

Maximizing length of the fourth and fifth digits helps maintain grip strength—a function of the ulnar side of the hand. Once the index finger is shortened proximal to the DIP joint, patients readily substitute the long finger when performing pad-to-pad pinch with the thumb. In those instances, preserving the length of a shortened index finger is less critical. These and other factors must be considered when managing a digital wound formed by ALM removal. For instance, exposed bone at the distal phalanx of the little finger might best be treated by flap coverage that preserves length, while an index finger proximal phalanx amputation stump can be managed appropriately by bone shortening and primary closure.

Reconstructive options at the hand include healing by secondary intention, primary repair, skin grafting, and flap reconstruction. Healing by secondary intention is a reasonable option for small soft tissue defects when bone or tendon is not exposed. Studies have shown that soft tissue defects at the tip of a digit treated by secondary intention ultimately provide durable coverage with tip sensation which is superior to sensory return after flap or graft coverage. Sizable skin deficits of the tip (>1.5 cm) are best treated by skin graft as secondary healing of such sizable areas may yield unstable, painful scar or contracture (Fig. 2a, b). As one climbs the "reconstructive ladder," the risk of soft tissue contracture is less of a problem. Contracture is a concern on the flexor side of the hand as well as at the interdigital web spaces. At those sites, flaps are preferred. If skin grafting must be performed, full-thickness grafts typically exhibit less soft tissue contracture. The ulnar border of the hand provides palmar skin to cover small defects. Larger full-thickness grafts may be harvested from the lower abdominal or groin creases.

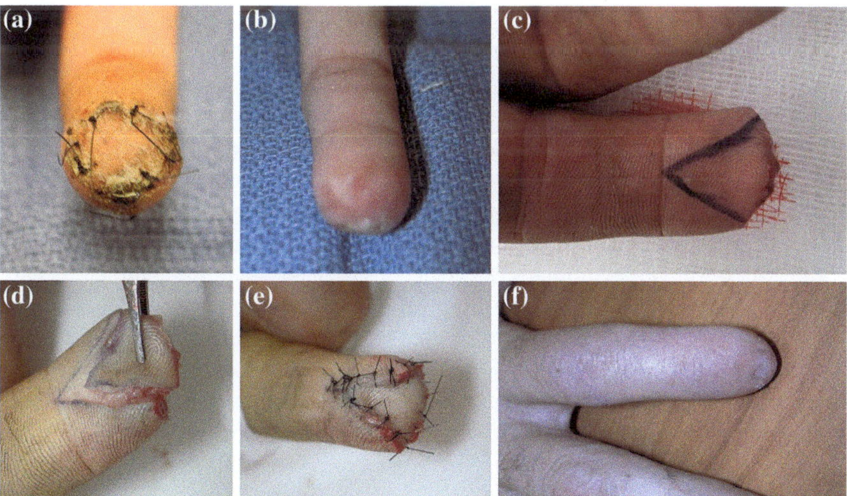

Fig. 2 Sizeable skin deficits of the tip are best treated by skin grafting, while the Atasoy flap is a good choice for smaller defects

Incisions at the palmar side of the hand as well as at the interdigital web space must be planned carefully, and if the reconstructive surgeon is not performing the primary resection he should assist the resecting surgeon in planning the resection. Flexion creases should not be violated, and incisions at the web spaces should parallel digits. The dorsum of the hand is much more forgiving, and incisions at the dorsum may be oriented in any direction and over any extensor crease.

While a multitude of flaps have been described to manage hand defects, several are true workhorses for these reconstructive problems. The "Atasoy" flap described in 1970 provides easy, reliable coverage of fingertip amputations through a "V to Y" advancement of triangular tissue from the volar surface of the distal phalanx (Fig. 2c–f) [18]. This technique provides sensate, durable coverage with palmar tissue. However, its use in melanoma may be limited by the flap's restriction to relatively small defects with preserved ample volar tissue. The "cross finger flap" describes the transfer of skin and subcutaneous tissue from the dorsum of a digit to a defect at a neighboring ray [19, 20]. The resultant open areas are treated with a skin graft. Roughly three weeks following the first procedure, a secondary operation is performed to divide and insert the flap (Fig. 3a–d). Fairly large defects may be treated with this flap, although the tissue is insensate. For defects at the volar distal phalanx of the thumb, an innervated cross finger flap from the dorsum of the index finger proximal phalanx may be considered (Fig. 3e–h) [20]. A thenar flap allows for the staged transfer of palmar skin to the tip of the index or long fingers, though available tissue is somewhat limited and remains insensate. Many other types of reconstructive flaps have been described for reconstruction of defects in the hands, and for more complex cases, staged distant flaps or the microsurgical transfer of tissue remains an option [21, 22].

Tumor ablation at the nail bed always yields a defect with exposed distal phalanx. Flap coverage is preferred to handle such cases. However, the "Bridging Phenomenon" of skin grafts teaches that areas of full-thickness graft up to 1 cm in diameter may survive over areas of poor vascularity such as bone provided that the periphery of the graft is sitting on a well-perfused surface. Therefore, full-thickness grafts of skin or even germinal matrix from the lower extremity remain an option for nail bed defects. A reverse cross finger flap from the dorsum of a neighboring middle phalanx remains the best option for sizeable nail bed defects. The exposed undersurface of the flap is treated with a skin graft or germinal matrix graft [22].

Regardless of the technique used to reconstruct the hand after tumor ablation prompt, active and passive motion must be initiated as soon as possible. Supervision by a certified hand therapist is essential to provide the best functional outcome [17]. Movement at joints distant to the operative site is also important as stiffness will develop in normal joints that remain immobile for even a few weeks. Secondary procedures may be necessary to treat joint contracture. Debulking procedures and scar revisions may help to restore normal appearance to the hand, an exposed part of the body.

While treating melanoma remains a challenge for the oncologic surgeon, the complexity of hand anatomy and function complicate surgical treatment and its outcome. To yield optimal results, patients with melanoma of the hand must be

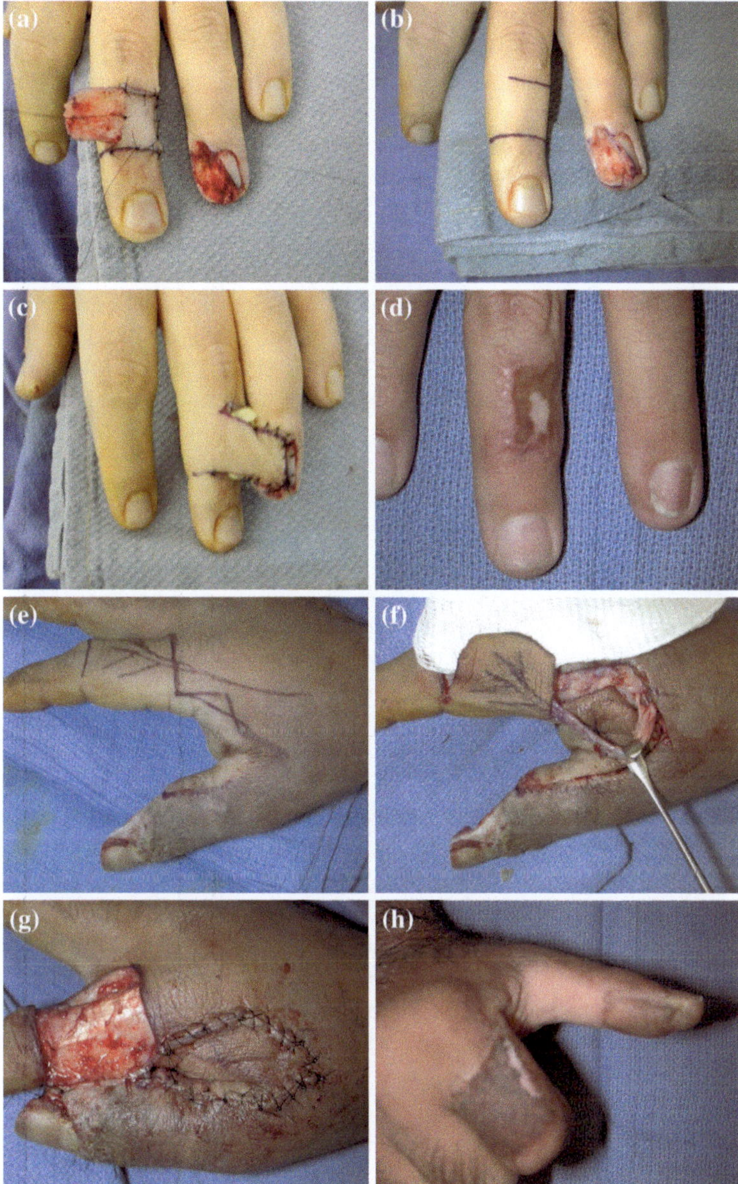

Fig. 3 Cross finger flaps

cared for by a team including an oncologic surgeon, a hand surgeon, an oncologist, a radiation oncologist, and a hand therapist.

7 Treatment of Metastatic Disease

Many of the new therapeutic approaches aimed at metastatic melanoma are either targeted at signaling pathways activated by specific driver mutations (BRAF, NRAS, PTEN, and others), or designed to activate or enhance the immune response to the tumor. Almost all of the new therapeutic options that are now available were designed for, and tested in, patients with SSM/NM [23, 24]. Because of the genetic and etiological differences between ALM and SSM/NM, it is difficult to extrapolate findings from recent clinical trials of agents such as vemurafenib or ipilimumab in patients with melanoma. However, some data do exist, and newer therapies are finding their way into the treatment of patients with advanced ALM [23]. Another treatment option for patients with ALM is to target *KIT*, as it is often mutated or amplified in ALM [4]. Targeted therapies using imatinib or sunitinib have been used in patients with advanced ALM, though responses have been mixed and further data are needed to confirm efficacy in this population [25, 26].

8 Prognosis

Studies have been done examining melanoma-specific survival rates for patients with different subtypes of melanoma. After controlling for primary tumor thickness and stage, patients with ALM appear to have a worse prognosis overall (five- and ten-year melanoma-specific survival rates of 80.3 and 67.5 %, respectively), than patients with superficial spreading and nodular melanomas (five- and ten-year melanoma-specific survival rates of 91.3 and 87.5 %, respectively [$p < 0.001$]) [1]. There does not appear to be a difference in prognosis between male and female patients, but light-skinned Hispanic patients and patients from Asian or Pacific Island populations appear to have a worse prognosis than other patients with ALM. It is possible that delay of diagnosis and thicker tumors at presentation may account for these population differences [1]. This difference in prognosis between ALM and other cutaneous melanomas highlights the need for better patient screening during physical examinations and increased effort in patient education specially targeting vulnerable populations, so that these lesions can be picked up as early in their course as possible.

References

1. Bradford PT, Goldstein AM, McMaster ML, Tucker MA (2009) Acral lentiginous melanoma: incidence and survival patterns in the United States, 1986–2005. Arch Dermatol 145:427–434. doi:10.1001/archdermatol.2008.609
2. Piliang MP (2011) Acral lentiginous melanoma. Clin Lab Med 31:281–288. doi:10.1016/j.cll.2011.03.005
3. Zell JA et al (2008) Survival for patients with invasive cutaneous melanoma among ethnic groups: the effects of socioeconomic status and treatment. J Clin Oncol Official J Am Soc Clin Oncol 26:66–75. doi:10.1200/JCO.2007.12.3604

4. Zebary A et al (2013) KIT, NRAS, BRAF and PTEN mutations in a sample of Swedish patients with acral lentiginous melanoma. J Dermatol Sci 72:284–289. doi:10.1016/j.jdermsci.2013.07.013
5. Nagore E, Pereda C, Botella-Estrada R, Requena C, Guillen C (2009) Acral lentiginous melanoma presents distinct clinical profile with high cancer susceptibility. Cancer Causes Control CCC 20:115–119. doi:10.1007/s10552-008-9221-y
6. Soon SL et al (2003) Acral lentiginous melanoma mimicking benign disease: the Emory experience. J Am Acad Dermatol 48:183–188. doi:10.1067/mjd.2003.63
7. Stubblefield J, Kelly B (2014) Melanoma in non-caucasian populations. Surg Clin North Am 94:1115–1126, ix. doi:10.1016/j.suc.2014.07.008
8. Durbec F, Martin L, Derancourt C, Grange F (2012) Melanoma of the hand and foot: epidemiological, prognostic and genetic features. A systematic review. Br J Dermatol 166:727–739. doi:10.1111/j.1365-2133.2011.10772.x
9. Perrin C, Michiels JF, Pisani A, Ortonne JP (1997) Anatomic distribution of melanocytes in normal nail unit: an immunohistochemical investigation. Am J Dermatopathol 19:462–467
10. Bastian BC (2014) The molecular pathology of melanoma: an integrated taxonomy of melanocytic neoplasia. Ann Rev Pathol 9:239–271. doi:10.1146/annurev-pathol-012513-104658
11. Bennett DC (2008) How to make a melanoma: what do we know of the primary clonal events? Pigment Cell Melanoma Res 21:27–38. doi:10.1111/j.1755-148X.2007.00433.x
12. Egger ME et al (2012) Unique prognostic factors in acral lentiginous melanoma. Am J Surg 204:874–879; discussion 879–880. doi:10.1016/j.amjsurg.2012.05.013
13. Evans GR, Friedman J, Shenaq J, Mosser S (1997) Plantar flap reconstruction for acral lentiginous melanoma. Ann Surg Oncol 4:575–578
14. Savarese I et al (2014) Acral lentiginous melanoma treated with topical imiquimod cream: possible cooperation between drug and tumour cells. Clin Exp Dermatol. doi:10.1111/ced.12469
15. Sue GR, Hanlon A, Lazova R, Narayan D (2014) Use of imiquimod for residual acral melanoma. BMJ Case Report. doi:10.1136/bcr-2014-203826
16. Sureda N et al (2011) Conservative surgical management of subungual (matrix derived) melanoma: report of seven cases and literature review. Br J Dermatol 165:852–858. doi:10.1111/j.1365-2133.2011.10477.x
17. Goitz RJ, Westkaemper JG, Tomaino MM, Sotereanos DG (1997) Soft-tissue defects of the digits. Coverage considerations. Hand Clin 13:189–205
18. Atasoy E, Ioakimidis E, Kasdan ML, Kutz JE, Kleinert HE (1970) Reconstruction of the amputated finger tip with a triangular volar flap. A new surgical procedure. J Bone Joint Surg 52:921–926
19. Curtis RM (1957) Cross-finger pedicle flap in hand surgery. Ann Surg 145:650–655
20. Gokrem S, Tuncali D, Terzioglu A, Toksoy K, Aslan G (2007) The thin cross finger skin flap. J Hand Surg Eur 32:417–420. doi:10.1016/j.jhsb.2007.02.010
21. Chen HC, Buchman MT, Wei FC (1999) Free flaps for soft tissue coverage in the hand and fingers. Hand Clin 15:541–554
22. O'Neill PJ, Litts C (2004) Hand and forearm reconstruction after skin cancer ablation. Clin Plast Surg 31:113–119
23. Miller DM, Flaherty KT, Tsao H (2014) Current status and future directions of molecularly targeted therapies and immunotherapies for melanoma. Semin Cutan Med Surg 33:60–67
24. Naidoo J, Page DB, Wolchok JD (2014) Immune modulation for cancer therapy. Br J Cancer 111:2214–2219. doi:10.1038/bjc.2014.348
25. Hodi FS et al (2013) Imatinib for melanomas harboring mutationally activated or amplified KIT arising on mucosal, acral, and chronically sun-damaged skin. J Clin Oncol Official J Am Soc Clin Oncol 31:3182–3190. doi:10.1200/JCO.2012.47.7836
26. Minor DR et al (2012) Sunitinib therapy for melanoma patients with KIT mutations. Clin Cancer Res Official J Am Assoc Cancer Res 18:1457–1463. doi:10.1158/1078-0432.CCR-11-1987

Pediatric Melanoma and Atypical Melanocytic Neoplasms

Radhika Sreeraman Kumar, Jane L. Messina, Damon Reed, Fariba Navid and Vernon K. Sondak

Abstract

Melanoma is uncommon in the pediatric age range, but is increasing in frequency and often presents with atypical features compared to the classic ABCDE criteria common to adult melanoma cases. Moreover, many melanocytic neoplasms in childhood pose diagnostic challenges to the pathologist, and sometimes cannot be unequivocally classified as benign nevi or melanoma. This chapter addresses the evaluation and management of pediatric patients with melanoma and atypical melanocytic neoplasms, including the roles of and unresolved questions surrounding sentinel lymph node biopsy, completion lymphadenectomy, adjuvant therapy, and treatment of advanced disease.

R. Sreeraman Kumar
Department of Radiation Oncology, Moffitt Cancer Center, Tampa, FL, USA

J.L. Messina
Department of Anatomic Pathology, Moffitt Cancer Center, Tampa, FL, USA

J.L. Messina · D. Reed · V.K. Sondak (✉)
Department of Cutaneous Oncology, Moffitt Cancer Center, 12902 Magnolia Drive, Tampa, FL 33612, USA
e-mail: vernon.sondak@moffitt.org

J.L. Messina
Department of Pathology and Cell Biology, University of South Florida Morsani College of Medicine, Tampa, FL, USA

D. Reed
Department of Oncologic Sciences, University of South Florida Morsani College of Medicine, Tampa, FL, USA

F. Navid
Department of Oncology, St. Jude Children's Research Hospital, Memphis, TN, USA

H.L. Kaufman and J.M. Mehnert (eds.), *Melanoma*,
Cancer Treatment and Research 167, DOI 10.1007/978-3-319-22539-5_15

Keywords
Melanoma · Sentinel node biopsy · Pediatrics · Adolescent and young adult (AYA) oncology · Atypical melanocytic neoplasms

Contents

V.K. Sondak
Department of Oncologic Sciences and Surgery, University of South Florida Morsani College of Medicine, Tampa, FL, USA

J.L. Messina
Department of Oncologic Sciences, University of South Florida Morsani College of Medicine, Tampa, FL, USA

J.L. Messina
Department of Dermatology, University of South Florida Morsani College of Medicine, Tampa, FL, USA

D. Reed
Adolescent and Young Adult (AYA) Program, Sarcoma Department, Moffitt Cancer Center, Tampa, FL, USA

D. Reed
Department of Hematology/Oncology, All Children's Hospital Johns Hopkins Medicine, St. Petersburg, FL, USA

1 Introduction

1.1 Definition

Pediatric melanoma is defined as a malignant melanocytic lesion in a child from birth to age of 18 or 21 years, depending on the cutoff employed for defining adulthood. In this chapter, unless otherwise specified when quoting studies using different age cutoffs, we consider pediatric cases to be under the age of 21 years. Pediatric melanoma can be further subclassified according to the specific age range at presentation (congenital, infantile, prepubertal childhood versus postpubertal adolescence; see Fig. 1), histologic subtype, presence or absence of precursor lesions, and by using the standard clinical and pathologic staging criteria applied to adult cases. A major issue in any discussion of pediatric melanoma is the difficulty frequently encountered in establishing whether or not a histologically abnormal melanocytic lesion is in fact unequivocally malignant. While some of the difficulty may stem from a relative hesitancy to diagnose melanoma in young children, there are clearly a number of abnormal melanocytic lesions that are difficult or impossible to reliably categorize as benign or malignant using currently available histopathologic criteria. The broad but concise term *atypical melanocytic neoplasm* is our

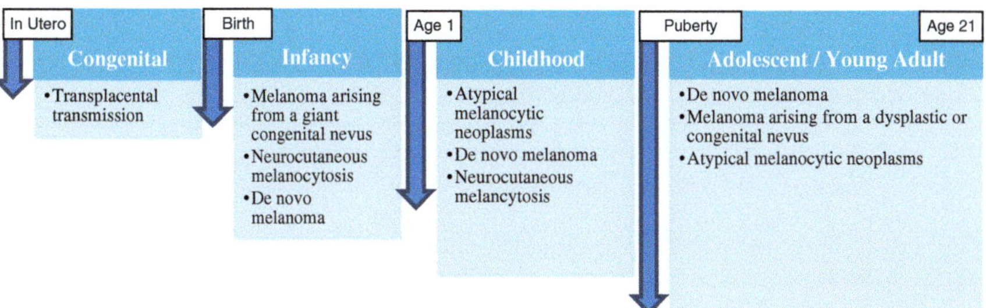

Fig. 1 Pediatric melanoma presentations in different age ranges. The length of the arrow is roughly proportional to the relative frequency of melanoma (and/or atypical melanocytic neoplasms) occurring in each interval, so melanoma occurring in utero due to transplacental transmission from the mother or presenting in the first year of life is least common, but pediatric melanoma becomes progressively more common in subsequent years, especially postpuberty

preferred name for this broad class of lesions, which like pediatric melanoma may be further subclassified based on histologic appearance and potential for recurrence and metastasis [71, 95].

1.2 Epidemiology

Pediatric melanoma accounts for 1–4 % of all cases of melanoma and 1–3 % of all pediatric malignancies [7]. It is the most common primary malignant tumor of the skin in patients younger than 20 years of age. Though the incidence of melanoma in children younger than 10 years has remained stable, the incidence of adolescent melanoma is increasing at a rate of 2.9 % per year in the USA over the past 3 decades [7, 101], with similar trends reflected throughout the world [1, 47].

There were estimated to be 450 new cases of melanoma diagnosed in children younger than 21 years in the USA in 2014 [105]. There is a slight female predominance, and the increase in incidence of melanoma is highest in female adolescents. While Caucasian children account for the majority of new diagnoses, the incidence continues to rise in the Hispanic and Native American populations [93].

1.3 Comparison with Adult Melanoma

Compared to adults, children present with thicker primary lesions and a higher incidence of sentinel lymph node metastases [44, 49, 61]. Melanoma in a child is more likely to arise from a precursor lesion such as a nevus and have an atypical clinical presentation that does not follow the typical ABCDEs of melanoma (Table 1), as well as to show unusual pathologic features [26, 35]. Specifically, lesions are more frequently non-pigmented and often have histologic features reminiscent of a Spitz nevus, so-called spitzoid features [86]. They are also more often of nodular histology. Non-whites, such as Hispanics and Asians, are overrepresented compared to adult melanoma [7]. Despite the later stage at presentation, pediatric melanoma appears to have a more favorable prognosis than adult melanoma of a similar stage [49, 61]. The overall survival in children with melanoma ranges from 70 to 80 % at 10 years [8].

Table 1 Comparison of "ABCDE" characteristics of adult and pediatric melanoma

	Hallmarks of adult melanoma	Alternative characteristics of pediatric melanoma
A	Asymmetry	Amelanotic
B	Border irregularity	Bump/bleeding
C	Color variation	Colorless/uniform color
D	Diameter	De novo/any diameter
E	Evolution	Evolution

Adapted from Cordoro et al. [26]

1.4 Classification and Risk Factors

1.4.1 General Risk Factors

The risk factors for pediatric melanoma differ slightly depending on age at presentation. Sun exposure, tanning bed use, and fair skin are more relevant risk factors in postpubertal patients, while prepubertal patients may be slightly more likely to have genetic risk factors [105, 111].

1.4.2 Congenital/Neonatal Melanoma: In Utero to 1 Year

Congenital and neonatal melanoma is very rare [112], and the available information is based on a small number of case reports. The incidence of congenital and neonatal melanoma has not increased appreciably over the past 30 years [7, 8].

Transplacental Transmission

Melanoma is one of the malignancies recognized to be able to spread from mother to fetus via transplacental transmission. Placental metastasis of melanoma is extremely rare, and fewer than 30 cases have been reported in the literature [3, 5, 90, 104]. The risk factors described to date include maternal diagnosis of node-positive disease greater than 3 years prior to pregnancy, metastatic melanoma manifesting in the mother during the third trimester, maternal age less than 30 years, primiparity, birth at greater than 36 weeks' gestation, and male fetal gender [5, 96]. Of the reported cases of placental metastatic melanoma, 60–67 % of infants were alive 18 months after birth [3, 96]. Fetal transmission across the placenta is even more rare, with eight cases reported to date [3, 117, 121]. Patients are often diagnosed at birth or within twelve months of birth. The prognosis is dismal, with six of the eight reported cases dying in the first year of life. There have been two reported cases of spontaneous regression [121]. Karyotyping has been performed on two cases of male fetal metastatic melanoma, showing an XX karyotype in both cases [117, 121]. If transplacental melanoma transmission is suspected, karyotyping analysis or fluorescence in situ hybridization (FISH) can be used in males for confirmation of the tumor's origin. New assays are available to quantify the copy number of sex chromosomes in genomic DNA purified from a fetal tumor biopsy specimen suspected to be of material origin [94]. Because the development of placental metastases has been noted in even early-stage melanoma patients, thorough sectioning and histologic examination of the placenta is advocated in all patients with a history of invasive melanoma.

Melanoma in a Giant Pigmented Nevus

Congenital melanocytic nevi (CMN) are melanocytic proliferations that present at or very shortly after birth. By definition, they are benign and are categorized by projected adult size: small (<1.5 cm in diameter), medium (1.5–20 cm), and large (>20 cm) [114]. The distinction between large and giant CMN has been inconsistent, with some defining giant CMN by various body surface area measurements instead of projected adult size [4]. A more recent classification system, which takes into account nevus size as well as satellite nevus counts and physical features such as color, surface change, and hypertrichosis, classifies giant CMN as either 40–60 cm (G1) or >60 cm (G2) [92]. Giant CMN are more likely to give rise to pediatric melanoma, but estimates of risk vary markedly [130]. A 2006 meta-analysis of 6571 CMN patients found that 0.7 % developed melanoma at a mean age of 15.5 years [56]. The relatively early onset of melanoma in the setting of giant CMN is the basis for advocating surgical removal of these lesions early in life. Small and medium CMN have a reported lifetime risk of malignant transformation of 2–5 %, but most cases of melanoma arising in these lesions are diagnosed 6 in adulthood. CMN in axial locations are more likely to develop melanoma than CMN in the extremities [28].

Neurocutaneous Melanoma

Neurocutaneous melanoma is extremely rare. It arises in the setting of neurocutaneous melanocytosis, which can include both benign and malignant proliferations of melanocytes in the central nervous system associated with a giant CMN or with more than three small to medium CMN. 6–11 % of patients with giant CMN develop symptomatic neurocutaneous melanocytosis [4, 51]. Neurologic symptoms such as headache, vomiting, seizures, neuropsychiatric disturbance, or myelopathy typically present by age 10 and are associated with increased intracranial pressure and mass effect present on imaging [51]. 40–60 % of patients with neurocutaneous melanocytosis develop melanoma. These patients have a poor prognosis due to the difficulty of resection, limited treatment options, and risk of leptomeningeal infiltration [52, 99]. Genomic studies have suggested that NRAS mosaicism, in particular postzygotic mutations in codon 61, is associated with the onset of neurocutaneous melanocytosis [54].

De Novo/Sporadic Melanoma

De novo lesions are exceedingly rare among melanomas diagnosed within the first year of life, with fourteen cases reported to date [6, 112]. Of these, three children have succumbed to the disease. At present, there are no known risk factors. Diagnosis is challenging, because of some histologic overlap with giant CMN. Recently, comparative genomic hybridization (CGH) of two cases of de novo congenital melanoma was used to establish the diagnosis, revealing multiple chromosomal aberrations [112].

1.4.3 Childhood Melanoma: 1 Year to Puberty

While age cutoffs of 10–12 have been used in most studies to divide childhood from adolescent melanoma, it is likely that the most relevant biologic cutoff is to separate melanomas that arise before and after puberty. Tanner stage may be a more accurate method of distinguishing between childhood and postpubertal adolescence, when hormone-driven changes in melanocyte physiology likely occur. However, in retrospective reviews, determining whether a given child has or has not gone through puberty is quite difficult, hence the need to use clinical surrogates; a cutoff of either

10 or 12 remains appropriate for retrospective reviews or clinical trials that aim to separate childhood melanoma from adolescent cases.

De Novo/Sporadic Melanoma

The majority of childhood melanomas are sporadic and unassociated with congenital nevi or genetic syndromes. The risk factors in these cases have not been well established but likely include UV radiation exposure, fair skin, and multiple nevi [111]. However, compared to adolescent melanoma patients, prepubertal patients are more likely to be non-Caucasian and for this and other reasons, the specific role of UV exposure in this group remains quite unclear [57].

Arising from Giant CMN and Dysplastic Nevi

Similar to neonatal melanoma, childhood melanomas can also arise from giant CMN. One-third of childhood melanomas originate from giant CMN or another precursor lesion, including common and dysplastic nevi [2, 4, 28, 29, 57, 61, 85, 87, 99, 114].

Genetic Syndromes

Genetic mutations that confer sensitivity to DNA damage, alterations in cell cycle tumor suppressors such as p53, and mutations in other tumor suppressor genes are associated with a greater risk of melanoma in children, adolescents, and adults.

Xeroderma Pigmentosum

Xeroderma pigmentosum is an autosomal recessive genetic disorder of nucleotide excision repair, which makes affected individuals exquisitely sensitive to DNA damage by UV radiation. Affected patients will generally develop non-melanoma skin cancer at a median age of 8 years, while melanoma occurs in approximately 5–13 % of xeroderma pigmentosum patients by age 21 [17, 85].

Familial Melanoma Syndromes

Familial melanoma syndromes are not particularly well characterized in adults and even less so in children. Recent genomic studies identified mutations in *CDKN2A* or *CDK4* that can lead to multiple and recurrent melanomas. *CDKN2A* is the most common high-risk melanoma susceptibility locus; mutations in this gene are also associated with dysplastic (atypical) nevus syndrome, >100 nevi, nevi of buttocks/feet, multiple primary melanomas, and pancreatic cancer risk [15]. However, such germline mutations have been found to be present in less than 5 % of childhood melanomas [13, 79]. Other less common familial melanoma syndromes, such as those caused by germline *BAP-1*, *BRCA2*, and *MC1R* mutations, are generally associated with development of melanoma in adulthood rather than childhood.

1.4.4 Adolescent and Young Adult Melanoma

Adolescent and young adult melanoma encompasses patients from puberty to age 21. This is the segment of the pediatric population with the highest incidence of a diagnosis of melanoma. Moreover, it is the segment in which the incidence rate is rising most rapidly, particularly in teenage girls [125]. The risk factors are thought to be similar to those for adults: ultraviolet radiation exposure, tanning bed use, fair skin, family history of melanoma, and the presence of multiple and atypical nevi [29, 35, 57, 60, 61, 81, 125]. Other risk factors include xeroderma pigmentosum and germline mutations involving cell cycle mediators (see Sections "Xeroderma Pigmentosum" and "Familial Melanoma Syndromes" above).

2 Clinical Presentation

2.1 General

Pediatric melanoma presents with distinct clinical manifestations in comparison with adult melanoma [35, 44, 61]. In up to 60 % of childhood and 40 % of adolescent melanomas, the classical "ABCD" hallmarks of diagnosis in adults are not seen. In comparison with the traditional criteria of **a**symmetry, **b**order irregularity, **c**olor variation, **d**iameter ≥6 mm, pediatric patients were found to have more symmetric, raised, and amelanotic lesions with bleeding, uniform or no color, a diameter <6 mm, and de novo lesions. Therefore, a new set of criteria for diagnosis has been proposed for pediatric melanoma: amelanotic, bump/bleeding, uniform or no color, and de novo/any diameter (see Table 1) [26]. These new criteria, however, have neither been prospectively validated nor yet shown to decrease the ratio of normal to malignant lesions subjected to biopsy.

2.2 Congenital/Neonatal Melanoma

Since congenital melanomas arise in the setting of maternal metastatic melanoma, this potential risk is of great concern to pregnant patients with melanoma and their doctors. Congenital melanoma is often first recognized on the basis of a finding of gross or microscopic involvement of the placenta by metastatic melanoma. Thus, for pregnant women with a history of invasive melanoma, and especially for those with known stage III or IV melanoma, we advocate that the placenta should be submitted for gross and microscopic pathologic analysis, supplemented as necessary with immunohistochemical staining for melanocyte lineage antigens. The absence of placental involvement with melanoma is reassuring, while a finding of melanoma cells on the fetal side of the placenta is very concerning for potential maternal–fetal spread. Virtually all cases of neonatal melanoma arising from maternal transmission have manifested before 12 months of age [3, 117].

Neonates with melanoma that is not related to maternal–fetal transmission generally present with a history of a progressive nodule or nodules within a large congenital melanocytic lesion, or with neurologic symptoms or symptoms of increased intracranial pressure in the case of neurocutaneous melanocytosis.

2.3 Childhood Melanoma: Age 1–Puberty

Due to the rarity of melanoma in this age group, there are few series describing a typical clinical presentation. In addition to the lack of conventional ABCD criteria, affected patients are more likely to have darker skin phototypes (Fitzpatrick type III or IV), extremity location of primary, and a high overall number of nevi [26].

2.4 Adolescent and Young Adult Melanoma: Puberty–18

Over three-quarters of pediatric melanoma arise in this subgroup of patients. As with younger patients, atypical presentations such as lack of visible pigmentation (pink/red/flesh-colored), or a symmetric papular or nodular appearance are reported more commonly than in adult melanoma. Cordoro et al. [26] found that the most common prebiopsy diagnosis in this age group was pyogenic granuloma.

3 Initial Clinical and Pathologic Workup

Recognizing the relatively non-specific presentation and the rarity of pediatric melanoma, the potential for delay in diagnosis is quite high. Suspicious pigmented lesions in childhood should ideally be biopsied and evaluated by a dermatopathologist with expertise in evaluating these cases. Clinical history, including history of a congenital nevus or other precursor lesion in the area biopsied, patient age, extent of biopsy (complete excision, shave biopsy, partial excision/punch), patient demographics, color and size of the lesion, and a photograph of the lesion, can all be helpful to the pathologist, emphasizing the value of a close collaboration between clinician and pathologist in dealing with pediatric pigmented lesions of all types. Not uncommonly in our experience, skin lesions in children are initially considered to be warts and thus may be treated with a variety of topical agents prior to being referred for biopsy, and information about this can also be potentially helpful to the pathologist.

The preferred biopsy method is complete excision with a narrow margin of normal skin, which allows for more complete pathologic evaluation of the lesion, including its relationship to neighboring skin and subcutis. Formalin fixation is sufficient for all routine and specialized specimen evaluation methods, including FISH and CGH, the latter two of which are increasingly being utilized as adjuncts in the evaluation of pediatric melanocytic lesions, as discussed subsequently.

Initial histopathologic evaluation of biopsy specimens, especially those demonstrating histologically challenging, ambiguous melanocytic proliferations, may include a variety of commercially available immunohistochemical stains. Commonly used stains include assessment of proliferative activity, either using proliferation index with Ki-67 [78] or assessing mitotic count with phosphohistone H3 [21, 78]. Melanocytic maturation can be demonstrated by progressive loss of HMB-45 staining as dermal depth of melanocytes increases in benign and Spitz nevi compared to melanoma [68]. Complete loss of p16 expression by immunohistochemistry indicates homozygous (biallelic) deletion of *p16/CDKN2A* and may be seen in either atypical Spitz tumor or melanoma, but only rarely if at all in Spitz nevi [25, 65, 128]. Loss of BAP-1 expression has been demonstrated in a subset of histologically challenging, spitzoid-appearing benign and malignant melanocytic proliferations that may occur sporadically or in inherited form [124]. Recently, the presence of kinase fusions involving ALK, ROS-1, NTRK-1, BRAF, or RET has been found in up to 40 % of lesions with spitzoid histology, but has not yet been shown to be indicative of the malignant potential of these lesions [123].

4 Pathologic Classification

4.1 Spectrum of Melanocytic Neoplasia

There is a broad spectrum of melanocytic neoplasia in children, ranging from congenital to acquired, dysplastic, Spitz, blue, and deep penetrating nevi, pigmented epithelioid melanocytoma, and melanoma. Across this spectrum, there are lesions which do not neatly fit into any one diagnostic category, and these lesions have been given a variety of appellations, including borderline tumors, melanocytic tumors of uncertain malignant potential (MELTUMP), spitzoid tumors of uncertain malignant potential (STUMP), and atypical Spitz tumor. Multiple observational, retrospective, and prospective studies have sought to evaluate the natural history of these atypical neoplasms [11, 22, 28, 38, 66, 74, 107], but significant uncertainty remains and diagnostic agreement between even expert dermatopathologists is far less than 100 % [37]. For the purposes of this chapter, we refer to these diagnostically challenging lesions as "atypical melanocytic neoplasms."

Of these, the atypical spitzoid neoplasms are the most common. The term spitzoid refers to lesions with some but not all of the features of a typical (benign) Spitz nevus. It is often difficult to identify spitzoid lesions with the potential for recurrence and distant metastasis, as no consistent, distinctive factors have been identified that categorize malignant potential.

Multiple studies have attempted to identify tumor markers to characterize the malignant potential of atypical melanocytic neoplasms. CGH and FISH have been most consistently used when some but not all of the features of either melanoma or a benign lesion like a Spitz nevus are present in a given case [82]. Initial FISH results using probes targeting chromosomes 6p25 (the locus of gene *RREB1*), 6q23

(*MYB*), Cep6 (the centromere of chromosome 6), and 11q13 (*CCND1*) showed a sensitivity of 86.7 % and specificity of 95.4 % in diagnosis of melanoma compared to benign nevi, although false-positive diagnoses in tetraploid cases were an issue [39]. The second-generation FISH test targets 6p25, 11q13, 9p21 (*CDKN2A*), and 8q24 (*cMYC*) and has a higher accuracy with histologically unequivocal melanocytic neoplasms [38]. However, when used in the setting of diagnostically challenging spitzoid melanocytic proliferations, the sensitivity is less than 70 % [66, 79], so this test is not reliable as the sole arbiter of a malignant or benign diagnosis. It may be useful as a diagnostic adjunct: in one series of 64 patients with atypical Spitz tumors analyzed by FISH, 9 of the 11 patients who developed advanced disease or died had deletion of 9p21, which results in loss of *p16/CDKN2A* [38].

CGH assesses for gains and losses of portions of genetic material across the entire spectrum of 23 chromosome pairs. In one series, while 96 % of melanomas had chromosomal gains or losses, only 13 % of atypical melanocytic neoplasms had abnormalities. While most benign nevi have normal karyotypes, 15 % of Spitz nevi showed an increase in copy number of chromosome 11p at the *HRAS* locus, versus 70 % of atypical spitzoid neoplasms [12]. In contrast, melanoma in pediatric and adult cases rarely shows an *HRAS* mutation. Loss of *BAP1* on 3p21 is associated with the development of melanocytic tumors with spitzoid features, and a recent screening of a database of ambiguous melanocytic tumors showed that 6.7 % of cases had 3p21 loss [129]. Kinase fusions involving ALK, ROS-1, NTRK-1, BRAF, and RET are found in up to 51 % of melanocytic tumors with spitzoid morphology. Although the presence of a fusion protein is not informative about the biologic potential of the lesion, some may confer sensitivity to tyrosine kinase inhibitors [16, 123]. There are further studies investigating the role of epigenetics and hypermethylation as biomarkers of melanoma and treatment response. Mutations of the *TERT* promoter, which increase telomerase activity, were recently found in 4 of 58 atypical spitzoid tumors, and all 4 cases with a *TERT* mutation developed metastases and died of disease [59]. Most recently, microRNA studies have been conducted and may show promise as adjuncts for evaluating histologically ambiguous lesions [43, 58].

Involvement of lymph nodes draining the site of an atypical lesion could potentially indicate its malignant nature; patients with diagnostically challenging lesions may be offered a sentinel lymph node biopsy for this purpose (see Sect. 4.3).

4.2 A Proposed Nomenclature for Categorization of Pediatric Melanocytic Neoplasia

Compounding the difficulty making a firm diagnosis of benign or malignant lesions is the lack of a standard terminology so that clinicians can understand exactly what the pathologist is trying to convey about the nature of the lesion in question. This in turn makes it difficult for clinicians to communicate to the patient or patient's family about the nature of the lesion, the risk for metastasis and death, and the

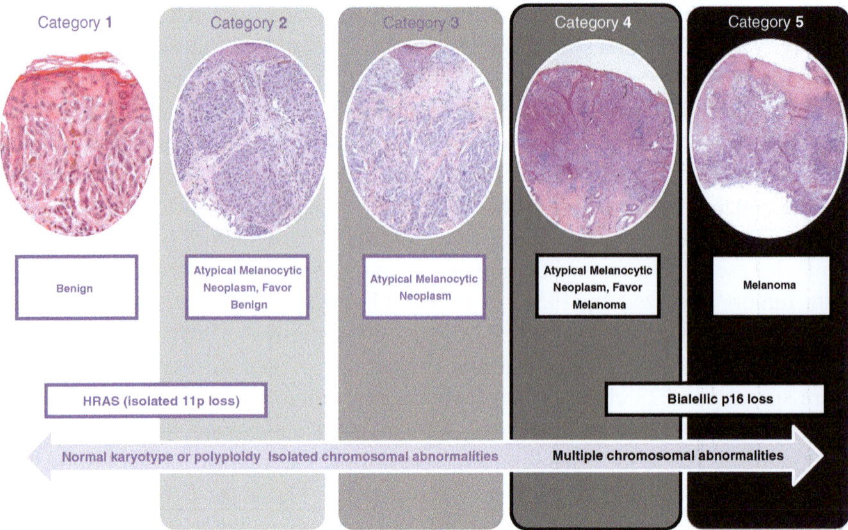

Fig. 2 Spectrum of melanocytic neoplasms in children. We have adopted a 1–5 scale that reflects the histologic appearance of the primary lesion (depicted) as well as molecular/genetic information derived from comparative genomic hybridization or fluorescence in situ hybridization, and can also reflect the findings of sentinel node biopsy in appropriate cases. Only a few molecular abnormalities, however, definitively characterize as lesion as likely benign (isolated 11p loss) or malignant (biallelic p21 loss). This numerical scale facilitates communication not only between the pathologist and the clinician, but also between the clinician and the patient and family. Importantly, the categorization can evolve as additional clinical, pathologic, and molecular information becomes available. (Modified from Sreeraman Kumar et al. [108].)

available treatment options. In an effort to add a degree of objectivity to this process, we have adopted a five-point system for categorizing melanocytic lesions from clearly benign at one end of the spectrum to clearly malignant at the other (Fig. 2). This system is derived from the original "BiRADS" reporting system for categorizing the results of mammography [30] and is similar to a proposal for categorizing dysplastic nevi [91]. We have found this system useful in our conversations between pathologist and clinician and between clinician and patient/family, and also for conveying the process whereby the initial uncertainty about a lesion can lessen or even resolve entirely as additional pathologic material is analyzed or new clinical details emerge [106].

4.2.1 Category 1: Benign

Lesions in this category possess classic histopathologic features of an unequivocally benign lesion. In the pediatric age groups, examples include Spitz nevi, pigmented spindle cell nevi of Reed, blue nevi, deep penetrating nevi, CMN, proliferative nodules in congenital nevi, melanocytic nevi, dysplastic melanocytic nevi, and speckled lentiginous nevi. There is no additional evaluation needed, but to prevent recurrence complete excision is generally warranted, if not already achieved with the initial biopsy.

4.2.2 Category 2: Atypical Melanocytic Neoplasm, Favor Benign

Lesions in this category possess most but not all of the classic histopathologic features of one of the unequivocally benign lesions mentioned above. Some non-typical features are seen, but not to the extent that the pathologist feels that the lesion may represent a melanoma. Examples of such features include focal areas of proliferation/mitoses, focal increases in cellularity, or isolated foci of cellular atypia. At times, an unequivocal diagnosis cannot be made due to an incomplete biopsy that does not allow full evaluation of the lesion. Hence, these lesions should all be completely excised and the re-excision specimen evaluated to ensure that no more concerning features are seen in areas of the lesion not sampled in the initial biopsy material, but beyond that no further evaluation or management is generally warranted.

4.2.3 Category 3: Atypical Melanocytic Neoplasm, Not Amenable to Further Classification

These are lesions with atypical features indicating possible metastatic potential, but which lack features that allow the pathologist to definitively classify the lesion as most likely malignant or benign. Many different terms have been proffered to describe these lesions, such as STUMP, spitzoid atypical melanocytic proliferation of uncertain significance (SAMPUS), and MELTUMP. However, these terms—while adequately capturing the inherent uncertainty of behavior—do not convey to the clinician whether there are any features that are more or less suggestive of malignancy. There are also some melanocytic lesions that are recognized diagnostic entities but for which the likelihood of malignancy is simply unknown, such as pigmented epithelioid melanocytoma, atypical cellular blue nevus, and some BAP-1 deleted melanocytic neoplasms (seen in patients with germline deletions of *BAP1*). CGH and/or FISH can be particularly helpful in these lesions. For example, an atypical spitzoid lesion in Category 3 by histopathologic criteria that had a single chromosomal aberration in chromosome 11p might be appropriately categorized as an atypical Spitz nevus, favor benign (Category 2), while an identical appearing lesion with multiple chromosomal gains and losses and FISH abnormalities in a high percentage of cells would be considered very concerning for melanoma, potentially more appropriately reported as atypical spitzoid lesion, favor spitzoid melanoma (Category 4).

Lesions in Category 3 should always be completely excised, and the re-excision specimen carefully examined for hints in any residual neoplasm that could allow for a more definitive diagnosis. Furthermore, sentinel node biopsy *may* be offered for some lesions in this category, with the recognition that the finding of lesional cells in the sentinel node may or may not allow for a reclassification as unequivocally malignant (see below).

4.2.4 Category 4: Atypical Melanocytic Neoplasm, Favor Malignant

These are lesions with substantial atypical features indicating the possibility of metastatic potential, but which lack sufficient features that allow the pathologist to definitively classify the lesion as malignant. As indicated above, there may be overlap between lesions in this category and those mentioned in Category 3, hence our feeling that simply labeling all these as "lesions of uncertain malignant potential" fails to adequately convey to the clinician a high enough degree of concern. Examples include Spitz-like neoplasms with high dermal cellularity, deep dermal or subcutaneous extension, high mitotic rate in the deep dermis, asymmetry and/or necrosis [118], or atypical cellular blue neoplasms that are large, with necrosis and/or increased mitoses $>2/\text{mm}^2$ [9]. These are lesions with metastatic potential, and there are well-described cases of such lesions eventually leading to recurrence, metastasis, and death (and of course ultimate reclassification into Category 5). Excision to negative margins should always be performed, and these lesions should be treated in an identical manner to an unequivocal melanoma of similar depth. For us, this includes sentinel node biopsy for most Category 4 lesions 1 mm or thicker. CGH and/or FISH can be helpful, and if markedly abnormal may provide sufficient evidence for the pathologist to render an outright malignant diagnosis (Category 5). Similarly, in most cases of Category 4 neoplasms, findings of lesional cells in the sentinel node, especially in the nodal parenchyma or growing in an expansile fashion, should be considered to represent evidence that the lesion is indeed malignant.

4.2.5 Category 5: Melanoma

Lesions in this category possess classic histopathologic features of an unequivocal melanoma. A greater percentage of melanomas in the pediatric population are spitzoid or nevoid in appearance, which adds to the difficulty in making an outright diagnosis of malignancy. Desmoplastic, lentigo maligna, and subungual melanomas are less common in children than in adults (Table 2) [8].

4.3 Further Evaluation and Reclassification of Atypical Melanocytic Neoplasms

It is not uncommon that additional information becomes available regarding a lesion that could not be categorized unequivocally as either benign or malignant on initial biopsy, and in some cases this new information allows for a definitive diagnosis. Virtually all lesions in Category 2, 3, or 4 should be completely excised to negative margins, and the re-excision examined by an experienced dermatopathologist for additional diagnostic clues unavailable in the initial biopsy specimen. As discussed above, further investigation with CGH and/or FISH as well as sentinel node biopsy should be considered in selected cases, and at times can allow a definitive diagnosis. Finally, long-term follow-up can result in reclassification of a benign or atypical

Table 2 Distribution of histologic subtypes of pediatric melanoma as reported in several large single-institution series

Author (number of cases)						
Histologic subtype	Paradela [87] (n = 128)	Livestro [61] (n = 73)	Aldrink [2] (n = 136)	Han [44] (n = 62)	Cordoro [26] (n = 60)	Total (n = 461)
Superficial spreading	48 %	62 %	49 %	47 %	9 %	45 %
Nodular	34 %	12 %	21 %	23 %	30 %	25 %
Acral lentiginous	4 %	1 %	4 %	0	0	2 %
Spitzoid	Not separately reported[a]	Not reported	2 %	4 %	13 %	3 %
Other/NOS/unclassified	14 %	25 %	24 %	26 %	48 %	5 %

Only cases deemed to be melanoma are included; cases of atypical melanocytic neoplasms, if reported in that series, are excluded. This could lead to an underestimation of some histologic subtypes, particularly spitzoid melanomas, which are often characterized as "atypical" rather than unequivocally malignant

Abbreviation: *NOS* not otherwise specified

[a] 36 % of cases had Spitzoid cytologic features

lesion to malignant based on the development of regional or distant spread or death from melanoma. Whenever management decisions are made based on an initial biopsy specimen, especially when that specimen represents a less-than-complete sampling of the lesion, the possibility that subsequent information will alter the diagnosis should be kept firmly in mind. Patients and families need to understand the uncertainties involved with the diagnosis of pediatric melanocytic lesions, and the possibility that a lesion initially felt to be most likely benign can subsequently prove to be malignant. Conversely, they as well as their physicians should also understand that a malignant diagnosis is not synonymous with death from melanoma: most patients with unequivocal melanoma diagnosed before age 21 are in fact cured with appropriate treatment.

5 Diagnostic and Treatment Paradigms for Pediatric Melanoma and Atypical Melanocytic Neoplasms

5.1 Preoperative Staging Workup

In patients diagnosed with unequivocal melanoma at initial biopsy, further evaluation begins with a thorough physical examination, including an assessment of the presence of any residual pigmented lesion at the primary site and examination of the regional lymph nodes. In patients with enlarged or difficult to examine regional lymph nodes, ultrasonography can be helpful, and if appropriate, ultrasound-guided fine needle aspiration can be carried out in an effort to establish the diagnosis of stage III melanoma preoperatively. Because of the risks associated with ionizing radiation in children and adolescents [70, 89], CT or PET/CT scans should be used preoperatively only for well-defined indications: patients with clinically positive lymph nodes in whom biopsy establishes a diagnosis of stage III melanoma and those with signs or symptoms suspicious of metastatic disease should generally have further radiologic evaluation prior to surgery, while most other cases should not. For patients with atypical lesions (Category 2, 3, or 4), outside of a careful evaluation of the regional lymph nodes that may include ultrasonography in selected cases, preoperative radiologic imaging is not indicated. Routine use of laboratory tests is not indicated in pediatric patients with atypical or malignant lesions, except as needed to evaluate symptoms or ensure the safe conduct of planned surgery.

5.2 Wide Excision

Surgery is the mainstay of treatment for localized cutaneous melanoma and for atypical melanocytic lesions of all histologic types and in all categories of suspicion. If the initial biopsy of a Category 1 or 2 lesion has positive margins, complete excision is recommended. For Category 4 or 5 lesions (suspected or diagnosed melanoma), and likely for most Category 3 lesions, wide excision is indicated even if the initial biopsy had negative margins. The optimum margin of excision for pediatric melanoma has never been established, as children were excluded from randomized trials evaluating margin width in cutaneous melanoma. Pediatric melanoma seems to have a lower risk of local recurrence when compared with adult melanoma of the same thickness [61]. For older children, we advocate wide excision of the primary site utilizing standard adult guidelines for excision margin widths, namely 1 cm margins for lesions ≤1 mm in thickness at all sites, for tumors 1–2 mm in thickness in areas where a wider margin would require a skin graft or result in severe deformity, and for all tumors on the head and neck or distal extremities, and 2 cm margins for most thicker lesions. In children younger than 14, we utilize a 1 cm margin for melanomas of all thicknesses and in all primary sites and have not seen local recurrences with that approach [44, 126]. For Category 2 and 3 lesions, a maximum 1 cm margin is taken regardless of thickness or age. Whatever the initial excision margin employed, the goal of surgery is to achieve a final negative histologic margin. In those rare cases where a re-excision specimen is found to have residual neoplasm at the excision margin, further re-excision is indicated. If narrow re-excision of a Category 2 or 3 lesion uncovers residual tumor diagnostic of melanoma, wider excision may be warranted.

5.3 Indications for Sentinel Lymph Node Biopsy

The role of sentinel lymph node biopsy in pediatric melanoma and atypical melanocytic neoplasms remains controversial. Sentinel lymph node biopsy is a well-tolerated procedure that allows for surgical staging and can inform further treatment decisions. The majority of pediatric patients with melanoma are node negative and have an excellent prognosis [8, 42, 49, 60, 74, 83, 87]. These patients can be followed with routine surveillance and are at low risk of recurrence, and the reassurance value of a negative sentinel node biopsy should not be underestimated. In many cases, however, the sentinel lymph node or nodes contain cells identical to the primary tumor—in fact, the incidence of a positive sentinel node is similar in patients with pediatric melanoma and atypical melanocytic neoplasms and higher than in adults with melanomas of similar thickness [95]. Conversely, the prognosis of sentinel node-positive pediatric cases appears to be substantially better than that for adults. We will address the role of sentinel lymph node biopsy in pediatric melanoma and atypical melanocytic neoplasms separately.

5.3.1 Indications for Sentinel Node Biopsy in Pediatric Melanoma

As in adults [73, 127], there is a strong argument for sentinel lymph node biopsy as a prognostic tool for pediatric melanoma, as recurrence and death are more likely to occur in sentinel node-positive cases [8, 14, 19, 44, 49, 71, 72, 75, 116]. The long-term consequences of removal of one or a few lymph nodes from a basin in a child are relatively few, albeit not zero [84]. In cases of pediatric melanoma ≥1 mm in thickness, well over 30 % of patients with clinically negative nodes will be found to have at least one positive sentinel lymph node (Table 3), and we routinely advocate the use of sentinel lymph node biopsy in pediatric patients with melanomas ≥1 mm in thickness in the absence of specific contraindications. As in adults [40], the indications for sentinel lymph node biopsy in thin melanoma (<1 mm) remain unclear. Lesions thicker than 0.75 mm, those with ulceration, and those with mitotic activity (mitotic rate $\geq 1/\text{mm}^2$) are most commonly considered for sentinel node biopsy in adults with thin melanoma [45, 127], and we employ these same criteria for older children with thin melanoma. Thin melanomas are rarely diagnosed in younger children [109], which further limits our knowledge about relative indications for sentinel node biopsy, and we employ sentinel node biopsy only very selectively for children under 14 with melanomas <1 mm.

5.3.2 Indications for Sentinel Node Biopsy in Pediatric Atypical Melanocytic Neoplasms

Recent editorials advocated for a limited role for sentinel lymph node biopsy in the absence of a definite diagnosis of melanoma, given the unclear prognostic value of a positive finding and the potential for overtreatment [21, 24, 50]. It can be difficult to differentiate metastatic melanoma from benign nodal nevus cells because lesional cells from benign melanocytic neoplasms such as Spitz and cellular blue nevi can also be found within regional lymph nodes. Patients with unequivocally benign nevi can have benign collections of nodal melanocytes (termed "nodal nevi") up to 22 % of the time. However, in patients with atypical melanocytic neoplasms, the collections of melanocytes are often seen in the parenchyma of the lymph node, similar to melanoma. Although it is generally considered that multiple positive

Table 3 Results of sentinel lymph node biopsy in pediatric patients with clinically node-negative melanoma as reported in several large single-institution series

Author	# of patients undergoing sentinel lymph node biopsy	% positive sentinel lymph node biopsies	% of sentinel node-positive cases undergoing completion lymphadenectomy	% of completion lymphadenectomy cases with positive non-sentinel nodes	Median follow-up	Overall survival	Notes
Gibbs [42]	2	100 %	100 %	0	62 months	100 %	No local or distant recurrence
Pacella [83]	4	50 %	100 %	0	14 months	100 %	All patients received adjuvant interferon
Toro [116]	12	25 %	100 %	33 %	11.7 months	92 %	1 death in the patient with positive non-sentinel nodes. There were no other recurrences
Butter [19]	4	50 %	50 %	0	Not reported	75 %	1 death in a node-negative patient who developed nodal metastasis at 8 months, underwent chemotherapy and interferon and died at 26 months

(continued)

Table 3 (continued)

Author	# of patients undergoing sentinel lymph node biopsy	% positive sentinel lymph node biopsies	% of sentinel node-positive cases undergoing completion lymphadenectomy	% of completion lymphadenectomy cases with positive non-sentinel nodes	Median follow-up	Overall survival	Notes
Ferrari [35]	4	50 %	100 %	Not reported	122 months	Not reported	
Roaten [97]	15	33 %	100 %	Not reported	33 months	100 %	
Shah [103]	10	60 %	100 %	33 %	26 months	100 %	5 patients received adjuvant interferon, 1 patient developed recurrence and is alive
Livestro [61]	16	44 %	100 %	14 %	5.4 years	94 %	1 node-positive patient developed a recurrence and died of disease
Aldrink [2]	18	39 %	100 %	29 %	8.5 years	100 %	4 patients lost to follow-up; no recurrence rate reported
Howman-Giles [49]	55	25 %	93 %	15 %	60 months	Overall: 94.1 % Node negative: 100 % Node positive: 79 %	3 deaths in the node-positive deaths, 1 node-negative patient alive with recurrence at 51 months

(continued)

Table 3 (continued)

Author	# of patients undergoing sentinel lymph node biopsy	% positive sentinel lymph node biopsies	% of sentinel node-positive cases undergoing completion lymphadenectomy	% of completion lymphadenectomy cases with positive non-sentinel nodes	Median follow-up	Overall survival	Notes
Berk [14]	10	20 %	100 %	50 %	24.5 months	90 %	1 node-positive patient developed nodal recurrence and liver metastases
Paradela [87]	69	45 %	74 %	10 %	45.4 months	Overall: 91 % Node negative: 90 % Node positive: 93 %	4 distant recurrences resulted in death: 2 node-positive patients and 2 node-negative patients
Tcheung [115]	4	50 %	100 %	Not reported	9.9 years	100 %	
Moore-Olufemi [72]	57	35 %	Not reported	Not reported	4.64 years	Overall: 88 % Node positive: 68 % Node negative: 94 %	7 deaths: 2 with positive CLND, 2 in patients with negative SLNB and 3 with positive SLNB and negative CLND

(continued)

Table 3 (continued)

Author	# of patients undergoing sentinel lymph node biopsy	% positive sentinel lymph node biopsies	% of sentinel node-positive cases undergoing completion lymphadenectomy	% of completion lymphadenectomy cases with positive non-sentinel nodes	Median follow-up	Overall survival	Notes
Han [44]	62	29 %	78 %	14 %	60 months	Overall: 85.5 % Node positive: 72 % Node negative: 91 %	Node-positive: 8 patients with recurrence: 4 locoregional and 1 distant and 1 unknown Node-negative: 5 patients with recurrence: 2 locoregional, 2 distant, and 1 unknown
Hung [50]	7	57 %	75 %	0 %	84 months	100 %	1 patient with positive SLNB developed an in-transit metastasis. All patients with positive SLNB received adjuvant interferon therapy

(continued)

Table 3 (continued)

Author	# of patients undergoing sentinel lymph node biopsy	% positive sentinel lymph node biopsies	% of sentinel node-positive cases undergoing completion lymphadenectomy	% of completion lymphadenectomy cases with positive non-sentinel nodes	Median follow-up	Overall survival	Notes
Mu [75]	244	25 %	78 %	Not reported	34 months	87 %	
Paradela [86]	69 (44 non-spitzoid, 25 spitzoid)	39 % (non-spitzoid 30 %, spitzoid 56 %)	Not reported	Not reported	Not reported	Not reported	
Parida [88]	29	41 %	100 %	Not reported	21.5 months	Node negative: 100 % Not reported for node positive	None of the SLNB negative patients had nodal recurrences
Averbook [8]	180	30 %	91 %	37 %		97 %	
Total (n)[a]	691	33 % (227)	66 % (151)	9 % (15)	–	94 %[b] (588)	

Only cases deemed to be melanoma are included; cases of atypical melanocytic neoplasms, if reported in that series, are excluded

Abbreviation: *CLND* completion lymph node dissection; *SLNB* sentinel lymph node biopsy

[a]Total provided for studies with all available information, excluding the Averbook registry data due to potential duplication of case reporting

[b]Excludes patients without available follow-up data

nodes, expansile tumor deposits, and the presence of necrosis or nodal effacement support a diagnosis of malignancy, there have been no studies that define a threshold of nodal involvement that is diagnostic for malignancy. Moreover, clinical studies have shown few or even no recurrences for atypical melanocytic neoplasms with positive sentinel nodes, at median follow-up intervals of 2–4 years (Table 4) [18, 20, 36, 41, 62, 64, 66, 71, 76, 102, 113, 120], and some small series of atypical melanocytic neoplasms managed with excision alone had no evidence of recurrent disease [22]. All these facts argue for a cautious approach to sentinel node biopsy in pediatric atypical melanocytic neoplasms, but a contrary case can also be made.

In fact, we have encountered numerous cases where patients with pediatric atypical neoplasms developed recurrence and even died of metastatic malignancy, often many years or even decades after initial diagnosis. Even in unequivocal pediatric melanoma, many of the recurrences and deaths from disease occur more than five years after initial diagnosis (Fig. 3) [44], so studies with relatively short (and often incomplete) follow-up must be viewed with a healthy degree of skepticism. Perhaps the strongest argument in favor of sentinel node biopsy for pediatric atypical neoplasms is the uncertainty associated with the diagnosis itself. It is well recognized that experienced pathologists will disagree in a substantial portion of cases in which at least one pathologist has rendered a diagnosis of atypical melanocytic neoplasm. Importantly, even cases with documented fatal outcomes have been called atypical or benign by at least some experienced pathologists when shown blinded cases [10, 37]. Hence, some cases that represent melanoma are not identified as such based on the initial biopsy. While the significance of atypical cells in the sentinel node is not always clear in these patients, there are cases where the presence of expansile nodules of tumor cells reveals a diagnosis of malignancy that might otherwise have been missed. Conversely, as alluded to previously, the finding of a negative sentinel node or nodes can help reassure the patient and family that—despite uncertainty about whether the lesion may be melanoma—everything possible has been done to make a diagnosis and the patient has been treated appropriately if the diagnosis is in fact melanoma. Recurrences in the nodal basin and distant metastatic disease are very uncommon in patients with pediatric atypical neoplasms after negative sentinel lymph node biopsy (see Table 4), and most such patients can be safely observed without any additional surgical or adjuvant therapy [46, 71].

5.4 Surgical Management of the Sentinel Node-Positive Nodal Basin

The management of the pediatric melanoma patient with a positive sentinel lymph node is contentious, and key principles are largely drawn by analogy to the adult literature. Completion lymphadenectomy, by definition a radical lymph node dissection after a positive sentinel node biopsy, is the current standard of care

Table 4 Results of sentinel lymph node biopsy in pediatric patients with clinically node-negative atypical melanocytic neoplasms as reported in several large single-institution series

Author	# of patients undergoing sentinel lymph node biopsy	% positive sentinel lymph node biopsies	% of sentinel node-positive cases undergoing completion lymphadenectomy	% of completion lymphadenectomy cases with positive non-sentinel nodes	Median follow-up	Overall survival/recurrence	Comments
Lohmann [62][a]	10	50 %	100 %	20 %		100 %	
Su [113]	12	50 %	100 %	17 %	12 months	100 %	
Gamblin [36]	10	30 %	100 %	33 %	Node negative: 28.1 months Node positive: 49 months	100 %	All node-positive patients received interferon
Urso [120]	5	40 %	50 %	100 %	5 months	100 %	
Murali [76]	9	55 %	100 %	0	10.7 months	100 %	
Ludgate [64]	57	47 %	100 %	3.4 %	Node positive: 43.8 months Node negative: 28.6 months	100 % in patients undergoing SLNB	89 % of node-positive patients received interferon
Busam [18]	11	55 %	Not reported	Not reported	47 months	100 %	

(continued)

Table 4 (continued)

Author	# of patients undergoing sentinel lymph node biopsy	% positive sentinel lymph node biopsies	% of sentinel node-positive cases undergoing completion lymphadenectomy	% of completion lymphadenectomy cases with positive non-sentinel nodes	Median follow-up	Overall survival/recurrence	Comments
Ghazi [41][a]	27	22 %	66 %	0	Node negative: 14 months Node positive: 31 months	100 % in patients undergoing SLNB	1 death in patient who had clinically positive nodes
Sepehr [102]	2	0	Not applicable	Not applicable	30 months	100 %	
Mills [71]	24	29 %	86 %	17 %	4.1 years	100 %	
Total (n)	167	40 % (67)	97 % (65)	9 % (6)	–	100 %	

Only cases deemed to be atypical are included; cases of melanoma, if reported in that series, are excluded. This could lead to an underestimation of the outcome for cases initially characterized as "atypical" rather than malignant, because some cases might subsequently be reclassified as malignant and excluded from analysis

Abbreviation: *SLNB* sentinel lymph node biopsy

[a]Includes some patients >21 years of age

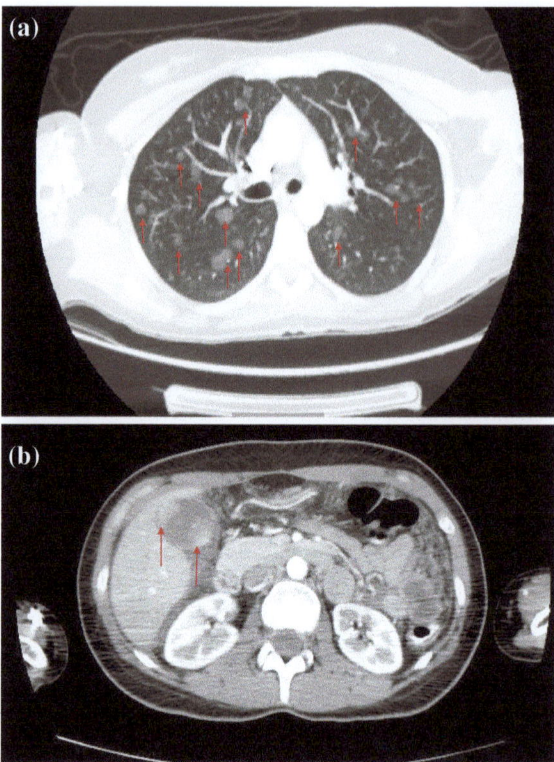

Fig. 3 Late recurrence of melanoma initially presenting in childhood. This patient was initially diagnosed at age 14 with a 3.4 mm ulcerated melanoma on her back. One sentinel lymph node in the ipsilateral axilla had a microscopic focus of metastatic disease. Twelve years later, she returned with abdominal pain and a new cutaneous lesion. **a** CT scan of the thorax demonstrated multiple pulmonary metastases, some of which are denoted with *red arrows*. **b** CT scan of the upper abdomen demonstrated mass lesions in the gallbladder (*arrows*), biopsy proven to represent metastatic melanoma. She subsequently developed brain metastases and died of disease nearly 14 years after her original biopsy

recommendation for adult patients [127], although involved non-sentinel nodes are found on histologic examination in only about 10 % of lymphadenectomy specimens (see Table 3) [67, 77, 98]. Only limited data are available on the rates of non-sentinel node involvement in pediatric melanoma, but what data are available suggests that the rate may [49, 61, 103, 116] or may not [119] be lower than that in adults. Virtually, no data are available on the in-basin recurrence rates for pediatric patients who do not undergo completion lymphadenectomy.

In our experience, the rates of lymphedema are lower for pediatric patients undergoing radical lymphadenectomy compared to adults, and dysesthesias and numbness that can be troublesome in adults are rarely consequential in children. However, the increased risk of infection that accompanies lymphadenectomy can be a problem, particularly for younger children, and younger patients likely are also at some increased risk for motor nerve injuries that can have lifelong consequences. On the other hand, teenagers and young adults can be non-compliant with the close follow-up that is usually recommended for sentinel node-positive patients who do not undergo completion lymphadenectomy. Hence, our recommendation for completion lymphadenectomy is individualized based on a number of factors: the number and site(s) of sentinel nodes involved with tumor, the extent of tumor involvement within those nodes, the findings on the preoperative lymphoscintigraphy (which may presage the likelihood of non-sentinel node involvement [131]), and particularly the age of the child. For a very young child, even a few years of delay in performing a lymphadenectomy can decrease the short- and long-term consequences of that procedure, as long as the patient has been carefully followed and treated promptly after recurrence is manifest. Teenagers and older patients need to be carefully assessed to be sure they will be compliant with a close follow-up regimen, and if not, they may be best served by a completion lymphadenectomy. All patients who are observed without completion lymphadenectomy after a positive sentinel node biopsy in our practice are recommended to undergo ultrasound surveillance of the positive basin at least two to three times per year for the first several years, and then every six to twelve months thereafter for a minimum of five years, and are counseled to return promptly if they develop lymphadenopathy or other evidence of recurrence.

5.5 Surgical Management of the Clinically Node-Positive Nodal Basin

In contrast to patients with micrometastatic disease in a sentinel node, pediatric patients with clinically detectable lymph node involvement should undergo radical lymphadenectomy of the involved basin(s) unless there is clear evidence of distant metastatic disease. In general, identical surgical principles are utilized in children and adults to determine the extent of the lymphadenectomy, and like in adults, the relative indications for pelvic ("deep") node dissection in inguinal node-positive cases remain unclear. The only absolute indication for pelvic node dissection in pediatric melanoma is pathologic or radiologic evidence of involvement of one or more iliac or obturator nodes, but deep node dissection should be considered for cases with large or multiple involved inguinal nodes even in the absence of abnormal pelvic nodes on preoperative scanning. Most adult studies indicate that inclusion of the external iliac and obturator nodes with an inguinofemoral node dissection does not increase long-term morbidity [33, 100], and our experience in pediatric patients supports this.

5.6 Adjuvant Systemic Therapy

While systemic adjuvant therapy has been widely used in the adult melanoma population for stage III and even selected high-risk stage II patients [55], there is a dearth of information in the pediatric population, given both the rarity of the disease and the exclusion of children from most melanoma clinical trials.

5.6.1 Interferon-α2b

Three single-institution studies have retrospectively evaluated the feasibility of using high-dose interferon-α2b in stage III resected pediatric melanoma [23, 80, 103]. Patients were noted to tolerate the therapy well, requiring fewer dose modifications than typically reported in adult studies. In one study involving five patients with resected stage III disease, dose modification was required during the induction phase in two patients due to myelosuppression and during the maintenance phase in two patients for abnormal liver function tests, while depression and major mood change were observed in two other patients [103]. A prospective study of high-dose interferon in 15 sentinel node-positive patients (eight of whom were initially diagnosed with atypical melanocytic neoplasms but subsequently reclassified as melanoma) found that all 15 patients were able to complete induction therapy, and only one patient failed to complete maintenance therapy due to toxicity (coming off therapy five weeks before scheduled completion). Two patients developed recurrent disease during maintenance, one of whom was resected to a disease-free state and continued on therapy. The other patient as well as one patient who recurred after the end of therapy died of metastatic melanoma [80].

Although interferon-α2b is well tolerated in children, subcutaneous injection of the medication three times weekly is inconvenient. Pegylated interferon-α2b (peginterferon) can be administered once a week and has pharmacokinetic and pharmacodynamic properties more favorable for maintenance therapy than standard interferon [27]. It has been approved for use in the adjuvant therapy of node-positive melanoma [31, 32, 48]. However, the approved regimen involves five years of therapy, which limits patient acceptance. We have successfully substituted peginterferon for standard maintenance interferon, administering it once weekly at 3 mcg/kg for 48 weeks after a "standard" one-month IV induction phase. A current pediatric clinical trial (NCT00539591) is comparing the pharmacokinetics, feasibility, and quality-of-life impact of subcutaneous peginterferon 1 mcg/kg/week for 48 weeks with that of conventional interferon during maintenance therapy. Results favoring the use of peginterferon once weekly would certainly increase the convenience of therapy in children.

Recently, cooperative group phase III studies investigating the role of adjuvant interferon in patients with node-positive melanoma have begun including children under 18 years of age. SWOG trial S0008 (NCT00006237), ECOG E1697 (NCT00003641), and E1609 (NCT012734338) are examples. No results specific for pediatric patients have as yet been presented from any of these studies, but they hold promise to increase our knowledge base about adjuvant interferon in pediatric melanoma.

5.6.2 Other Adjuvant Therapy Agents Under Evaluation

New agents for treating unresectable metastatic melanoma (see Sect. 5.7 below) merit evaluation as adjuvant therapy in an effort to improve on the risk–benefit ratio of interferon in adults and children. E1609 compares high-dose interferon to two doses of ipilimumab (monoclonal antibody blocking CTLA-4) and includes children age 15 and older. This will likely provide the first opportunity to evaluate new agents in the adjuvant therapy of melanoma.

5.7 Metastatic Disease

5.7.1 Systemic Therapy

Pediatric patients with metastatic melanoma should strongly consider enrollment in a clinical trial given the limited knowledge specifically about this patient population. There are currently several trials evaluating drugs that have been proven to increase survival in the adult stage IV melanoma population, such as ipilimumab, vemurafenib or dabrafenib (BRAF inhibitors), or anti-PD1 antibodies. Like with adult melanoma, knowing the *BRAF* mutation status of the melanoma is paramount to making decisions about treatment for stage IV disease. The overall distribution of *BRAF* mutant melanomas in the pediatric melanoma population is not known, but it appears that adolescents and young adults with histologically conventional melanoma have a higher rate of *BRAF* V600E mutations than seen in the adult melanoma population [69]. Melanomas in children, especially those arising in congenital nevi, predominantly lack *BRAF* mutations and hence are currently not candidates for molecularly targeted therapy [63]. As in adults, immunotherapy is appropriate first-line therapy for pediatric melanoma patients whose tumor lacks a *BRAF* mutation and even for some *BRAF* mutant melanoma cases with relatively low tumor burden and few or no symptoms [53]. Interleukin-2, ipilimumab, and the anti-PD1 inhibitors pembrolizumab and nivolumab are currently commercially available, but there is little or no published experience regarding safety and efficacy of any of these agents in children under 16.

5.7.2 Palliative Radiation

Radiation therapy in the pediatric population is reserved for palliation of metastatic disease, particularly brain metastases, or rarely for the treatment of unresectable regional disease. Advances in radiation techniques such as image guidance, stereotactic radiation therapy, intensity-modulated radiation, and proton beam radiation have allowed for more conformal treatment, allowing for increased sparing of normal tissue that likely has particular value in the pediatric population [110]. Fractionated techniques have been shown to be safe in children [122], suggesting that with modern techniques, radiation therapy can be used on a case-by-case basis as an effective method of palliation of metastases in children.

6 Prognosis and Follow-up

While there are no established follow-up guidelines specifically for pediatric melanoma, early detection of recurrence may allow for surgical intervention and/or a more favorable outcome, and of course sun protection and screening for second primary cutaneous malignancies is important in melanoma patients of all ages.

6.1 Follow-up

A study comparing pediatric patients with positive and negative sentinel lymph nodes found that recurrence occurred only in patients with node-positive disease and could occur more than five years from diagnosis due to the long natural history of the disease [44]. To date, there are no specific recommendations or guidelines for the follow-up of pediatric melanoma patients after surgery.

6.2 Prognosis of Pediatric Melanoma Based on Stage of Disease

Stage of disease is one of the primary determinants of overall survival in pediatric melanoma just as in adults, with localized disease having a more favorable prognosis. Available evidence suggests that prognosis is likely better for pediatric melanoma patients diagnosed when prepubertal versus postpubertal [35, 57], but this is not reflected in current staging systems.

6.2.1 Stage I–II: Localized Disease

Early-stage, localized pediatric melanoma portends an excellent prognosis with multiple series reporting from 94 to 100 % overall survival over 10 years for stage I disease and from 79 to 100 % for stage II disease, with a disease-free survival of more than 70 % [8, 34, 57, 109]. Ulceration and increase in tumor thickness are associated with a less favorable prognosis and a higher local recurrence rate and a decreased overall survival, as in adult melanoma.

6.2.2 Stage III: Regional Metastatic Disease

Metastatic disease to regional lymph nodes is associated with decreases in overall survival and disease-free survival in comparison with localized disease. Pediatric melanoma patients have a more favorable prognosis than adults with similar staged disease, with 70–77 % overall survival at 10 years [8, 34, 57].

6.2.3 Stage IV: Distant Metastatic Disease

Distant metastases are associated with a poor prognosis, with 40 % overall survival at 5 years and 0 % at 10 years reported in a large registry series [8].

6.3 Prognosis of Atypical Melanocytic Neoplasms

Atypical melanocytic neoplasms, as described in Sects. 4.1 and 4.2 above, are diverse and heterogeneous both histopathologically and molecularly and likely in terms of their prognosis as well. While most patients with atypical melanocytic neoplasms have an excellent prognosis, deaths from melanoma have occurred in children whose initial lesion could not—even in retrospect—be characterized as clearly malignant. Atypical lesions with certain specific high-risk features are more likely to develop recurrent or metastatic melanoma. Prior studies have shown that atypical melanocytic neoplasms with diameter greater than 1 cm, extension into the subcutaneous tissue, ulceration and higher numbers of mitoses per high-powered field, and those arising in children greater than 10 years of age are associated with increased risk of metastases [107]. In addition, recent studies show that lesions with 9p21 deletions have an increased risk of recurrence and metastasis [38]. However, the prognostic significance of sentinel lymph node biopsy remains controversial in these atypical neoplasms, as described in Sect. 5.3.2 above.

7 Future Directions and Challenges

Our understanding of the natural history and epidemiology of pediatric melanoma is limited by the relatively small number of patients, variations in pathologic diagnosis, and incomplete data about the cases that do occur. While one multicenter patient registry has been published [8], most studies are single-institution studies with small patient numbers. Unresolved questions about the utility of sentinel lymph node biopsy, completion lymphadenectomy, adjuvant therapy, and treatment of advanced disease will only be better elucidated with greater national and international collaboration and a commitment to prospective evaluations and clinical trials. For pediatric patients with unresectable disease or metastasis, access to the latest biologic treatments is limited by their age. As the incidence of pediatric melanoma continues to rise, the need for improved prognostication and age-specific treatment and follow-up guidelines are sorely needed.

References

1. AIRTUM Working Group, COM AIEOP Working Group (2013) Italian cancer figures, report 2012: cancer in children and adolescents. Epidemiol Prev 37:1–225
2. Aldrink JH, Selim MA, Diesen DL, Johnson J, Pruitt SK, Tyler DS, Seigler HF (2009) Pediatric melanoma: a single-institution experience of 150 patients. J Pediatr Surg 44:1514–1521

3. Alexander A, Samlowski WE, Grossman D, Bruggers CS, Harris RM, Zone JJ, Noyes RD, Bowen GM, Leachman SA (2003) Metastatic melanoma in pregnancy: risk of transplacental metastases in the infant. J Clin Oncol 21:2179–2186
4. Alikhan A, Ibrahimi OA, Eisen DB (2012) Congenital melanocytic nevi: where are we now? Part I. Clinical presentation, epidemiology, pathogenesis, histology, malignant transformation, and neurocutaneous melanosis. J Am Acad Dermatol 67:495
5. Anderson JF, Kent S, Machin GA (1989) Maternal malignant melanoma with placental metastasis: a case report with literature review. Pediatr Pathol 9:35–42
6. Asai J, Takenaka H, Ikada S, Soga F, Kishimoto S (2004) Congenital malignant melanoma: a case report. Br J Dermatol 151:693–697
7. Austin MT, Xing Y, Hayes-Jordan AA, Lally KP, Cormier JN (2013) Melanoma incidence rises for children and adolescents: an epidemiologic review of pediatric melanoma in the United States. J Pediatr Surg 48:2207–2213
8. Averbook BJ, Lee SJ, Delman KA, Gow KW, Zager JS, Sondak VK, Messina JL, Sabel MS, Pittelkow MR, Ecker PM, Markovic SN, Swetter SM, Leachman SA, Testori A, Curiel-Lewandrowski C, Go RS, Jukic DM, Kirkwood JM (2013) Pediatric melanoma: analysis of an international registry. Cancer 119:4012–4019
9. Barnhill RL, Argenyi Z, Berwick M, Duray PH, Erickson L, Guitart J, Horenstein MG, Lowe L, Messina J, Paine S, Piepkorn MW, Prieto V, Rabkin MS, Schmidt B, Selim A, Shea CR, Trotter MJ (2008) Atypical cellular blue nevi (cellular blue nevi with atypical features): lack of consensus for diagnosis and distinction from cellular blue nevi and malignant melanoma ("malignant blue nevus"). Am J Surg Path 32:36–44
10. Barnhill RL, Argenyi ZB, From L, Glass LF, Maize JC, Mihm MC Jr, Rabkin MS, Ronan SG, White WL, Piepkorn M (1999) Atypical Spitz nevi/tumors: lack of consensus for diagnosis, discrimination from melanoma, and prediction of outcome. Hum Pathol 30:513–520
11. Barnhill RL (2006) The Spitzoid lesion: rethinking Spitz tumors, atypical variants, 'Spitzoid melanoma' and risk assessment. Mod Pathol 19:S21–S33
12. Bastian BC, Olshen AB, LeBoit PE, Pinkel D (2003) Classifying melanocytic tumors based on DNA copy number changes. Am J Pathol 163:1765–1770
13. Berg P, Wennberg AM, Tuominen R, Sander B, Rozell BL, Platz A, Hansson J (2004) Germline CDKN2A mutations are rare in child and adolescent cutaneous melanoma. Melanoma Res 14:251–255
14. Berk DR, LaBuz E, Dadras SS, Johnson DL, Swetter SM (2010) Melanoma and melanocytic tumors of uncertain malignant potential in children, adolescents and young adults–the Stanford experience 1995–2008. Pediatr Dermatol 27:244–254
15. Bis S, Tsao H (2013) Melanoma genetics: the other side. Clin Dermatol 31:148–155
16. Botton T, Yeh I, Bastian BC (2014) Melanoma BRAF fusions—letter. Clin Cancer Res 20:6631
17. Bradford PT, Goldstein AM, Tamura D, Khan SG, Ueda T, Boyle J, Oh KS, Imoto K, Inui H, Moriwaki S, Emmert S, Pike KM, Raziuddin A, Plona TM, DiGiovanna JJ, Tucker MA, Kraemer KH (2011) Cancer and neurologic degeneration in xeroderma pigmentosum: long term follow-up characterises the role of DNA repair. J Med Genet 48:168–176
18. Busam KJ, Murali R, Pulitzer M, McCarthy SW, Thompson JF, Shaw HM, Brady MS, Coit DG, Dusza S, Wilmott J, Kayton M, Laquaglia M, Scolyer RA (2009) Atypical spitzoid melanocytic tumors with positive sentinel lymph nodes in children and teenagers, and comparison with histologically unambiguous and lethal melanomas. Am J Surg Pathol 33:1386–1395
19. Butter A, Hui T, Chapdelaine J, Beaunoyer M, Flageole H, Bouchard S (2005) Melanoma in children and the use of sentinel lymph node biopsy. J Pediatr Surg 40:797–800
20. Caraco C, Mozzillo N, Di Monta G, Botti G, Anniciello AM, Marone U, Di Cecilia ML, Staibano S, De Rosa G (2012) Sentinel lymph node biopsy in atypical Spitz nevi: is it useful? Eur J Surg Oncol 38:932–935

21. Casper DJ, Ross KI, Messina JL, Sondak VK, Bodden CN, McCardle TW, Glass LF (2010) Use of anti-phosphohistone H3 immunohistochemistry to determine mitotic rate in thin melanoma. Am J Dermatopathol 32:650–654
22. Cerrato F, Wallins JS, Webb ML, McCarty ER, Schmidt BA, Labow BI (2012) Outcomes in pediatric atypical Spitz tumors treated without sentinel lymph node biopsy. Pediatr Dermatol 29:448–453
23. Chao MM, Schwartz JL, Wechsler DS, Thornburg CD, Griffith KA, Williams JA (2005) High-risk surgically resected pediatric melanoma and adjuvant interferon therapy. Pediatr Blood Cancer 44:441–448
24. Coit DG, Ernstoff MS, Busam KJ (2013) Is pediatric melanoma always malignant? Cancer 119:3910–3913
25. Conway C, Beswick S, Elliott F, Chang YM, Randerson-Moor J, Harland M, Affleck P, Marsden J, Sanders DS, Boon A, Knowles MA, Bishop DT, Newton-Bishop JA (2010) Deletion at chromosome arm 9p in relation to BRAF/NRAS mutations and prognostic significance for primary melanoma. Genes Chromosomes Cancer 49:425–438
26. Cordoro KM, Gupta D, Frieden IJ, McCalmont T, Kashani-Sabet M (2013) Pediatric melanoma: results of a large cohort study and proposal for modified ABCD detection criteria for children. J Am Acad Dermatol 68:913–925
27. Daud AI, Xu C, Hwu WJ, Urbas P, Andrews S, Papadopoulos NE, Floren LC, Yver A, Deconti RC, Sondak VK (2011) Pharmacokinetic/pharmacodynamic analysis of adjuvant pegylated interferon alpha-2b in patients with resected high-risk melanoma. Cancer Chemother Pharmacol 67:657–666
28. DeDavid M, Orlow SJ, Provost N, Marghoob AA, Rao BK, Huang CL, Wasti Q, Kopf AW, Bart RS (1997) A study of large congenital melanocytic nevi and associated malignant melanomas: review of cases in the New York University Registry and the world literature. J Am Acad Dermatol 36:409–416
29. Downard CD, Rapkin LB, Gow KW (2007) Melanoma in children and adolescents. Surg Oncol 16:215–220
30. D'Orsi CJ, Bassett W, Geig SA, Jackson VP, Kopans DB, Linver MN et al (2003) ACR BI-RADS mammography. In: ACR Breast Imaging Reporting and Data System, Breast Imaging Atlas. 4th ed, pp 193–198
31. Eggermont AM, Suciu S, Santinami M, Testori A, Kruit WH, Marsden J, Punt CJ, Sales F, Gore M, Mackie R, Kusic Z, Dummer R, Hauschild A, Musat E, Spatz A, Keilholz U, Group EM (2008) Adjuvant therapy with pegylated interferon alfa-2b versus observation alone in resected stage III melanoma: final results of EORTC 18991, a randomised phase III trial. Lancet 372:117–126
32. Eggermont AM, Suciu S, Testori A, Kruit WH, Marsden J, Punt CJ, Santinami M, Sales F, Schadendorf D, Patel P, Dummer R, Robert C, Keilholz U, Yver A, Spatz A (2012) Ulceration and stage are predictive of interferon efficacy in melanoma: results of the phase III adjuvant trials EORTC 18952 and EORTC 18991. Eur J Cancer 48:218–225
33. Faries MB, Thompson JF, Cochran A, Elashoff R, Glass EC, Mozzillo N, Nieweg OE, Roses DF, Hoekstra HJ, Karakousis CP, Reintgen DS, Coventry BJ, Wang HJ, Morton DL (2010) The impact on morbidity and length of stay of early versus delayed complete lymphadenectomy in melanoma: results of the Multicenter Selective Lymphadenectomy Trial (I). Ann Surg Oncol 17:3324–3329
34. Ferrari A, Bisogno G, Cecchetto G, Santinami M, Maurichi A, Bono A, Vajna De Pava M, Pierani P, Bertolini P, Rossi CR, De Salvo GL (2014) Cutaneous melanoma in children and adolescents: the Italian rare tumors in pediatric age project experience. J Pediatr 164:376–382
35. Ferrari A, Bono A, Baldi M, Collini P, Casanova M, Pennacchioli E, Terenziani M, Marcon I, Santinami M, Bartoli C (2005) Does melanoma behave differently in younger children than in adults? A retrospective study of 33 cases of childhood melanoma from a single institution. Pediatrics 115:649–654

36. Gamblin TC, Edington H, Kirkwood JM, Rao UN (2006) Sentinel lymph node biopsy for atypical melanocytic lesions with spitzoid features. Ann Surg Oncol 13:1664–1670
37. Gerami P, Busam K, Cochran A, Cook MG, Duncan LM, Elder DE, Fullen DR, Guitart J, LeBoit PE, Mihm MC Jr, Prieto VG, Rabkin MS, Scolyer RA, Xu X, Yun SJ, Obregon R, Yazdan P, Cooper C, Weitner BB, Rademaker A, Barnhill RL (2014) Histomorphologic assessment and interobserver diagnostic reproducibility of atypical spitzoid melanocytic neoplasms with long-term follow-up. Am J Surg Pathol 38:934–940
38. Gerami P, Cooper C, Bajaj S, Wagner A, Fullen D, Busam K, Scolyer RA, Xu X, Elder DE, Abraham RM, Prieto VG, Guitart J, Liu P, Pestova E, Barnhill RL (2013) Outcomes of atypical Spitz tumors with chromosomal copy number aberrations and conventional melanomas in children. Am J Surg Pathol 37:1387–1394
39. Gerami P, Wass A, Mafee M, Fang Y, Pulitzer MP, Buzam KJ (2009) Flourescence in situ hybridization for distinguishing nevoid melanomas from mitotically active nevi. Am J Surg Pathol 33:1783–1788
40. Gershenwald JE, Coit DG, Sondak VK, Thompson JF (2012) The challenge of defining guidelines for sentinel lymph node biopsy in patients with thin primary cutaneous melanomas. Ann Surg Oncol 19:3301–3303
41. Ghazi B, Carlson GW, Murray DR, Gow KW, Page A, Durham M, Kooby DA, Parker D, Rapkin L, Lawson DH, Delman KA (2010) Utility of lymph node assessment for atypical spitzoid melanocytic neoplasms. Ann Surg Oncol 17:2471–2475
42. Gibbs P, Moore A, Robinson W, Walsh P, Golitz L, Gonzalez R (2000) Pediatric melanoma: are recent advances in the management of adult melanoma relevant to the pediatric population. J Pediatr Hematol Oncol 22:428–432
43. Grignol V, Fairchild ET, Zimmerer JM, Lesinski GB, Walker MJ, Magro CM, Kacher JE, Karpa VI, Clark J, Nuovo G, Lehman A, Volinia S, Agnese DM, Croce CM, Carson WE 3rd (2011) miR-21 and miR-155 are associated with mitotic activity and lesion depth of borderline melanocytic lesions. Br J Cancer 105:1023–1029
44. Han D, Zager JS, Han G, Marzban SS, Puleo CA, Sarnaik AA, Reed D, Messina JL, Sondak VK (2012) The unique clinical characteristics of melanoma diagnosed in children. Ann Surg Oncol 19:3888–3895
45. Han D, Zager JS, Shyr Y, Chen H, Berry LD, Iyengar S, Djulbegovic M, Weber JL, Marzban SS, Sondak VK, Messina JL, Vetto JT, White RL, Pockaj B, Mozzillo N, Charney KJ, Avisar E, Krouse R, Kashani-Sabet M, Leong SP (2013) Clinicopathologic predictors of sentinel lymph node metastasis in thin melanoma. J Clin Oncol 31:4387–4393
46. Han D, Turner LM, Reed DR, Messina JL, Sondak VK (2013) The prognostic significance of lymph node metastasis in pediatric melanoma and atypical melanocytic proliferations. Expert Rev Dermatol 8:103–106
47. Helvind NM, Holmich LR, Smith S, Glud M, Andersen KK, Dalton SO, Drzewiecki KT (2015) Incidence of in situ and invasive melanoma in Denmark from 1985–2012. JAMA Dermatol
48. Herndon TM, Demko SG, Jiang X, He K, Gootenberg JE, Cohen MH, Keegan P, Pazdur R (2012) U.S. Food and Drug Administration Approval: peginterferon-alfa-2b for the adjuvant treatment of patients with melanoma. Oncologist 17:1323–1328
49. Howman-Giles R, Shaw HM, Scolyer RA, Murali R, Wilmott J, McCarthy SW, Uren RF, Thompson JF (2010) Sentinel lymph node biopsy in pediatric and adolescent cutaneous melanoma patients. Ann Surg Oncol 17:138–143
50. Hung T, Piris A, Lobo A, Mihm MC Jr, Sober AJ, Tsao H, Tanabe KK, Duncan LM (2013) Sentinel lymph node metastasis is not predictive of poor outcome in patients with problematic spitzoid melanocytic tumors. Hum Pathol 44:87–94
51. Jain P, Kannan L, Kumar A, Sigamani E, Suri V, Basheer N, Suri A, Gulati S (2013) Symptomatic neurocutaneous melanosis in a child. JAMA Neurol 70:516
52. Kadonaga JN, Frieden IJ (1991) Neurocutaneous melanosis: Definition and review of the literature. J Am Acad Dermatol 24:747–755

53. Kaufman HL, Kirkwood JM, Hodi FS, Agarwala S, Amatruda T, Bines SD, Clark JI, Curti B, Ernstoff MS, Gajewski T, Gonzalez R, Hyde LJ, Lawson D, Lotze M, Lutzky J, Margolin K, McDermott DF, Morton D, Pavlick A, Richards JM, Sharfman W, Sondak VK, Sosman J, Steel S, Tarhini A, Thompson JA, Titze J, Urba W, White R, Atkins MB (2013) The Society for Immunotherapy of Cancer consensus statement on tumour immunotherapy for the treatment of cutaneous melanoma. Nat Rev Clin Oncol 10:588–598
54. Kinsler VA, Thomas AC, Ishida M, Bulstrode NW, Loughlin S, Hing S, Chalker J, McKenzie K, Abu-Amero S, Slater O, Chanudet E, Palmer R, Morrogh D, Stanier P, Healy E, Sebire NJ, Moore GE (2013) Multiple congenital melanocytic nevi and neurocutaneous melanosis are caused by postzygotic mutations in codon 61 of NRAS. J Invest Dermatol 133:2229–2236
55. Kirkwood JM, Strawderman MH, Ernstoff MS, Smith TJ, Borden EC, Blum RH (1996) Interferon alfa-2b adjuvant therapy of high-risk resected cutaneous melanoma: the Eastern Cooperative Oncology Group trial EST 1684. J Clin Oncol 14:7–17
56. Krengel S, Hauschild A, Schafer T (2006) Melanoma risk in congenital melanocytic naevi: a systematic review. B J Dermatol 155:1–8
57. Lange JR, Pallis BE, Chang DC, Soong SJ, Balch CM (2007) Melanoma in children and teenagers: an analysis of patients from the National Cancer Data Base. J Clin Oncol 25:1363–1368
58. Latchana N, Martin del Campo S, Grignol V, Carson M, Clark J, Peters S, Carson W III (2014) Classifications of indeterminate melanomas by microRNA profiling. Perspectives in Melanoma XVIII, Dublin, Ireland
59. Lee S, Barnhill RL, Dummer R, Dalton J, Wu J, Pappo A, Bahrami A (2015) *TERT* promoter mutations are predictive of aggressive clinical behavior in patients with spitzoid melanocytic neoplasms. Sci Rep 5:11200
60. Lewis KG (2008) Trends in pediatric melanoma mortality in the United States, 1968 through 2004. Dermatol Surg 34:152–159
61. Livestro DP, Kaine EM, Michaelson JS, Mihm MC, Haluska FG, Muzikansky A, Sober AJ, Tanabe KK (2007) Melanoma in the young: differences and similarities with adult melanoma. A case-matched controlled analysis. Cancer 110:614–624
62. Lohmann CM, Coit DG, Brady MS, Berwick M, Busam KJ (2002) Sentinel lymph node biopsy in patients with diagnostically controversial spitzoid melanocytic tumors. Am J Surg Pathol 26:47–55
63. Lu C, Zhang J, Nagahawatte P, Easton J, Lee S, Liu Z, Ding L, Wyczalkowski MA, Valentine M, Navid F, Mulder H, Tatevossian RG, Dalton J, Davenport J, Yin Z, Edmonson M, Rusch M, Wu G, Li Y, Parker M, Hedlund E, Shurtleff S, Raimondi S, Bhavin V, Donald Y, Mardis ER, Wilson RK, Evans WE, Ellison DW, Pounds S, Dyer M, Downing JR, Pappo A, Bahrami A (2015) The genomic landscape of childhood and adolescent melanoma. J Invest Dermatol 135:816–823
64. Ludgate MW, Fullen DR, Lee J, Lowe L, Bradford C, Geiger J, Schwartz J, Johnson TM (2009) The atypical Spitz tumor of uncertain biologic potential: a series of 67 patients from a single institution. Cancer 115:631–641
65. Mason A, Wititsuwannakul J, Klump VR, Lott J, Lazova R (2012) Expression of p16 alone does not differentiate between Spitz nevi and Spitzoid melanoma. J Cutan Pathol 39:1062–1074
66. McCormack CJ, Conyers RK, Scolyer RA, Kirkwood J, Speakman D, Wong N, Kelly JW, Henderson MA (2014) Atypical Spitzoid neoplasms: a review of potential markers of biological behavior including sentinel node biopsy. Melanoma Res 24:437–447
67. McMasters KM, Wong SL, Edwards MJ, Chao C, Ross MI, Noyes RD, Viar V, Cerrito PB, Reintgen DS (2002) Frequency of nonsentinel lymph node metastasis in melanoma. Ann Surg Oncol 9:137–141

68. McNutt NS, Urmacher C, Hakimian J, Hoss DM, Lugo J (1995) Nevoid malignant melanoma: morphologic patterns and immunohistochemical reactivity. J Cutan Pathol 22:502–517
69. Menzies AM, Haydu LE, Visintin L, Carlino MS, Howle JR, Thompson JF, Kefford RF, Scolyer RA, Long GV (2012) Distinguishing clinicopathologic features of patients with V600E and V600K BRAF-mutant metastatic melanoma. Clin Cancer Res 18:3242–3249
70. Miglioretti DL, Johnson E, Williams A, Greenlee RT, Weinmann S, Solberg LI, Feigelson HS, Roblin D, Flynn MJ, Vanneman N, Smith-Bindman R (2013) The use of computed tomography in pediatrics and the associated radiation exposure and estimated cancer risk. JAMA Pediatr 167:700–707
71. Mills OL, Marzban S, Zager JS, Sondak VK, Messina JL (2012) Sentinel node biopsy in atypical melanocytic neoplasms in childhood: a single institution experience in 24 patients. J Cutan Pathol 39:331–336
72. Moore-Olufemi S, Herzog C, Warneke C, Gershenwald JE, Mansfield P, Ross M, Prieto V, Lally KP, Hayes-Jordan A (2011) Outcomes in pediatric melanoma: comparing prepubertal to adolescent pediatric patients. Ann Surg 253:1211–1215
73. Morton DL, Thompson JF, Cochran AJ, Mozzillo N, Nieweg OE, Roses DF, Hoekstra HJ, Karakousis CP, Puleo CA, Coventry BJ, Kashani-Sabet M, Smithers BM, Paul E, Kraybill WG, McKinnon JG, Wang HJ, Elashoff R, Faries MB (2014) Final trial report of sentinel-node biopsy versus nodal observation in melanoma. N Engl J Med 370:599–609
74. Moscarella E, Zalaudek I, Cerroni L, Sperduti I, Catricala C, Smolle J, Hofmann-Wellenhof R, Sgambato A, Pellacani G, Argenziano G (2012) Excised melanocytic lesions in children and adolescents—a 10-year survey. Br J Dermatol 167:368–373
75. Mu E, Lange JR, Strouse JJ (2012) Comparison of the use and results of sentinel lymph node biopsy in children and young adults with melanoma. Cancer 118:2700–2707
76. Murali R, Sharma RN, Thompson JF, Stretch JR, Lee CS, McCarthy SW, Scolyer RA (2008) Sentinel lymph node biopsy in histologically ambiguous melanocytic tumors with spitzoid features (so-called atypical spitzoid tumors). Ann Surg Oncol 15:302–309
77. Murali R, Desilva C, Thompson JF, Scolyer RA (2010) Non-sentinel node risk score (N-SNORE): a scoring system for accurately stratifying risk of non-sentinel node positivity in patients with cutaneous melanoma with positive sentinel lymph nodes. J Clin Oncol 28:4441–4449
78. Nasr MR, El-Zammar O (2008) Comparison of pHH3, Ki-67, and survivin immunoreactivity in benign and malignant melanocytic lesions. Am J Dermatopathol 30:117–122
79. Navid F (2012) Genetic alterations in childhood melanoma. Am Soc Clin Oncol Educ Book 2012:589–592
80. Navid F, Furman WL, Fleming M, Rao BN, Kovach S, Billups CA, Cain AM, Amonette R, Jenkins JJ, Pappo AS (2005) The feasibility of adjuvant interferon alpha-2b in children with high-risk melanoma. Cancer 103:780–787
81. Neier M, Pappo A, Navid F (2012) Management of melanomas in children and young adults. J Pediatr Hematol Oncol 34(Suppl 2):S51–S54
82. North JP, Garrido MC, Kolaitis NA, LeBoit PE, McCalmont TH, Bastian BC (2014) Fluorescence in situ hybridization as an ancillary tool in the diagnosis of ambiguous melanocytic neoplasms: a review of 804 cases. Am J Surg Pathol 38:824–831
83. Pacella SJ, Lowe L, Bradford C, Marcus BC, Johnson T, Rees R (2003) The utility of sentinel lymph node biopsy in head and neck melanoma in the pediatric population. Plast Reconstr Surg 112:1257–1265
84. Palmer PE 3rd, Warneke CL, Hayes-Jordan AA, Herzog CE, Hughes DP, Lally KP, Austin MT (2013) Complications in the surgical treatment of pediatric melanoma. J Pediatr Surg 48:1249–1253
85. Pappo AS (2003) Melanoma in children and adolescents. Eur J Cancer 39:2651–2661

86. Paradela S, Fonseca E, Pita-Fernandez S, Prieto VG (2013) Spitzoid and non-spitzoid melanoma in children: a prognostic comparative study. J Eur Acad Dermatol Venereol 27:1214–1221
87. Paradela S, Fonseca E, Pita-Fernandez S, Kantrow SM, Diwan AH, Herzog C, Prieto VG (2010) Prognostic factors for melanoma in children and adolescents: a clinicopathologic, single-center study of 137 patients. Cancer 116:4334–4344
88. Parida L, Morrisson GT, Shammas A, Hossain AK, McCarville MB, Gerstle JT, Charron M, Rao BN, Shulkin BL (2012) Role of lymphoscintigraphy and sentinel lymph node biopsy in the management of pediatric melanoma and sarcoma. Pediatr Surg Int 28:571–578
89. Pearce MS, Salotti JA, Little MP, McHugh K, Lee C, Kim KP, Howe NL, Ronckers CM, Rajaraman P, Sir Craft AW, Parker L, Berrington de Gonzalez A (2012) Radiation exposure from CT scans in childhood and subsequent risk of leukaemia and brain tumours: a retrospective cohort study. Lancet 380:499–505
90. Perret-Court A, Fernandez C, Monestier S, Millet V, Tasei AM (2010) Placental metastasis of melanoma: a new case and literature review. Ann Pathol 30:143–146
91. Piepkorn MW, Barnhill RL, Elder DE, Knezevich SR, Carney PA, Reisch LM, Elmore JG (2014) The MPATH-Dx reporting schema for melanocytic proliferations and melanoma. J Am Acad Dermatol 70:131–141
92. Price HN, O'Haver J, Marghoob A, Badger K, Etchevers H, Krengel S (2015) Practical application of the new classification scheme for congenital melanocytic nevi. Pediatr Dermatol 32:23–27
93. Rajput A, Faizi SA, Nir I, Morris KT, Fahy B, Russell J, Wiggins C (2014) Pediatric melanoma in New Mexico American Indians, Hispanics, and non-Hispanic whites, 1981–2009. Am J Surg 207:412–416
94. Raso A, Mascelli S, Nozza P, Biassoni R, Negri F, Garaventa A, Tarantino V, Garre ML, Cama A, Capra V (2010) Detection of transplacental melanoma metastasis using quantitative PCR. Diagn Mol Pathol 19:78–82
95. Reed D, Kudchadkar R, Zager JS, Sondak VK, Messina JL (2013) Controversies in the evaluation and management of atypical melanocytic proliferations in children, adolescents, and young adults. J Natl Compr Canc Netw 11:679–686
96. Richardson SK, Tannous ZS, Mihm MC Jr (2002) Congenital and infantile melanoma: review of the literature and report of an uncommon variant, pigment-synthesizing melanoma. J Am Acad Dermatol 47:77–90
97. Roaten JB, Partrick DA, Pearlman D, Gonzalez RJ, Gonzalez R, McCarter MD (2005) Sentinel Lymph node biopsy for melanoma and other melanocytic tumors in adolescents. J Pediatr Surg Jan 40(1):232–235
98. Rossi CR, De Salvo GL, Bonandini E, Mocellin S, Foletto M, Pasquali S, Pilati P, Lise M, Nitti D, Rizzo E, Montesco MC (2008) Factors predictive of nonsentinel lymph node involvement and clinical outcome in melanoma patients with metastatic sentinel lymph node. Ann Surg Oncol 15:1202–1210
99. Ruiz-Maldonado R, Tamayo L, Laterza AM, Duran C (1992) Giant pigmented nevi: clinical, histopathologic, and therapeutic considerations. J Pediatr 120:906–911
100. Sarnaik AA, Puleo CA, Zager JS, Sondak VK (2009) Limiting the morbidity of inguinal lymphadenectomy for metastatic melanoma. Cancer Control 16:240–247
101. Senerchia AA, Ribeiro KB, Rodriguez-Galindo C (2014) Trends in incidence of primary cutaneous malignancies in children, adolescents, and young adults: a population-based study. Pediatr Blood Cancer 61:211–216
102. Sepehr A, Chao E, Trefrey B, Blackford A, Duncan LM, Flotte TJ, Sober A, Mihm MC Jr, Tsao H (2011) Long-term outcome of Spitz-type melanocytic tumors. Arch Dermatol 147:1173–1179
103. Shah NC, Gerstle JT, Stuart M, Winter C, Pappo A (2006) Use of sentinel lymph node biopsy and high-dose interferon in pediatric patients with high-risk melanoma: the Hospital for Sick Children experience. J Pediatr Hematol Oncol 28:496–500

104. Shuhaila A, Rohaizak M, Phang KS, Mahdy ZA (2008) Maternal melanoma with placental metastasis. Singapore Med J 49:e71–72
105. Slade AD, Austin MT (2014) Childhood melanoma: an increasingly important health problem in the USA. Curr Opin Pediatr 26:356–361
106. Sondak VK, Reed D, Messina JL (2015) A comprehensive approach to pediatric atypical melanocytic neoplasms, with comment on the role of sentinel lymph node biopsy. Crit Rev Oncog (in press)
107. Spatz A, Calonje E, Handfield-Jones S, Barnhill RL (1999) Spitz tumors in children: a grading system for risk stratification. Arch Dermatol 135:282–285
108. Sreeraman Kumar R, Messina JL, Sondak VK, Reed DR (2015) Treating melanoma in adolescents and young adults: challenges and solutions. Clinical Oncol Adolesc Young Adults (in press)
109. Stanelle EJ, Busam JK, Rich BS, Christison-Lagay ER, Dunkel IJ, Marghoob AA, Halpern A, Coit DG, La Quaglia MP (2015) Early-stage non-Spitzoid cutaneous melanoma in patients younger than 22 years of age at diagnosis: long-term follow-up and survival analysis. J Pediatr Surg 50:1019–1023
110. Stinauer MA, Kavanagh BD, Schefter TE, Gonzalez R, Flaig T, Lewis K, Robinson W, Chidel M, Glode M, Raben D (2011) Stereotactic body radiation therapy for melanoma and renal cell carcinoma: impact of single fraction equivalent dose on local control. Radiat Oncol 6:34
111. Strouse JJ, Fears TR, Tucker MA, Wayne AS (2005) Pediatric melanoma: risk factor and survival analysis of the Surveillance, Epidemiology and End Results database. J Clin Oncol 23:4735–4741
112. Su A, Low L, Li X, Zhou S, Mascarenhas L, Barnhill RL (2014) De novo congenital melanoma: analysis of 2 cases with array comparative genomic hybridization. Am J Dermatopathol 36:915–919
113. Su LD, Fullen DR, Sondak VK, Johnson TM, Lowe L (2003) Sentinel lymph node biopsy for patients with problematic spitzoid melanocytic lesions: a report on 18 patients. Cancer 97:499–507
114. Tannous ZS, Mihm MC Jr, Sober AJ, Duncan LM (2005) Congenital melanocytic nevi: clinical and histopathologic features, risk of melanoma, and clinical management. J Am Acad Dermatol 52:197–203
115. Tcheung WJ, Marcello JE, Puri PK, Abernethy AP, Nelson KC (2011) Evaulation of 39 cases of pediatric cutaneous head and neck melanoma. J Am Acad Dermatol 65:e37–42
116. Toro J, Ranieri JM, Havlik RJ, Coleman JJ 3rd, Wagner JD (2003) Sentinel lymph node biopsy in children and adolescents with malignant melanoma. J Pediatr Surg 38:1063–1065
117. Trumble ER, Smith RM, Pearl G, Wall J (2005) Transplacental transmission of metastatic melanoma to the posterior fossa. Case report. J Neurosurg 103:191–193
118. Urso C (2005) A new perspective for Spitz tumors? Am J Dermatopathol 27:364–366
119. Urso C, Borgognoni L, Doria M, Tinacci G, Zini E (2009) Non-sentinel lymph node involvement in a patient with an atypical Spitz tumor and a positive sentinel node. Report of a case and review of the literature. J Cutan Pathol 36:586–590
120. Urso C, Borgognoni L, Saieva C, Ferrara G, Tinacci G, Begliomini B, Reali UM (2006) Sentinel lymph node biopsy in patients with "atypical Spitz tumors." A report on 12 cases. Hum Pathol 37:816–823
121. Valenzano Menada M, Moioli M, Garaventa A, Nozza P, Foppiano M, Trimarchi N, Fulcheri E (2010) Spontaneous regression of transplacental metastases from maternal melanoma in a newborn: case report and review of the literature. Melanoma Res 20:443–449
122. Weintraub D, Yen CP, Xu Z, Savage J, Williams B, Sheehan J (2012) Gamma knife surgery of pediatric gliomas. J Neurosurg Pediatr 10:471–477
123. Wiesner T, He J, Yelensky R, Esteve-Puig R, Botton T, Yeh I, Lipson D, Otto G, Brennan K, Murali R, Garrido M, Miller VA, Ross JS, Berger MF, Sparatta A, Palmedo G, Cerroni L,

Busam KJ, Kutzner H, Cronin MT, Stephens PJ, Bastian BC (2014) Kinase fusions are frequent in Spitz tumours and spitzoid melanomas. Nat Comm 5:3116

124. Wiesner T, Obenauf AC, Murali R, Fried I, Griewank KG, Ulz P, Windpassinger C, Wackernagel W, Loy S, Wolf I, Viale A, Lash AE, Pirun M, Socci ND, Rutten A, Palmedo G, Abramson D, Offit K, Ott A, Becker JC, Cerroni L, Kutzner H, Bastian BC, Speicher MR (2011) Germline mutations in BAP1 predispose to melanocytic tumors. Nat Genet 43:1018–1021
125. Wong JR, Harris JK, Rodriguez-Galindo C, Johnson KJ (2013) Incidence of childhood and adolescent melanoma in the United States: 1973–2009. Pediatrics 131:846–854
126. Wong JY, Sondak VK (2012) Unanswered questions about margin recommendations for primary cutaneous melanoma. J Natl Compr Canc Netw 10:357–365
127. Wong SL, Balch CM, Hurley P, Agarwala SS, Akhurst TJ, Cochran A, Cormier JN, Gorman M, Kim TY, McMasters KM, Noyes RD, Schuchter LM, Valsecchi ME, Weaver DL, Lyman GH (2012) Sentinel lymph node biopsy for melanoma: American Society of Clinical Oncology and Society of Surgical Oncology joint clinical practice guideline. J Clin Oncol 30:2912–2918
128. Yazdan P, Cooper C, Sholl LM, Busam K, Rademaker A, Weitner BB, Obregon R, Guitart J, Gerami P (2014) Comparative analysis of atypical Spitz tumors with heterozygous versus homozygous 9p21 deletions for clinical outcomes, histomorphology, BRAF mutation, and p16 expression. Am J Surg Path 38:638–645
129. Yeh I, Mully TW, Wiesner T, Vemula SS, Mirza SA, Sparatta AJ, McCalmont TH, Bastian BC, LeBoit PE (2014) Ambiguous melanocytic tumors with loss of 3p21. Am J Surg Path 38:1088–1095
130. Zaal LH, Mooi WJ, Klip H, van der Horst CM (2005) Risk of malignant transformation of congenital melanocytic nevi: a retrospective nationwide study from The Netherlands. Plast Reconstr Surg 116:1902–1909
131. van der Ploeg IM, Valdes Olmos RA, Kroon BB, Nieweg OE (2008) Tumor-positive sentinel node biopsy of the groin in clinically node-negative melanoma patients: superficial or superficial and deep lymph node dissection? Ann Surg Oncol 15:1485–1491

Novel Treatments in Development for Melanoma

Chantale Bernatchez, Zachary A. Cooper, Jennifer A. Wargo, Patrick Hwu and Gregory Lizée

Abstract

The past several years can be considered a renaissance era in the treatment of metastatic melanoma. Following a 30-year stretch in which oncologists barely put a dent in a very grim overall survival (OS) rate for these patients, things have rapidly changed course with the recent approval of three new melanoma drugs by the FDA. Both oncogene-targeted therapy and immune checkpoint blockade approaches have shown remarkable efficacy in a subset of melanoma patients and have clearly been game-changers in terms of clinical impact. However, most patients still succumb to their disease, and thus, there remains an urgent need to improve upon current therapies. Fortunately, innovations in molecular medicine have led to many silent gains that have greatly increased our understanding of the nature of cancer biology as well as the complex interactions between tumors and the immune system. They have also allowed for the first time a detailed understanding of an individual patient's cancer at the genomic and proteomic level. This information is now starting to be employed at all stages of cancer treatment, including diagnosis, choice of drug therapy, treatment monitoring, and analysis of resistance mechanisms upon recurrence. This new era of personalized medicine will foreseeably lead to paradigm shifts in immunotherapeutic treatment approaches such as individualized cancer vaccines and adoptive transfer of genetically modified T cells. Advances in xenograft technology will also allow for the testing of drug combinations using in vivo models, a truly necessary development as the number of new drugs needing to be

C. Bernatchez · Z.A. Cooper · J.A. Wargo · P. Hwu (✉) · G. Lizée
University of Texas MD Anderson Cancer Center, Houston, TX, USA
e-mail: phwu@mdanderson.org

H.L. Kaufman and J.M. Mehnert (eds.), *Melanoma*,
Cancer Treatment and Research 167, DOI 10.1007/978-3-319-22539-5_16

tested is predicted to skyrocket in the coming years. This chapter will provide an overview of recent technological developments in cancer research, and how they are expected to impact future diagnosis, monitoring, and development of novel treatments for metastatic melanoma.

Keywords
Targeted therapy · Immunotherapy · Personalized medicine

Abbreviations

TCGA	The cancer genome atlas
PDX	Patient-derived xenograft
BTLA	B and T lymphocyte attenuator
CAR	Chimeric antigen receptor
CTL	Cytotoxic T lymphocyte
CTLA-4	Cytotoxic T-lymphocyte-associated protein 4
DC	Dendritic cell
DLT	Dose-limiting toxicity
IL-2	Interleukin-2
IFA	Incomplete Freund's adjuvant
Mart-1	Melanoma antigen recognized by T-cells 1
MAGE-A3	Melanoma-associated antigen 3
NY-ESO1	Cancer/testis antigen 1
TAA	Tumor-associated antigen
TCR	T-cell receptor
TGFbDNRII	Transforming growth factor-beta dominant-negative receptor II
TIL	Tumor-infiltrating lymphocyte
PD-1	Programmed cell death protein 1
WES	Whole exome sequencing
MHC	Major histocompatibility complex
HLA	Human leukocyte antigen
APC	Antigen-presenting cell
TLR	Toll-like receptor
REP	Rapid expansion process
Tregs	Regulatory T cells
Tscm	Stem cell memory-like T cells
AICD	Activation-induced cell death
CEA	Carcinoembryonic
GD2	Disialoganglioside
ERBB2	Erb-b2 receptor tyrosine kinase 2
MAPK	Mitogen-activated protein kinase

Contents

1 Introduction

Thanks to numerous scientific developments over the past two decades (as outlined in previous chapters), patients with metastatic melanoma currently have access to far more effective treatment options than at any time in the past. The recent FDA approval of three new agents to treat this deadly disease has brought hope to many patients and has also validated the effectiveness of both oncogene-targeted and immunotherapeutic approaches [1–6]. There are now dozens of ongoing clinical trials designed to test the effectiveness of several novel agents, in addition to many others testing combinations of agents likely to show therapeutic synergy. Although ongoing, certain drug combinations have shown unprecedented response and overall survival (OS) rates. This has lent much credence to the idea that the cure to cancer will ultimately lie in strategic combinations of agents that can target tumor cells in multiple ways, thus attenuating the chances of selecting for the re-emergence of resistant clones. Indeed, several tumor-intrinsic mechanisms of resistance have already been documented for the mutant BRAF inhibitor vemurafenib, and a large percentage of patients still recur or progress with disease, even on the most promising combination regimens [7–10].

While the initial forays into the molecular era of tumor biology and immunology brought us promising targets such as mutated BRAF, CTLA-4, and PD-1, continued advanced efforts in proteomic and genomic profiling have revealed an enormous complexity of molecular interactions, not only within tumor cells and infiltrating immune cells, but also in the critical cross talk between these cells [11–14]. With recent advances in molecular profiling, it is now possible to obtain vast amounts of information from an individual patient's tumor for an affordable cost [15–18]. Fortunately, concurrent advances in computing and bioinformatics methodology have allowed researchers to keep pace and enable navigation of these tremendously complex data landscapes that could only be imagined in the first years of the twenty-first century. Such analyses will facilitate not only the development of a higher order of understanding of tumor biology and immunology, but will be sure to revolutionize the future of patient diagnosis, treatment selection, and ability to monitor clinical responses.

The process has already begun in earnest. Table 1 lists some of the advanced molecular assays that are currently used to perform molecular profiling of tumors. Some of these assays are already CLIA-certified and commercially available, while others are still in the earlier stages of development. As we will discuss throughout this chapter, these technologies will enable the expansion of our current arsenal of treatments, allowing for the refinement of current capabilities and the development

Table 1 Analytical methods that will influence the future diagnosis and treatment of cancer

Assay	Purpose	Material tested	Quantity required
Whole exome sequencing	Detection of somatic mutations	Blood and tumor DNA	250 ng[a]
MIP array	Gene copy number	Tumor DNA	100 ng[a]
RNAseq	Quantitative transcriptome analysis	Tumor RNA	250 ng
FusionPlex array	Detection of known genetic fusions	Tumor RNA	100 ng[a]
Micro-RNA	Micro-RNA profiling	Tumor miRNA	1 ug
Reverse-phase protein array (RPPA)	Phospho-protein profiling, pathway activation, biomarkers	Tumor lysate	5 mg[a]
Mass-spec-based proteomics	Tumor proteomics profiling, CAR target identification	Tumor lysate	50 mg
Mass-spec MHC-I peptide elution	Immunopeptidome analysis, ID of T-cell targets	Tumor peptides	200 mg
Multiplex IHC staining	Tumor microenvironment biomarker assessment	Tumor biopsy	One tumor section for up to 8 biomarkers[a]
Tumor-infiltrating lymphocytes (TILs)	Generation of tumor-specific T cells	Tumor biopsy	50 mg[b]
TCR sequencing and cloning	TCR CDR3 diversity analysis, development of TCR-based therapeutics	Tumor biopsy DNA	20 ng[a]
Patient-derived xenograft (PDX)	Establish tumor cell line or xenogeneic tumor model	Tumor biopsy	10 mg[b]
HLA peptide-binding prediction algorithms	Determine peptide epitope binding of TAA to patient-specific HLA alleles	Amino acid sequence information	N/A

[a]FFPE tissue OK
[b]Requires fresh tumor

of completely novel approaches for the treatment of melanoma. Section 1 will discuss how these methods can be used to discover patient-specific immunogenic peptide antigens, information that can in turn be readily used to facilitate the development of personalized vaccines for cancer patients. In Sect. 2, we will focus on the future of T-cell-based immunotherapies, including the adoptive transfer of antigen-specific, laboratory-expanded endogenous cytotoxic T lymphocytes (CTLs), and genetically modified (TCR or CAR) T cells. Section 3 will focus on the future of oncogene-targeted, checkpoint blockade, and other novel treatment approaches, and how the next-generation technologies will be employed to improve clinical diagnosis, treatment, monitoring, and patient outcomes.

2 Creating Ultra-Personalized Cancer Vaccines and Immunotherapeutics

2.1 Identification of Mutated Tumor-Associated Antigens

CTL can kill tumor cells upon recognition of specific peptide fragments presented at the cell surface by MHC class I (MHC-I) molecules, encoded by the HLA-A, HLA-B, and HLA-C genes in humans. These peptide fragments are derived from proteins made within cells, and their constitutive display to $CD8^{+}$ CTL forms the basis of immunosurveillance [19–23]. This system may have initially evolved to combat viral infections; thus, CTL is very sensitive to changes in the peptide repertoire displayed by MHC-I on cells of the body, which enables the detection of intracellular viruses and clearance of virally infected cells. In a similar fashion, CTL can recognize and respond to subtle changes in the peptide repertoire of tumor cells that arise due to genomic instability [24, 25]. Accumulation of mutations within the genome of cancer cells leads to amino acid sequence alterations in proteins that can potentially be presented by MHC-I molecules at the cell surface as mutated peptide antigens. Targeting such mutated tumor-associated antigens (TAA) with T-cell-based immunotherapies has at least two significant advantages: (1) a high level of tumor specificity, since somatic mutations would not be expressed by any other cells of the body, and (2) increased immunogenicity, since the immune system would be much less likely to be tolerized by prior exposure to such neo-antigens in vivo [26].

Next-generation DNA and RNA sequencing have always held the promise of achieving deeper levels of understanding of cancer. However, since techniques such as whole exome sequencing (WES) and RNAseq (Table 1) have become more widely available, it is now possible to perform a complete mutational analysis on an individual person's tumor within weeks at an affordable cost. In order to identify mutated antigens in individual patients that could be targeted with T-cell-based immunotherapies, WES is typically performed on both a tumor sample and a normal peripheral blood sample from the same patient (Table 1). This allows for comparison of the normal, germline exome with that of the tumor, which will likely have accumulated genetic changes during the course of tumorigenesis [27].

Bioinformatics analysis yields mutation calls in codons, which are categorized as being either synonymous (not changing the amino acid of the encoded protein) or non-synonymous (resulting in an amino acid alteration). Non-synonymous mutations could become the source of mutated peptides being displayed as potential targets on the tumor cell surface, so these mutations are of most interest. The resulting amino acid changes are analyzed by specialized HLA-binding algorithms, which can predict with very good accuracy whether a peptide has the biochemical characteristics required for binding to a given HLA allele [28–30]. If a mutation results in a peptide that is predicted to bind to an HLA molecule expressed by the cancer patient, it is considered a good potential candidate T-cell target.

A number of laboratories have reported the utility of this method, both in cancer patients and in animal tumor models [31–34]. In fact, emerging evidence suggests that spontaneous antitumor immune responses may be preferentially directed toward mutated antigens. This has been demonstrated in mouse models in which T-cells spontaneously elicited against carcinogen-induced, immunogenic murine tumors were shown to be specific for a single tumor-specific mutation [33]. In this model, mutation-specific $CD8^+$ T cells were both necessary and sufficient to eradicate tumors. In humans, the success of checkpoint blockade therapy (discussed further below) has been associated with mutational burden, suggesting that enhanced immune responses resulting from therapy are also directed toward tumor-specific mutations [35]. Furthermore, WES analysis of metastatic melanoma patient tumors has demonstrated that both $CD4^+$ and $CD8^+$ tumor-infiltrating lymphocytes (TILs) can show recognition and functional reactivity to peptides derived from mutated tumor antigens [31, 32]. Although cause and effect cannot be definitively proven, many of these patients experienced objective clinical responses upon adoptive transfer of these expanded TIL, as discussed further below. Collectively, these results highlight the immunogenicity of mutated antigens and demonstrate why targeting these antigens is such a promising approach.

Although targeting mutated TAA has many advantages, there are also some limitations to this approach. One important issue that has arisen from the data is that very few mutations seem to be immunogenic in terms of generating spontaneous immunity. For example, $CD8^+$ TIL from melanoma patients that have undergone objective responses to adoptive TIL therapy appear to recognize only 2–4 % of predicted mutated epitopes, and the frequency is significantly lower when assessing $CD4^+$ TIL reactivity [31, 32]. However, it is very possible that a higher frequency of mutated epitopes is actually presented on tumor cells but does not generate spontaneous immunity, and these could still be targeted. Mutational loads also differ significantly between tumor types, with environmentally induced cancers such as lung cancer (tobacco) or melanoma (sunlight) appearing at the high end of the scale (containing 200–1000 somatic mutations) and most hematopoietic malignancies showing significantly fewer (typically <20 mutations) [36]. This mutation load is an important factor when one considers that not all mutated genes are transcribed and expressed as proteins; in this context, RNAseq analysis is useful for confirmation of gene expression (Table 1). In addition, only about half of somatic mutations are non-synonymous. Furthermore, antigen processing machinery and the particular

HLA alleles expressed by the tumor also play important roles in determining whether a mutated antigen will actually be expressed at the cell surface in the context of MHC-I molecules. For these reasons, it has been estimated that a tumor containing 200 somatic mutations will likely only present 2–5 mutated peptides at the cell surface [26]. This implies that while it may be possible to identify and target mutated epitopes in melanoma and lung cancer, mutated epitopes may be too few to reliably target in most other cancers. Another disadvantage of this approach is that most mutated epitopes constitute patient-specific "passenger" mutations which have limited usefulness for other cancer patients. Conversely, oncogenic "driver" mutations presented as immunogenic peptides would likely constitute ideal shared targets, particularly since expression of the mutated protein is presumed to be essential for maintaining the malignant phenotype. Examples of such frequently occurring mutations include codon 12 mutations to KRAS (expressed by >90 % of pancreatic cancers and ~30 % of lung cancers) and *V600E* mutations to BRAF (expressed by nearly half of cutaneous melanomas) [37–40]. Regardless of the mutation type, identification of mutated tumor-associated epitopes from individual patients remains a critical goal of tumor immunologists, and one that is certainly feasible now that next-generation sequencing technologies have become more widely available.

2.2 Identification of Non-mutated Tumor-Associated Antigens

Non-mutated or "self" antigens can also constitute viable targets for T-cell-based immunotherapy. These antigens fall into three broad categories: differentiation antigens, cancer testis antigens, and antigens overexpressed in tumors compared with normal tissues. Potential autoimmune toxicities are always a chief concern with this approach, but the tissue-restricted nature of these antigens provides some level of tumor specificity. The best studied of these are the melanoma/melanocyte differentiation antigens, which include MART-1, gp100, tyrosinase, and tyrosinase-related proteins (TRP)-1 and (TRP)-2, among others. Expression of these antigens is highly restricted to melanocytes and melanomas that arise from these cells. Consequently, autoimmune side effects of targeting these antigens typically include vitiligo caused by melanocyte destruction in the skin, and uveitis caused by T-cell recognition of melanocytes located near the retina [41, 42]. Cancer testis antigens are genes whose expression is normally highly restricted to testis tissues, but that are also frequently expressed by tumor cells. They include NY-ESO1, and the MAGE and GAGE genes, along with many others [43, 44]. Tumor antigens that are highly overexpressed in cancers include amplified genes such as *MDM2*, *KIT*, or endogenous retrovirally (*ERV*) encoded sequences [45–47].

Direct elution of MHC-I bound peptides from the surface of tumor cells combined with advanced mass spectrometry (MS) allows for global immunopeptidome analysis, in which it is now feasible to directly identify several hundreds to thousands of TAA from each patient tumor [48–51]. The vast majority of these peptides are non-mutated self-antigens; it has proven quite challenging to identify mutated peptides using this method, even from melanoma cell lines containing a relatively high mutation load [52]. This may reflect inadequate sensitivity of the detection method or may be indicative of immuno-editing, in which the most immunogenic tumor cell variants are "edited out" or culled in favor of antigen-loss variants [53, 54]. Since the biggest concern in targeting non-mutated antigens is the induction of off-target autoimmune side effects, it is very important to understand whether a given tumor-associated peptide is expressed in normal tissues, and which normal tissues they are. Currently, the GTex Portal public database provides RNAseq data from $\sim$50 different human tissues derived from dozen of donors (www.gtexportal.org). Although RNA data do not provide any direct information regarding antigen presentation in these normal tissues, RNA transcript levels often correlate with protein expression levels, allowing for an indirect assessment of how likely a peptide is to be expressed. Thus, the source gene for every tumor-associated peptide detected by MS can be vetted to reduce risk and ensure that RNA transcript expression levels in essential tissues such as heart, brain, lung, liver, colon, and kidney are very low to absent. In addition, The Cancer Genome Atlas (TCGA) database contains RNAseq data from thousands of patients with many different cancer etiologies, allowing for the identification of genes that are overexpressed in tumors as compared to normal tissues (http://cancergenome.nih.gov and http://www.cbioportal.org/). In practice, the majority of peptides detected by MS are derived from source genes that are either ubiquitously expressed or expressed at substantial levels in essential tissues, and are thus deemed inappropriate to target. However, peptides derived from differentiation, cancer testis, or overexpressed tumor antigens can also be routinely detected by MS in most patient tumors, suggesting that this method could be very powerful for enabling the design of individualized immunotherapies, particularly for patients bearing cancers with low mutation loads.

Despite the mechanisms of central and peripheral T-cell tolerance against self-antigens in vivo, spontaneous immune responses against non-mutated tumor antigens are not uncommon. In fact, the first studies of antitumor reactivity in melanoma TIL revealed that MART-1 and gp100 were frequent targets of the antitumor immune response and thus were among the first tumor antigens documented [55]. Subsequently, many studies in patients with different cancers have shown that $CD8^+$ T-cell reactivity can be detected against several other non-mutated tumor antigens, and these T cells can increase to significant numbers following vaccination, as will be discussed below. It is also possible to break tolerance against some non-mutated antigens using in vitro T-cell expansion methods that include culturing peripheral blood cells with specific peptide antigen and γ-chain cytokines including interleukin (IL)-2, IL-7, and IL-21 [56].

One important advantage of targeting non-mutated tumor antigens is that many of these can be shared between cancer patients with matching HLA types. Antitumor immune responses in melanoma patients that express HLA-A*0201 have been very well-characterized over the past two decades; thus, several shared antigenic peptides have been identified that have been targets in a number of clinical trials involving vaccination and/or adoptive T-cell transfer [57–60]. An important challenge is extending this knowledge of targetable peptide antigens to patients with other HLA types. Since HLA genes are among the most polymorphic genes known and since each allele has a unique peptide-binding preference, there still exists a large catalog of human tumor antigens that have yet to be documented. However, once a suitable tumor antigen target has been identified in a given patient, other peptides from the same source gene can be analyzed for potential binding to other HLA alleles. In this context, HLA peptide-binding prediction algorithms such as NetMHC3.4 have proven very useful for expanding the targetable peptide universe [61]. Although only a small subset of predicted binders are actually processed and presented by HLA molecules on tumor cells, such predictive algorithms can substantially reduce the number of potential candidate epitopes to screen. Predictive algorithms are now available for >100 HLA alleles, and despite criticisms of false negatives and variable prediction quality for different alleles, they provide a very important level of quality control for screening tumor-associated peptides detected by MS. These algorithms can also be used in conjunction with MS analyses to uncover previously unknown tumor antigens. For example, to discover NY-ESO1 peptides that are presented by a relatively rare HLA allele such as HLA-A*2501, the tumor antigen source protein and/or HLA allele can be overexpressed in a tumor cell line and subjected to peptide elution and MS analysis. In parallel, HLA-binding algorithms can be used to predict which NY-ESO1 peptides are likely to bind to HLA-A*2501; these peptides can be synthesized and characterized by MS in order to analyze their natural fragmentation profiles and HPLC retention times. Performing targeted MS analysis on the peptides eluted from the cell line can then provide high-confidence identification for any matching peptides [62, 63]. Thus, while comparison of RNAseq gene expression data from normal tissues and tumor (i.e., TCGA or patient-derived) can identify appropriate non-mutated tumor-associated proteins to target, HLA prediction algorithms and MS analysis can be used to hone in on the exact peptide sequences from these proteins that are actually presented by individual cancer patients.

2.3 Cancer Vaccines

Few approaches to treating cancer have raised as many hopes as that of cancer vaccines. Over the past 10 years, patient vaccination trials ongoing or completed have totaled well over a thousand (https://www.clinicaltrials.gov). Unfortunately, the reality had not yet come close to reaching the promise, as a meta-analysis of cancer vaccine trials performed at multiple institutions over nearly a decade showed a paltry collective objective response rate of <5 % [64, 65]. Although select vaccine trials have shown a survival benefit in some cancers, overall the results have been highly disappointing. In light of this, what is the future of cancer vaccines? Can they be improved upon to the point of demonstrating consistent clinical benefit for patients, or should this approach be dropped? Despite the disappointing results, it can be argued that cancer vaccine approaches of the past have been sub-optimal for at least three reasons: (1) use of weak or even deleterious vaccine adjuvants, (2) targeting of weakly immunogenic TAAs/sub-optimal antigen presentation, and (3) selection of inappropriate patient populations. A re-assessment of the collective human and animal vaccine data suggests a number of important ways immunization approaches could be improved going forward, as outlined below.

Extensive studies have now been performed in several animal tumor models to answer the question of which factors are most important for eliciting tumor-specific $CD8^+$ T-cell responses in the context of vaccination. Much information has been gleaned from studies of antiviral immune responses, in which enormous numbers of viral-specific T cells are naturally generated in 1–2 weeks in the course of successfully clearing the virus. Natural viral vectors genetically engineered to express TAAs are generally very potent at inducing antitumor $CD8^+$ T-cell responses, but their effectiveness can be rapidly blunted by antibody-mediated humoral immunity directed against the viral vectors [66, 67]. Nonetheless, this is a promising treatment approach that is being actively explored [68–71]. Many cancer vaccinologists have focused efforts instead on recapitulating the endogenous signals that lead to successful antiviral immune responses in order to improve antitumor immunity. Since dendritic cells (DCs) are the most potent antigen-presenting cell known for activating naïve T-cell responses, the most effective vaccines will likely either employ these cells directly (grown ex vivo and infused for vaccination) or will be designed to activate endogenous DCs in situ [72–74].

Many cancer vaccine trials have employed incomplete Freund's adjuvant (IFA), a mineral oil-like substance that forms a long-lived depot in the body when injected along with antigenic peptides or proteins [75–77]. While IFA does serve to protect peptides from degradation, thus prolonging antigen presentation, it also preferentially attracts primed $CD8^+$ T cells back to the vaccination site, thus effectively sequestering them from the tumors [78, 79]. These basic insights have cast hundreds of IFA-based cancer vaccine trials in a new light and suggest that alternative adjuvants must be explored in future vaccine formulations. In addition, we now know that tumor antigen presentation by non-professional APCs can actively blunt $CD8^+$ T-cell activation and promote tolerance. Thus, immunizing directly with processed TAA peptide epitopes may actually be detrimental to the generation of effective TAA-specific immunity [80]. Restricting TAA presentation to DCs in vivo can be achieved by immunizing with long peptides that require APC-specific processing in order to be presented [81, 82]. However, DCs still require specific activation signals in order to become mature and thus licensed to prime naïve $CD8^+$ T cells [72, 83]. Two signals most important for optimal DC activation are toll-like receptor (TLR) signaling and CD40 signaling. TLR ligands derived from viral or bacterial pathogens are potent mediators of DC activation and directly bridge the gap from innate to adaptive immunity [84]. CD40 signaling is normally provided to DCs in vivo by $CD4^+$ T-helper cells, but use of CD40-specific antibodies can substitute for this signal, proving very effective at inducing CD4-independent antitumor CTL responses [85]. In DCs, concurrent signaling of TLR with CD40 leads to the expression of costimulatory molecules including CD86 and CD70 that are critical for naïve CD8+ T-cell activation [86]. This combination of signals has proven to be effective at inducing tumor regressions in multiple murine tumor models and in some cases induce complete cures [87–89]. Remarkably, vanishingly few cancer vaccine trials in humans have employed strategies utilizing this combination. It is critical that future vaccination approaches relying on activating endogenous DCs be mindful of the signals required to achieve optimal activation and T-cell priming.

Due to the potential induction of T-cell tolerance, in the context of cancer vaccines TAA presentation is best left to professional APCs, of which DCs are the prototype. Accordingly, autologous DC-based cancer vaccines have proven to be one of the most effective approaches for generating antitumor CTL responses both in mouse and human studies [72, 90]. They possess all of the natural components required for the priming of an effective T-cell-mediated immune response and also hold the important advantage over viral vaccines that they do not induce neutralizing immunity after repeated immunizations [91]. DC vaccines are usually derived from peripheral blood monocytes that have been differentiated into DCs in vitro. Following differentiation, DCs are typically activated with various maturation signals for 1–2 days, then loaded with antigenic peptides, recombinant proteins, or tumor cell lysates just prior to immunization. The latter two antigen-loading strategies are designed to be useful for all patients, regardless of HLA type or knowledge of antigenic peptides. However, the protein-loading approach relies on the relatively inefficient process of cross-presentation, resulting in very low levels of antigenic peptides being presented at the DC surface [92]. The tumor cell lysate approach suffers from the same drawback, but is compounded even further by the fact that the DCs are required to process and cross-present thousands of different tumor-associated proteins simultaneously. In light of the fact that the majority of tumor-associated proteins are not tumor specific, it seems unlikely that this approach will be capable of generating effective tumor-specific immune responses. This has also been borne out in dozens of clinical trials using autologous or genetically modified allogeneic tumor cell lysates as vaccines, which consistently demonstrate relatively weak antigen-specific T-cell priming and only anecdotal clinical responses [64, 93]. By contrast, DCs pulsed with known minimal peptide epitopes have been shown to be very potent at generating TAA-specific CTL responses in mice that were associated with significant protection from tumor challenge and tumor regressions in some murine tumor models [91, 94, 95]. Peptide-pulsed DC vaccination of human cancer patients has also been successful at generating significant antigen-specific CD8+ T-cell responses as measured in peripheral blood, but objective clinical responses to DC vaccination remain rare [72, 96, 97]. This may be due in part to the very limited number of shared tumor antigens that have been tested clinically. As discussed above, it is now possible to use WES, MS, and bioinformatics technologies to routinely identify patient-specific tumor antigens. Clearly, it will soon be possible to prepare personalized autologous DC vaccines pulsed with multiple individualized peptides, including the most immunogenic mutated and non-mutated antigens, in order to raise effective antitumor immunity against multiple tumor targets. This individualized approach has not been tested directly, but will likely represent an improvement over the "one size fits all" philosophy that most vaccine trials have historically employed. As discussed further below, if DC vaccines are not capable of inducing tumor regressions directly, they can still raise the precursor frequency of TAA-specific T cells in the peripheral blood of cancer patients that could in turn be expanded further in vitro for adoptive transfer.

The clinical data are very clear that while adoptive T-cell transfer is certainly capable of inducing objective tumor regressions in advanced cancer patients with bulky tumors (as detailed further below), cancer vaccines are not [98]. The failure of cancer vaccines to facilitate regressions in patients with clinically evident disease may be blamed partly on unrealistic expectations for this treatment modality: Although many vaccine approaches have been successful at generating detectable tumor antigen-specific T cells in patient peripheral blood, these immune responses are typically not of sufficient magnitude to impact solid tumors containing trillions of cancer cells. Although some issues regarding sub-optimal T-cell trafficking to tumor sites remain unresolved, it may be more useful to consider moving cancer vaccines into the setting of patients in remission or with no evidence of disease following first-line treatment, but who are nonetheless at high risk for recurrence. In this patient population, tumor burdens are presumably low enough that immune responses raised by vaccines may be capable of clearing these residual tumor cells, thus effectively preventing recurrence altogether. These types of vaccine trials typically need longer periods of time to assess efficacy, and possibly high numbers of patients to observe a statistically significant effect. The increased time and associated costs have likely dissuaded many of these types of trials from being performed. However, in light of the long list of failed vaccine trials in cancer patients with advanced disease, it is likely imperative that the context be shifted to a different patient population where such immunization approaches may have a more realistic chance to succeed.

3 Adoptive T-Cell Transfer

T cells reactive against melanoma TAA exist in melanoma patients. Their proportion in the circulation is relatively low, but they are greatly enriched in the tumor tissue. Different methodologies have been developed to either isolate those cells from the blood or to expand tumor-specific T cells from the tumor tissue ex vivo for re-infusion into the patient (Fig. 1). Moreover, new technologies have emerged now allowing conversion of any T cell into tumor-specific T cells by genetically controlling T-cell receptor (TCR) gene expression, or to endow T cells with defined characteristics such as response to chemokines or production of specific cytokines. Recent advances in our understanding of immunology coupled with technological breakthroughs have made way for the development of very powerful new immunotherapy strategies.

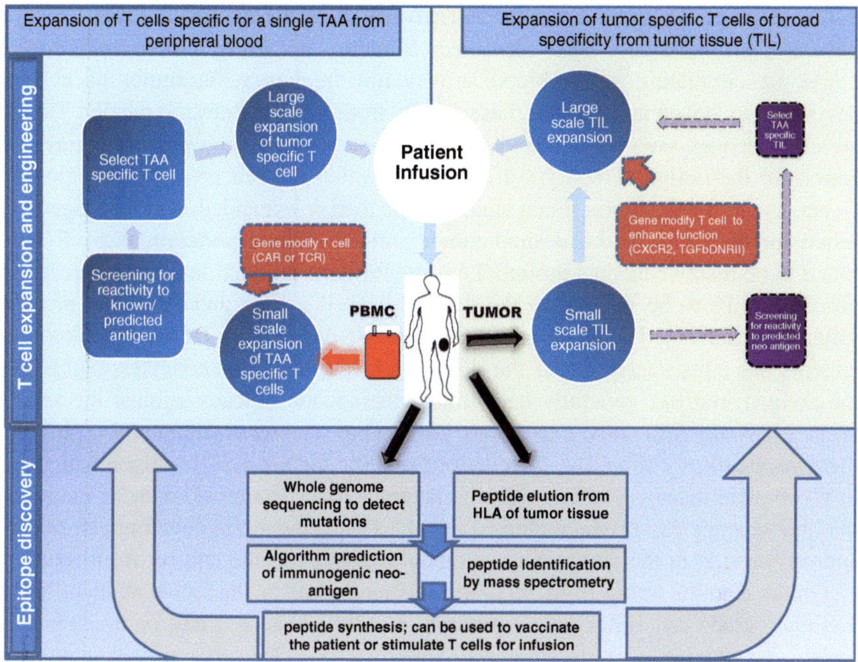

Fig. 1 Epitope discovery engine and T-cell therapy for melanoma. Two approaches to epitope discovery are depicted (*bottom panel*). To identify neo-antigens arising from mutations (*left side*), the whole genome sequencing of the tumor tissue is first performed. Mutated sequences are then interrogated for the coding of immunogenic peptides through the use of algorithms to predict peptides binding to the patient's HLA molecules. The second approach consists of rather eluting peptides off of fresh tumor tissue or cultured tumor lines by immunoprecipitation of the HLA molecules and further eluting the peptide under acidic conditions followed by identification of the peptides by mass spectrometry (*right side*). Peptides found or predicted by these approaches could potentially be synthesized and used directly to vaccinate patients with the proper adjuvant. TAA-derived peptides can also be used to derive peptide-specific T-cell lines from the patient's blood (*upper left panel*). Peptide-specific T cells can be selectively enriched and further expanded to large scale for infusion back to the patient. Alternatively, T cells can be grown directly from tumor tissue. Screening for neo-antigen specificities is an optional step of TIL therapy, signified by the dotted lines, since the TIL product is already enriched for tumor-reactive T cells (*upper right panel*). During their expansion, T cells can be genetically modified. Typically, a defined T-cell specificity is conferred to peripheral blood T cells by transferring a TCR or CAR molecule to ensure uniform tumor targeting, while genes enhancing functionality are rather expressed in TIL

3.1 Use of Naturally Occurring Tumor-Specific T Cells

Tumors are visible to the immune system since tumor-reactive T cells are detected in the blood and accumulate in the tumor tissue. Clinical regression of tumors can be obtained when such cells are isolated, expanded, and re-infused to the patient. The first part of this section will discuss the use of naturally occurring tumor-reactive T cells from the blood, while the last section will focus on the tumor tissue as a source of tumor-reactive T cells.

3.1.1 Tumor Antigen-Specific Peripheral Blood-Derived T Cells

Several TAA have now been identified. Naturally occurring T cells specific for TAAs are circulating in the blood at very low frequency. Strategies have been developed to isolate and expand these T cells from a blood draw. Typically, T cells are expanded ex vivo by repeated re-stimulation with cognate peptide antigen to enrich for the desired T-cell specificity, after which the cell product is single cell cloned by limiting dilution. Each single cell is then re-expanded, and its progeny is tested for reactivity to the desired tumor antigen. Clonal populations of T cells found to be reactive against desired TAA are further expanded in a rapid expansion process (REP) to be infused to the patient. This is a long and laborious process (often 3–4 months). The transfer of melanoma TAA-specific $CD8^+$ T-cell clones to patients has consistently led to the destruction of normal melanocytes expressing the antigen, but has generally had limited therapeutic efficacy against the tumor tissue [99–102] with some exceptions [103]. One case report definitely highlights the clinical efficacy of a $CD4^+$ T-cell clone specific for NY-ESO1 antigen which led to a complete response in a melanoma patient [104]. Therefore, there is evidence that this strategy can produce clinical benefit. Obstacles to the development of this approach reside in the complexity of manufacturing and the choice of antigen.

On the manufacturing front, technical advances such as the recent availability of a clinical grade cell sorter now permits to rapidly isolate a T-cell population uniformly recognizing a single antigen of interest [105]. This advance alleviates the cumbersome step of single-cell cloning. The major difference in the end product generated with this approach is the polyclonality of the expanded T cells. Focusing on a polyclonal population may insure the selection of a diversified T-cell repertoire of varied affinities against the antigen of choice. Also of critical importance is the development of a robust T cell expansion process ensuring that a population of T cells reactive to the antigen of choice can reliably be expanded from every patient enrolled for therapy. The removal of Tregs through CD25 depletion of the blood product before stimulation for T-cell expansion coupled with the in vitro use of Interleukin 21 (IL-21) during the culture led to improved outgrowth of TAA-specific $CD8^+$ T cells with a less differentiated phenotype [56]. Clinical trials are now testing the therapeutic efficacy of polyclonal TAA-specific autologous T cells grown with IL-21.

So far, the TAAs that have been targeted with autologous T cells have mainly been proteins whose expression is much higher in tumors compared with normal tissue such as Melan-A/Mart-1 or gp100 for melanoma. However, the fact that those proteins are also expressed in some normal tissues has led to measurable toxicity. For example, targeting of melanocyte differentiation antigens has led to autoimmune attack of normal melanocytes of the skin, eye, and ear, leading to vitiligo, uveitis, and hearing loss (reversible with local steroid administration). The lack of tumor targeting might be attributable to expression of the antigens on a large number of normal melanocytes, thus diverting the T cells. Lower affinity T cells are expected to be found for epitopes normally expressed in the host as a product of thymic selection. As discussed above, the discovery of neo-antigens arising from mutations in tumor tissue unveils a new class of TAA that has the potential of specific and powerful targeting of tumors. Targeting such antigens uniquely expressed in the tumor would circumvent the toxicity issue. Presumably, a larger repertoire of higher affinity T cells recognizing "foreign" determinants should exist in the periphery because these T cells would not have been subjected to negative selection. Mouse models have demonstrated the effectiveness of mutation-reactive T cells in tumor clearance [33, 106]. T-cells specific for mutations found in the tumor also exist in cancer patients [107, 108]. Furthermore, the ex vivo expansion and transfer of T cells recognizing tumor mutations have led to clinical regressions in cancer patients, validating this approach [109, 110].

3.1.2 Broad-Spectrum Tumor-Specific T Cells: TIL

Tumor-infiltrating lymphocytes (TILs) are T cells found within tumor tissue. In mice, it was observed that TILs are 50–100 times more effective against tumor targets than lymphokine-activated killer (LAK) cells expanded from the blood [111]. TILs have a poor ability to kill tumor cells right after isolation from tumor tissue, but this function is recovered with ex vivo culture in media containing interleukin-2 (IL-2) [112]. Based on this observation, clinical trials using autologous ex vivo expanded TIL were conducted in metastatic melanoma patients. Poor persistence of the transferred T cells and transient clinical responses were initially reported [113, 114]. The clinical response rate was later substantially augmented by adding pre-infusion host conditioning. With chemotherapy-induced transient lymphodepletion as host preconditioning and high-dose bolus IL-2 as cytokine support, the therapy reached a 38–51 % clinical response rate. Increased T-cell persistence post-transfer was measured and produced durable responses, with a 10–20 % reported complete response rate [115–119]. Two studies performed on a small number of patients measured a 20–30 % objective clinical response when infusing lower TIL numbers and substituting high-dose bolus IL-2 with low-dose IL-2 administered subcutaneously in TIL therapy regimen [120, 121]. Although the need for lymphodepletion preconditioning and IL-2 support to infused T cells is fairly well-established, the extent of lymphodepletion or the dose of IL-2 needed have not been precisely determined. Most studies err on the side of caution and administer high doses of both lymphodepletion and IL-2 to maximize the potential of T cells to engraft and proliferate—but often at the expense of high but manageable toxicities for the patient. This has limited the use of TIL therapy to patients that are fit enough to sustain these toxicities. To extend the use of TIL to a broader patient population, including possibly patients from other cancer types, milder regimens will likely need to be rigorously evaluated.

The final infusion products used in TIL therapy remain largely uncharacterized. The infused cells consist of a combination of $CD8^+$ and $CD4^+$ T cells recognizing the autologous tumor to varying degrees. High-throughput TCR sequencing of T cells from cancer patients shows that T-cell clones present in tumor tissue are distinct from T-cell clones found in the blood or adjacent normal tissue [122]. These data reinforce the concept that the T-cell population within tumor tissue is selectively enriched for tumor-specific T cells. However, very little is known about what antigens are recognized by melanoma TIL. Less than 5 % HLA-A2 positive TIL have been shown to recognize HLA-A2-restricted epitopes derived from known shared TAAs [123]. Recent studies suggest that epitopes derived from mutations found in the tumor are recognized by a proportion of TIL in a majority of melanoma patients. However, due to the unique mutation profile and HLA subtypes found in each patient, screening for those epitopes has been challenging. Since melanoma is known to have a high mutational load, much effort is being devoted to the development of methods to find and expand mutation-specific T cells for clinical use [36, 124]. A number of recent studies have shown the prevalence and clinical effectiveness of TIL recognizing mutations in melanoma [31, 32, 110, 125]. Although some cases have been documented, it remains to be seen how often this type of spontaneous immunity occurs in other cancers [125].

Better clinical outcome has been linked to the infusion of TIL products with higher content of $CD8^+$ T cells [118, 126, 127]. However, a randomized study was done to compare unselected TIL products to CD8-enriched TIL products, and no significant differences were observed in the clinical outcome of patients between the 2 arms [128]. This study demonstrated that $CD8^+$ TILs are sufficient to produce clinical benefit but showed no value in enriching for them. Moreover, a recent study clearly demonstrated the clinical effectiveness of a CD4 TIL clone recognizing a mutated tumor-associated antigen [125]. CD4 T cells are known to produce cytokines and provide costimulation to help CD8 T-cell expansion and function. Although CD4 help is needed for CD8 priming and memory formation, it is not clear whether memory $CD8^+$ T cells, such as the antigen-experienced T cells found within tumors, require CD4 help for further expansion and anti-tumor function. A recent study asked this very question using a mouse melanoma tumor model and demonstrated that the cotransfer of tumor-specific $CD4^+$ and $CD8^+$ T cells was beneficial for $CD8^+$ T cell persistence and function [129]. These data support the idea that both CD8 and CD4 TIL can mediate tumor regressions and emphasize the value of keeping a CD4 TIL population in the infusion product.

Aside from tumor antigen specificity, other characteristics of TIL have been linked to better clinical outcomes. For example, T-cell differentiation status is known to impact functionality. Several studies have demonstrated the superior value of transferring less differentiated cells to obtain maximal proliferation potential and persistence. The goal of adoptive T-cell therapy is to transfer not only cells with tumor specificity, but cells that will engraft and create a long-lived memory pool to provide sustained tumor control. Only a small fraction of differentiating T cells will form a durable memory pool. A subpopulation of very early memory T cells has recently been identified as having stem cell memory-like characteristics (Tscm) in which the cells have the ability to self-renew and differentiate into all memory and effector T-cell types [130]. Cell culture conditions to generate Tscm cells from the naïve T-cell repertoire have been described, making it possible to derive Tscm cells in vitro [131]. Other strategies found to revert the T-cell phenotype from effector to memory are inhibition of the AKT or the

Wnt/β-catenin pathways [132–134]. Increased expression of B and T lymphocyte attenuator (BTLA) on infused CD8$^+$ TIL also favors better clinical outcome [118]. BTLA confers better proliferative capacity in response to IL-2, better resistance to activation-induced cell death (AICD), and marks CD8$^+$ TIL at an earlier differentiation status [135]. It will be important to refine the pedigree of the desired T cells, thus allowing for the generation of a defined T-cell product with reproducibly high antitumor potency.

The technical ability to control both T-cell specificity and differentiation status could conceivably yield a very powerful treatment regimen. Ultimately, a combination of better tumor specificity and improved T-cell fitness will be the key to improving the clinical effectiveness of ACT therapy. A number of new technologies will help to translate these scientific discoveries into the clinic. For example, clinical grade cell sorting technology is now available (MACSQuant Tyto, Miltenyi), allowing for sorting of freshly isolated TIL of a defined specificity using tetramers, or to sorting of activated T cells based on the surface expression of activation markers such as CD137 or PD-1 as a means of enriching for tumor-reactive cells. Trials are ongoing to test efficacy of CD137-sorted TIL (NCT02111863). Alternatively, an anti-CD137 can be added to early TIL culture to favor expansion of tumor-reactive CD8$^+$ TIL [136]. Advances in our understanding of the characteristics of the most effective tumor-reactive T cells coupled with these technological advances will ultimately lead to the generation of more effective TIL products in the near future.

TIL therapy has now been performed on over 400 melanoma patients and reported in publications from 6 institutions worldwide [115, 117, 118, 119, 120, 121]. A major limitation to the dissemination of this therapy is that current methodologies for TIL expansion are labor intensive and often cost-prohibitive. Industrialization of the process will be needed in order to scale up treatments for a large number of patients. The challenge that lies ahead will be to make use of the technological advances to streamline the process of TIL generation. Once final culture conditions are locked, a fully automated and closed cell culture system will need to be adopted for this treatment to make it past the level of "boutique" therapy that it is today. A number of bioreactor types or scalable cell culture systems have been tested so far and found to be suitable for TIL clinical manufacturing [137–139]. For the time being, those systems all have some shortcomings and nothing has yet provided a fully automated TIL production solution. Academia and industry will have to work together to develop a TIL product that is both potent and cost-effective.

As mentioned above, TIL therapy has now been explored in cancer types outside of melanoma. TIL have been grown and studied in other solid tumor types, including ovarian and colorectal cancers [23, 140, 141, 142, 143, 144] and even used to successfully treat a patient with metastatic cholangiocarcinoma [125]. Knowledge from longstanding experience with melanoma TIL is being used to tackle translation of this therapy to other tumor types. The field is bound to rapidly evolve in the next few years, as researchers uncover the nature of T cells infiltrating other tumor types and assess the suitability of TIL therapy for these cancers.

3.2 Engineering T Cells

T cells can be genetically engineered to target the antigen of choice. Two approaches have been tested in this regard, utilizing gene therapy to introduce TCRs or chimeric antigen receptors (CARs).

3.2.1 TCR-Transduced T Cells

The first strategy consists of cloning the TCR alpha and beta chain genes of a T-cell recognizing the antigen of choice with reasonable affinity and then inducing its expression in patient T-cells isolated from the blood. The TCR gene-modified cells are then expanded ex vivo and re-introduced into the patient. The resulting population of T cells uniformly recognizes one TAA in an HLA-restricted manner, which limits the applicability of this approach to patients sharing the restricting HLA allele. A major limitation so far with this approach has been in identifying appropriate TAA with expression patterns restricted to the tumor tissue, in order to avoid off-target toxicities.

For example, an HLA-A*0201-restricted MART-1-specific TCR obtained from $CD8^+$ TIL isolated from a melanoma patient with a complete response to TIL therapy was used to gene-modify T cells for adoptive transfer into other HLA-A*0201-positive melanoma patients. Results from this study showed a lower response rate than the use of bulk TIL populations, with only 2/15 patients responding (13 %) compared to a reported 50 % response rate of TIL therapy [59]. A subsequent trial using a TCR with dramatically improved affinity for the TAA (MART-1 or gp100) demonstrated better clinical efficacy (30 % for MART-1 TCR, 19 % for gp100 TCR), but also a substantial increase in autoimmune manifestations of uveitis and hearing loss due to the destruction of melanocytes of the eye and ear (41.7 %) [145]. Similarly, the transfer of autologous T cells transduced with an affinity-enhanced TCR recognizing the carcinoembryonic (CEA) antigen in 3 colorectal cancer patients produced dose-limiting toxicities in all 3 patients due to the induction of severe transient colitis [146]. The cancer–testis antigen melanoma-associated antigen A3 (MAGE-A3) has also been targeted with TCR-transduced T cells using a TCR that had been genetically engineered to enhance functional avidity for a MAGE-A3 peptide presented in the context of HLA-A*0201 molecule [147]. Clinical responses were seen in 5 patients out of 9, with two durable responses of more than one year. Unexpectedly, 3 patients treated experienced serious neurotoxicity which led to two treatment-related deaths. Brain tissue was later found to express low levels of MAGE-A12, resulting in the presentation of an epitope also recognized by the TCR. Another trial utilizing MAGE-A3 affinity-enhanced TCR-transduced T cells recognizing a peptide in the context of HLA-A*0101 found lethal cardiotoxicity in the first 2 patients infused [148]. In this case, the toxicity was found to be caused by cross-recognition by the transduced TCR of a structurally related peptide derived from titin, a very large protein expressed by a subset of muscle cells in the heart.

These clinical examples involving transfer of autologous T cells modified to express engineered TCRs with “supra-physiological” affinity for a defined TAA has clearly demonstrated specific activity in vivo but definitively suffers from demonstrated “on-target, off-tumor” toxicity. The strong reactivity found to a peptide from a completely different protein expressed in the heart certainly highlights the significant risk and potential clinical importance of TCR cross-reactivity, particularly since the target peptide only shared 5 out of 9 amino acids with the TAA being targeted. Although algorithms exist to predict binding of peptides to HLA molecules, the level of degeneracy permitted by a given TCR on recognition of cognate peptide is unclear for a majority of HLA molecules. A recent study showed that one TCR from a patient-derived $CD8^+$ T-cell clone involved in the pathology of autoimmune type 1 diabetes may be able to bind up to 1×10^6 related but distinct peptides [149]. In this work, a decamer peptide differing from the index peptide at 7 out of 10 amino acids was over 100-fold more potent at eliciting T-cell activation. Manipulating TCR affinity to achieve supra-physiological levels has clearly resulted in unanticipated toxicities. As discussed in Sect. 1, refinement of peptide-binding prediction tools as well as the development of improved in vitro screening methods and bioinformatics tools like gene expression data from normal tissues is currently being employed to make this approach safer.

The therapeutic value of this approach could potentially be greatly augmented with the use of safer TAA strictly not expressed by essential normal tissues; thus, the identification of shared TAA with better toxicity profiles is clearly warranted. Recent data showing high clinical response rates in cancer patients following the transfer of TCR-transduced T cells targeting the cancer germline antigen NY-ESO1 and the absence of toxicity associated with the transferred cells support this concept [150]. NY-ESO1 might be a good prototype antigen since it is normally only found on germline tissues that do not express HLA molecules and therefore cannot be targeted by T cells in an antigen-dependent manner. The treatment led to objective clinical responses in 11/18 (61 %) of synovial cell sarcoma patients and in 11/20 (55 %) melanoma patients, including 5 complete remissions lasting at least 2 years. Encouragingly, NY-ESO1 is but one of many examples of cancer–testis antigens that may be safely and efficiently targeted by TCR-transduced T cells in future.

3.2.2 Chimeric Antigen Receptor (CAR)-Modified T Cells

The second approach for retargeting of T cells is to introduce a completely engineered antigen receptor: The CAR has been designed to effectively combine the high-affinity antigen recognition domain of an antibody with the efficient killing machinery of a T cell. This was accomplished by creating a molecule that links the variable domains of an antibody to the intracellular signaling domains of the TCR complex. Thus, the recognition afforded by CAR is HLA-independent and is directed at a protein expressed on the surface of tumor cells. CAR T cells have a very low threshold of activation as antibodies have affinities in the range of 10^{-6}–10^{-9} M, two to three logs higher than the typical TCR affinity range of 10^{-4}–10^{-6} M.

Early studies of CAR-modified T cells for ovarian cancer immunotherapy utilized an antibody to a folate-binding protein linked to the intracellular domain of the common gamma chain of the Fc receptor for the immunoglobulins IgE and IgG [151]. Although in vitro and in vivo studies demonstrated good activation and tumor killing by CAR T cells upon antigen exposure, a phase I clinical study reported poor persistence of the cells in the circulation post-infusion, correlating with poor migration to tumor tissue, and no clinical benefit [152]. In subsequent generations of CARs, the Fc gamma receptor component was replaced by the intracellular domain of the TCR molecule and intracellular domains of costimulatory molecules such as CD27, CD28, 4-1BB, or OX-40 were added. This resulted in greatly improved persistence of the transferred CAR T cells and significant clinical benefit began to emerge. B-cell malignancies in particular have been effectively targeted by second-generation CAR T-cell therapy incorporating the signaling domains of either CD28 or 4-1BB molecule. Thus, B-cell acute lymphoblastic leukemia, chronic lymphocytic leukemia, and diffuse large B-cell lymphoma have been successfully treated with the use of CAR T cells recognizing CD19, with reported complete remissions in 50–90 % of the patients [153–157]. The only solid tumor with reported objective clinical responses to CAR T-cell therapy is in pediatric glioblastoma using CAR T cells specific for the Ganglioside 2 (GD2) molecule, with 3/11 patients with active disease at infusion experiencing complete remissions. The complete response was short-lived for one patient but durable for the two others, lasting over 60 months in one case and over 21 months for the third patient [158]. Importantly, GD2 CAR T-cell administration did not induce any severe or dose-limiting toxicity (DLT) in the glioblastoma patients. More recently, the infusion of T cells transiently expressing a CAR specific for mesothelin using a RNA expression system was reported to be safe in 2 patients and also showed evidence of clinical efficacy [159]. The transient expression of CAR on T cells required the repeated injections of T cells. This was developed as a safety measure to prevent toxicity if off-target damage should arise, but in one patient, it actually caused the development of IgE antibodies against the murine antibody portion of the CAR molecule, leading unexpectedly to an anaphylactic reaction and cardiac arrest within minutes following the third cell infusion [160]. This event took place 49 days after the first infusion. The toxicity was manageable, and the patient fully recovered, but this experience has led to the realization that CAR T cells using murine antibodies can be immunogenic. This also raises important concerns regarding potential recognition and clearance of CAR-modified T cells by the immune system, which would greatly limit their persistence. Future studies shall determine which environmental factors such as chemotherapy preconditioning regimens and post-infusion cytokine support matter for CAR T-cell persistence. Features of CAR construct ameliorating persistence, and function should also emerge from future trials and will dictate what cosignaling intracellular components should be used to endow the best qualities to CAR T cells.

Second- and third-generation CAR T cells are probably the most powerful effector T cells currently in use and must be employed with caution. For hematologic malignancies treated with CAR-modified T cells targeting CD19, the CAR

T-cell infusion led to the rapid eradication of all cells expressing the target molecule for a high proportion of patients. Therapy-related toxicities often accompany this rapid and powerful tumor killing. Cytokine release syndrome (CRS) is characterized by high fevers, hypotension, and hypoxia and is due to the release of soluble factors in the blood by the activated CAR T and other immune cells. The importance of the CRS has been directly linked to tumor burden and correlates with CAR T-cell expansion [156]. This potentially serious side effect can be managed with the administration of the interleukin-6 receptor antagonist tocilizumab [161]. In the case of CD19 CAR T cells, the recognition of cognate antigen on normal B cells also leads to B-cell aplasia and reduction in circulating levels of immunoglobulin, which can be managed by the infusion of gammaglobulins. Other CAR T cells targeting antigens later found to be expressed even at very low levels on essential organs caused significant toxicity. For example, CAR T cells directed at the ERBB2 protein infused into a colon cancer patient reacted against minimal levels of the protein expressed by the lung, causing respiratory distress within 15 min of infusion. The patient later developed severe hypotension which progressively evolved and caused the patient's death 5 days later [162]. A very large number of ERBB2 CAR T cells were infused into this patient (10^{10}), which is clearly a cause for exploring safer levels of infusion product in early trials. Dose-limiting liver toxicity has also been observed at much lower CAR T cell doses of $0.2–2.1 \times 10^9$ in 4/8 renal cell carcinoma patients treated with CAR T cells recognizing carboxy-anhydrase-IX (CAIX) [163]. Targeting of the liver was thought to be due to low-level CAIX expression in bile duct epithelial cells. Pretreatment of a second group of patients with anti-CAIX antibody prevented liver toxicity, suggesting the liver damage was an "on-target" "off-tumor" effect.

The success of CAR-modified T-cell therapy has so far mainly been limited to hematological malignancies, while its efficacy in solid tumors remains unclear. Preclinical testing of potential targets for melanoma is currently underway [164, 165].

3.2.3 Enhancing T-Cell Function

Anti-tumor potential is not only defined by the ability of the T cell to recognize and kill tumor targets but also by its ability to persist, traffic to tumor tissues, and perform its function in an environment that is highly immunosuppressive. T cells can also be genetically modified to enhance those characteristics.

IL-2 is an essential growth factor for T cells. Systemic or subcutaneous administration of IL-2 post-T-cell infusion has been found to promote persistence of the transferred cells [102]. Avenues have been explored to alleviate the need for IL-2 supplementation since it is associated with significant toxicity. The insertion of the IL-2 gene in T cells increased their survival to IL-2 withdrawal in vitro but failed to alter the fate or function of the T cells in vivo post-adoptive transfer [166]. Modification of the T cells to express IL-12 has been found to sustain effector function and eliminate the need for lymphodepleting preconditioning or further cytokine support in a mouse model of melanoma [167, 168]. A dose escalation clinical trial in metastatic melanoma patients testing the infusion of TIL modified to express IL-12 only upon TCR triggering reported a 63 % clinical response rate (10/16 patients) at the highest cell dose tested ($0.1–3.0 \times 10^9$ gene-modified cells) [169]. Unfortunately, responses were short-lived probably due to the acknowledged lack of persistence of the engineered T cells, disappearing within one month of the infusion. IL-12-mediated toxicities prevented the infusion of higher cell doses and may have contributed to the rapid disappearance of T cells as well. Thus far, genetic engineering of TIL has not increased the efficacy of TIL therapy; however, only a few genes have been tested. A host of other genes are now being targeted in clinical and preclinical settings and offer hope to increase the efficacy of TIL therapy.

In mouse models of melanoma and EBV-positive lymphoma, T cells made resistant to the inhibition of transforming growth factor beta (TGFb) through the expression of a dominant negative form of the TGFb receptor 2 (DNRII) mediated better tumor regressions [170, 171]. Our group is currently testing this approach in humans, with the insertion of TGFb DNRII in TIL for the treatment of melanoma (NCT01955460). Another focus of our research is to enhance T-cell migration to tumor sites. Although melanoma tumors express the chemokine CXCL-1, very few T cells or TIL express its ligand, CXCR2 [172, 173]. We have found that introducing CXCR2 into TIL favors their localization at the tumor sites post-infusion in a mouse model [174]. A clinical study is now enrolling patients to test this hypothesis (NCT01740557).

Additionally, preclinical data have shown that the overexpression of microRNA155 (miR-155) in $CD8^+$ T cells augments the responsiveness to cytokines sharing the γc subunit of the IL-2 receptor such as IL-7, IL-15, and IL-21. Furthermore, the use of anti-tumor $CD8^+$ T cells overexpressing miR-155 has demonstrated enhanced T-cell persistence and effector function without the need for host lymphodepletion or exogenous cytokine supplementation post-cell infusion in mice [175]. The expression of mir155 in TIL may favor their persistence post-infusion and alleviate the need for toxic host conditioning and high-dose IL-2 regimen.

As discussed further below, combinations of multiple therapies will likely ultimately benefit cancer patients the most. The challenge will be to determine which therapies should be combined to potentiate clinical responses in each individual patient's case. In preclinical models, it has been shown that responses to adoptive T-cell therapy are greatly enhanced by combination with checkpoint blockade or targeted therapy, particularly anti-PD-1 and BRAF inhibitor [176, 177]. These likely represent the first of many combination therapies to be developed in the coming years.

4 Novel Strategies in Targeted and Immunotherapies

4.1 Limitations of Current Targeted Therapy and Immunotherapy Regimens

With the advances in understanding key oncogenic driver mutations in melanoma, the development of drugs that can target these mutations has been one of the most significant recent therapeutic developments. Mutations in the *BRAF* gene occur in

~50 % of melanoma patients [178] and numerous therapeutics have been developed to target this constitutively active protein [179]. Agents targeting BRAF-mutant melanoma have demonstrated a significant increase in progression-free (PFS) and OS [180–183]. However, the therapeutic response to the blockade of constitutively activated mutant *BRAF* is transient, with most patients progressing on treatment ~6 months after initiation [181, 182, 184]. This has led to therapeutic strategies combining BRAF inhibitors with other modalities. One example of this is the addition of a MEK inhibitor which targets a second node within the same MAP kinase pathway and has extended the median time of disease progression to 10 months [185]. Additionally, combining oncogene-targeted agents with the use of immunotherapy has been another area of tremendous promise. Monoclonal antibodies targeting the immunomodulatory molecules CTLA-4 and PD-1 were approved by the FDA in 2011 and 2014, respectively. Ipilimumab (α-CTLA-4) showed clinical benefit with an overall response rate (ORR) in 10.9 % of patients, and 60 % of these patients benefitted from durable responses lasting greater than 2 years [186–188]. More recently, Topalian et al. reported results of a phase I trial of 296 patients with either advanced melanoma or other solid tumors including non-small-cell lung cancer, prostate cancer, renal cell carcinoma, and colorectal cancer, in which the checkpoint blocking antibody α-PD-1 (BMS-936558, nivolumab) achieved a 28 % response rate in melanoma patients, with durable responses lasting greater than one year in half of responding patients [183]. Furthermore, α-PD-1 therapy was associated with a lower rate of grade 3 or 4 adverse events compared with ipilimumab.

4.2 Rationale for Combining Immunotherapy and Targeted Therapy

Single-agent treatments employing either oncogene-targeted therapies or immunotherapies have drawbacks, namely lack of a durable responses and low response rate, respectively. There is mounting preclinical and clinical evidence suggesting the potential of combining immunotherapy and targeted therapy. The potential role of oncogenic BRAF in immune escape was initially reported by Sumimoto and colleagues [189], and blocking BRAF signaling through MAPK pathway inhibition in vitro led to an increase in melanocyte differentiation antigens (MDAs) up to 100-fold [190]. This increased MDA expression led to an increase in reactivity to antigen-specific T lymphocytes, an effect further substantiated through studies in patients with metastatic melanoma treated with BRAF inhibitors. Results show a similar increase in MDAs as well as a significant increase in intratumoral $CD8^+$ T cells and clonality 10–14 days after initiation of BRAF inhibition [191–193]. These findings were also associated with a decrease in IL-6 and IL-8, tumor-associated fibroblast-secreted IL-1α, and stromal VEGF [177, 192, 194]. Equally important is the increase in the immunomodulatory molecules PD-1 and PD-L1 10–14 days following initiation of *BRAF* inhibition, suggesting a potential immune-based mechanism of resistance. PD-L1 expression has also been suggested as a mechanism of resistance to BRAF inhibitors as BRAF-resistant cell lines express higher PD-L1 and the addition of MEK inhibitors has a suppressive effect on PD-L1 expression [195]. The increase in PD-L1 expression following BRAF inhibition may be due to infiltrating T-cell IFN-γ secretion [196]. These data suggest that addition of immunotherapy and specifically immune checkpoint blockade may enhance the anti-tumoral response when combined with a BRAF inhibitor.

Several preclinical studies have also explored the potential of combining BRAF inhibition with immunotherapy, with all [11, 177, 197, 198] but one [199] suggesting an added benefit. These studies suggest that combinations of immune checkpoint blockade, adoptive cell transfer, and other immunotherapies improve clinical benefit after addition to BRAF inhibitors. These preclinical models may facilitate decision making in the sequencing and timing of clinical trials; however, they are limited by the number of immune competent preclinical melanoma models, and further development of these is clearly needed.

Based on preclinical research, translating these ideas into the patient-care setting has been a high priority. An initial phase I study tested the combination of the BRAF inhibitor vemurafenib with the CTLA-4-targeting drug ipilimumab and was terminated early due to hepatotoxicity [200]. This phase I study had a first cohort of six patients who received a full dose of vemurafenib at 960 mg orally twice daily for one month as a single agent prior to administration of ipilimumab at the FDA-approved dose of 3 mg/kg intravenously. DLTs of grade 3 transaminase elevations were noted in four patients within 2–5 weeks after the first dose of ipilimumab [200]. A second cohort of patients was then started on lower dose vemurafenib (720 mg by mouth twice daily) with full dose ipilimumab; however, hepatotoxicity was again observed with grade 3 transaminase elevations in two patients and grade 2 elevation in a single patient [200]. Of note, all hepatic adverse events were asymptomatic and reversible either with temporary discontinuation of both study drugs or with administration of glucocorticoids [200].

Exploring this strategy has been continued as an ongoing targeted and immunotherapy trial utilizes the BRAF inhibitor dabrafenib with or without the MEK inhibitor trametinib, combined with ipilimumab in patients with BRAF V600E/K-mutated metastatic melanoma (NCT01767454). At the American Society of Clinical Oncology (ASCO) meeting in June 2014, 12 patients had been enrolled on the doublet of ipilimumab with dabrafenib and 7 patients were enrolled on triplet therapy. There were no DLTs in the doublet arm of dabrafenib 150 mg by mouth twice daily and ipilimumab 3 mg/kg; thus, a dose expansion of 30 additional patients is ongoing. While hepatotoxicity was observed in the doublet arm, there were no grade 3 or 4 toxicities noted which is likely explained by the lower propensity of hepatotoxicity seen with dabrafenib compared to vemurafenib [201]. In the triplet cohort, there were two cases of colitis associated with colon perforation in the first 7 treated patients. Both of these patients required extensive courses of steroids, and one patient did require surgery for management of the colon perforation. These toxicities were seen despite the use of low-dose dabrafenib 100 mg twice daily and trametinib 1 mg daily [201], and accrual of patients in this cohort was suspended due to toxicity. Data of the estimated duration of benefit from doublet therapy are immature and not yet reported. Numerous other clinical trials combining targeted therapy with immunotherapies such as α-PD-L1 (NCT02027961, NCT01656642), IL-2 or IFN-α (NCT01754376, NCT01683188, NCT01603212, NCT01959633, NCT01943422), or T cells (NCT00338377, NCT01585415, NCT01659151) are underway and currently accruing patients.

The sequence and timing of combination therapy is an important consideration, as there is some evidence that the immune response to BRAF inhibitors is early and transient. This suggests that there is a short window of opportunity to add immunotherapies, while T cells are primed early on in the course of BRAF inhibition. This combination of therapy must be delicately balanced with toxicity as demonstrated by previous clinical trials though whether this toxicity is specific to vemurafenib and ipilimumab is uncertain at this point.

Additionally, it is uncertain whether adding immunotherapies to a backbone of combined BRAF/MEK inhibitors will be as effective, as the MAPK pathway is critical for T-cell activation. The effect of MEK inhibitor monotherapy on tumor-infiltrating T cells in patients has also not been well evaluated and is a critical point as MEK inhibitors may be more widely applicable in combinations of targeted therapy and immunotherapy for *NRAS*-mutant melanoma and for other cancer types. Studies have been performed in peripheral blood lymphocytes of melanoma patients on MEK inhibitors and show a modest decrease in T-cell function at therapeutic doses [202]. Additionally, MEK-mediated phosphorylation of ERK has been demonstrated to decrease progressively across stages of T-cell memory differentiation suggesting a larger effect of MEK inhibitors on naïve T cells than effector memory or late effector memory cells [203]. Recently, it was also suggested that treating with a combination of BRAF inhibitors with MEK inhibitors may offset the deleterious in vitro effects of MEK alone [204]. However, in vivo murine studies suggest that "timing is everything" and that MEK inhibitors may demonstrate synergy with immune checkpoint blockade in the treatment of *RAS*-mutant cancer if both are given concurrently or if MEK inhibitors were given as a lead into anti-PD1. Conversely, all mice treated with PD1 lead into MEK inhibition showed anti-tumor effect but minimal long-term survival benefit [204]. Preclinical and clinical studies investigating both timing and sequence of targeted therapy and immunotherapy are necessary to optimize clinical effectiveness of these new combinations and are currently underway.

Currently, there are many new targeted and immunotherapies on the forefront of development for the treatment of melanoma. Many of these potential therapies continue to target the MAPK pathway as the majority of melanomas harbor activating mutations in *BRAF* or *NRAS*. An unexpected side effect of first-generation BRAF inhibitors includes the paradoxical activation of the *RAS* pathway leading to the potential for *RAS*-induced cancers. A next-generation "paradox-breaker" selective RAF inhibitor has now been developed and demonstrates inhibition of RAF-signaling in BRAF-mutant cell lines without paradoxical effects in wild-type cells as well as further blockade of the RAF pathway in BRAF-mutant cells with acquired resistance [205]. Targeting additional nodes in the MAPK pathway have also gained traction as strategies of delaying resistance to BRAF-targeted therapy. Recently, the antitumor activity of ERK inhibitors was demonstrated in

BRAF-mutant, *NRAS*-mutant, and wild-type melanomas, while synergistic effects were demonstrated when combined with vemurafenib in BRAF-mutant melanomas in vitro [206]. The use of ERK inhibitors in monotherapy is now being explored, and the addition of ERK inhibitors has been suggested by many groups in overcoming resistance to BRAF inhibitors [207]. NF1 mutations in melanoma, which are present in 25 % of BRAF and NRAS WT melanomas [178], have recently also been shown to be important in melanomagenesis and acquired resistance to BRAF inhibitors. In recent studies, NF1 could be successfully targeted in mouse models with a combination of MEK and PI3K/mTOR inhibitors [208] or a combination of irreversible RAF inhibition and MEK inhibition [209].

In addition to further targeting of the MAPK pathway, many studies have shown an active role of the PI3K-AKT pathway as loss of PTEN in melanoma represents a high prevalence de novo and plays a role in resistance to MAPK pathway inhibitors [210]. Early in vitro and in vivo studies of isoform-specific or pan-PI3K, mTOR, and AKT inhibitors have been tested and shown anti-tumor effects in vitro and in vivo [211–213]. Additionally, PI3K isoform-specific inhibitors are being utilized to achieve significant pathway inhibition as melanoma cells with PTEN loss were demonstrated to be more dependent on the PI3K catalytic subunit p110β than the p110α subunit [214, 215]. Clinical testing of two different p110β-selective inhibitors (GSK2636771, SAR260301) is now underway.

The cell-cycle pathway, specifically the p-16-cyclin D-CDK4/6-retinoblastoma protein pathway (CDK4 pathway), is another pathway having been targeted as melanoma has a high frequency of genomic alterations in this pathway [178, 216], and these incidents may transform melanocytes [217]. Recently, selective CDK4 inhibitors entered clinical trials including palbociclib which is the most extensively evaluated compound in patients. Additionally, numerous CDK4/6 inhibitors are in clinical development and have shown selectivity for CDK4 in preclinical studies and include LEE011, LY2835219, and P276-00 [218–222]. Recent studies have demonstrated that the combination of these inhibitors with BRAF inhibitors may overcome resistance [223, 224].

Other potential targeted therapies include histone deacetylase (HDAC) inhibitors which have been shown to synergistically act with BRAF inhibitors [225, 226] and may delay resistance to therapy [227]. HSP90 inhibitors are also a potential future therapy and have shown added benefit when studied with BRAF inhibition monotherapy or BRAF and MEK inhibition both in vitro and in vivo [228, 229] as they allow proteasomal degradation of the destabilized BRAF protein. Additionally, HSP90 inhibitors have also shown efficacy in non-BRAF melanoma mouse models, having demonstrated anti-tumor activity in an *NRAS* mouse model through the inhibition of Wee1, AKT, and CDK4 [230].

In addition to the development of new targeted therapies, the recent success of anti-PD-1 and anti-PD-L1 promotes the potential for future drugs targeting immunomodulatory molecules. These molecules range from additional immune checkpoint molecules such as TIM-3 and LAG-3 to activation targets such as OX-40 and CD28. These molecules and others [231] are all being extensively investigated as monotherapies and in combination with other targeted therapies.

All of these potential targeted and immunotherapies show great promise; however, for maximal response, it is becoming more apparent that maximal clinical efficacy may occur through optimizing different combinations of therapies which may include any number of targeted radiation and immunotherapies. This optimization will require a deeper understanding of both the genomic and immunologic properties of melanomas.

5 Future Directions

The successes of immunotherapy and targeted therapy approaches have vastly changed the landscape of melanoma clinical management in the last 5 years. New therapies with impressive clinical response rates that significantly prolong the life of patients are now available, providing proof of principle that these approaches are well worth pursuing. Consequently, these new FDA approvals have opened up entirely new classes of drugs that are being actively explored for other cancers.

Counteracting normal T-cell checkpoint mechanisms turned out to be a winning strategy, with the approval of two biologics in this new class of drug: anti-CTLA-4 and anti-PD-1 antibodies. This has spurred interest in the development and clinical testing of antibodies to either activate or block any and all known negative or positive T-cell costimulatory molecules, with many new agents entering phase I trials soon. In parallel, the remarkably high clinical effectiveness of a small molecule specifically targeting mutated BRAF molecule sent waves of hope to metastatic melanoma patients that were otherwise facing a very grim prognosis. The short response period for most patients followed by sometimes dramatic recurrences has now prompted an enormous emphasis on research to find mechanisms of resistance.

Overall, the sands are rapidly shifting in terms of clinical management of melanoma. The availability of drugs that can induce potent clinical responses in a large fraction of the patient population allows for an adequate study of resistance to therapy. With the historically low and transient response rates afforded by chemotherapy and radiotherapy or the very low numbers of long-term responders to IL-2, this was not previously possible. The increased availability of biological material from a significant number of responding and non-responding patients combined with powerful technological analyses will hopefully reveal the characteristics of the tumor or the host immune system most conducive to response to therapy. Therefore, understanding response and resistance to therapy with the use of longitudinal tissue and blood sampling (Fig. 2) to help better guide clinical decisions is an important focus of interest for the future. This strategy is highly aligned with the idea of personalized medicine. Large-scale tumor and immune cell characterization are under way through various national or local efforts. A good example is the TCGA, which aims to define the genomic and molecular features of a large number of tumor samples and has accumulated samples from 11,000 patients from 33 cancers types and completed the WES of over 1000 tumor samples as of 2014 (http://cancergenome.nih.gov/). Understanding the mutational landscape of an individual's tumor will eventually allow for tailoring of treatment modalities to target pathways affected by genetic alterations mapped to the individual. Response of a patient's tumor to the chosen drug can also now be directly interrogated in mice. Indeed, patient-derived xenografts (PDX) can often be successfully established in a mouse, which allows the in vivo screening of drugs on a patient's growing tumor. Although PDXs cannot be made for every patient, the development of a characterized set of patient-derived tumor lines and their use for in vitro high-throughput screening of compounds as well as xenografts in vivo confirmatory studies may help elucidate general sensitivity of specific genetic alterations to given drug candidates. The derivation of tumor lines from patients who do not respond or are rendered resistant to the therapy will represent a unique opportunity to elucidate mechanisms of resistance. This translational research can only be performed through close proximity between the laboratory and the clinic and is essential to uncover markers of susceptibility to available active drugs. Currently in the clinic, great strides have been made to personalize treatments through the guidance of molecular and immune profiling, and there is a strong drive to pursue this personalization of treatment throughout the course of therapy (Fig. 2).

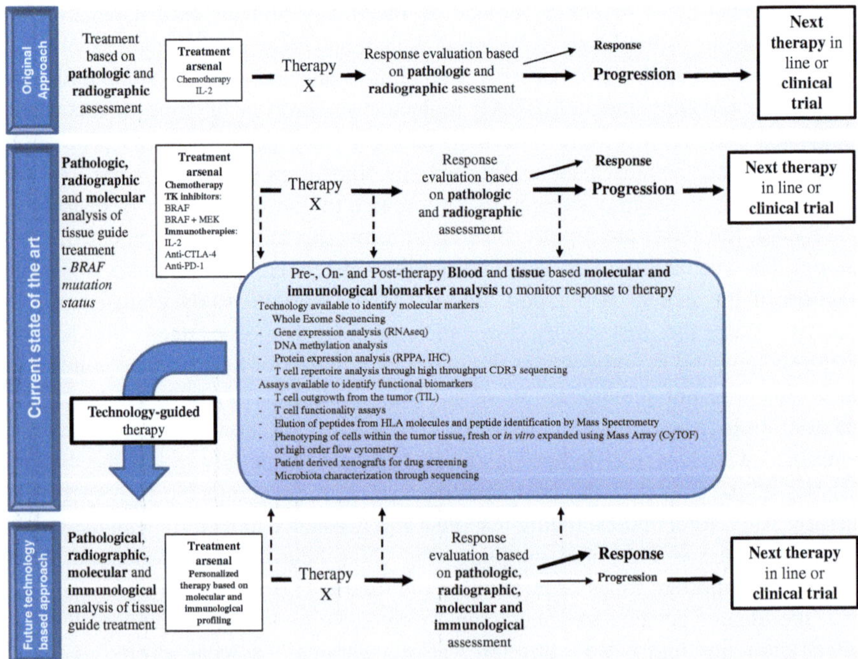

Fig. 2 Integrating longitudinal tissue and blood sampling into clinical practice. Depiction of the past and current approaches to melanoma patient clinical management (*top* and *middle panel*, respectively). The current approach integrates multiple molecular, immunologic, and functional assessments to pinpoint biomarkers of response or resistance to therapy that will be used to stratify patients and guide therapy in the future and hopefully improve response to therapy (*bottom panel*)

Recent successes of cancer immunotherapy have convincingly demonstrated the importance of immune surveillance in durable tumor control. Any new drug being developed now needs to be assessed for its impact on the immune system and the potential synergy with immunotherapy approaches. Although cancer immunotherapy has developed slowly, with many difficulties in priming productive anti-tumoral responses through vaccination, we now have a better grasp on how to ensure a productive and prolonged immune response through "releasing the brakes" on endogenous T cells or transferring the right subset of long-lived effector T cells. Between the new effective immunotherapy modalities approved or in development and the increasing list of effective targeted agents available, the possibilities for combination therapy are rapidly becoming vast.

Biomarkers of response are still needed to better stratify patients and provide guidance about how to sequence the available treatment modalities to realize the best clinical benefit for every patient while ensuring optimal safety. The discovery and validation of reliable biomarkers will require the involvement of leaders with a wide variety of expertise (cancer biologists, immunologists, molecular biologists, bioinformatics specialists, chemists) and will include many of the next-generation technologies listed in Table 1. Major collaborative efforts between researchers and clinical investigators will also be required to ensure the success of this endeavor. Encouragingly, many of these large-scale collaborations are already underway, making the future of melanoma patient clinical care look very bright indeed.

References

1. Stadler S, Weina K, Gebhardt C, Utikal J (2014) New therapeutic options for advanced non-resectable malignant melanoma. Adv Med Sci 60(1):83–88. doi:10.1016/j.advms.2014.12.002
2. Page DB, Postow MA, Callahan MK, Allison JP, Wolchok JD (2014) Immune modulation in cancer with antibodies. Annu Rev Med 65:185–202. doi:10.1146/annurev-med-092012-112807
3. Ott PA, Hodi FS, Robert C (2013) CTLA-4 and PD-1/PD-L1 blockade: new immunotherapeutic modalities with durable clinical benefit in melanoma patients. Clin Cancer Res Official J Am Assoc Cancer Res 19(19):5300–5309. doi:10.1158/1078-0432.CCR-13-0143
4. Kwong LN, Davies MA (2014) Targeted therapy for melanoma: rational combinatorial approaches. Oncogene 33(1):1–9. doi:10.1038/onc.2013.34
5. Samatar AA, Poulikakos PI (2014) Targeting RAS-ERK signalling in cancer: promises and challenges. Nat Rev Drug Discov 13(12):928–942. doi:10.1038/nrd4281
6. Kaufman HL (2015) Precision immunology: the promise of immunotherapy for the treatment of cancer. J Clin Oncol Official J Am Soc Clin Oncol. doi:10.1200/JCO.2014.59.6023
7. Aris M, Barrio MM (2015) Combining immunotherapy with oncogene-targeted therapy: a new road for melanoma treatment. Front Immunol 6:46. doi:10.3389/fimmu.2015.00046
8. Chen G, Davies MA (2014) Targeted therapy resistance mechanisms and therapeutic implications in melanoma. Hematol Oncol Clin North Am 28(3):523–536. doi:10.1016/j.hoc.2014.03.001
9. Menzies AM, Long GV (2014) Systemic treatment for BRAF-mutant melanoma: where do we go next? Lancet Oncol 15(9):e371–e381. doi:10.1016/S1470-2045(14)70072-5

10. Das Thakur M, Stuart DD (2014) Molecular pathways: response and resistance to BRAF and MEK inhibitors in BRAF(V600E) tumors. Clin Cancer Res Official J Am Assoc Cancer Res 20(5):1074–1080. doi:10.1158/1078-0432.CCR-13-0103
11. Knight DA, Ngiow SF, Li M, Parmenter T, Mok S, Cass A, Haynes NM, Kinross K, Yagita H, Koya RC, Graeber TG, Ribas A, McArthur GA, Smyth MJ (2013) Host immunity contributes to the anti-melanoma activity of BRAF inhibitors. J Clin Investig 123(3):1371–1381. doi:10.1172/JCI66236
12. Croci DO, Zacarias Fluck MF, Rico MJ, Matar P, Rabinovich GA, Scharovsky OG (2007) Dynamic cross-talk between tumor and immune cells in orchestrating the immunosuppressive network at the tumor microenvironment. Cancer Immunol Immunother CII 56(11): 1687–1700. doi:10.1007/s00262-007-0343-y
13. Khalili JS, Liu S, Rodriguez-Cruz TG, Whittington M, Wardell S, Liu C, Zhang M, Cooper ZA, Frederick DT, Li Y, Joseph RW, Bernatchez C, Ekmekcioglu S, Grimm E, Radvanyi LG, Davis RE, Davies MA, Wargo JA, Hwu P, Lizee G (2012) Oncogenic BRAF (V600E) promotes stromal cell-mediated immunosuppression via induction of interleukin-1 in melanoma. Clin Cancer Res Official J Am Assoc Cancer Res 18(19):5329–5340. doi:10.1158/1078-0432.CCR-12-1632
14. Qian BZ, Pollard JW (2010) Macrophage diversity enhances tumor progression and metastasis. Cell 141(1):39–51. doi:10.1016/j.cell.2010.03.014
15. Agwa E, Ma PC (2013) Overview of various techniques/platforms with critical evaluation of each. Curr Treat Options Oncol 14(4):623–633. doi:10.1007/s11864-013-0259-z
16. Ow TJ, Sandulache VC, Skinner HD, Myers JN (2013) Integration of cancer genomics with treatment selection: from the genome to predictive biomarkers. Cancer 119(22):3914–3928. doi:10.1002/cncr.28304
17. Patel LR, Nykter M, Chen K, Zhang W (2013) Cancer genome sequencing: understanding malignancy as a disease of the genome, its conformation, and its evolution. Cancer Lett 340(2):152–160. doi:10.1016/j.canlet.2012.10.018
18. Bennett NC, Farah CS (2014) Next-generation sequencing in clinical oncology: next steps towards clinical validation. Cancers 6(4):2296–2312. doi:10.3390/cancers6042296
19. Yewdell JW, Bennink JR (1992) Cell biology of antigen processing and presentation to major histocompatibility complex class I molecule-restricted T lymphocytes. Adv Immunol 52:1–123
20. Joffre OP, Segura E, Savina A, Amigorena S (2012) Cross-presentation by dendritic cells. Nat Rev Immunol 12(8):557–569. doi:10.1038/nri3254
21. Peaper DR, Cresswell P (2008) Regulation of MHC class I assembly and peptide binding. Annu Rev Cell Dev Biol 24:343–368. doi:10.1146/annurev.cellbio.24.110707.175347
22. Lizee G, Basha G, Jefferies WA (2005) Tails of wonder: endocytic-sorting motifs key for exogenous antigen presentation. Trends Immunol 26(3):141–149. doi:10.1016/j.it.2005.01.005
23. Mlecnik B, Bindea G, Pages F, Galon J (2011) Tumor immunosurveillance in human cancers. Cancer Metastasis Rev 30(1):5–12. doi:10.1007/s10555-011-9270-7
24. Roberts SA, Gordenin DA (2014) Hypermutation in human cancer genomes: footprints and mechanisms. Nat Rev Cancer 14(12):786–800
25. Overwijk WW, Wang E, Marincola FM, Rammensee HG, Restifo NP (2013) Mining the mutanome: developing highly personalized Immunotherapies based on mutational analysis of tumors. J Immunother Cancer 1:11. doi:10.1186/2051-1426-1-11
26. Heemskerk B, Kvistborg P, Schumacher TN (2013) The cancer antigenome. EMBO J 32 (2):194–203. doi:10.1038/emboj.2012.333
27. Burrell RA, Swanton C (2014) The evolution of the unstable cancer genome. Curr Opin Genet Dev 24:61–67. doi:10.1016/j.gde.2013.11.011
28. Lundegaard C, Lund O, Buus S, Nielsen M (2010) Major histocompatibility complex class I binding predictions as a tool in epitope discovery. Immunology 130(3):309–318. doi:10.1111/j.1365-2567.2010.03300.x

29. Liao WW, Arthur JW (2011) Predicting peptide binding affinities to MHC molecules using a modified semi-empirical scoring function. PLoS ONE 6(9):e25055. doi:10.1371/journal.pone.0025055
30. Fritsch EF, Rajasagi M, Ott PA, Brusic V, Hacohen N, Wu CJ (2014) HLA-binding properties of tumor neoepitopes in humans. Cancer Immunol Res 2(6):522–529. doi:10.1158/2326-6066.CIR-13-0227
31. Robbins PF, Lu YC, El-Gamil M, Li YF, Gross C, Gartner J, Lin JC, Teer JK, Cliften P, Tycksen E, Samuels Y, Rosenberg SA (2013) Mining exomic sequencing data to identify mutated antigens recognized by adoptively transferred tumor-reactive T cells. Nat Med 19(6):747–752. doi:10.1038/nm.3161
32. Linnemann C, van Buuren MM, Bies L, Verdegaal EM, Schotte R, Calis JJ, Behjati S, Velds A, Hilkmann H, Atmioui DE, Visser M, Stratton MR, Haanen JB, Spits H, van der Burg SH, Schumacher TN (2015) High-throughput epitope discovery reveals frequent recognition of neo-antigens by CD4+ T cells in human melanoma. Nat Med 21(1):81–85. doi:10.1038/nm.3773
33. Matsushita H, Vesely MD, Koboldt DC, Rickert CG, Uppaluri R, Magrini VJ, Arthur CD, White JM, Chen YS, Shea LK, Hundal J, Wendl MC, Demeter R, Wylie T, Allison JP, Smyth MJ, Old LJ, Mardis ER, Schreiber RD (2012) Cancer exome analysis reveals a T-cell-dependent mechanism of cancer immunoediting. Nature 482(7385):400–404. doi:10.1038/nature10755
34. Yadav M, Jhunjhunwala S, Phung QT, Lupardus P, Tanguay J, Bumbaca S, Franci C, Cheung TK, Fritsche J, Weinschenk T, Modrusan Z, Mellman I, Lill JR, Delamarre L (2014) Predicting immunogenic tumour mutations by combining mass spectrometry and exome sequencing. Nature 515(7528):572–576. doi:10.1038/nature14001
35. Snyder A, Makarov V, Merghoub T, Yuan J, Zaretsky JM, Desrichard A, Walsh LA, Postow MA, Wong P, Ho TS, Hollmann TJ, Bruggeman C, Kannan K, Li Y, Elipenahli C, Liu C, Harbison CT, Wang L, Ribas A, Wolchok JD, Chan TA (2014) Genetic basis for clinical response to CTLA-4 blockade in melanoma. N Engl J Med 371(23):2189–2199. doi:10.1056/NEJMoa1406498
36. Lawrence MS, Stojanov P, Polak P, Kryukov GV, Cibulskis K, Sivachenko A, Carter SL, Stewart C, Mermel CH, Roberts SA, Kiezun A, Hammerman PS, McKenna A, Drier Y, Zou L, Ramos AH, Pugh TJ, Stransky N, Helman E, Kim J, Sougnez C, Ambrogio L, Nickerson E, Shefler E, Cortes ML, Auclair D, Saksena G, Voet D, Noble M, DiCara D, Lin P, Lichtenstein L, Heiman DI, Fennell T, Imielinski M, Hernandez B, Hodis E, Baca S, Dulak AM, Lohr J, Landau DA, Wu CJ, Melendez-Zajgla J, Hidalgo-Miranda A, Koren A, McCarroll SA, Mora J, Lee RS, Crompton B, Onofrio R, Parkin M, Winckler W, Ardlie K, Gabriel SB, Roberts CW, Biegel JA, Stegmaier K, Bass AJ, Garraway LA, Meyerson M, Golub TR, Gordenin DA, Sunyaev S, Lander ES, Getz G (2013) Mutational heterogeneity in cancer and the search for new cancer-associated genes. Nature 499(7457):214–218. doi:10.1038/nature12213
37. Davies H, Bignell GR, Cox C, Stephens P, Edkins S, Clegg S, Teague J, Woffendin H, Garnett MJ, Bottomley W, Davis N, Dicks E, Ewing R, Floyd Y, Gray K, Hall S, Hawes R, Hughes J, Kosmidou V, Menzies A, Mould C, Parker A, Stevens C, Watt S, Hooper S, Wilson R, Jayatilake H, Gusterson BA, Cooper C, Shipley J, Hargrave D, Pritchard-Jones K, Maitland N, Chenevix-Trench G, Riggins GJ, Bigner DD, Palmieri G, Cossu A, Flanagan A, Nicholson A, Ho JW, Leung SY, Yuen ST, Weber BL, Seigler HF, Darrow TL, Paterson H, Marais R, Marshall CJ, Wooster R, Stratton MR, Futreal PA (2002) Mutations of the BRAF gene in human cancer. Nature 417(6892):949–954. doi:10.1038/nature00766
38. Sharkey MS, Lizee G, Gonzales MI, Patel S, Topalian SL (2004) CD4(+) T-cell recognition of mutated B-RAF in melanoma patients harboring the V599E mutation. Cancer Res 64(5):1595–1599

39. Miglio U, Oldani A, Mezzapelle R, Veggiani C, Paganotti A, Garavoglia M, Boldorini R (2014) KRAS mutational analysis in ductal adenocarcinoma of the pancreas and its clinical significance. Pathol Res Pract 210(5):307–311. doi:10.1016/j.prp.2014.01.011
40. Warren RL, Holt RA (2010) A census of predicted mutational epitopes suitable for immunologic cancer control. Hum Immunol 71(3):245–254. doi:10.1016/j.humimm.2009.12.007
41. Phan GQ, Rosenberg SA (2013) Adoptive cell transfer for patients with metastatic melanoma: the potential and promise of cancer immunotherapy. Cancer Control J Moffitt Cancer Cent 20(4):289–297
42. Kawakami Y, Robbins PF, Rosenberg SA (1996) Human melanoma antigens recognized by T lymphocytes. Keio J Med 45(2):100–108
43. Chen YT, Old LJ (1999) Cancer-testis antigens: targets for cancer immunotherapy. Cancer J Sci Am 5(1):16–17
44. Meek DW, Marcar L (2012) MAGE-A antigens as targets in tumour therapy. Cancer Lett 324(2):126–132. doi:10.1016/j.canlet.2012.05.011
45. Rycaj K, Plummer JB, Yin B, Li M, Garza J, Radvanyi L, Ramondetta LM, Lin K, Johanning GL, Tang DG, Wang-Johanning F (2015) Cytotoxicity of human endogenous retrovirus K-specific T cells toward autologous ovarian cancer cells. Clin Cancer Res Official J Am Assoc Cancer Res 21(2):471–483. doi:10.1158/1078-0432.CCR-14-0388
46. Gordan JD, Vonderheide RH (2002) Universal tumor antigens as targets for immunotherapy. Cytotherapy 4(4):317–327. doi:10.1080/146532402760271091
47. Asai T, Storkus WJ, Mueller-Berghaus J, Knapp W, DeLeo AB, Chikamatsu K, Whiteside TL (2002) In vitro generated cytolytic T lymphocytes reactive against head and neck cancer recognize multiple epitopes presented by HLA-A2, including peptides derived from the p53 and MDM-2 proteins. Cancer Immun 2:3
48. Hunt DF, Henderson RA, Shabanowitz J, Sakaguchi K, Michel H, Sevilir N, Cox AL, Appella E, Engelhard VH (1992) Characterization of peptides bound to the class I MHC molecule HLA-A2.1 by mass spectrometry. Science 255(5049):1261–1263
49. Singh-Jasuja H, Emmerich NP, Rammensee HG (2004) The Tubingen approach: identification, selection, and validation of tumor-associated HLA peptides for cancer therapy. Cancer Immunol Immunother CII 53(3):187–195. doi:10.1007/s00262-003-0480-x
50. Rammensee HG, Falk K, Rotzschke O (1993) Peptides naturally presented by MHC class I molecules. Annu Rev Immunol 11:213–244. doi:10.1146/annurev.iy.11.040193.001241
51. Bassani-Sternberg M, Barnea E, Beer I, Avivi I, Katz T, Admon A (2010) Soluble plasma HLA peptidome as a potential source for cancer biomarkers. Proc Natl Acad Sci USA 107 (44):18769–18776. doi:10.1073/pnas.1008501107
52. Rammensee HG, Singh-Jasuja H (2013) HLA ligandome tumor antigen discovery for personalized vaccine approach. Expert Rev Vaccines 12(10):1211–1217. doi:10.1586/14760584.2013.836911
53. Khong HT, Restifo NP (2002) Natural selection of tumor variants in the generation of "tumor escape" phenotypes. Nat Immunol 3(11):999–1005. doi:10.1038/ni1102-999
54. Schreiber RD, Old LJ, Smyth MJ (2011) Cancer immunoediting: integrating immunity's roles in cancer suppression and promotion. Science 331(6024):1565–1570. doi:10.1126/science.1203486
55. Kawakami Y, Rosenberg SA (1997) Immunobiology of human melanoma antigens MART-1 and gp100 and their use for immuno-gene therapy. Int Rev Immunol 14(2–3):173–192
56. Li Y, Yee C (2008) IL-21 mediated Foxp3 suppression leads to enhanced generation of antigen-specific CD8+ cytotoxic T lymphocytes. Blood 111(1):229–235. doi:10.1182/blood-2007-05-089375
57. Walter S, Weinschenk T, Stenzl A, Zdrojowy R, Pluzanska A, Szczylik C, Staehler M, Brugger W, Dietrich PY, Mendrzyk R, Hilf N, Schoor O, Fritsche J, Mahr A, Maurer D, Vass V, Trautwein C, Lewandrowski P, Flohr C, Pohla H, Stanczak JJ, Bronte V, Mandruzzato S, Biedermann T, Pawelec G, Derhovanessian E, Yamagishi H, Miki T,

Hongo F, Takaha N, Hirakawa K, Tanaka H, Stevanovic S, Frisch J, Mayer-Mokler A, Kirner A, Rammensee HG, Reinhardt C, Singh-Jasuja H (2012) Multipeptide immune response to cancer vaccine IMA901 after single-dose cyclophosphamide associates with longer patient survival. Nat Med 18(8):1254–1261. doi:10.1038/nm.2883

58. Mittendorf EA, Clifton GT, Holmes JP, Schneble E, van Echo D, Ponniah S, Peoples GE (2014) Final report of the phase I/II clinical trial of the E75 (nelipepimut-S) vaccine with booster inoculations to prevent disease recurrence in high-risk breast cancer patients. Ann Oncol Official J Eur Soc Med Oncol/ESMO 25(9):1735–1742. doi:10.1093/annonc/mdu211
59. Morgan RA, Dudley ME, Wunderlich JR, Hughes MS, Yang JC, Sherry RM, Royal RE, Topalian SL, Kammula US, Restifo NP, Zheng Z, Nahvi A, de Vries CR, Rogers-Freezer LJ, Mavroukakis SA, Rosenberg SA (2006) Cancer regression in patients after transfer of genetically engineered lymphocytes. Science 314(5796):126–129. doi:10.1126/science.1129003
60. Gnjatic S, Jager E, Chen W, Altorki NK, Matsuo M, Lee SY, Chen Q, Nagata Y, Atanackovic D, Chen YT, Ritter G, Cebon J, Knuth A, Old LJ (2002) CD8(+) T cell responses against a dominant cryptic HLA-A2 epitope after NY-ESO-1 peptide immunization of cancer patients. Proc Natl Acad Sci USA 99(18):11813–11818. doi:10.1073/pnas.142417699
61. Lundegaard C, Lund O, Nielsen M (2008) Accurate approximation method for prediction of class I MHC affinities for peptides of length 8, 10 and 11 using prediction tools trained on 9mers. Bioinformatics 24(11):1397–1398. doi:10.1093/bioinformatics/btn128
62. Yi Z, Luo M, Carroll CA, Weintraub ST, Mandarino LJ (2005) Identification of phosphorylation sites in insulin receptor substrate-1 by hypothesis-driven high-performance liquid chromatography-electrospray ionization tandem mass spectrometry. Anal Chem 77(17):5693–5699. doi:10.1021/ac050760y
63. Kalkum M, Lyon GJ, Chait BT (2003) Detection of secreted peptides by using hypothesis-driven multistage mass spectrometry. Proc Natl Acad Sci USA 100(5):2795–2800. doi:10.1073/pnas.0436605100
64. Rosenberg SA, Yang JC, Restifo NP (2004) Cancer immunotherapy: moving beyond current vaccines. Nat Med 10(9):909–915. doi:10.1038/nm1100
65. Robin C, Beckerich F, Cordonnier C (2015) Immunization in cancer patients: where we stand. Pharmacol Res Official J Ital Pharmacol Soc 92C:23–30. doi:10.1016/j.phrs.2014.10.002
66. Lindsey KR, Gritz L, Sherry R, Abati A, Fetsch PA, Goldfeder LC, Gonzales MI, Zinnack KA, Rogers-Freezer L, Haworth L, Mavroukakis SA, White DE, Steinberg SM, Restifo NP, Panicali DL, Rosenberg SA, Topalian SL (2006) Evaluation of prime/boost regimens using recombinant poxvirus/tyrosinase vaccines for the treatment of patients with metastatic melanoma. Clin Cancer Res Official J Am Assoc Cancer Res 12(8):2526–2537. doi:10.1158/1078-0432.CCR-05-2061
67. Irvine KR, Chamberlain RS, Shulman EP, Surman DR, Rosenberg SA, Restifo NP (1997) Enhancing efficacy of recombinant anticancer vaccines with prime/boost regimens that use two different vectors. J Natl Cancer Inst 89(21):1595–1601
68. Kaufman HL, Kim DW, Kim-Schulze S, DeRaffele G, Jagoda MC, Broucek JR, Zloza A (2014) Results of a randomized phase I gene therapy clinical trial of nononcolytic fowlpox viruses encoding T cell costimulatory molecules. Hum Gene Ther 25(5):452–460. doi:10.1089/hum.2013.217
69. Pulido J, Kottke T, Thompson J, Galivo F, Wongthida P, Diaz RM, Rommelfanger D, Ilett E, Pease L, Pandha H, Harrington K, Selby P, Melcher A, Vile R (2012) Using virally expressed melanoma cDNA libraries to identify tumor-associated antigens that cure melanoma. Nat Biotechnol 30(4):337–343. doi:10.1038/nbt.2157
70. Adair RA, Roulstone V, Scott KJ, Morgan R, Nuovo GJ, Fuller M, Beirne D, West EJ, Jennings VA, Rose A, Kyula J, Fraser S, Dave R, Anthoney DA, Merrick A, Prestwich R, Aldouri A, Donnelly O, Pandha H, Coffey M, Selby P, Vile R, Toogood G, Harrington K, Melcher AA (2012) Cell carriage, delivery, and selective replication of an oncolytic virus in tumor in patients. Science Transl Med 4(138):138ra177

71. Durantez M, Lopez-Vazquez AB, de Cerio AL, Huarte E, Casares N, Prieto J, Borras-Cuesta F, Lasarte JJ, Sarobe P (2009) Induction of multiepitopic and long-lasting immune responses against tumour antigens by immunization with peptides, DNA and recombinant adenoviruses expressing minigenes. Scand J Immunol 69(2):80–89. doi:10.1111/j.1365-3083.2008.02202.x
72. Lizee G, Overwijk WW, Radvanyi L, Gao J, Sharma P, Hwu P (2013) Harnessing the power of the immune system to target cancer. Annu Rev Med 64:71–90. doi:10.1146/annurev-med-112311-083918
73. Banchereau J, Steinman RM (1998) Dendritic cells and the control of immunity. Nature 392(6673):245–252. doi:10.1038/32588
74. Benteyn D, Heirman C, Bonehill A, Thielemans K, Breckpot K (2015) mRNA-based dendritic cell vaccines. Expert Rev Vaccines 14(2):161–176. doi:10.1586/14760584.2014.957684
75. Powell DJ Jr, Rosenberg SA (2004) Phenotypic and functional maturation of tumor antigen-reactive CD8+ T lymphocytes in patients undergoing multiple course peptide vaccination. J Immunother 27(1):36–47
76. Bettinotti MP, Panelli MC, Ruppe E, Mocellin S, Phan GQ, White DE, Marincola FM (2003) Clinical and immunological evaluation of patients with metastatic melanoma undergoing immunization with the HLA-Cw* 0702-associated epitope MAGE-A12:170-178. Int J Cancer J Int du Cancer 105(2):210–216. doi:10.1002/ijc.11045
77. Hailemichael Y, Overwijk WW (2013) Peptide-based anticancer vaccines: the making and unmaking of a T-cell graveyard. Oncoimmunology 2(7):e24743. doi:10.4161/onci.24743
78. Hailemichael Y, Dai Z, Jaffarzad N, Ye Y, Medina MA, Huang XF, Dorta-Estremera SM, Greeley NR, Nitti G, Peng W, Liu C, Lou Y, Wang Z, Ma W, Rabinovich B, Sowell RT, Schluns KS, Davis RE, Hwu P, Overwijk WW (2013) Persistent antigen at vaccination sites induces tumor-specific CD8(+) T cell sequestration, dysfunction and deletion. Nat Med 19 (4):465–472. doi:10.1038/nm.3105
79. Salerno EP, Shea SM, Olson WC, Petroni GR, Smolkin ME, McSkimming C, Chianese-Bullock KA, Slingluff CL Jr (2013) Activation, dysfunction and retention of T cells in vaccine sites after injection of incomplete Freund's adjuvant, with or without peptide. Cancer Immunol Immunother CII 62(7):1149–1159. doi:10.1007/s00262-013-1435-5
80. Bijker MS, van den Eeden SJ, Franken KL, Melief CJ, Offringa R, van der Burg SH (2007) CD8+ CTL priming by exact peptide epitopes in incomplete Freund's adjuvant induces a vanishing CTL response, whereas long peptides induce sustained CTL reactivity. J Immunol 179(8):5033–5040
81. van Poelgeest MI, Welters MJ, van Esch EM, Stynenbosch LF, Kerpershoek G, van Persijn van Meerten EL, van den Hende M, Lowik MJ, Berends-van der Meer DM, Fathers LM, Valentijn AR, Oostendorp J, Fleuren GJ, Melief CJ, Kenter GG, van der Burg SH (2013) HPV16 synthetic long peptide (HPV16-SLP) vaccination therapy of patients with advanced or recurrent HPV16-induced gynecological carcinoma, a phase II trial. J Transl Med 11:88. doi:10.1186/1479-5876-11-88
82. Steinman RM, Witmer-Pack M, Inaba K (1993) Dendritic cells: antigen presentation, accessory function and clinical relevance. Adv Exp Med Biol 329:1–9
83. Smith CM, Wilson NS, Waithman J, Villadangos JA, Carbone FR, Heath WR, Belz GT (2004) Cognate CD4(+) T cell licensing of dendritic cells in CD8(+) T cell immunity. Nat Immunol 5(11):1143–1148. doi:10.1038/ni1129
84. Iwasaki A, Medzhitov R (2004) Toll-like receptor control of the adaptive immune responses. Nat Immunol 5(10):987–995. doi:10.1038/ni1112
85. O'Sullivan B, Thomas R (2003) CD40 and dendritic cell function. Crit Rev Immunol 23(1–2): 83–107
86. Bullock TN, Yagita H (2005) Induction of CD70 on dendritic cells through CD40 or TLR stimulation contributes to the development of CD8+ T cell responses in the absence of CD4+ T cells. J Immunol 174(2):710–717

87. Van Deusen KE, Rajapakse R, Bullock TN (2010) CD70 expression by dendritic cells plays a critical role in the immunogenicity of CD40-independent, CD4+ T cell-dependent, licensed CD8+ T cell responses. J Leukoc Biol 87(3):477–485. doi:10.1189/jlb.0809535
88. Fehres CM, Bruijns SC, van Beelen AJ, Kalay H, Ambrosini M, Hooijberg E, Unger WW, de Gruijl TD, van Kooyk Y (2014) Topical rather than intradermal application of the TLR7 ligand imiquimod leads to human dermal dendritic cell maturation and CD8+ T-cell cross-priming. Eur J Immunol 44(8):2415–2424. doi:10.1002/eji.201344094
89. Rosalia RA, Cruz LJ, van Duikeren S, Tromp AT, Silva AL, Jiskoot W, de Gruijl T, Lowik C, Oostendorp J, van der Burg SH, Ossendorp F (2015) CD40-targeted dendritic cell delivery of PLGA-nanoparticle vaccines induce potent anti-tumor responses. Biomaterials 40:88–97. doi:10.1016/j.biomaterials.2014.10.053
90. Steinman RM, Banchereau J (2007) Taking dendritic cells into medicine. Nature 449 (7161):419–426. doi:10.1038/nature06175
91. Lou Y, Wang G, Lizee G, Kim GJ, Finkelstein SE, Feng C, Restifo NP, Hwu P (2004) Dendritic cells strongly boost the antitumor activity of adoptively transferred T cells in vivo. Cancer Res 64(18):6783–6790. doi:10.1158/0008-5472.CAN-04-1621
92. Yewdell JW, Norbury CC, Bennink JR (1999) Mechanisms of exogenous antigen presentation by MHC class I molecules in vitro and in vivo: implications for generating CD8+ T cell responses to infectious agents, tumors, transplants, and vaccines. Adv Immunol 73:1–77
93. Keenan BP, Jaffee EM (2012) Whole cell vaccines–past progress and future strategies. Semin Oncol 39(3):276–286. doi:10.1053/j.seminoncol.2012.02.007
94. Yamada A, Sasada T, Noguchi M, Itoh K (2013) Next-generation peptide vaccines for advanced cancer. Cancer Sci 104(1):15–21. doi:10.1111/cas.12050
95. Melief CJ (2008) Cancer immunotherapy by dendritic cells. Immunity 29(3):372–383. doi:10.1016/j.immuni.2008.08.004
96. Thurner B, Haendle I, Roder C, Dieckmann D, Keikavoussi P, Jonuleit H, Bender A, Maczek C, Schreiner D, von den Driesch P, Brocker EB, Steinman RM, Enk A, Kampgen E, Schuler G (1999) Vaccination with mage-3A1 peptide-pulsed mature, monocyte-derived dendritic cells expands specific cytotoxic T cells and induces regression of some metastases in advanced stage IV melanoma. J Exp Med 190(11):1669–1678
97. Nestle FO, Farkas A, Conrad C (2005) Dendritic-cell-based therapeutic vaccination against cancer. Curr Opin Immunol 17(2):163–169. doi:10.1016/j.coi.2005.02.003
98. Restifo NP, Dudley ME, Rosenberg SA (2012) Adoptive immunotherapy for cancer: harnessing the T cell response. Nat Rev Immunol 12(4):269–281. doi:10.1038/nri3191
99. Chandran SS, Paria BC, Srivastava AK, Rothermel LD, Stephens DJ, Dudley ME, Somerville RP, Wunderlich JR, Sherry RM, Yang JC, Rosenberg SA, Kammula US (2014) Persistence of CTL clones targeting melanocyte differentiation antigens was insufficient to mediate significant melanoma regression in humans. Clin Cancer Res Official J Am Assoc Cancer Res. doi:10.1158/1078-0432.CCR-14-2208
100. Dudley ME, Wunderlich J, Nishimura MI, Yu D, Yang JC, Topalian SL, Schwartzentruber DJ, Hwu P, Marincola FM, Sherry R, Leitman SF, Rosenberg SA (2001) Adoptive transfer of cloned melanoma-reactive T lymphocytes for the treatment of patients with metastatic melanoma. J Immunother 24(4):363–373
101. Dudley ME, Wunderlich JR, Yang JC, Hwu P, Schwartzentruber DJ, Topalian SL, Sherry RM, Marincola FM, Leitman SF, Seipp CA, Rogers-Freezer L, Morton KE, Nahvi A, Mavroukakis SA, White DE, Rosenberg SA (2002) A phase I study of nonmyeloablative chemotherapy and adoptive transfer of autologous tumor antigen-specific T lymphocytes in patients with metastatic melanoma. J Immunother 25(3):243–251
102. Yee C, Thompson JA, Byrd D, Riddell SR, Roche P, Celis E, Greenberg PD (2002) Adoptive T cell therapy using antigen-specific CD8+ T cell clones for the treatment of patients with metastatic melanoma: in vivo persistence, migration, and antitumor effect of

transferred T cells. Proc Natl Acad Sci USA 99(25):16168–16173. doi:10.1073/pnas.242600099

103. Khammari A, Labarriere N, Vignard V, Nguyen JM, Pandolfino MC, Knol AC, Quereux G, Saiagh S, Brocard A, Jotereau F, Dreno B (2009) Treatment of metastatic melanoma with autologous Melan-A/MART-1-specific cytotoxic T lymphocyte clones. J Invest Dermatol 129(12):2835–2842. doi:10.1038/jid.2009.144
104. Hunder NN, Wallen H, Cao J, Hendricks DW, Reilly JZ, Rodmyre R, Jungbluth A, Gnjatic S, Thompson JA, Yee C (2008) Treatment of metastatic melanoma with autologous CD4+ T cells against NY-ESO-1. N Engl J Med 358(25):2698–2703. doi:10.1056/NEJMoa0800251
105. Pollack SM, Jones RL, Farrar EA, Lai IP, Lee SM, Cao J, Pillarisetty VG, Hoch BL, Gullett A, Bleakley M, Conrad EU 3rd, Eary JF, Shibuya KC, Warren EH, Carstens JN, Heimfeld S, Riddell SR, Yee C (2014) Tetramer guided, cell sorter assisted production of clinical grade autologous NY-ESO-1 specific CD8(+) T cells. J Immunother Cancer 2(1):36. doi:10.1186/s40425-014-0036-y
106. Gubin MM, Zhang X, Schuster H, Caron E, Ward JP, Noguchi T, Ivanova Y, Hundal J, Arthur CD, Krebber WJ, Mulder GE, Toebes M, Vesely MD, Lam SS, Korman AJ, Allison JP, Freeman GJ, Sharpe AH, Pearce EL, Schumacher TN, Aebersold R, Rammensee HG, Melief CJ, Mardis ER, Gillanders WE, Artyomov MN, Schreiber RD (2014) Checkpoint blockade cancer immunotherapy targets tumour-specific mutant antigens. Nature 515(7528):577–581. doi:10.1038/nature13988
107. Robbins PF, El-Gamil M, Li YF, Kawakami Y, Loftus D, Appella E, Rosenberg SA (1996) A mutated beta-catenin gene encodes a melanoma-specific antigen recognized by tumor infiltrating lymphocytes. J Exp Med 183(3):1185–1192
108. Pieper R, Christian RE, Gonzales MI, Nishimura MI, Gupta G, Settlage RE, Shabanowitz J, Rosenberg SA, Hunt DF, Topalian SL (1999) Biochemical identification of a mutated human melanoma antigen recognized by CD4(+) T cells. J Exp Med 189(5):757–766
109. Huang J, El-Gamil M, Dudley ME, Li YF, Rosenberg SA, Robbins PF (2004) T cells associated with tumor regression recognize frameshifted products of the CDKN2A tumor suppressor gene locus and a mutated HLA class I gene product. J Immunol 172(10):6057–6064
110. Lu YC, Yao X, Li YF, El-Gamil M, Dudley ME, Yang JC, Almeida JR, Douek DC, Samuels Y, Rosenberg SA, Robbins PF (2013) Mutated PPP1R3B is recognized by T cells used to treat a melanoma patient who experienced a durable complete tumor regression. J Immunol 190(12):6034–6042. doi:10.4049/jimmunol.1202830
111. Rosenberg SA, Spiess P, Lafreniere R (1986) A new approach to the adoptive immunotherapy of cancer with tumor-infiltrating lymphocytes. Science 233(4770):1318–1321
112. Topalian SL, Muul LM, Solomon D, Rosenberg SA (1987) Expansion of human tumor infiltrating lymphocytes for use in immunotherapy trials. J Immunol Methods 102(1):127–141
113. Rosenberg SA, Aebersold P, Cornetta K, Kasid A, Morgan RA, Moen R, Karson EM, Lotze MT, Yang JC, Topalian SL et al (1990) Gene transfer into humans–immunotherapy of patients with advanced melanoma, using tumor-infiltrating lymphocytes modified by retroviral gene transduction. N Engl J Med 323(9):570–578. doi:10.1056/NEJM199008303230904
114. Rosenberg SA, Packard BS, Aebersold PM, Solomon D, Topalian SL, Toy ST, Simon P, Lotze MT, Yang JC, Seipp CA et al (1988) Use of tumor-infiltrating lymphocytes and interleukin-2 in the immunotherapy of patients with metastatic melanoma. A preliminary report. N Engl J Med 319(25):1676–1680. doi:10.1056/NEJM198812223192527
115. Besser MJ, Shapira-Frommer R, Treves AJ, Zippel D, Itzhaki O, Hershkovitz L, Levy D, Kubi A, Hovav E, Chermoshniuk N, Shalmon B, Hardan I, Catane R, Markel G, Apter S, Ben-Nun A, Kuchuk I, Shimoni A, Nagler A, Schachter J (2010) Clinical responses in a phase II study using adoptive transfer of short-term cultured tumor infiltration lymphocytes in metastatic melanoma patients. Clin Cancer Res Official J Am Assoc Cancer Res 16(9):2646–2655. doi:10.1158/1078-0432.CCR-10-0041

116. Dudley ME, Wunderlich JR, Robbins PF, Yang JC, Hwu P, Schwartzentruber DJ, Topalian SL, Sherry R, Restifo NP, Hubicki AM, Robinson MR, Raffeld M, Duray P, Seipp CA, Rogers-Freezer L, Morton KE, Mavroukakis SA, White DE, Rosenberg SA (2002) Cancer regression and autoimmunity in patients after clonal repopulation with antitumor lymphocytes. Science 298(5594):850–854. doi:10.1126/science.1076514
117. Dudley ME, Wunderlich JR, Yang JC, Sherry RM, Topalian SL, Restifo NP, Royal RE, Kammula U, White DE, Mavroukakis SA, Rogers LJ, Gracia GJ, Jones SA, Mangiameli DP, Pelletier MM, Gea-Banacloche J, Robinson MR, Berman DM, Filie AC, Abati A, Rosenberg SA (2005) Adoptive cell transfer therapy following non-myeloablative but lymphodepleting chemotherapy for the treatment of patients with refractory metastatic melanoma. J Clin Oncol Official J Am Soc Clin Oncol 23(10):2346–2357. doi:10.1200/JCO.2005.00.240
118. Radvanyi LG, Bernatchez C, Zhang M, Fox PS, Miller P, Chacon J, Wu R, Lizee G, Mahoney S, Alvarado G, Glass M, Johnson VE, McMannis JD, Shpall E, Prieto V, Papadopoulos N, Kim K, Homsi J, Bedikian A, Hwu WJ, Patel S, Ross MI, Lee JE, Gershenwald JE, Lucci A, Royal R, Cormier JN, Davies MA, Mansaray R, Fulbright OJ, Toth C, Ramachandran R, Wardell S, Gonzalez A, Hwu P (2012) Specific lymphocyte subsets predict response to adoptive cell therapy using expanded autologous tumor-infiltrating lymphocytes in metastatic melanoma patients. Clin Cancer Res Official J Am Assoc Cancer Res 18(24):6758–6770. doi:10.1158/1078-0432.CCR-12-1177
119. Pilon-Thomas S, Kuhn L, Ellwanger S, Janssen W, Royster E, Marzban S, Kudchadkar R, Zager J, Gibney G, Sondak VK, Weber J, Mule JJ, Sarnaik AA (2012) Efficacy of adoptive cell transfer of tumor-infiltrating lymphocytes after lymphopenia induction for metastatic melanoma. J Immunother 35(8):615–620. doi:10.1097/CJI.0b013e31826e8f5f
120. Ellebaek E, Iversen TZ, Junker N, Donia M, Engell-Noerregaard L, Met O, Holmich LR, Andersen RS, Hadrup SR, Andersen MH, thor Straten P, Svane IM (2012) Adoptive cell therapy with autologous tumor infiltrating lymphocytes and low-dose Interleukin-2 in metastatic melanoma patients. J Transl Med 10:169. doi:10.1186/1479-5876-10-169
121. Ullenhag GJ, Sadeghi AM, Carlsson B, Ahlstrom H, Mosavi F, Wagenius G, Totterman TH (2012) Adoptive T-cell therapy for malignant melanoma patients with TILs obtained by ultrasound-guided needle biopsy. Cancer Immunol Immunother CII 61(5):725–732. doi:10.1007/s00262-011-1182-4
122. Sherwood AM, Emerson RO, Scherer D, Habermann N, Buck K, Staffa J, Desmarais C, Halama N, Jaeger D, Schirmacher P, Herpel E, Kloor M, Ulrich A, Schneider M, Ulrich CM, Robins H (2013) Tumor-infiltrating lymphocytes in colorectal tumors display a diversity of T cell receptor sequences that differ from the T cells in adjacent mucosal tissue. Cancer Immunol Immunother CII 62(9):1453–1461. doi:10.1007/s00262-013-1446-2
123. Kvistborg P, Shu CJ, Heemskerk B, Fankhauser M, Thrue CA, Toebes M, van Rooij N, Linnemann C, van Buuren MM, Urbanus JH, Beltman JB, Thor Straten P, Li YF, Robbins PF, Besser MJ, Schachter J, Kenter GG, Dudley ME, Rosenberg SA, Haanen JB, Hadrup SR, Schumacher TN (2012) TIL therapy broadens the tumor-reactive CD8(+) T cell compartment in melanoma patients. Oncoimmunology 1(4):409–418
124. Lu YC, Yao X, Crystal JS, Li YF, El-Gamil M, Gross C, Davis L, Dudley ME, Yang JC, Samuels Y, Rosenberg SA, Robbins PF (2014) Efficient identification of mutated cancer antigens recognized by T cells associated with durable tumor regressions. Clin Cancer Res Official J Am Assoc Cancer Res 20(13):3401–3410. doi:10.1158/1078-0432.CCR-14-0433
125. Tran E, Turcotte S, Gros A, Robbins PF, Lu YC, Dudley ME, Wunderlich JR, Somerville RP, Hogan K, Hinrichs CS, Parkhurst MR, Yang JC, Rosenberg SA (2014) Cancer immunotherapy based on mutation-specific CD4+ T cells in a patient with epithelial cancer. Science 344(6184):641–645. doi:10.1126/science.1251102
126. Besser MJ, Shapira-Frommer R, Itzhaki O, Treves AJ, Zippel DB, Levy D, Kubi A, Shoshani N, Zikich D, Ohayon Y, Ohayon D, Shalmon B, Markel G, Yerushalmi R, Apter S, Ben-Nun A, Ben-Ami E, Shimoni A, Nagler A, Schachter J (2013) Adoptive transfer of

tumor-infiltrating lymphocytes in patients with metastatic melanoma: intent-to-treat analysis and efficacy after failure to prior immunotherapies. Clin Cancer Res Official J Am Assoc Cancer Res 19(17):4792–4800. doi:10.1158/1078-0432.CCR-13-0380

127. Dudley ME, Gross CA, Langhan MM, Garcia MR, Sherry RM, Yang JC, Phan GQ, Kammula US, Hughes MS, Citrin DE, Restifo NP, Wunderlich JR, Prieto PA, Hong JJ, Langan RC, Zlott DA, Morton KE, White DE, Laurencot CM, Rosenberg SA (2010) CD8+ enriched "young" tumor infiltrating lymphocytes can mediate regression of metastatic melanoma. Clinical Cancer Res Official J Am Assoc Cancer Res 16(24):6122–6131. doi:10.1158/1078-0432.CCR-10-1297
128. Dudley ME, Gross CA, Somerville RP, Hong Y, Schaub NP, Rosati SF, White DE, Nathan D, Restifo NP, Steinberg SM, Wunderlich JR, Kammula US, Sherry RM, Yang JC, Phan GQ, Hughes MS, Laurencot CM, Rosenberg SA (2013) Randomized selection design trial evaluating CD8+ -enriched versus unselected tumor-infiltrating lymphocytes for adoptive cell therapy for patients with melanoma. J Clin Oncol Official J Am Soc Clin Oncol 31(17):2152–2159. doi:10.1200/JCO.2012.46.6441
129. Church SE, Jensen SM, Antony PA, Restifo NP, Fox BA (2014) Tumor-specific CD4+ T cells maintain effector and memory tumor-specific CD8+ T cells. Eur J Immunol 44(1):69–79. doi:10.1002/eji.201343718
130. Gattinoni L, Lugli E, Ji Y, Pos Z, Paulos CM, Quigley MF, Almeida JR, Gostick E, Yu Z, Carpenito C, Wang E, Douek DC, Price DA, June CH, Marincola FM, Roederer M, Restifo NP (2011) A human memory T cell subset with stem cell-like properties. Nat Med 17(10):1290–1297. doi:10.1038/nm.2446
131. Cieri N, Camisa B, Cocchiarella F, Forcato M, Oliveira G, Provasi E, Bondanza A, Bordignon C, Peccatori J, Ciceri F, Lupo-Stanghellini MT, Mavilio F, Mondino A, Bicciato S, Recchia A, Bonini C (2013) IL-7 and IL-15 instruct the generation of human memory stem T cells from naive precursors. Blood 121(4):573–584. doi:10.1182/blood-2012-05-431718
132. Crompton JG, Sukumar M, Roychoudhuri R, Clever D, Gros A, Eil RL, Tran E, Hanada K, Yu Z, Palmer DC, Kerkar SP, Michalek RD, Upham T, Leonardi A, Acquavella N, Wang E, Marincola FM, Gattinoni L, Muranski P, Sundrud MS, Klebanoff CA, Rosenberg SA, Fearon DT, Restifo NP (2015) Akt inhibition enhances expansion of potent tumor-specific lymphocytes with memory cell characteristics. Cancer Res 75(2):296–305. doi:10.1158/0008-5472.CAN-14-2277
133. Forget MA, Huon Y, Reuben A, Grange C, Liberman M, Martin J, Mes-Masson AM, Arbour N, Lapointe R (2012) Stimulation of Wnt/ss-catenin pathway in human CD8+ T lymphocytes from blood and lung tumors leads to a shared young/memory phenotype. PLoS ONE 7(7):e41074. doi:10.1371/journal.pone.0041074
134. Gattinoni L, Zhong XS, Palmer DC, Ji Y, Hinrichs CS, Yu Z, Wrzesinski C, Boni A, Cassard L, Garvin LM, Paulos CM, Muranski P, Restifo NP (2009) Wnt signaling arrests effector T cell differentiation and generates CD8+ memory stem cells. Nat Med 15(7):808–813. doi:10.1038/nm.1982
135. Cara L Haymaker, Richard C Wu, Ritthipichai K, Bernatchez C, Forget MA, Chen JQ, Liu H, Wang E, Marincola F, Hwu P, Radvanyi LG (2015) BTLA marks a less-differentiated tumor-infiltrating lymphocyte subset in melanoma with enhanced survival properties. OncoImmunology, Vol. 4(8), doi: 10.1080/2162402X.2015.1014246
136. Chacon J, Sarnaik A, Chen J, Creasy C, Kale C, Robinson J, Weber J, Hwu P, Pilon-Thomas S, Radvanyi LG (2014) Manipulating the tumor microenvironment ex vivo for enhanced expansion of tumor-infiltrating lymphocytes for adoptive cell therapy. Clinical Cancer Res Official J Am Assoc Cancer Res. doi:10.1158/1078-0432.CCR-14-1934
137. Donia M, Larsen SM, Met O, Svane IM (2014) Simplified protocol for clinical-grade tumor-infiltrating lymphocyte manufacturing with use of the Wave bioreactor. Cytotherapy 16(8):1117–1120. doi:10.1016/j.jcyt.2014.02.004

138. Jin J, Sabatino M, Somerville R, Wilson JR, Dudley ME, Stroncek DF, Rosenberg SA (2012) Simplified method of the growth of human tumor infiltrating lymphocytes in gas-permeable flasks to numbers needed for patient treatment. J Immunother 35(3):283–292. doi:10.1097/CJI.0b013e31824e801f
139. Somerville RP, Devillier L, Parkhurst MR, Rosenberg SA, Dudley ME (2012) Clinical scale rapid expansion of lymphocytes for adoptive cell transfer therapy in the WAVE(R) bioreactor. J Transl Med 10:69. doi:10.1186/1479-5876-10-69
140. Friedman KM, Devillier LE, Feldman SA, Rosenberg SA, Dudley ME (2011) Augmented lymphocyte expansion from solid tumors with engineered cells for costimulatory enhancement. J Immunother 34(9):651–661. doi:10.1097/CJI.0b013e31823284c3
141. Turcotte S, Gros A, Hogan K, Tran E, Hinrichs CS, Wunderlich JR, Dudley ME, Rosenberg SA (2013) Phenotype and function of T cells infiltrating visceral metastases from gastrointestinal cancers and melanoma: implications for adoptive cell transfer therapy. J Immunol 191(5):2217–2225. doi:10.4049/jimmunol.1300538
142. Ye Q, Loisiou M, Levine BL, Suhoski MM, Riley JL, June CH, Coukos G, Powell DJ Jr (2011) Engineered artificial antigen presenting cells facilitate direct and efficient expansion of tumor infiltrating lymphocytes. J Transl Med 9:131. doi:10.1186/1479-5876-9-131
143. Fujita K, Ikarashi H, Takakuwa K, Kodama S, Tokunaga A, Takahashi T, Tanaka K (1995) Prolonged disease-free period in patients with advanced epithelial ovarian cancer after adoptive transfer of tumor-infiltrating lymphocytes. Clin Cancer Res Official J Am Assoc Cancer Res 1(5):501–507
144. deLeeuw RJ, Kroeger DR, Kost SE, Chang PP, Webb JR, Nelson BH (2015) CD25 identifies a subset of CD4+ FoxP3- TIL that are exhausted yet prognostically favorable in human ovarian cancer. Cancer Immunol Res 3(3):245–253. doi:10.1158/2326-6066.CIR-14-0146
145. Johnson LA, Morgan RA, Dudley ME, Cassard L, Yang JC, Hughes MS, Kammula US, Royal RE, Sherry RM, Wunderlich JR, Lee CC, Restifo NP, Schwarz SL, Cogdill AP, Bishop RJ, Kim H, Brewer CC, Rudy SF, VanWaes C, Davis JL, Mathur A, Ripley RT, Nathan DA, Laurencot CM, Rosenberg SA (2009) Gene therapy with human and mouse T-cell receptors mediates cancer regression and targets normal tissues expressing cognate antigen. Blood 114(3):535–546. doi:10.1182/blood-2009-03-211714
146. Parkhurst MR, Yang JC, Langan RC, Dudley ME, Nathan DA, Feldman SA, Davis JL, Morgan RA, Merino MJ, Sherry RM, Hughes MS, Kammula US, Phan GQ, Lim RM, Wank SA, Restifo NP, Robbins PF, Laurencot CM, Rosenberg SA (2011) T cells targeting carcinoembryonic antigen can mediate regression of metastatic colorectal cancer but induce severe transient colitis. Mol Ther J Am Soc Gene Ther 19(3):620–626. doi:10.1038/mt.2010.272
147. Chinnasamy N, Wargo JA, Yu Z, Rao M, Frankel TL, Riley JP, Hong JJ, Parkhurst MR, Feldman SA, Schrump DS, Restifo NP, Robbins PF, Rosenberg SA, Morgan RA (2011) A TCR targeting the HLA-A*0201-restricted epitope of MAGE-A3 recognizes multiple epitopes of the MAGE-A antigen superfamily in several types of cancer. J Immunol 186(2):685–696. doi:10.4049/jimmunol.1001775
148. Linette GP, Stadtmauer EA, Maus MV, Rapoport AP, Levine BL, Emery L, Litzky L, Bagg A, Carreno BM, Cimino PJ, Binder-Scholl GK, Smethurst DP, Gerry AB, Pumphrey NJ, Bennett AD, Brewer JE, Dukes J, Harper J, Tayton-Martin HK, Jakobsen BK, Hassan NJ, Kalos M, June CH (2013) Cardiovascular toxicity and titin cross-reactivity of affinity-enhanced T cells in myeloma and melanoma. Blood 122(6):863–871. doi:10.1182/blood-2013-03-490565
149. Wooldridge L, Ekeruche-Makinde J, van den Berg HA, Skowera A, Miles JJ, Tan MP, Dolton G, Clement M, Llewellyn-Lacey S, Price DA, Peakman M, Sewell AK (2012) A single autoimmune T cell receptor recognizes more than a million different peptides. J Biol Chem 287(2):1168–1177. doi:10.1074/jbc.M111.289488
150. Robbins PF, Kassim SH, Tran TL, Crystal JS, Morgan RA, Feldman SA, Yang JC, Dudly ME, Wunderlich JR, Sherry RM, Kammula US, Hughes MS, Restifo NP, Raffeld M,

Lee CR, Li YF, El-Gamil M, Rosenberg SA (2014) A pilot trial using lymphocytes genetically engineered with an NY-ESO-1-reactive T cell receptor: long term follow up and correlates with response. Clin Cancer Res Official J Am Assoc Cancer Res. doi:10.1158/1078-0432.CCR-14-2708

151. Hwu P, Shafer GE, Treisman J, Schindler DG, Gross G, Cowherd R, Rosenberg SA, Eshhar Z (1993) Lysis of ovarian cancer cells by human lymphocytes redirected with a chimeric gene composed of an antibody variable region and the Fc receptor gamma chain. J Exp Med 178(1):361–366
152. Kershaw MH, Westwood JA, Parker LL, Wang G, Eshhar Z, Mavroukakis SA, White DE, Wunderlich JR, Canevari S, Rogers-Freezer L, Chen CC, Yang JC, Rosenberg SA, Hwu P (2006) A phase I study on adoptive immunotherapy using gene-modified T cells for ovarian cancer. Clin Cancer Res Official J Am Assoc Cancer Res 12(20 Pt 1):6106–6115. doi:10.1158/1078-0432.CCR-06-1183
153. Brentjens RJ, Davila ML, Riviere I, Park J, Wang X, Cowell LG, Bartido S, Stefanski J, Taylor C, Olszewska M, Borquez-Ojeda O, Qu J, Wasielewska T, He Q, Bernal Y, Rijo IV, Hedvat C, Kobos R, Curran K, Steinherz P, Jurcic J, Rosenblat T, Maslak P, Frattini M, Sadelain M (2013) CD19-targeted T cells rapidly induce molecular remissions in adults with chemotherapy-refractory acute lymphoblastic leukemia. Sci Transl Med 5(177):177ra138. doi:10.1126/scitranslmed.3005930
154. Davila ML, Riviere I, Wang X, Bartido S, Park J, Curran K, Chung SS, Stefanski J, Borquez-Ojeda O, Olszewska M, Qu J, Wasielewska T, He Q, Fink M, Shinglot H, Youssif M, Satter M, Wang Y, Hosey J, Quintanilla H, Halton E, Bernal Y, Bouhassira DC, Arcila ME, Gonen M, Roboz GJ, Maslak P, Douer D, Frattini MG, Giralt S, Sadelain M, Brentjens R (2014) Efficacy and toxicity management of 19-28z CAR T cell therapy in B cell acute lymphoblastic leukemia. Sci Transl Med 6(224):224ra225. doi:10.1126/scitranslmed.3008226
155. Kalos M, Levine BL, Porter DL, Katz S, Grupp SA, Bagg A, June CH (2011) T cells with chimeric antigen receptors have potent antitumor effects and can establish memory in patients with advanced leukemia. Sci Transl Med 3(95):95ra73. doi:10.1126/scitranslmed.3002842
156. Lee DW, Kochenderfer JN, Stetler-Stevenson M, Cui YK, Delbrook C, Feldman SA, Fry TJ, Orentas R, Sabatino M, Shah NN, Steinberg SM, Stroncek D, Tschernia N, Yuan C, Zhang H, Zhang L, Rosenberg SA, Wayne AS, Mackall CL (2014) T cells expressing CD19 chimeric antigen receptors for acute lymphoblastic leukaemia in children and young adults: a phase 1 dose-escalation trial. Lancet. doi:10.1016/S0140-6736(14)61403-3
157. Maude SL, Frey N, Shaw PA, Aplenc R, Barrett DM, Bunin NJ, Chew A, Gonzalez VE, Zheng Z, Lacey SF, Mahnke YD, Melenhorst JJ, Rheingold SR, Shen A, Teachey DT, Levine BL, June CH, Porter DL, Grupp SA (2014) Chimeric antigen receptor T cells for sustained remissions in leukemia. N Engl J Med 371(16):1507–1517. doi:10.1056/NEJMoa1407222
158. Louis CU, Savoldo B, Dotti G, Pule M, Yvon E, Myers GD, Rossig C, Russell HV, Diouf O, Liu E, Liu H, Wu MF, Gee AP, Mei Z, Rooney CM, Heslop HE, Brenner MK (2011) Antitumor activity and long-term fate of chimeric antigen receptor-positive T cells in patients with neuroblastoma. Blood 118(23):6050–6056. doi:10.1182/blood-2011-05-354449
159. Beatty GL, Haas AR, Maus MV, Torigian DA, Soulen MC, Plesa G, Chew A, Zhao Y, Levine BL, Albelda SM, Kalos M, June CH (2014) Mesothelin-specific chimeric antigen receptor mRNA-engineered T cells induce anti-tumor activity in solid malignancies. Cancer Immunol Res 2(2):112–120. doi:10.1158/2326-6066.CIR-13-0170
160. Maus MV, Haas AR, Beatty GL, Albelda SM, Levine BL, Liu X, Zhao Y, Kalos M, June CH (2013) T cells expressing chimeric antigen receptors can cause anaphylaxis in humans. Cancer Immunol Res 1(1):26–31. doi:10.1158/2326-6066.CIR-13-0006
161. Maude SL, Barrett D, Teachey DT, Grupp SA (2014) Managing cytokine release syndrome associated with novel T cell-engaging therapies. Cancer J 20(2):119–122. doi:10.1097/PPO.0000000000000035

162. Morgan RA, Yang JC, Kitano M, Dudley ME, Laurencot CM, Rosenberg SA (2010) Case report of a serious adverse event following the administration of T cells transduced with a chimeric antigen receptor recognizing ERBB2. Mol Ther J Am Soc Gene Ther 18(4):843–851. doi:10.1038/mt.2010.24
163. Brentjens R, Yeh R, Bernal Y, Riviere I, Sadelain M (2010) Treatment of chronic lymphocytic leukemia with genetically targeted autologous T cells: case report of an unforeseen adverse event in a phase I clinical trial. Mol Ther J Am Soc Gene Ther 18(4):666–668. doi:10.1038/mt.2010.31
164. Beard RE, Zheng Z, Lagisetty KH, Burns WR, Tran E, Hewitt SM, Abate-Daga D, Rosati SF, Fine HA, Ferrone S, Rosenberg SA, Morgan RA (2014) Multiple chimeric antigen receptors successfully target chondroitin sulfate proteoglycan 4 in several different cancer histologies and cancer stem cells. J Immunother Cancer 2:25. doi:10.1186/2051-1426-2-25
165. Burns WR, Zhao Y, Frankel TL, Hinrichs CS, Zheng Z, Xu H, Feldman SA, Ferrone S, Rosenberg SA, Morgan RA (2010) A high molecular weight melanoma-associated antigen-specific chimeric antigen receptor redirects lymphocytes to target human melanomas. Cancer Res 70(8):3027–3033. doi:10.1158/0008-5472.CAN-09-2824
166. Heemskerk B, Liu K, Dudley ME, Johnson LA, Kaiser A, Downey S, Zheng Z, Shelton TE, Matsuda K, Robbins PF, Morgan RA, Rosenberg SA (2008) Adoptive cell therapy for patients with melanoma, using tumor-infiltrating lymphocytes genetically engineered to secrete interleukin-2. Hum Gene Ther 19(5):496–510. doi:10.1089/hum.2007.0171
167. Kerkar SP, Muranski P, Kaiser A, Boni A, Sanchez-Perez L, Yu Z, Palmer DC, Reger RN, Borman ZA, Zhang L, Morgan RA, Gattinoni L, Rosenberg SA, Trinchieri G, Restifo NP (2010) Tumor-specific CD8+ T cells expressing interleukin-12 eradicate established cancers in lymphodepleted hosts. Cancer Res 70(17):6725–6734. doi:10.1158/0008-5472.CAN-10-0735
168. Pegram HJ, Lee JC, Hayman EG, Imperato GH, Tedder TF, Sadelain M, Brentjens RJ (2012) Tumor-targeted T cells modified to secrete IL-12 eradicate systemic tumors without need for prior conditioning. Blood 119(18):4133–4141. doi:10.1182/blood-2011-12-400044
169. Zhang L, Morgan RA, Beane JD, Zheng Z, Dudley ME, Kassim SH, Nahvi AV, Ngo LT, Sherry RM, Phan GQ, Hughes MS, Kammula US, Feldman SA, Toomey MA, Kerkar SP, Restifo NP, Yang JC, Rosenberg SA (2015) Tumor Infiltrating lymphocytes genetically engineered with an inducible gene encoding interleukin-12 for the immunotherapy of metastatic melanoma. Clin Cancer Res Official J Am Assoc Cancer Res. doi:10.1158/1078-0432.CCR-14-2085
170. Foster AE, Dotti G, Lu A, Khalil M, Brenner MK, Heslop HE, Rooney CM, Bollard CM (2008) Antitumor activity of EBV-specific T lymphocytes transduced with a dominant negative TGF-beta receptor. J Immunother 31(5):500–505. doi:10.1097/CJI.0b013e318177092b
171. Zhang L, Yu Z, Muranski P, Palmer DC, Restifo NP, Rosenberg SA, Morgan RA (2013) Inhibition of TGF-beta signaling in genetically engineered tumor antigen-reactive T cells significantly enhances tumor treatment efficacy. Gene Ther 20(5):575–580. doi:10.1038/gt.2012.75
172. Kershaw MH, Wang G, Westwood JA, Pachynski RK, Tiffany HL, Marincola FM, Wang E, Young HA, Murphy PM, Hwu P (2002) Redirecting migration of T cells to chemokine secreted from tumors by genetic modification with CXCR2. Hum Gene Ther 13(16):1971–1980. doi:10.1089/10430340260355374
173. Sapoznik S, Ortenberg R, Galore-Haskel G, Kozlovski S, Levy D, Avivi C, Barshack I, Cohen CJ, Besser MJ, Schachter J, Markel G (2012) CXCR1 as a novel target for directing reactive T cells toward melanoma: implications for adoptive cell transfer immunotherapy. Cancer Immunol Immunother CII 61(10):1833–1847. doi:10.1007/s00262-012-1245-1
174. Peng W, Ye Y, Rabinovich BA, Liu C, Lou Y, Zhang M, Whittington M, Yang Y, Overwijk WW, Lizee G, Hwu P (2010) Transduction of tumor-specific T cells with CXCR2 chemokine receptor improves migration to tumor and antitumor immune responses. Clin

Cancer Res Official J Am Assoc Cancer Res 16(22):5458–5468. doi:10.1158/1078-0432.CCR-10-0712

175. Ji Y, Wrzesinski C, Yu Z, Hu J, Gautam S, Hawk NV, Telford WG, Palmer DC, Franco Z, Sukumar M, Roychoudhuri R, Clever D, Klebanoff CA, Surh CD, Waldmann TA, Restifo NP, Gattinoni L (2015) miR-155 augments CD8+ T-cell antitumor activity in lymphoreplete hosts by enhancing responsiveness to homeostatic gammac cytokines. Proc Natl Acad Sci USA 112(2):476–481. doi:10.1073/pnas.1422916112
176. Peng W, Liu C, Xu C, Lou Y, Chen J, Yang Y, Yagita H, Overwijk WW, Lizee G, Radvanyi L, Hwu P (2012) PD-1 blockade enhances T-cell migration to tumors by elevating IFN-gamma inducible chemokines. Cancer Res 72(20):5209–5218. doi:10.1158/0008-5472.CAN-12-1187
177. Liu C, Peng W, Xu C, Lou Y, Zhang M, Wargo JA, Chen JQ, Li HS, Watowich SS, Yang Y, Tompers Frederick D, Cooper ZA, Mbofung RM, Whittington M, Flaherty KT, Woodman SE, Davies MA, Radvanyi LG, Overwijk WW, Lizee G, Hwu P (2013) BRAF inhibition increases tumor infiltration by T cells and enhances the antitumor activity of adoptive immunotherapy in mice. Clin Cancer Res Official J Am Assoc Cancer Res 19(2):393–403. doi:10.1158/1078-0432.CCR-12-1626
178. Hodis E, Watson IR, Kryukov GV, Arold ST, Imielinski M, Theurillat JP, Nickerson E, Auclair D, Li L, Place C, Dicara D, Ramos AH, Lawrence MS, Cibulskis K, Sivachenko A, Voet D, Saksena G, Stransky N, Onofrio RC, Winckler W, Ardlie K, Wagle N, Wargo J, Chong K, Morton DL, Stemke-Hale K, Chen G, Noble M, Meyerson M, Ladbury JE, Davies MA, Gershenwald JE, Wagner SN, Hoon DS, Schadendorf D, Lander ES, Gabriel SB, Getz G, Garraway LA, Chin L (2012) A landscape of driver mutations in melanoma. Cell 150(2):251–263. doi:10.1016/j.cell.2012.06.024
179. Holderfield M, Deuker MM, McCormick F, McMahon M (2014) Targeting RAF kinases for cancer therapy: BRAF-mutated melanoma and beyond. Nat Rev Cancer 14(7):455–467. doi:10.1038/nrc3760
180. Flaherty KT, Puzanov I, Kim KB, Ribas A, McArthur GA, Sosman JA, O'Dwyer PJ, Lee RJ, Grippo JF, Nolop K, Chapman PB (2010) Inhibition of mutated, activated BRAF in metastatic melanoma. N Engl J Med 363(9):809–819. doi:10.1056/NEJMoa1002011
181. Chapman PB, Hauschild A, Robert C, Haanen JB, Ascierto P, Larkin J, Dummer R, Garbe C, Testori A, Maio M, Hogg D, Lorigan P, Lebbe C, Jouary T, Schadendorf D, Ribas A, O'Day SJ, Sosman JA, Kirkwood JM, Eggermont AM, Dreno B, Nolop K, Li J, Nelson B, Hou J, Lee RJ, Flaherty KT, McArthur GA (2011) Improved survival with vemurafenib in melanoma with BRAF V600E mutation. N Engl J Med 364(26):2507–2516. doi:10.1056/NEJMoa1103782
182. Hauschild A, Grob JJ, Demidov LV, Jouary T, Gutzmer R, Millward M, Rutkowski P, Blank CU, Miller WH Jr, Kaempgen E, Martin-Algarra S, Karaszewska B, Mauch C, Chiarion-Sileni V, Martin AM, Swann S, Haney P, Mirakhur B, Guckert ME, Goodman V, Chapman PB (2012) Dabrafenib in BRAF-mutated metastatic melanoma: a multicentre, open-label, phase 3 randomised controlled trial. Lancet 380(9839):358–365. doi:10.1016/S0140-6736(12)60868-X
183. Topalian SL, Hodi FS, Brahmer JR, Gettinger SN, Smith DC, McDermott DF, Powderly JD, Carvajal RD, Sosman JA, Atkins MB, Leming PD, Spigel DR, Antonia SJ, Horn L, Drake CG, Pardoll DM, Chen L, Sharfman WH, Anders RA, Taube JM, McMiller TL, Xu H, Korman AJ, Jure-Kunkel M, Agrawal S, McDonald D, Kollia GD, Gupta A, Wigginton JM, Sznol M (2012) Safety, activity, and immune correlates of anti-PD-1 antibody in cancer. N Engl J Med 366(26):2443–2454. doi:10.1056/NEJMoa1200690
184. Sullivan RJ, Flaherty KT (2013) Resistance to BRAF-targeted therapy in melanoma. Eur J Cancer 49(6):1297–1304. doi:10.1016/j.ejca.2012.11.019
185. Flaherty KT, Infante JR, Daud A, Gonzalez R, Kefford RF, Sosman J, Hamid O, Schuchter L, Cebon J, Ibrahim N, Kudchadkar R, Burris HA 3rd, Falchook G, Algazi A, Lewis K, Long GV, Puzanov I, Lebowitz P, Singh A, Little S, Sun P, Allred A, Ouellet D,

Kim KB, Patel K, Weber J (2012) Combined BRAF and MEK inhibition in melanoma with BRAF V600 mutations. N Engl J Med 367(18):1694–1703. doi:10.1056/NEJMoa1210093
186. Brahmer JR, Tykodi SS, Chow LQ, Hwu WJ, Topalian SL, Hwu P, Drake CG, Camacho LH, Kauh J, Odunsi K, Pitot HC, Hamid O, Bhatia S, Martins R, Eaton K, Chen S, Salay TM, Alaparthy S, Grosso JF, Korman AJ, Parker SM, Agrawal S, Goldberg SM, Pardoll DM, Gupta A, Wigginton JM (2012) Safety and activity of anti-PD-L1 antibody in patients with advanced cancer. N Engl J Med 366(26):2455–2465. doi:10.1056/NEJMoa1200694
187. Hodi FS, O'Day SJ, McDermott DF, Weber RW, Sosman JA, Haanen JB, Gonzalez R, Robert C, Schadendorf D, Hassel JC, Akerley W, van den Eertwegh AJ, Lutzky J, Lorigan P, Vaubel JM, Linette GP, Hogg D, Ottensmeier CH, Lebbe C, Peschel C, Quirt I, Clark JI, Wolchok JD, Weber JS, Tian J, Yellin MJ, Nichol GM, Hoos A, Urba WJ (2010) Improved survival with ipilimumab in patients with metastatic melanoma. N Engl J Med 363(8):711–723. doi:10.1056/NEJMoa1003466
188. Topalian SL, Sznol M, McDermott DF, Kluger HM, Carvajal RD, Sharfman WH, Brahmer JR, Lawrence DP, Atkins MB, Powderly JD, Leming PD, Lipson EJ, Puzanov I, Smith DC, Taube JM, Wigginton JM, Kollia GD, Gupta A, Pardoll DM, Sosman JA, Hodi FS (2014) Survival, durable tumor remission, and long-term safety in patients with advanced melanoma receiving nivolumab. J Clin Oncol Official J Am Soc Clin Oncol 32(10):1020–1030. doi:10.1200/JCO.2013.53.0105
189. Sumimoto H, Imabayashi F, Iwata T, Kawakami Y (2006) The BRAF-MAPK signaling pathway is essential for cancer-immune evasion in human melanoma cells. J Exp Med 203 (7):1651–1656. doi:10.1084/jem.20051848
190. Boni A, Cogdill AP, Dang P, Udayakumar D, Njauw CN, Sloss CM, Ferrone CR, Flaherty KT, Lawrence DP, Fisher DE, Tsao H, Wargo JA (2010) Selective BRAFV600E inhibition enhances T-cell recognition of melanoma without affecting lymphocyte function. Cancer Res 70(13):5213–5219. doi:10.1158/0008-5472.CAN-10-0118
191. Cooper ZA, Frederick DT, Juneja VR, Sullivan RJ, Lawrence DP, Piris A, Sharpe AH, Fisher DE, Flaherty KT, Wargo JA (2013) BRAF inhibition is associated with increased clonality in tumor-infiltrating lymphocytes. Oncoimmunology 2(10):e26615. doi:10.4161/onci.26615
192. Frederick DT, Piris A, Cogdill AP, Cooper ZA, Lezcano C, Ferrone CR, Mitra D, Boni A, Newton LP, Liu C, Peng W, Sullivan RJ, Lawrence DP, Hodi FS, Overwijk WW, Lizee G, Murphy GF, Hwu P, Flaherty KT, Fisher DE, Wargo JA (2013) BRAF inhibition is associated with enhanced melanoma antigen expression and a more favorable tumor microenvironment in patients with metastatic melanoma. Clin Cancer Res Official J Am Assoc Cancer Res 19(5):1225–1231. doi:10.1158/1078-0432.CCR-12-1630
193. Wilmott JS, Long GV, Howle JR, Haydu LE, Sharma RN, Thompson JF, Kefford RF, Hersey P, Scolyer RA (2012) Selective BRAF inhibitors induce marked T-cell infiltration into human metastatic melanoma. Clin Cancer Res Official J Am Assoc Cancer Res 18 (5):1386–1394. doi:10.1158/1078-0432.CCR-11-2479
194. Khalili JS, Liu S, Rodriguez-Cruz TG, Whittington M, Wardell S, Liu C, Zhang M, Cooper ZA, Frederick DT, Li Y, Zhang M, Joseph RW, Bernatchez C, Ekmekcioglu S, Grimm E, Radvanyi LG, Davis RE, Davies MA, Wargo JA, Hwu P, Lizee G (2012) Oncogenic BRAF(V600E) promotes stromal cell-mediated immunosuppression via induction of interleukin-1 in melanoma. Clin Cancer Res Official J Am Assoc Cancer Res 18 (19):5329–5340. doi:10.1158/1078-0432.CCR-12-1632
195. Jiang X, Zhou J, Giobbie-Hurder A, Wargo J, Hodi FS (2013) The activation of MAPK in melanoma cells resistant to BRAF inhibition promotes PD-L1 expression that is reversible by MEK and PI3K inhibition. Clin Cancer Res Official J Am Assoc Cancer Res 19(3):598–609. doi:10.1158/1078-0432.CCR-12-2731
196. Spranger S, Spaapen RM, Zha Y, Williams J, Meng Y, Ha TT, Gajewski TF (2013) Up-regulation of PD-L1, IDO, and T(regs) in the melanoma tumor microenvironment is

driven by CD8(+) T cells. Sci Transl Med 5(200):200ra116. doi:10.1126/scitranslmed.3006504

197. Cooper ZA, Juneja VR, Sage PT, Frederick DT, Piris A, Mitra D, Lo JA, Hodi FS, Freeman GJ, Bosenberg MW, McMahon M, Flaherty KT, Fisher DE, Sharpe AH, Wargo JA (2014) Response to BRAF inhibition in melanoma is enhanced when combined with immune checkpoint blockade. Cancer Immunol Res 2(7):643–654. doi:10.1158/2326-6066.CIR-13-0215
198. Koya RC, Mok S, Otte N, Blacketor KJ, Comin-Anduix B, Tumeh PC, Minasyan A, Graham NA, Graeber TG, Chodon T, Ribas A (2012) BRAF inhibitor vemurafenib improves the antitumor activity of adoptive cell immunotherapy. Cancer Res 72(16):3928–3937. doi:10.1158/0008-5472.CAN-11-2837
199. Hooijkaas A, Gadiot J, Morrow M, Stewart R, Schumacher T, Blank CU (2012) Selective BRAF inhibition decreases tumor-resident lymphocyte frequencies in a mouse model of human melanoma. Oncoimmunology 1(5):609–617. doi:10.4161/onci.20226
200. Ribas A, Hodi FS, Callahan M, Konto C, Wolchok J (2013) Hepatotoxicity with combination of vemurafenib and ipilimumab. N Engl J Med 368(14):1365–1366. doi:10.1056/NEJMc1302338
201. Puzanov I, Callahan M, Linette GP, Patel S, Luke J, Sosman JA, Wolchok J, Hamid O, Minor D, Orford K, Hug B, Ma B, Matthys G, Hoos A (2014) Phase I study of the BRAF inhibitor dabrafenib (D)± the MEK inhibitor trametinib (T) in combination with ipilimumab (I) for V600E/K mutation-positive unresectable or metastatic melanoma (MM). In: 2014 ASCO Annual Meeting
202. Vella LJ, Pasam A, Dimopoulos N, Andrews M, Knights A, Puaux AL, Louahed J, Chen W, Woods K, Cebon JS (2014) MEK inhibition, alone or in combination with BRAF inhibition, affects multiple functions of isolated normal human lymphocytes and dendritic cells. Cancer Immunol Res 2(4):351–360. doi:10.1158/2326-6066.CIR-13-0181
203. Shindo T, Kim TK, Benjamin CL, Wieder ED, Levy RB, Komanduri KV (2013) MEK inhibitors selectively suppress alloreactivity and graft-versus-host disease in a memory stage-dependent manner. Blood 121(23):4617–4626. doi:10.1182/blood-2012-12-476218
204. Liu L, Mayes PA, Eastman S, Shi H, Yadavilli S, Zhang T, Yang J, Seestaller-Wehr L, Zhang SY, Hopson C, Tsvetkov L, Jing J, Zhang S, Smothers J, Hoos A (2015) The BRAF and MEK Inhibitors Dabrafenib and Trametinib: effects on immune function and in combination with immunomodulatory antibodies targeting PD1, PD-L1 and CTLA-4. Clin Cancer Res Official J Am Assoc Cancer Res. doi:10.1158/1078-0432.CCR-14-2339
205. Basile KJ, Le K, Hartsough EJ, Aplin AE (2014) Inhibition of mutant BRAF splice variant signaling by next-generation, selective RAF inhibitors. Pigment Cell Melanoma Res 27 (3):479–484. doi:10.1111/pcmr.12218
206. Wong DJ, Robert L, Atefi MS, Lassen A, Avarappatt G, Cerniglia M, Avramis E, Tsoi J, Foulad D, Graeber TG, Comin-Anduix B, Samatar A, Lo RS, Ribas A (2014) Antitumor activity of the ERK inhibitor SCH722984 against BRAF mutant, NRAS mutant and wild-type melanoma. Mol Cancer 13:194. doi:10.1186/1476-4598-13-194
207. Shtivelman E, Davies MQ, Hwu P, Yang J, Lotem M, Oren M, Flaherty KT, Fisher DE (2014) Pathways and therapeutic targets in melanoma. Oncotarget 5(7):1701–1752
208. Maertens O, Johnson B, Hollstein P, Frederick DT, Cooper ZA, Messiaen L, Bronson RT, McMahon M, Granter S, Flaherty K, Wargo JA, Marais R, Cichowski K (2013) Elucidating distinct roles for NF1 in melanomagenesis. Cancer Discov. doi:10.1158/2159-8290.CD-12-0313
209. Whittaker SR, Theurillat JP, Van Allen E, Wagle N, Hsiao J, Cowley GS, Schadendorf D, Root DE, Garraway LA (2013) A genome-scale RNA interference screen implicates NF1 loss in resistance to RAF inhibition. Cancer Discov 3(3):350–362. doi:10.1158/2159-8290.CD-12-0470
210. Kwong LN, Davies MA (2013) Navigating the therapeutic complexity of PI3K pathway inhibition in melanoma. Clin Cancer Res Official J Am Assoc Cancer Res 19(19):5310–5319. doi:10.1158/1078-0432.CCR-13-0142

211. Deng W, Gopal YN, Scott A, Chen G, Woodman SE, Davies MA (2012) Role and therapeutic potential of PI3K-mTOR signaling in de novo resistance to BRAF inhibition. Pigment Cell Melanoma Res 25(2):248–258. doi:10.1111/j.1755-148X.2011.00950.x
212. Aziz SA, Jilaveanu LB, Zito C, Camp RL, Rimm DL, Conrad P, Kluger HM (2010) Vertical targeting of the phosphatidylinositol-3 kinase pathway as a strategy for treating melanoma. Clin Cancer Res Official J Am Assoc Cancer Res 16(24):6029–6039. doi:10.1158/1078-0432.CCR-10-1490
213. Marsh Durban V, Deuker MM, Bosenberg MW, Phillips W, McMahon M (2013) Differential AKT dependency displayed by mouse models of BRAFV600E-initiated melanoma. J Clin Investig 123(12):5104–5118. doi:10.1172/JCI69619
214. Wee S, Wiederschain D, Maira SM, Loo A, Miller C, deBeaumont R, Stegmeier F, Yao YM, Lengauer C (2008) PTEN-deficient cancers depend on PIK3CB. Proc Natl Acad Sci USA 105(35):13057–13062. doi:10.1073/pnas.0802655105
215. Jia S, Liu Z, Zhang S, Liu P, Zhang L, Lee SH, Zhang J, Signoretti S, Loda M, Roberts TM, Zhao JJ (2008) Essential roles of PI(3)K-p110beta in cell growth, metabolism and tumorigenesis. Nature 454(7205):776–779. doi:10.1038/nature07091
216. Curtin JA, Fridlyand J, Kageshita T, Patel HN, Busam KJ, Kutzner H, Cho KH, Aiba S, Brocker EB, LeBoit PE, Pinkel D, Bastian BC (2005) Distinct sets of genetic alterations in melanoma. N Engl J Med 353(20):2135–2147. doi:10.1056/NEJMoa050092
217. Sheppard KE, McArthur GA (2013) The cell-cycle regulator CDK4: an emerging therapeutic target in melanoma. Clin Cancer Res Official J Am Assoc Cancer Res 19(19):5320–5328. doi:10.1158/1078-0432.CCR-13-0259
218. Leonard JP, LaCasce AS, Smith MR, Noy A, Chirieac LR, Rodig SJ, Yu JQ, Vallabhajosula S, Schoder H, English P, Neuberg DS, Martin P, Millenson MM, Ely SA, Courtney R, Shaik N, Wilner KD, Randolph S, Van den Abbeele AD, Chen-Kiang SY, Yap JT, Shapiro GI (2012) Selective CDK4/6 inhibition with tumor responses by PD0332991 in patients with mantle cell lymphoma. Blood 119(20):4597–4607. doi:10.1182/blood-2011-10-388298
219. Joshi KS, Rathos MJ, Mahajan P, Wagh V, Shenoy S, Bhatia D, Chile S, Sivakumar M, Maier A, Fiebig HH, Sharma S (2007) P276-00, a novel cyclin-dependent inhibitor induces G1-G2 arrest, shows antitumor activity on cisplatin-resistant cells and significant in vivo efficacy in tumor models. Mol Cancer Ther 6(3):926–934. doi:10.1158/1535-7163.MCT-06-0614
220. Joshi KS, Rathos MJ, Joshi RD, Sivakumar M, Mascarenhas M, Kamble S, Lal B, Sharma S (2007) In vitro antitumor properties of a novel cyclin-dependent kinase inhibitor, P276-00. Mol Cancer Ther 6(3):918–925. doi:10.1158/1535-7163.MCT-06-0613
221. Tate SC, Cai S, Ajamie RT, Burke T, Beckmann RP, Chan EM, De Dios A, Wishart GN, Gelbert LM, Cronier DM (2014) Semi-mechanistic pharmacokinetic/pharmacodynamic modeling of the antitumor activity of LY2835219, a new cyclin-dependent kinase 4/6 inhibitor, in mice bearing human tumor xenografts. Clin Cancer Res Official J Am Assoc Cancer Res 20(14):3763–3774. doi:10.1158/1078-0432.CCR-13-2846
222. Dickson MA (2014) Molecular pathways: CDK4 inhibitors for cancer therapy. Clin Cancer Res Official J Am Assoc Cancer Res 20(13):3379–3383. doi:10.1158/1078-0432.CCR-13-1551
223. Yadav V, Chen SH, Yue YG, Buchanan S, Beckmann RP, Peng SB (2014) Co-targeting BRAF and cyclin dependent kinases 4/6 for BRAF mutant cancers. Pharmacol Ther. doi:10.1016/j.pharmthera.2014.12.003
224. Yadav V, Burke TF, Huber L, Van Horn RD, Zhang Y, Buchanan SG, Chan EM, Starling JJ, Beckmann RP, Peng SB (2014) The CDK4/6 inhibitor LY2835219 overcomes vemurafenib resistance resulting from MAPK reactivation and cyclin D1 upregulation. Mol Cancer Ther 13(10):2253–2263. doi:10.1158/1535-7163.MCT-14-0257
225. Lai F, Jin L, Gallagher S, Mijatov B, Zhang XD, Hersey P (2012) Histone deacetylases (HDACs) as mediators of resistance to apoptosis in melanoma and as targets for combination

therapy with selective BRAF inhibitors. Adv Pharmacol 65:27–43. doi:10.1016/B978-0-12-397927-8.00002-6

226. Lai F, Guo ST, Jin L, Jiang CC, Wang CY, Croft A, Chi MN, Tseng HY, Farrelly M, Atmadibrata B, Norman J, Liu T, Hersey P, Zhang XD (2013) Cotargeting histone deacetylases and oncogenic BRAF synergistically kills human melanoma cells by necrosis independently of RIPK1 and RIPK3. Cell Death Dis 4:e655. doi:10.1038/cddis.2013.192
227. Johannessen CM, Johnson LA, Piccioni F, Townes A, Frederick DT, Donahue MK, Narayan R, Flaherty KT, Wargo JA, Root DE, Garraway LA (2013) A melanocyte lineage program confers resistance to MAP kinase pathway inhibition. Nature 504(7478):138–142. doi:10.1038/nature12688
228. Smyth T, Paraiso KH, Hearn K, Rodriguez-Lopez AM, Munck JM, Haarberg HE, Sondak VK, Thompson NT, Azab M, Lyons JF, Smalley KS, Wallis NG (2014) Inhibition of HSP90 by AT13387 delays the emergence of resistance to BRAF inhibitors and overcomes resistance to dual BRAF and MEK inhibition in melanoma models. Mol Cancer Ther 13 (12):2793–2804. doi:10.1158/1535-7163.MCT-14-0452
229. Paraiso KH, Haarberg HE, Wood E, Rebecca VW, Chen YA, Xiang Y, Ribas A, Lo RS, Weber JS, Sondak VK, John JK, Sarnaik AA, Koomen JM, Smalley KS (2012) The HSP90 inhibitor XL888 overcomes BRAF inhibitor resistance mediated through diverse mechanisms. Clin Cancer Res Official J Am Assoc Cancer Res 18(9):2502–2514. doi:10.1158/1078-0432.CCR-11-2612
230. Haarberg HE, Paraiso KH, Wood E, Rebecca VW, Sondak VK, Koomen JM, Smalley KS (2013) Inhibition of Wee1, AKT, and CDK4 underlies the efficacy of the HSP90 inhibitor XL888 in an in vivo model of NRAS-mutant melanoma. Mol Cancer Ther 12(6):901–912. doi:10.1158/1535-7163.MCT-12-1003
231. Pardoll DM (2012) The blockade of immune checkpoints in cancer immunotherapy. Nat Rev Cancer 12(4):252–264. doi:10.1038/nrc3239

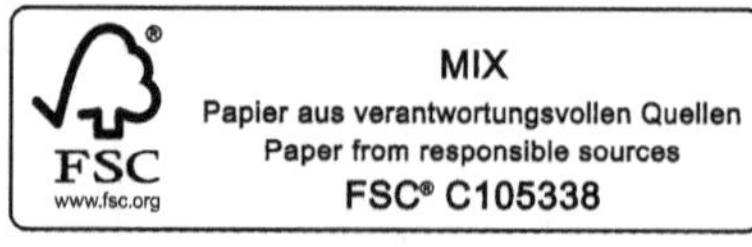

If you have any concerns about our products,
you can contact us on
ProductSafety@springernature.com

In case Publisher is established outside the EU,
the EU authorized representative is:
Springer Nature Customer Service Center GmbH
Europaplatz 3, 69115 Heidelberg, Germany

Printed by Libri Plureos GmbH
in Hamburg, Germany